Clinical Handbook of Psychotropic Drugs

25th edition

T0077180

Ric M. Procyshyn, BScPharm, MSc, PharmD, PhD[A, B] (Principal Editor)
Kalyna Z. Bezchlibnyk-Butler, BScPhm, FCSHP (Co-Editor)
David D. Kim, BSc, MSc, PhD[B, C] (Co-Editor)

The Editors wish to acknowledge contributions from the following chapter co-editors:

Alasdair M. Barr, PhD[B, C] (Drugs of Abuse)
Agnieszka K. Biala, MPharm, PhD[D] (Sex-Drive Depressants)
Andrius Baskys, MD, PhD[E] (Drugs for Treatment of Dementia, Pharmacogenetic Information for Common Psychotropic Drugs)
Vincent Dagenais-Beaulé, MSc, PharmD[F] (Antipsychotics)
Lynda Eccott, BSc, MScPharm[G] (Natural Health Products)
Dean Elbe, BScPharm, PharmD, BCPP[H] (Drugs for ADHD)
Katelyn Halpape, BSP, ACPR, PharmD, BCPP[I] (Mood Stabilizers)
Rahim Janmohamed, BScPharm[J] (Treatment of Substance Use Disorders)
Reza Rafizadeh, BScPharm, RPh, ACPR, BCPP[K] (Treatment of Substance Use Disorders)
Christian G. Schütz, MD, PhD, MPH, FRCPC[L] (Treatment of Substance Use Disorders)
Amy Soubolsky, BSP, MScPharm[I] (Mood Stabilizers) Fidel Vila-Rodriguez, MD, PhD, FRCPC, FAPA[A] (Electroconvulsive Therapy, Repetitive Transcranial Magnetic Stimulation)
Vivian Yih, BScPharm, PharmD[M] (Antidepressants)
Bree Zehm, PharmD[N] (Antidepressants)
Tony Zhou, PharmD, ACPR[O] (Anxiolytics, Hypnotics/Sedatives)

[A] Department of Psychiatry, University of British Columbia, Vancouver, BC, Canada; [B] British Columbia Mental Health & Substance Use Services Research Institute, Vancouver, BC, Canada; [C] Department of Anesthesiology, Pharmacology & Therapeutics, University of British Columbia, Vancouver, BC, Canada; [D] Biala & Co., Vancouver, BC, Canada; [E] Specialty Center, WesternU Health, Western University of Health Sciences, Pomona, CA, USA; [F] Department of Clinical Pharmacy, Jewish General Hospital, Lady Davis Institute for Medical Research & Faculty of Pharmacy, Université de Montréal, Montréal, QC, Canada; [G] Faculty of Pharmaceutical Sciences, University of British Columbia, Vancouver, BC, Canada; [H] Healthy Minds Centre, BC Children's Hospital, Vancouver, BC, Canada; [I] College of Pharmacy and Nutrition, University of Saskatchewan, Saskatoon, SK, Canada; [J] British Columbia Centre on Substance Use, Interdisciplinary Addiction Fellowship Program, Vancouver, BC, Canada; [K] Lower Mainland Pharmacy Services and Faculty of Pharmaceutical Sciences, University of British Columbia, Vancouver, BC, Canada; [L] BC Mental Health and Substance Use Services, Provincial Health Service Authority, Vancouver, BC, Canada; [M] Fraser Health Authority Mental Health and Substance Use Tertiary Older Adult Program, Vancouver, BC, Canada; [N] Department of Pharmacy, Island Health, Victoria, BC, Canada; [O] Lower Mainland Pharmacy Services and Surrey Memorial Hospital, Surrey, BC, Canada

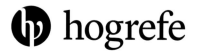

Library of Congress Cataloging-in-Publication Data

is available via the Library of Congress Marc Database under the
LC Control Number 2023933864

National Library of Canada Cataloguing-in-Publication Data

Main entry under title:

Clinical handbook of psychotropic drugs
21st rev. ed.
Includes bibliographical references and index

ISBN 978-0-88937-474-4

1. Psychotropic drugs – Handbooks, manuals, etc.
I. Bezchlibnyk-Butler, Kalyna Z., 1947–.
II. Jeffries, J. Joel, 1939–.
RM315.C55   2015   615'.788   C93-094102-0

PUBLISHING OFFICES
USA: Hogrefe Publishing Corporation, 44 Merrimac Street, Suite 207, Newburyport, MA 01950
            Phone (978) 255-3700, E-mail customersupport@hogrefe.com
EUROPE: Hogrefe Publishing GmbH, Merkelstr. 3, 37085 Göttingen, Germany
            Phone +49 551 99950-0, Fax +49 551 99950-111; E-mail publishing@hogrefe.com

SALES & DISTRIBUTION
USA: Hogrefe Publishing, Customer Services Department,
            30 Amberwood Parkway, Ashland, OH 44805
            Phone (800) 228-3749, Fax (419) 281-6883; E-mail customerservice@hogrefe.com
UK: Hogrefe Publishing, c/o Marston Book Services Ltd.,
            160 Eastern Ave., Milton Park, Abingdon, OX14 4SB, UK
            Phone +44 1235 465577, Fax +44 1235 465556; E-mail direct.orders@marston.co.uk
EUROPE: Hogrefe Publishing, Merkelstr. 3, 37085 Göttingen, Germany
            Phone +49 551 99950-0, Fax +49 551 99950-111; E-mail publishing@hogrefe.com

OTHER OFFICES
CANADA: Hogrefe Publishing, 82 Laird Drive, East York, Ontario, M4G 3V1
SWITZERLAND: Hogrefe Publishing, Länggass-Strasse 76, 3012 Bern

Printed and bound in the USA

25th edition

ISBN 978-0-88937-632-8 (print), 978-1-61676-632-0 (pdf)
https://doi.org/10.1027/00632-000

The authors and publisher have made every effort to ensure that drug selections and dosages suggested in this text are in accord with current recommendations and practice at the time of publication. However, due to changing government regulations, continuing research, and changing information concerning drug therapy and reactions, the reader is urged to check the package insert for each drug for any change in indications and dosage, or for added precautions. The authors and publisher disclaim any responsibility for any consequences which may follow from the use of information presented in this book.

INTRODUCTION

The *Clinical Handbook of Psychotropic Drugs* is a user-friendly and practical resource guide for health care practitioners working in any setting where psychotropic drugs are utilized. Its content is derived from various forms of published literature (including randomized controlled trials, scientific data such as pharmacokinetic trials, cohort trials, case series, and case reports) as well as from leading clinical experts. The handbook is continually updated as the scientific literature evolves, so we can provide current evidence-based and clinically relevant information to optimize patient care. New sections, periodically added, reflect changes in therapy and in current practice.

For this 25th edition, we have again revised and updated the book throughout and added a number of new treatments and formulations. In the antidepressants chapter, we have added a new section on the NMDA receptor antagonist/CYP2D6 inhibitor combination product (dextromethorphan/bupropion), and the dementia chapter has a new section on lecanemab, a new fast-track FDA-approved treatment for Alzheimer's disease. The revised clozapine monitoring tables in the antipsychotics chapter now also contain monitoring requirements for patients with or without non-benign ethnic neutropenia. In the chapter on substance use disorder, we have added a rapid micro-induction method for buprenorphine that allows treatment to start without waiting for the patient to be in withdrawal.

As in previous editions, charts and tables of comparisons are employed to enable the reader to have quick access to information.

Both American and Canadian trade names are used in the text. Though plasma levels are given in SI units, conversion rates to Imperial US units are available in the text.

Given that changes may occur in a medication's indications, and differences are seen among countries, specific "indications" listed in this text as "approved" should be viewed in conjunction with product monographs approved in your jurisdiction of interest.

Dose comparisons and plasma levels are based on scientific data. However, it is important to note that some patients will respond to doses outside the reported ranges. Age, sex, and the medical condition of the patient must always be taken into consideration when prescribing any psychotropic agent.

Patient Information Sheets for most drug categories are provided as printable pdf files to facilitate education/counselling of patients receiving these medications. For details, please see p. 474.

For those who like the convenience of electronic resources, the *Clinical Handbook of Psychotropic Drugs* is also available as an online version that provides even quicker access to all the information in the handbook, with some added extras: (1) An auto-completion powered search function, (2) browse features for generic names, trade names, indications, and interacting agents, (3) column-selector enhancement of comparison charts (dosages, side effects, pharmacokinetics, interactions, etc.) that allows you to choose which information is displayed, and (4) hundreds of additional references. Further details on this can be found at https://chpd.hogrefe.com/

On behalf of the editors, I would like to express my abundant gratitude to each of the contributors. The *Clinical Handbook of Psychotropic Drugs* would not be possible if it were not for their collective expertise, investment of time, and commitment to patient care. Over the years, many readers have asked challenging questions and provided useful feedback regarding the content and format of the handbook. This input is critical to keeping this handbook current, accurate, and relevant. Please feel free to e-mail me at the address below with your comments and questions.

Ric M. Procyshyn
E-mail: rprocyshyn@bcmhs.bc.ca

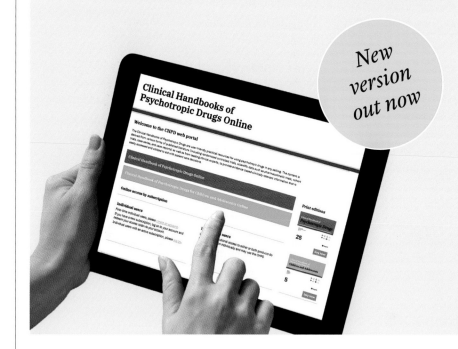
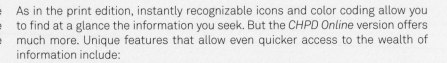
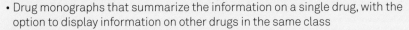
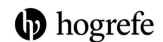

TABLE OF CONTENTS

ANTIDEPRESSANTS

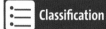 **Classification**

- Antidepressants can be classified as follows:

Pharmacological Class	Examples	Page
Cyclic Antidepressants [*]		
Selective Serotonin Reuptake Inhibitors (SSRIs)	Citalopram, escitalopram, fluoxetine, fluvoxamine, paroxetine, sertraline	See p. 3
Norepinephrine Dopamine Reuptake Inhibitor (NDRI)	Bupropion	See p. 19
Selective Serotonin-Norepinephrine Reuptake Inhibitor (SNRIs)	Desvenlafaxine, duloxetine, levomilnacipran, venlafaxine	See p. 25
Serotonin-2 Antagonists/Serotonin Reuptake Inhibitors (SARIs)	Nefazodone, trazodone	See p. 33
Serotonin-1A Partial Agonist/Serotonin Reuptake Inhibitor (SPARI)	Vilazodone	See p. 40
Serotonin Modulator and Stimulator (SMS)	Vortioxetine	See p. 44
Noradrenergic/Specific Serotonergic Agent (NaSSA)	Mirtazapine	See p. 49
Nonselective Cyclic Agents (Mixed Reuptake Inhibitor/Receptor Blockers)	Amitriptyline, desipramine, imipramine, maprotiline, nortriptyline	See p. 54
Monoamine Oxidase Inhibitors		
Reversible MAO-A Inhibitor (RIMA)	Moclobemide	See p. 64
Irreversible MAO (A&B) Inhibitors (MAOIs)	Phenelzine, tranylcypromine	See p. 67
Irreversible MAO-B Inhibitor	Selegiline	See p. 74
GABA$_A$ Receptor Positive Modulator	Brexanolone	See p. 77
NMDA Receptor Antagonist	Esketamine	See p. 80
NMDA Receptor Antagonist/CYP2D6 Inhibitor	Dextromethorphan/bupropion	See p. 84

[*] Cyclic antidepressants are currently classified according to their effect on brain neurotransmitters. These neurotransmitter effects determine the antidepressants' spectrum of activity and adverse effects (see table p. 89),

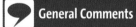 **General Comments**

- Antidepressants are associated with a small (2–3%) risk of hostility or suicidal ideation and associated behaviors in children, adolescents, and young adults (aged up to 24 years). Risk for suicide should be closely assessed and monitored during the initial weeks of antidepressant therapy
- In patients presenting with depression and a high risk of suicide, treatment selection should consider safety in overdose (i.e., consider using newer antidepressant agents rather than nonselective cyclic and MAOI antidepressants). Prescription quantities should be consistent with safe patient care
- Some antidepressants are associated with restlessness or psychomotor agitation prior to seeing any change in core symptoms of depression. On average, all antidepressants are equally efficacious at reducing symptoms of depression though some randomized double-blind, controlled trials and systematic reviews suggest otherwise. Overall effects of antidepressants are modest when the effects of publication bias are considered. Compared to placebo, the effect size of antidepressant treatment is reported as 0.31
- Based on the most comprehensive network meta-analysis and systematic review thus far involving 21 antidepressants, only agomelatine, escitalopram, and vortioxetine demonstrated superior efficacy combined with better acceptability/tolerability when used as initial treatment for Major depressive disorder (MDD).[1] However, the authors make it clear that there are important limitations to these results – they may only help inform as to initial treatment choice, they do not reflect longer term tolerability or benefit with respect to functionality, and they do not account for individual factors which are typically used to help guide treatment selection in clinical practice

- A systematic review and network meta-analysis (42 RCTs with 18,998 patients) comparing efficacy of treatment using the (self-rated) Sheehan Disability Scale in patients with MDD found duloxetine to be the most effective on functional outcomes. Other antidepressants ranked by efficacy were paroxetine, levomilnacipran, venlafaxine, quetiapine, desvenlafaxine, agomelatine, escitalopram, amitriptyline, bupropion, sertraline, vortioxetine, and fluoxetine
- Using the WHO Pharmacovigilance database, a significantly increased reporting odds ratio (ROR) for all subtypes of movement disorders was found for antidepressants in general, with the highest association for bruxism (ROR = 10.37) and lowest for tics (ROR = 1.49). Among the various classes of antidepressants, a significant association was observed for SSRIs for all subtypes of movement disorders except restless legs syndrome
- Prophylaxis of depression is most effective if the therapeutic dose is maintained; continued therapy with all classes of antidepressants has been shown to significantly reduce risk of relapse
- Different antidepressant classes may be combined in patients with a partial response or in refractory cases; however, combinations should be assessed for potential interactions such as serotonin syndrome; additional monitoring should be implemented when necessary
- Tolerance (tachyphylaxis or "poop-out" syndrome) has been reported in 10–20% of patients on antidepressants, despite adherence to therapy. Possible explanations include adaptations in the CNS, increased disease severity or pathogenesis, loss of placebo effect, unrecognized rapid-cycling, incorrect diagnosis, comorbid substance use, anxiety disorders, ADHD or eating disorders [Management: check compliance; adjust dosage; switch to an alternate antidepressant (p. 97) or utilize augmentation strategies (p. 99)]

| **Therapeutic Effects** | • Elevation of mood, improved appetite and sleep patterns, increased physical activity, improved clarity of thinking, better memory; decreased feelings of guilt, worthlessness, helplessness, inadequacy, decrease in delusional preoccupation and ambivalence |

Selective Serotonin Reuptake Inhibitors (SSRIs)

Product Availability*

Generic Name	Chemical Class	Neuroscience-based Nomenclature* (Pharmacological Target/Mode of Action)	Trade Name[A]	Dosage Forms and Strengths
Citalopram	Phthalane derivative	Serotonin/Reuptake inhibitor	Celexa	Tablets/capsules: 10 mg, 20 mg, 30 mg[C], 40 mg Oral solution[B]: 10 mg/5 mL
Escitalopram	Phthalane derivative	Serotonin/Reuptake inhibitor	Cipralex[C], Lexapro[B]	Tablets/capsules: 5 mg[B], 10 mg, 20 mg Oral solution: 5 mg/5 mL[B]
			Cipralex Meltz[C]	Orodispersible tablets: 10 mg, 20 mg
Fluoxetine	Bicyclic	Serotonin/Reuptake inhibitor	Prozac, Sarafem[B]	Capsules: 10 mg, 20 mg, 40 mg[B] Tablets[B]: 10 mg, 15 mg, 20 mg, 60 mg Oral solution: 20 mg/5 mL
			Prozac Weekly[B]	Delayed-release pellets 90 mg[B]
Fluoxetine/olanzapine	Bicyclic	Serotonin/Reuptake inhibitor Dopamine, serotonin/Antagonist	Symbyax	Capsules[B]: Fluoxetine 25 mg with 3 mg, 6 mg or 12 mg olanzapine; fluoxetine 50 mg with 6 mg or 12 mg olanzapine
Fluvoxamine[D]	Monocyclic	Serotonin/Reuptake inhibitor	Luvox	Tablets: 25 mg[B], 50 mg, 100 mg
			Luvox CR	Extended-release capsules[B]: 100 mg, 150 mg
Paroxetine hydrochloride	Phenylpiperidine	Serotonin/Reuptake inhibitor	Paxil	Tablets: 10 mg, 20 mg, 30 mg, 40 mg Oral suspension[B]: 10 mg/5 mL
			Paxil CR	Controlled-release tablets: 12.5 mg, 25 mg, 37.5 mg[B]

Selective Serotonin Reuptake Inhibitors (SSRIs) (cont.)

Generic Name	Chemical Class	Neuroscience-based Nomenclature* (Pharmacological Target/Mode of Action)	Trade Name(A)	Dosage Forms and Strengths
Paroxetine mesylate(B)	Phenylpiperidine	Serotonin/Reuptake inhibitor	Pexeva	Tablets(B): 10 mg, 20 mg, 30 mg, 40 mg
			Brisdelle	Capsules(B): 7.5 mg
Sertraline	Tetrahydronaphthylmethylamine	Serotonin/Reuptake inhibitor	Zoloft	Capsules/tablets: 25 mg, 50 mg, 100 mg, 150 mg(B), 200 mg(B)
				Oral solution: 20 mg/mL(B)

* Refer to Health Canada's Drug Product Database or the FDA's Drugs@FDA for the most current availability information   * Developed by a taskforce consisting of representatives from the American College of Neuropsychopharmacology (ACNP), the Asian College of Neuropsychopharmacology (AsCNP), the European College of Neuropsychopharmacology (ECNP), the International College of Neuropsychopharmacology (CINP), and the International Union of Basic and Clinical Pharmacology (IUPHAR) (see https://nbn2r.com), (A) Generic preparations may be available,   (B) Not marketed in Canada,   (C) Not marketed in the USA,   (D) Not approved for depression in the USA

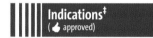

Indications‡
(👍 approved)

- 👍 Major depressive disorder (MDD)
- 👍 MDD, recurrent: Prophylaxis
- 👍 Bulimia nervosa (fluoxetine and sertraline)
- 👍 Obsessive-compulsive disorder (OCD) (fluvoxamine, fluoxetine, paroxetine, escitalopram, and sertraline)
- 👍 Panic disorder with or without agoraphobia (paroxetine, sertraline, fluoxetine)
- 👍 Social anxiety disorder (paroxetine, sertraline)
- 👍 Posttraumatic stress disorder (PTSD) (paroxetine, sertraline)
- 👍 Premenstrual dysphoric disorder (paroxetine, sertraline)
- 👍 Generalized anxiety disorder (GAD) (escitalopram, paroxetine)
- 👍 Depressive episodes associated with bipolar I disorder and treatment-resistant depression (fluoxetine/olanzapine combination – Symbyax)
- 👍 Moderate-to-severe vasomotor symptoms of menopause (low-dose paroxetine mesylate (LDPM); the only SSRI approved specifically for this indication in the US) – may be a first-choice alternative for women who are not suitable for, or refuse, hormone therapy
- Dysthymia
- Depression, atypical
- MDD in patients with comorbid medical disorder (i.e., poststroke depression and crying, myocardial infarction) or psychiatric illness; early use (within 1 month) may reduce occurrence of post-stroke depression (but not improve functional independence), consideration should be balanced with risk of adverse effects – there is currently no indication for routine use of SSRIs to promote stroke recovery; should weigh treatment risks and benefits in those at high risk of depression
- Prevention of peginterferon-α2a-associated depression in hepatitis C infected individuals without previous psychiatric illness
- Binge-eating disorder: Double-blind studies suggest efficacy of fluvoxamine and citalopram
- Borderline personality disorder: Treatment of self-injurious behavior, aggression, impulsive behavior, and behavior disturbances
- Neuropsychiatric symptoms of dementia – SSRIs effectively alleviate agitation, depressive symptoms, and care burden, and improve cognitive function
- Behavioral and cognitive symptoms of frontotemporal lobar degeneration (FTLD) – SSRIs specifically improve disinhibition, irritability, aggression, and aberrant motor activity
- Smoking cessation and withdrawal from drugs, including alcohol – variable response reported
- Chronic fatigue syndrome: Open label trials have shown 70% effectiveness but randomized controlled trials have not replicated this
- Body dysmorphic disorder (BDD) – recommended as a first-line medication for BDD, including delusional BDD. Relatively high doses may be needed and at least 12 weeks duration may be necessary to determine efficacy
- Postpartum depression – a review of randomized trials failed to show a superiority of SSRIs over other treatments
- Pervasive developmental disorder (autism) in adults (fluoxetine)[2] – limited evidence of efficacy

‡ Indications listed here do not necessarily apply to all SSRIs or all countries. Please refer to a country's regulatory database (e.g., US Food and Drug Administration, Health Canada Drug Product Database) for the most current availability information and indications

- Pain management (e.g., diabetic neuropathy, arthritis), phantom limb pain (fluoxetine, sertraline), Raynaud's phenomenon (fluoxetine), fibrositis, and fibromyalgia (fluoxetine) – data conflicting as to efficacy
- Trichotillomania, excoriation disorder (fluoxetine)
- Premature ejaculation (paroxetine may have better efficacy than fluoxetine or escitalopram; combination with phosphodiesterase-5 inhibitors may be more effective than monotherapy but this strategy has a higher risk of adverse effects)
- Enuresis, functional – data contradictory as to efficacy; case reports of bedwetting in children treated with SSRIs
- Schizophrenia, negative symptoms (fluoxetine)[3]
- Tardive dyskinesia: Case reports suggest fluvoxamine may be helpful due to its potent sigma-1 receptor agonist activity[4]
- Malignancy, cholestasis or chronic kidney disease-related pruritus unresponsive to standard treatment (paroxetine, sertraline)

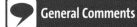

General Comments

- SSRIs have been associated with increased suicidal ideation, hostility, and psychomotor agitation in clinical trials involving children, adolescents, and young adults (up to 24 years old). This effect was not seen in those aged 24–65 and SSRIs were preventative for these concerns in those over the age of 65. Monitor all patients for worsening of depression and suicidal thinking
- In the STAR*D trial, patients with nonpsychotic major depressive disorder received 1–4 successive acute treatments with the initial treatment being citalopram. Approximately 30% of these patients reached remission after 10 weeks of therapy (average dose = 42 mg) and 50% had a response
- Response to SSRIs may be more delayed in OCD relative to depression or anxiety disorders; response is dose related, with better clinical responses associated with higher doses, although lower doses may be effective in preventing relapse

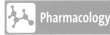

Pharmacology

- Exact mechanism of antidepressant action unknown; SSRIs, through inhibition of serotonin reuptake, increase concentrations of serotonin in the synapse, which causes downregulation of post-synaptic receptors (e.g., 5-HT$_{2A}$). Some SSRIs can also affect other neurotransmitters, e.g., some SSRIs also inhibit the reuptake of norepinephrine (i.e., fluoxetine, paroxetine), while others inhibit the reuptake of dopamine (i.e., sertraline) or antagonize muscarinic cholinergic receptors (paroxetine)

Dosing

- See p. 94
- SSRIs are thought to have a flat dose-response curve (i.e., most patients respond to the initial or even low doses, such as 5–10 mg of fluoxetine). Not recommended to increase dose until steady state has been reached first (4 weeks for fluoxetine and 1–2 weeks for other agents). The optimal dose balancing efficacy for depression and tolerability is at the lower end of the licensed dosing range (up to 40 mg fluoxetine equivalents) for a majority; however, dosing should be individualized, as there are limitations to available evidence and significant heterogeneity amongst individuals with depression. Those with anxiety disorders may have greater symptom improvement with doses at the higher end of the dosing range, although risk of side effects is greater[5]
- Patients maintained on fluoxetine 20 mg/day may be changed to Prozac Weekly 90 mg/week, starting 7 days after the last 20 mg/day dose
- Dosage should be decreased (by 50%) in patients with significant hepatic impairment, as plasma levels can increase up to 3-fold
- In kidney impairment, sertraline levels may increase by 50%; use 50% of the standard dose of paroxetine if CrCl is 10–50 mL/min, and 25% of the standard dose if CrCl is less than 10 mL/min
- Higher doses may be required in the treatment of OCD, eating disorders, and PTSD
- Lower starting dose may be effective for panic disorder and should be considered, as patients are more sensitive to stimulating effects
- Dosing interval of every 2 to 7 days has been used with fluoxetine in prophylaxis of depression; once weekly dosing used in maintenance treatment of panic disorder
- Intermittent dosing (during luteal phase of menstrual cycle) found effective for treatment of premenstrual dysphoric disorder
- Dosage of low-dose paroxetine mesylate for vasomotor symptoms associated with menopause is 7.5 mg daily given at bedtime

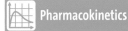

Pharmacokinetics

- See p. 94
- SSRIs are absorbed relatively slowly but completely (time to peak plasma concentration is 3–8 h); undergo little first-pass effect
- Highly bound to plasma protein (fluoxetine, paroxetine, and sertraline) and will displace other drugs from protein binding although this is rarely clinically significant (see Drug Interactions, p. 12)
- Metabolized primarily by the liver; all SSRIs affect CYP450 metabolizing enzyme (least: citalopram and escitalopram) and will affect the metabolism of other drugs metabolized by this system (see Drug Interactions, p. 12). Fluoxetine and paroxetine have been shown to decrease their own metabolism over time. Clearance of all SSRIs reduced in patients with liver cirrhosis

Selective Serotonin Reuptake Inhibitors (SSRIs) (cont.)

- Peak plasma level of sertraline is 30% higher when drug taken with food, as first-pass metabolism is reduced
- Fluoxetine as well as its active metabolite, norfluoxetine, have the longest half-lives (up to 70 h and 330 h, respectively); this has implications for reaching steady-state drug levels as well as for drug withdrawal and drug interactions
- Controlled-release paroxetine is enteric-coated and formulated for controlled dissolution; suggested to be better tolerated than the regular-release preparations in regards to GI effects, especially at start of therapy
- Once weekly dose of delayed-release fluoxetine 90 mg results in similar mean steady-state plasma concentration of fluoxetine and norfluoxetine, achieved with a daily dose of 10–20 mg; peak to trough differences vary (rates of nausea appear to be similar)

 Onset & Duration of Action
- SSRIs are long-acting drugs and can be given in a single daily dose, usually in the morning; of the SSRIs, fluvoxamine and paroxetine have the highest incidence of sedation and can be prescribed at night if necessary
- Therapeutic effect typically seen after 28 days (though some patients may respond sooner); most patients with depression respond to the initial (low) dose; increasing the dose too rapidly due to absence of therapeutic effect or adverse effects can result in higher doses than necessary being used and higher rate of adverse effects
- Tolerance to effects seen in some patients after months of treatment ("poop-out syndrome" or tachyphylaxis) (see p. 3)

 Adverse Effects
- The pharmacological and side effect profile of SSRIs is related to their in vivo affinity for and activity on neurotransmitters/receptors (see Table p. 89)
- For incidence of adverse effects at therapeutic doses see chart (p. 91)
- Incidence may be greater in early days of treatment; patients adapt to many side effects over time
- Rule out withdrawal symptoms of previous antidepressant – can be misattributed to side effects of current drug

CNS Effects
- Headache common, worsening of migraines [Management: acetaminophen prn]
- Seizures reported, primarily in patients with underlying seizure disorder (risk 0.04–0.3%); dose related
- Both activation and sedation can occur early in treatment
- Activation, excitement, impulse dyscontrol, anxiety, agitation, and restlessness; more frequent at higher doses [may respond to lorazepam]; psychosis or panic reactions may occur; isolated reports of antidepressants causing motor activation, aggression, depersonalization, **suicidal urges**, and potential to harm others. CAUTION in children and adolescents (see p. 10)
- Insomnia: Decreased REM sleep, prolonged sleep onset latency, reduced sleep efficacy, and increased awakenings with all SSRIs; increased dreaming, nightmares, sexual dreams and obsessions reported with fluoxetine [may respond to clonazepam or cyproheptadine 2–4 mg]; case reports of somnambulism with paroxetine
- Drowsiness – more common with fluvoxamine and paroxetine; prescribe bulk of dose at bedtime; sedation with fluoxetine may be related to high concentration of metabolite norfluoxetine
- Precipitation of hypomania or mania (between 10% and 25% of patients with a history of bipolar disorders – less frequent if patient receiving mood stabilizers); increased risk in patients with comorbid substance abuse
- Lethargy, apathy or amotivational syndrome (asthenia) reported – may be dose related and is reversible; more likely with SSRIs than SNRIs [prescribe bulk of dose at bedtime; amantadine (100–200 mg/day), bupropion, buspirone, modafinil (100–400 mg/day), or psychostimulant (e.g., methylphenidate 5–20 mg bid) or consider alternate agent]
- Case reports of cognitive impairment, decreased attention, and short-term memory impairment [early data suggest donepezil 2.5–10 mg/day may be of benefit]
- Case reports of visual hallucinations with fluoxetine, fluvoxamine, paroxetine, and sertraline
- Fine tremor [may respond to dose reduction or to propranolol]
- Akathisia [may respond to dose reduction, to propranolol or to a benzodiazepine]
- Dystonia, dyskinesia, parkinsonism or tics; more likely in older patients
- Increased extrapyramidal symptoms reported in patients with Parkinson's disease
- May induce or worsen extrapyramidal effects when given with antipsychotics (see Interactions p. 14)

- Case reports of tardive dyskinesia following chronic fluoxetine, sertraline, and paroxetine use; more likely in older patients
- Tinnitus
- Myoclonus (e.g., periodic leg movements during sleep); may increase spasticity; recurrence of restless legs syndrome
- Myoclonic tics may be seen in the face and shoulders
- Dysphasia, stuttering
- Impaired balance reported, especially in the elderly
- Nocturnal bruxism reported – may result in morning headache or lead to damage to teeth or bridgework [may respond to buspirone up to 50 mg/day]
- Paresthesias; may be caused by pyridoxine deficiency [Management: Pyridoxine 50–150 mg/day]; "electric-shock-like" sensations
- Joint pain
- Cerebrovascular disease and case reports of stroke (high doses of high-affinity SSRIs may increase risk of bleeding or vasospasm due to antiplatelet effect or serotonergic overstimulation)

| Anticholinergic Effects |
- Case reports of urinary retention, urgency, incontinence or cystitis
- Case report of acute angle closure with paroxetine in patient with narrow-angle glaucoma (paroxetine has the most anticholinergic activity of the SSRIs)

| Cardiovascular Effects |
- Citalopram and escitalopram cause dose-dependent QT interval prolongation. Citalopram not recommended to be prescribed at doses greater than 40 mg/day, and 20 mg/day in patients above age 60 (65 in Canada), in individuals with liver impairment, or if combined with CYP2C19 inhibitors. Similarly, the dose of escitalopram should be limited to 20 mg/day in individuals with liver impairment and to 10 mg/day if combined with CYP2C19 inhibitors. Citalopram use is discouraged in patients with congenital long QT syndrome. Patients with congestive heart failure, bradyarrhythmias, or predisposition to hypokalemia or hypomagnesemia because of concomitant illness or drugs are at higher risk of developing torsades de pointes
- In certain selected circumstances, a decision to exceed these dosing recommendations may occur; if so, consider the following recommendations: confirm there is no personal or family history of premature sudden cardiac death, QTc prolongation or structural and ischemic heart disease; a risk-benefit discussion should occur before commencing; review concomitant medications to ensure others may not contribute to QTc prolongation risk; and finally, perform an ECG prior to increasing dose and repeat ECG following dose increase when steady state has been reached – reconsider this dosing if absolute QTc more than 500 ms or change in QTc of more than 60 ms
- Slowing of sinus node reported with fluoxetine; caution in sinus node disease and in patients with serious left ventricular impairment; case reports of QT prolongation with fluoxetine (two mechanisms proposed: Direct blockade of the hERG potassium ion channels and disruption of hERG protein expression on the cell membrane)
- Rare reports of tachycardia, palpitations, hypertension, and atrial fibrillation
- Bradycardia
- Dizziness
- May cause coronary vasoconstriction; caution in patients with angina/ischemic heart disease
- Increased LDL cholesterol levels reported with paroxetine and sertraline
- In a meta-analysis of SSRIs in patients with depression and coronary heart disease, SSRIs were found to decrease depressive symptoms with no significant difference in mortality or readmission rates

| Hematological Effects |
- Bleeding disorders including petechiae, purpura (1% risk with fluoxetine); thrombocytopenia with fluoxetine; bruising, nosebleeds, GI bleeding, and post-surgery bleeding reported with all SSRI drugs; possible mechanisms include blockade of serotonin uptake by platelets, increased gastric acid secretion via increased vagal tone, and pharmacokinetic drug interactions. This risk is synergistic with nonsteroidal anti-inflammatory drugs (NSAIDs), antiplatelet drugs, and anticoagulants
- Very small absolute risk of intracranial hemorrhage (ICH) – insufficient evidence to recommend restricting SSRIs or modifying existing beneficial treatment; current American and European stroke guidelines make no recommendations for antidepressant use post-stroke and risk of ICH, though some authors recommend preferentially opting for initial treatment using antidepressants that only moderately or weakly inhibit serotonin reuptake in high-risk patients
- Rare blood dyscrasias including neutropenia and aplastic anemia

Selective Serotonin Reuptake Inhibitors (SSRIs) (cont.)

Endocrine & Metabolic Effects	<ul><li>Can induce SIADH with hyponatremia; can result in nausea, fatigue, headache, cognitive impairment, confusion, and seizures; risk increases with age (up to 32% incidence), female sex, low body weight, smoking and concomitant diuretic use; incidence reported as 0.071% according to data from a large drug surveillance program</li><li>Monitoring of serum sodium is suggested in the elderly, those with a history of hyponatremia or on other agents associated with hyponatremia, such as diuretics, or with comorbid conditions associated with hyponatremia, such as heart failure</li><li>Elevated prolactin – risk increased in females (up to 22% reported in women on fluoxetine); cases of galactorrhea reported; breast enlargement; case of gynecomastia in a male on paroxetine and citalopram</li><li>A recent meta-analysis suggests that there may be a small increased risk of type 2 diabetes mellitus as well as a short-term risk of acute pancreatitis, though the latter has not been replicated; plausible physiological mechanisms include impact on insulin secretion; may also be linked to weight increases with treatment. However, SSRIs are still recommended as first-line pharmacotherapy for depression with comorbid diabetes</li><li>One meta-analysis found that weight loss occurred with acute treatment with most of the SSRIs but this was not sustained with chronic treatment. Weight gain reported: Up to 18% of individuals gain more than 7% of body weight with chronic use – reported more frequently in females (more common with paroxetine)</li><li>Preliminary evidence that SSRIs slightly decrease thyroid function, but evidence quality is low and clinical magnitude of this effect unclear</li></ul>
GI Effects	<ul><li>Nausea; vomiting – generally decreases over time due to gradual desensitization of 5-HT$_3$ receptors [may respond to taking drug with meals or switching to the delayed/controlled-release preparation; cyproheptadine 2 mg or lactobacillus acidophilus (e.g., yogurt)]</li><li>Diarrhea, bloating – usually transient and dose-related; may be more frequent with fluoxetine 90 mg given weekly</li><li>Anorexia and weight loss frequently reported during early treatment – more pronounced in overweight patients and those with carbohydrate cravings</li><li>Weight gain reported, particularly with paroxetine</li><li>Higher risk of upper GI bleeding with SSRIs – impact on both platelet aggregation and gastric acid secretion; heightened risk in elderly, history of GI bleed, and if combined with NSAIDs or ASA as well as with other anticoagulants (see p. 13); concomitant use of proton pump inhibitors may reduce risk although more evidence is needed</li><li>Case reports of stomatitis with fluoxetine; glossodynia (burning mouth syndrome) reported during treatment with fluoxetine, sertraline</li></ul>
Urogenital & Sexual Effects	<ul><li>Sexual dysfunction should be well screened and managed because it is not always fully explored, could negatively impact treatment prognosis, and is a common cause of medication nonadherence[6]</li><li>A result of increased serotonergic transmission by way of the 5-HT$_{2A}$ receptor which results in reduced dopaminergic transmission, acetylcholine (ACh) blockade, and reduced nitric oxide levels – appears to be dose-related; risk increased with age and concomitant drug use</li><li>All three phases of the sexual cycle may be affected: Reduced interest and desire for sex; erectile dysfunction in men and diminished arousal in women; and difficulty in attaining orgasm in both sexes; reducing the dose is helpful in some (but not all) cases</li><li>Paroxetine may be more likely than other SSRIs to cause sexual dysfunction (up to 75% of patients)</li><li>The phosphodiesterase inhibitors such as sildenafil have been shown by double-blind randomized placebo-controlled trials to be effective in overcoming erectile dysfunction and orgasmic problems induced by SSRIs in men, and in reducing adverse sexual effects including reversal of anorgasmia in women, with similar adverse events to the general population</li><li>Decreased libido, impotence, ejaculatory disturbances occur relatively frequently [Management: Sildenafil (25–100 mg prn), amantadine (100–400 mg prn), bethanechol (10 mg tid or 10–50 mg prn), cyproheptadine (4–16 mg prn – sedation and/or loss of antidepressant response reported occasionally), neostigmine (7.5–15 mg prn), yohimbine (5.4–16.2 mg prn or 5.4 mg tid – may cause anxiety/agitation), buspirone (15–60 mg od or prn), bupropion (75–300 mg/day – results contradictory), or "drug holidays" (i.e., skip dose for 24 h prior to sexual activity; not effective with fluoxetine]</li><li>Anorgasmia or delayed orgasm [Management: Amantadine (100–400 mg prn); cyproheptadine (4–16 mg prn – sedation and/or loss of antidepressant response reported occasionally), buspirone (15–60 mg od or prn), bupropion (75–300 mg od – results contradictory); mirtazapine (15–45 mg od), yohimbine (5.4–10.8 mg od or prn – may cause anxiety/agitation); methylphenidate (5–40 mg od), dextroamphetamine (5–40 mg od), ginseng, sildenafil (25–150 mg prn)]</li></ul>

- Post-SSRI sexual dysfunction (PSSD) – onset follows cessation of serotonergic antidepressants; includes genital anesthesia, erectile dysfunction, and orgasmic/ejaculatory anhedonia; should be differentiated from depression-related sexual dysfunction
- Spontaneous orgasm with yawning
- Cases of priapism in both males and females reported with citalopram, fluoxetine, paroxetine, and sertraline

Hypersensitivity Reactions

- Rare
- Rash (up to 1% incidence), urticaria, psoriasis, pruritus, edema, photoallergy/photosensitivity (cross-sensitivity between SSRIs has been suggested); rare cases of Stevens-Johnson syndrome
- Serum sickness, toxic epidermal necrolysis (fluvoxamine)
- Rare reports of hypersensitivity pneumonitis

Other Adverse Effects

- Hepatic effects – infrequent, usually modest elevations in liver enzymes that are often self-limited and do not require dose modification or discontinuation although rare cases of acute failure and chronic hepatitis have been reported; onset varies, usually within 2–24 weeks and pattern of presentation has ranged from hepatocellular to cholestatic or mixed; immunoallergic features are uncommon
- Case reports of alopecia
- Rhinitis common
- Case reports of exacerbation of Raynaud's syndrome
- Sporadic cases of eosinophilic pneumonia, idiopathic pulmonary fibrosis, granulomatous lung disease, and diffuse alveolar damage
- Nocturia (in up to 16% of patients)
- When prescribing SSRIs, the increased risk of fractures must be considered, including risk of falls and potential fracture risk
- Amongst all SSRIs, sweating is most likely with paroxetine (a result of NE-reuptake inhibition) [Management: Daily showering, talcum powder; in severe cases: Drysol solution, oxybutynin up to 5 mg bid, clonidine 0.1 mg bid, guanfacine 2 mg at bedtime, benztropine 0.5 mg at bedtime; drug may need to be changed]

D/C Discontinuation Syndrome

- Unlikely if treatment duration has been less than 4 weeks
- Abrupt discontinuation of high doses may cause a syndrome consisting of *somatic symptoms:* Dizziness (exacerbated by movement), lethargy, nausea, vomiting, diarrhea, headache, fever, sweating, chills, malaise, incoordination, insomnia, vivid dreams; *neurological symptoms:* Myalgia, paresthesias; "electric-shock-like" sensations, dyskinesias, visual discoordination; *psychological symptoms:* Anxiety, agitation, crying, irritability, confusion, slowed thinking, disorientation; rarely aggression, impulsivity, hypomania, and depersonalization; cases of mania reported following antidepressant taper, despite adequate concomitant mood-stabilizing treatment
- Brain "zaps" (or electric-shock-like sensations), often associated with lateral eye movements, hearing static sounds, and feelings of dizziness/wooziness; occur most commonly with abrupt discontinuation of citalopram, escitalopram, paroxetine, and sertraline; usually transitory but may last for months
- Most likely to occur within 1–7 days after a short half-life drug is stopped or dose drastically reduced, and typically disappears within 3 weeks although cases of symptoms persisting for up to 1 year have been reported
- Reintroduction of treatment results in improvement of symptoms in 2–3 days
- Incidence (of 2–78%) is related to half-life of antidepressant – reported most frequently with paroxetine, least with fluoxetine; attributed to rapid decrease in 5-HT availability. With paroxetine, discontinuation symptoms may also be due to its ability to inhibit its own metabolism, causing a rapid decline in plasma levels if it is stopped rapidly
- Consider the effect drug discontinuation will have on the pharmacokinetics/pharmacodynamics (i.e., interactions) of any co-prescribed medication
- ☞ THEREFORE THESE MEDICATIONS SHOULD BE WITHDRAWN GRADUALLY AFTER PROLONGED USE. Taper antidepressant no more rapidly than by 25% per week (or nearest dose possible) and monitor for recurrence of depressive symptoms (except for fluoxetine, which can be tapered more rapidly due to its prolonged half-life)

Management

- Re-institute drug and taper more slowly
- Symptomatic management may be necessary if symptoms are severe or reintroduction of medication not prudent – ginger can mitigate nausea and disequilibrium effects
- Switching to fluoxetine (10–20 mg) also recommended to help in the withdrawal process; if the switch is successful, fluoxetine can usually be stopped after several weeks of treatment without discontinuation symptoms returning

Selective Serotonin Reuptake Inhibitors (SSRIs) (cont.)

- Benzodiazepines, anticholinergic/antihistaminergic or antipsychotic medications may also be considered for anxiety/agitation, acute dystonic reactions or hallucinations, respectively
- Consider utilizing a liquid or compounded formulation to allow for much smaller incremental dosing adjustments if necessary

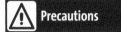 **Precautions**

- Monitor all patients for worsening depression and suicidal thinking especially at start of therapy or following an increase or decrease in dose; see comments under Pediatric Considerations, p. 10
- May impair the mental and physical ability to perform hazardous tasks (e.g., driving a car or operating machinery)
- May induce manic reactions in up to 20% of patients with bipolar disorder – reported more frequently with fluoxetine; because of risk of increased cycling, bipolar disorder is a relative contraindication unless a mood stabilizer is added
- ☞ **Use of SSRIs with other serotonergic agents may result in a hypermetabolic serotonin syndrome – usually occurs within 24 hours of medication initiation (but can occur within minutes to hours), overdose or change in dose. Symptoms include: Nausea, diarrhea, chills, sweating, dizziness, elevated temperature, elevated blood pressure, palpitations, increased muscle tone with twitching, tremor, myoclonic jerks, hyperreflexia, unsteady gait, restlessness, agitation, excitation, disorientation, confusion and delirium; may progress to rhabdomyolysis, coma, and death (see Interactions) [Management: Stop medication and administer supportive care, including benzodiazepines as necessary; cyproheptadine 4–16 mg may reduce duration of symptoms]. Residual symptoms such as muscle aches may last for up to 8 weeks in SSRIs with long half-lives**
- Fluoxetine, fluvoxamine, and paroxetine affect CYP450 and will inhibit the metabolism (and elevate the levels) of drugs metabolized by this system; sertraline will inhibit metabolism in higher doses (over 100 mg/day) (see Interactions, pp. 12–18)
- Combination of SSRIs with other cyclic antidepressants can lead to increased plasma level of other antidepressants. Combination therapy has been used in the treatment of resistant patients. Caution when switching from fluoxetine to another antidepressant (see Drug Interactions, p. 12). Caution when switching from one SSRI to another
- Treatment with medications that inhibit the serotonin transporter may be associated with abnormal bleeding, particularly when combined with NSAIDs, acetylsalicylic acid, or other medications that affect coagulation

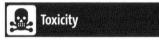 **Toxicity**

- SSRIs generally have a low probability of causing dose-related toxicity; symptoms include: Nausea, vomiting, tremor, myoclonus, irritability (one fatality reported with dose of 6000 mg of fluoxetine; seizure reported in adolescent after ingestion of 1880 mg)
- Rapid onset of seizures with QTc interval prolongation is common with citalopram; citalopram and escitalopram are more likely to cause cardiotoxicity than other SSRIs. Cardiac arrest and torsades de pointes have been reported with citalopram although toxicity has occurred in adults ingesting as little as 100–190 mg
- Altered mental state, QT prolongation, bradyarrhythmias, syncope, and seizures reported following an overdose of citalopram; fatal outcome in 6 patients with citalopram 840–3920 mg (some had also taken other sedative drugs or alcohol); fatalities reported with overdoses of citalopram and moclobemide when co-prescribed
- Case of serotonin syndrome reported after overdose of 8 g of sertraline

Management

- Treatment: Symptomatic and supportive
- Citalopram and escitalopram overdose – asymptomatic patients should have continuous ECG monitoring and monitoring of vital signs for 6 h; symptomatic patients until resolution of symptoms

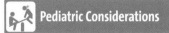 **Pediatric Considerations**

- For detailed information on the use of SSRIs in this population, please see the *Clinical Handbook of Psychotropic Drugs for Children and Adolescents*[8]
- No SSRIs are approved for use in pediatric depression in Canada
- Fluoxetine is approved for use in children and adolescents with depression (age 8–17) or OCD (age 7–17) in the USA
- Fluvoxamine and sertraline approved for the treatment of OCD (in children and adolescents over 7 years and over 6 years of age, respectively) (USA)
- Efficacy for major depressive disorder (MDD) in children and adolescents NOT demonstrated in controlled trials with sertraline, paroxetine, and citalopram; no data with fluvoxamine and escitalopram
- SSRIs are first-line psychopharmacological interventions for GAD and social anxiety disorder with accumulating data suggesting that they are associated with a greater magnitude of response, as well as a more rapid response relative to SNRIs

- CAUTION: Suicidal ideation and attempts (NOT completed suicides) are increased by antidepressants in people under the age of 24 (compared to placebo)
- SSRIs have been used in the treatment of depression, dysthymia, social phobia, anxiety, panic disorder, bulimia, OCD, autism, selective mutism, Tourette's syndrome, and ADHD; preliminary data suggest efficacy in some children with pervasive developmental disorders (autism) and selective mutism
- Children are more prone to behavioral adverse effects including: Agitation, restlessness (32–46%), activation, hypomania (up to 13%), insomnia (up to 21%), irritability, and social disinhibition (up to 25%)

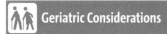 **Geriatric Considerations**

- Inconsistent reports of an association between dementia and antidepressant use, the nature of this association is unclear and there are a number of important confounding factors to consider when interpreting this data
- Overall, studies exploring efficacy in treating Alzheimer's disease comorbid with depression have had mixed results
- SSRIs are used (off-label) in the treatment of behavioral and psychological symptoms of dementia.[9, 10] Studies exploring benefits in reducing agitation have focused on citalopram and escitalopram – unknown whether these are more efficacious relative to other SSRIs
- SSRIs generally have a low risk of CNS, anticholinergic, and cardiovascular effects
- Initiate at a lower dose and increase more slowly; higher doses of fluoxetine have been associated with delirium
- Elderly patients may take longer to respond and may need trials of at least 12 weeks before treatment response noted; data contradictory as to efficacy in older patients
- Half-life of paroxetine increased by 170% and mean plasma level increased 4-fold in the elderly; clearance of sertraline decreased; citalopram plasma level and $T_{1/2}$ increased; C_{max}, AUC, and $T_{1/2}$ of escitalopram increased by 35%, 50%, and 50%, respectively
- Limit dose of citalopram and escitalopram to a maximum of 20 mg/day and 10 mg/day, respectively, due to risk of QT prolongation
- Monitor for drug-drug interactions (i.e., CYP450 inhibition/induction)
- Improvement as well as worsening in cognitive functioning in elderly depressed patients has been noted
- Impaired balance and falls reported; tend to occur early in treatment and are more likely with higher doses[11]; SSRIs increase fracture risk by causing a reduction in bone mineral density
- Both weight gain and weight loss reported; monitor for excessive weight loss in debilitated patients
- Extrapyramidal effects including dyskinesias and parkinsonism reported; they are not dose related and can develop with short-term or long-term use
- Monitor serum electrolytes (sodium and urea nitrogen levels); hyponatremia reported with all SSRIs (e.g., in 12% of elderly on paroxetine) usually within 2 weeks of drug initiation; can present with confusion, somnolence, fatigue, delirium, hallucinations, urinary incontinence, hypotension, and vomiting

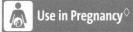 **Use in Pregnancy**◊

- Gestational exposure to SSRIs associated with significantly increased risk of post-partum hemorrhage (PPH), although increase is smaller than that associated with obstetric risk factors for PPH. That said, precautionary measures should be taken, such as administration of a uterotonic agent immediately after delivery to all women who have received SSRI treatment during the month preceding delivery and close monitoring for continued blood loss for the first 24 h following delivery
- Despite extensive studies on the effects of SSRIs in pregnancy, conflicting views on possible adverse effects on the course of pregnancy and on the newborn remain, likely because of the complex and confounding role of factors such as maternal illness itself and stress. Additionally, because depression in late pregnancy is a major predictor for potentially life-threatening postpartum depression, it is advisable to weigh the benefits of treatment against possible hazards. Overall, the consistent message at this time is that this is an individualized decision, but the risk associated with treatment discontinuation in those at high risk of relapse seems to outweigh the potential risks, as severe maternal illness may negatively affect the child's development[12]
- Teratogenicity – accumulating evidence suggests a generally small risk of congenital malformations and argues against a substantial teratogenic effect[13]
- In studies controlling for potential confounders, there was no significant detrimental effect of SSRIs on spontaneous abortions, intrauterine fetal death, preterm delivery, and intrauterine growth restriction

◊ See p. 473 for further information on drug use in pregnancy and effects on breast milk

Selective Serotonin Reuptake Inhibitors (SSRIs) (cont.)

- Studies show that prenatal exposure to SSRIs is associated with a small additional risk of persistent pulmonary hypertension in the newborn (PPHN) but clinical significance remains modest – symptoms may appear even several days after birth, but notably the clinical course is less severe relative to typical PPHN resulting from other causes. Of the SSRIs, sertraline appears to have the lowest risk but further studies are needed to confirm
- Neonatal abstinence syndrome (NAS), which includes poor neonatal adaption and neonatal withdrawal, is the most commonly reported adverse neonatal outcome associated with early-life SSRI exposure. Occurs in approximately 30% of exposed infants. Clinical findings include irritability, abnormal crying, tremor, jitteriness, lethargy, respiratory distress, poor muscle tone, and (rarely) convulsions. Symptoms peak within 2–4 days after birth, then typically dissipate within a few weeks
- At present, there is inadequate and inconsistent evidence for an association between SSRIs and autism spectrum disorder (ASD) in offspring, especially when controlling for confounding factors
- Higher plasma levels of paroxetine reported in infants whose mothers also received clonazepam
- Reports of prominent decreases in dose-adjusted levels of fluvoxamine particularly in the third trimester
- With the possible exception of paroxetine, available evidence isn't adequate to discern specific risks amongst the different SSRIs; prenatal exposure to escitalopram and fluvoxamine have been far less studied than other SSRIs
- Metabolic changes may necessitate dose adjustments over the course of pregnancy and after delivery

Breast Milk

- Although all SSRIs may be secreted in breast milk, concentrations are generally low and overall infant exposure relatively limited so SSRIs are all considered compatible; however, when initiating treatment during breastfeeding, sertraline and paroxetine are considered preferred agents as they have the most research combined with low to undetectable levels; fluoxetine is well researched but exhibits the highest breast milk concentrations and its long half-life increases risk of accumulation in the infant, making it less advisable in this scenario
- Mothers who are already stabilized on an SSRI at delivery should not be discouraged from breastfeeding, nor is there any evidence that would advise switching agents in the context of stable illness

 Nursing Implications

- Psychotherapy and education are also important in the treatment of depression
- Monitor therapy by watching for adverse effects and mood and activity level changes, including worsening of suicidal thoughts, especially at start of therapy or following an increase or decrease in dose
- Be aware that the medication reduces the degree of depression and may increase psychomotor activity; this may create concern about suicidal behavior
- Watch for increased bruising, nosebleeds, or evidence of GI bleed, especially in patients also taking ASA or NSAIDs, steroids or anticoagulants
- Excessive ingestion of caffeinated foods, drugs or beverages may increase anxiety and agitation and confuse the diagnosis
- Extended/controlled-release fluvoxamine, paroxetine and fluoxetine products, and delayed-release fluoxetine tablets should not be broken, crushed or chewed but swallowed whole, with water
- Sertraline should be given with food (increases peak plasma level); food reduces incidence of nausea with all SSRIs
- Ingestion of grapefruit juice while taking fluvoxamine and sertraline may increase the plasma level of these drugs
- SSRIs should not be stopped suddenly due to risk of precipitating withdrawal reactions

 Patient Instructions

- For detailed patient instructions on SSRI antidepressants, see the Patient Information Sheet (details p. 474)

Drug Interactions

- Clinically significant interactions are listed below
- For more interaction information on any given combination, also see the corresponding chapter for the second agent

Class of Drug	Example	Interaction Effects
α_2-adrenergic agonist	Tizanidine	Increased AUC of tizanidine (14- to 103-fold), increased C_{max} (5- to 32-fold), and half-life (3-fold) with fluvoxamine due to inhibition of metabolism via CYP1A2
Analgesic	Acetylsalicylic acid	Increased risk of upper GI bleed from 3.6-fold with SSRI alone to 5-fold in combination
Anorexiant	Phentermine	Case reports of mania and psychosis in combination
	Sibutramine	Reports of serotonin syndrome (see p. 10) Case report of hypomania with citalopram
Antiarrhythmic	Flecainide, mexiletine, propafenone	Increased plasma level of antiarrhythmic with fluoxetine and paroxetine due to inhibited metabolism via CYP2D6
	Lidocaine, quinidine	Increased plasma level of antiarrhythmic possible with fluoxetine, fluvoxamine, sertraline, and paroxetine due to inhibited metabolism via CYP3A4
Antibiotic	Clarithromycin	Case of delirium with fluoxetine; case of serotonin syndrome with citalopram
	Erythromycin	Increased plasma level of citalopram due to inhibited metabolism via CYP3A4 is possible – this can lead to QTc interval prolongation with citalopram and escitalopram; case of serotonin syndrome with sertraline in a 12-year-old
	Linezolid	Monitor for increased serotonergic effects due to linezolid's weak MAO inhibition
Anticoagulant	Apixaban, dabigatran, rivaroxaban	Increased risk of bleeding possible due to decreased platelet aggregation secondary to depletion of serotonin in platelets
	Warfarin	Increased risk of bleeding; increased prothrombin ratio or INR response due to decreased platelet aggregation secondary to depletion of serotonin in platelets 65% increase in plasma level of warfarin with fluvoxamine due to accumulation of R-warfarin through inhibited metabolism (via CYP1A2 and 3A4) and decreased clearance of S-isomer (via CYP2C9)
Anticonvulsant	Barbiturates	Barbiturate metabolism inhibited by fluoxetine; reduced plasma level of SSRIs due to enzyme induction by barbiturate
	Carbamazepine, phenobarbital, phenytoin	Decreased plasma level of SSRIs; half-life of paroxetine decreased by 28% Increased plasma level of carbamazepine or phenytoin due to inhibition of metabolism with fluoxetine and fluvoxamine; elevated phenytoin level with sertraline and paroxetine Increased nausea with fluvoxamine and carbamazepine
	Divalproex, Valproate, valproic acid	Increased plasma level of valproate (up to 50%) with fluoxetine Valproate may increase plasma level of fluoxetine
	Topiramate	Two case reports of angle-closure glaucoma in females on combination
Antidepressant NDRI	Bupropion	Additive antidepressant effect in refractory patients. Bupropion may reverse SSRI-induced sexual dysfunction. Case of hypersexual behavior in combination with fluoxetine Reports of unsteadiness and ataxia in elderly subjects in combination with paroxetine Cases of anxiety, panic, delirium, tremor, myoclonus, and seizure reported with fluoxetine due to inhibited metabolism of bupropion and/or fluoxetine (via CYP3A4 and 2D6), competition for protein binding, and additive pharmacological effects
SNRI	Duloxetine	Increased plasma level of duloxetine due to inhibition of metabolism via CYP1A2 by fluvoxamine; reported to reduce duloxetine plasma clearance by 77% in one study; avoid combination
	Venlafaxine	Reports that combination with SSRIs that inhibit CYP2D6 (e.g., paroxetine, fluoxetine) can result in increased levels of venlafaxine, with possible increase in blood pressure, anticholinergic effects, and serotonergic effects
SARI	Nefazodone, trazodone	Additive antidepressant effect Elevated plasma level of SARI; increased serotonergic effects Increased level of mCPP metabolite of trazodone and nefazodone with paroxetine (via inhibition of CYP2D6), resulting in increased anxiogenic potential

Selective Serotonin Reuptake Inhibitors (SSRIs) (cont.)

Class of Drug	Example	Interaction Effects
NaSSA	Mirtazapine	Combination reported to alleviate insomnia with low mirtazapine doses (less than 30 mg) and augment antidepressant response May mitigate SSRI-induced sexual dysfunction and "poop-out" syndrome Increased serotonergic effects possible Increased sedation and weight gain reported with combination Increased mirtazapine level (up to 4-fold) reported in combination with fluvoxamine due to inhibited metabolism
Nonselective cyclic	Amitriptyline, desipramine, imipramine	Elevated plasma level of cyclic antidepressant with fluoxetine, fluvoxamine, and paroxetine due to inhibition of oxidative metabolism; can occur with higher doses of sertraline Increased desipramine level (by 50%) with citalopram and escitalopram
	Clomipramine	Additive antidepressant effect in treatment-resistant patients Increased serotonergic effects
RIMA	Moclobemide	Combined therapy may have additive antidepressant effect in treatment-resistant patients; use caution and monitor for serotonergic effects; case reports of serotonin syndrome, especially with citalopram and escitalopram
Irreversible MAOI	Phenelzine, tranylcypromine	Hypermetabolic syndrome (serotonin syndrome – see p. 10) and death reported with combined use. Suggest waiting 5 weeks when switching from fluoxetine to MAOI and vice versa. Increased plasma level of tranylcypromine (by 15%) reported with paroxetine
Antiemetic (5-HT$_3$ antagonist)	Dolasetron, granisetron, ondansetron	Reports of serotonin syndrome with paroxetine and sertraline One case study suggests SSRIs may reduce the antiemetic effectiveness of 5-HT$_3$ antagonists due to the accumulation of serotonin from SSRIs overcoming the blockade by 5-HT$_3$ antagonists
	Alosetron	DO NOT USE with fluvoxamine as plasma level of alosetron increased 6-fold and half-life increased 3-fold due to inhibited metabolism via CYP1A2
Antifungal	Fluconazole, ketoconazole	Decreased C_{max} of ketoconazole by 21% with citalopram 2 cases of life-threatening serotonin syndrome reported with citalopram
	Terbinafine	Increased paroxetine exposure (AUC by 2.5-fold, C_{max} by 86%, half-life by 48%) via CYP2D6 inhibition by terbinafine
Antihistamine	Diphenhydramine	Increased plasma levels of fluoxetine and paroxetine possible due to inhibited metabolism via CYP2D6 Additive CNS effects
Antiparkinsonian	Benztropine	Increased plasma level of benztropine with paroxetine; case report of delirium associated with paroxetine combination
	Procyclidine	Increased plasma level of procyclidine with paroxetine (by 40%)
Antiplatelet	Clopidogrel	Increased risk of bleeding by (54%)
Antipsychotic	General	May worsen extrapyramidal effects and akathisia, especially if antidepressant added early in the course of antipsychotic therapy May be useful for negative symptoms of schizophrenia Increased plasma level of antipsychotic due to inhibition of metabolism via CYP1A2 (potent – fluvoxamine), 2D6 (potent – fluoxetine and paroxetine), and/or 3A4 (fluvoxamine). Monitor for increased antipsychotic adverse effects (e.g., sedation, orthostatic hypotension, EPS) when starting and antipsychotic efficacy when stopping SSRI. Adjust antipsychotic dose as needed. Alternatively, consider using an SSRI with no or weak effects on CYPs such as citalopram, escitalopram, and sertraline (at doses of 100 mg/day or less) or use an SSRI that does not affect the specific CYP enzyme which metabolizes the specific antipsychotic
First generation	Chlorpromazine, fluphenazine, haloperidol, perphenazine	Haloperidol levels: 20–35% higher with fluoxetine; 23–60% higher with fluvoxamine; 28% higher with sertraline Perphenazine peak levels 2- to 13-fold higher with paroxetine Case report of QT prolongation and patient collapsing with concurrent chlorpromazine and fluoxetine Increased EPS and akathisia

Class of Drug	Example	Interaction Effects
Second generation	Pimozide	Pimozide levels: 151% higher AUC and 62% higher peak level with paroxetine; 40% higher AUC and peak level with sertraline. Case reports of bradycardia with concurrent use of pimozide and fluoxetine Pimozide level also increased when combined with citalopram, escitalopram or fluvoxamine, increasing risk of QTc prolongation – DO NOT COMBINE
	Thioridazine	3-fold increase in thioridazine levels with fluvoxamine DO NOT COMBINE fluvoxamine, fluoxetine, sertraline or paroxetine with thioridazine due to risk of cardiac conduction disturbances
	Asenapine	Asenapine's C_{max} (+13%) and AUC (+29%) increased by fluvoxamine. Asenapine (a weak inhibitor of CYP2D6) increases paroxetine exposure by $\sim$2-fold. Reduce paroxetine dose by 50% if asenapine added
	Clozapine	Clozapine levels: With fluoxetine, 41–76% higher clozapine levels plus 38–45% higher norclozapine levels; one fatality reported; case report of acute myocarditis after addition of clozapine to fluoxetine and lithium. With fluvoxamine, 3–11-fold higher levels. With paroxetine, no change to 41% increase in clozapine plus 45% increase in norclozapine. With sertraline, 41–76% clozapine increase plus 45% norclozapine increase; one fatal arrhythmia reported but causality unclear
	Iloperidone	Iloperidone's AUC increased by $\sim$1.6- to 3-fold in the presence of fluoxetine or paroxetine. Reduce iloperidone dose by 50% if fluoxetine or paroxetine added
	Olanzapine	Olanzapine levels: With fluoxetine, 16% increase in peak concentration; not clinically significant. In the USA, olanzapine/fluoxetine available as a combination product. With fluvoxamine, 2.3- to 4-fold increase in olanzapine levels; consider use of an SSRI with less effect on CYP1A2 or use lower olanzapine doses and monitor for adverse effects (e.g., EPS, hypersalivation)
	Paliperidone, risperidone, ziprasidone	Case reports of dose-related mania when risperidone or ziprasidone added to SSRI Risperidone levels: With fluoxetine, 2.5- to 8-fold increased levels and case report of TD. With paroxetine, 3- to 9-fold higher levels and cases of serotonin syndrome; consider using an alternative SSRI. Case reports of serotonin syndrome and/or NMS with fluvoxamine and trazodone plus sertraline Case report of serotonin syndrome with ziprasidone and citalopram CAUTION with paliperidone and ziprasidone; possible additive prolongation of QT interval and associated life-threatening cardiac arrhythmias. Factors that further increase the risk include anorexia, bradycardia, hypokalemia, and hypomagnesemia
Third generation	Aripiprazole	44% increase in aripiprazole plasma level possible by fluoxetine or paroxetine, due to inhibited metabolism via CYP2D6. Reduce aripiprazole dose by 50%. No significant pharmacokinetic changes to escitalopram, fluoxetine, paroxetine, or sertraline. Case report of NMS with fluoxetine 20 mg/day and aripiprazole 30 mg/day. Case report of urinary obstruction with citalopram 10 mg/day and aripiprazole 20 mg/day; unknown if due to citalopram alone. Case reports of severe akathisia, acute dystonia, and myxedema coma with sertraline 200 mg/day and aripiprazole 10, 15, and 20 mg/day, respectively. Consider using an SSRI with no or weak effects on CYPs, such as citalopram and escitalopram
Antiretroviral		
Non-nucleoside reverse transcriptase inhibitor (NNRTI)	Efavirenz	Decreased plasma level of sertraline (39% decrease in AUC) via CYP3A4 induction; one case report of serotonin syndrome after initiation of efavirenz while taking fluoxetine
	Nevirapine	One study suggests nevirapine may decrease fluoxetine plasma levels, and fluvoxamine may increase nevirapine plasma levels
Protease inhibitor	Darunavir/ritonavir	Decreased plasma level of paroxetine (39% decrease in AUC) and sertraline (49% decrease in AUC)
	Fosamprenavir/ritonavir	Decreased plasma level of paroxetine (54% decrease in AUC)
	Ritonavir	Increased plasma level of sertraline due to competition for metabolism; moderate increase in level of fluoxetine and paroxetine. Serotonin syndrome reported in combination with high dose of fluoxetine. Note that ritonavir-boosted nirmatrelvir may be co-administered without dose adjustment[14] Cardiac and neurological side effects reported with fluoxetine due to elevated ritonavir level (19% increase in AUC)

Selective Serotonin Reuptake Inhibitors (SSRIs) (cont.)

Class of Drug	Example	Interaction Effects
Antitubercular	Rifampin	Case reports of SSRI withdrawal symptoms and decreased therapeutic efficacy of sertraline and citalopram due to CYP3A4 induction by rifampin
Anxiolytic Benzodiazepine	Alprazolam, bromazepam, diazepam	Increased plasma level of benzodiazepine metabolized by CYP3A4; alprazolam (by 100% with fluvoxamine and 46% with fluoxetine), bromazepam, triazolam, midazolam, and diazepam; small (13%) decrease in clearance of diazepam reported with sertraline Increased sedation, psychomotor and memory impairment Combination may increase risk of falls in the elderly
Buspirone	Buspirone	Anxiolytic effects of buspirone may be antagonized Increased plasma level of buspirone (3-fold increase in AUC) with fluvoxamine Case report of possible serotonin syndrome with fluoxetine
β-blocker	Metoprolol, propranolol	Decreased heart rate and syncope (additive effect) reported Increased side effects, lethargy, and bradycardia with fluoxetine, fluvoxamine, and paroxetine due to decreased metabolism of the β-blocker via CYP2D6 (5-fold increase in propranolol level reported with fluvoxamine) Increased metoprolol level with citalopram (by 100%) and with escitalopram (by 50%)
	Pindolol	Increased concentration of serotonin at postsynaptic sites; faster onset of therapeutic response Increased half-life of pindolol (by 28%) with fluoxetine; increased plasma level with paroxetine due to inhibited metabolism via CYP2D6
Caffeine		Increased caffeine levels with fluvoxamine due to inhibited metabolism via CYP1A2; half-life increased from 5 to 31 h Increased jitteriness and insomnia
Calcium channel blocker	Nifedipine, verapamil	Increased side effects (headache, flushing, edema) due to inhibited clearance of calcium channel blocker via CYP3A4 with fluoxetine, fluvoxamine, sertraline, and paroxetine
Cannabis/marijuana		Case report of mania in combination with fluoxetine possibly due to additive serotonin reuptake inhibition from the THC component of cannabis; caution with concurrent use due to risk of additive CNS effects
	Diltiazem	Bradycardia in combination with fluvoxamine
Cardiac glycoside	Digoxin	Decreased level (AUC) of digoxin (by 18%) reported with paroxetine
CNS depressant	Alcohol	Potentiation of CNS effects; low risk Rate of fluvoxamine absorption increased by ethanol
Corticosteroid	Prednisone	Increased risk of GI bleed
Cyclobenzaprine		Increased side effects of cyclobenzaprine with fluoxetine due to inhibited metabolism; observe for QT prolongation
DDAVP		Water intoxication and hyponatremia in rare cases
Ergot alkaloid	Dihydroergotamine	Increased serotonergic effects with intravenous use – AVOID. Oral, rectal, and subcutaneous routes can be used, with monitoring
	Ergotamine	Elevated ergotamine levels possible due to inhibited metabolism via CYP3A4 with fluoxetine and fluvoxamine
Ginkgo biloba		Possible increased risk of petechiae and bleeding due to combined anti-hemostatic effects
Grapefruit juice		Decreased metabolism via CYP3A4 of fluvoxamine and sertraline resulting in increased plasma levels
H$_2$ antagonist	Cimetidine	Inhibited metabolism and increased plasma level of sertraline (by 25%), paroxetine (by 50%), citalopram, and escitalopram
Hallucinogen	LSD	Recurrence or worsening of flashbacks reported with fluoxetine, sertraline, and paroxetine; conflicting studies suggest SSRIs may be associated with either an increase or decrease in subjective response to LSD

Class of Drug	Example	Interaction Effects
Hypnotic/sedative	Chloral hydrate	Increased sedation and side effects with fluoxetine and fluvoxamine due to inhibited metabolism of chloral hydrate
	Ramelteon	DO NOT COMBINE with fluvoxamine; increased C_{max} (70-fold) and AUC (190-fold) of ramelteon due to inhibited metabolism via CYP1A2
	Zolpidem	Case reports of hallucinations and delirium when combined with sertraline, fluoxetine, and paroxetine
		Administration of sertraline resulted in faster onset of action and increase in peak plasma concentration of zolpidem
Immunosuppressant	Cyclosporine	Decreased clearance of cyclosporine with sertraline due to competition for metabolism via CYP3A4
Insulin		Increased insulin sensitivity reported
Kava kava		Case report of lethargic state with paroxetine
Licorice		Increased serotonergic effects possible via MAO inhibition by licorice constituents
Lithium		Increased serotonergic effects
		Changes in lithium level and clearance reported
		Caution with fluoxetine and fluvoxamine; neurotoxicity and seizures reported
		Increased tremor and nausea reported with sertraline and paroxetine
		Additive antidepressant effect in treatment-resistant patients
L-tryptophan		May result in central and peripheral toxicity, hypermetabolic syndrome (serotonin syndrome – see p. 10)
MAO-B inhibitor	Rasagiline	Limited data; benefits of treating depression related to Parkinson's disease generally outweighs risks – may use MAO-B inhibitors cautiously with an SSRI as long as recommended doses are not exceeded and SSRI is slowly titrated with adequate monitoring; citalopram or sertraline are the preferred choices for initial SSRI selection
	Selegiline (L-deprenyl)	Case reports of serotonin syndrome (see p. 3), hypertension, and mania when combined with fluoxetine
		Risk of serotonin syndrome mostly theoretical – combination has been used for many years with very infrequent case reports
Melatonin		Increased levels of melatonin with fluvoxamine due to inhibited metabolism via CYP1A2 or 2C9 (12-fold increase in plasma melatonin levels reported); endogenous melatonin secretion increased
Methylene blue		Enhanced serotonergic effects through inhibition of MAO-A and B by methylene blue. Risk for serotonin syndrome (see Precautions p. 10)
Metoclopramide		Report of increased extrapyramidal effects with fluoxetine, fluvoxamine, paroxetine, and sertraline potentially via additive D_2 receptor antagonism by metoclopramide and inhibition of dopamine neurotransmission by SSRIs; case reports of serotonin syndrome with sertraline and fluoxetine potentially via the 5-HT$_3$ receptor blocking effect of metoclopramide
NSAID		Increased risk of upper GI bleed with combined use (risk increased 12-fold) CAUTION
Opioids and related drugs	Codeine, oxycodone, hydrocodone	Decreased analgesic effect with fluoxetine and paroxetine due to inhibited metabolism to active moiety – morphine, oxymorphone, and hydromorphone, respectively (interaction may be beneficial in the treatment of dependence by decreasing morphine and analog formation and opiate reinforcing properties)
	Dextromethorphan	Visual hallucinations reported with fluoxetine; fluoxetine and paroxetine may inhibit metabolism via CYP2D6; monitor for increased serotonergic effects
	Methadone	Elevated plasma level of methadone (by 10–100%) reported with fluvoxamine
	Morphine	Conflicting studies show fluoxetine antagonized and augmented analgesia from morphine
	Pentazocine	Report of excitatory toxicity (serotonergic) with fluoxetine and pentazocine
	Tramadol	Increased risk of seizures and serotonin syndrome
		Possible decreased analgesic effect with SSRIs that inhibit CYP2D6 (fluoxetine, paroxetine) due to decreased conversion to the active M1 metabolite
Phosphodiesterase type 5 (PDE5) inhibitor	Sildenafil	Possible enhanced hypotension due to inhibited metabolism of sildenafil via CYP3A4 with fluoxetine and fluvoxamine

Selective Serotonin Reuptake Inhibitors (SSRIs) (cont.)

Class of Drug	Example	Interaction Effects
Proguanil		The conversion of proguanil to its active metabolite, cycloguanil, is markedly inhibited by fluvoxamine (via CYP2C19 inhibition) in patients who have normal CYP2C19 activity
Proton pump inhibitor	Omeprazole	Increased plasma level of citalopram due to inhibited metabolism via CYP2C19
Selective norepinephrine reuptake inhibitor	Atomoxetine	Increased plasma level and half-life of atomoxetine due to inhibited metabolism via CYP2D6 (fluoxetine, paroxetine)
Smoking (tobacco)		Increased metabolism of fluvoxamine (by 25%) via CYP1A2
Statin	Lovastatin, simvastatin Pravastatin	Increased plasma level of statin with fluoxetine, fluvoxamine, sertraline, and paroxetine due to inhibited metabolism via CYP3A4 Synergistic effect on increasing blood glucose (paroxetine)
St. John's wort		May augment serotonergic effects – several reports of serotonin syndrome (see p. 10)
Stimulant	Amphetamine, methylphenidate	Potentiated effect in depression, dysthymia, and OCD, in patients with comorbid ADHD; may improve response in treatment-refractory paraphilias and paraphilia-related disorders Plasma level of antidepressant may be increased
Sulfonylurea	Glyburide, tolbutamide	Increased hypoglycemia reported in diabetics Increased plasma level of tolbutamide due to reduced clearance (up to 16%) with sertraline
Tamoxifen		Inhibitors of CYP2D6 (paroxetine, fluoxetine) appear to reduce the conversion of tamoxifen to its active metabolite (endoxifen) and may decrease the therapeutic efficacy of this drug
Theophylline		Increased plasma level of theophylline with fluvoxamine due to decreased metabolism via CYP1A2
Thyroid drug	Triiodothyronine (T_3-liothyronine)	Antidepressant effect potentiated Elevated serum thyrotropin (and reduced free thyroxine concentration) reported with sertraline; however, a newer study reports no clinically significant changes in thyroid function with fluoxetine or sertraline
Tolterodine		Decreased oral clearance of tolterodine (by up to 93%) with fluoxetine (a CYP2D6 inhibitor) – interaction not considered clinically significant unless patient is also taking a CYP3A4 inhibitor
Triptan	Rizatriptan, sumatriptan	Inadequate data available to determine the risk of serotonin syndrome with the addition of a triptan to SSRIs. However, given the seriousness of serotonin syndrome, caution is warranted

Norepinephrine Dopamine Reuptake Inhibitor (NDRI)

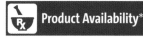 **Product Availability***

Generic Name	Chemical Class	Neuroscience-based Nomenclature* (Pharmacological Target/Mode of Action)	Trade Name(A)	Dosage Forms and Strengths
Bupropion	Monocyclic (aminoketone)	Norepinephrine, dopamine/Reuptake inhibitor (NET, DAT), releaser (NE, DA)	Aplenzin(B) Wellbutrin(B) Wellbutrin SR, Zyban(D) Wellbutrin XL, Forfivo(B)	Extended-release tablets(B): 174 mg, 348 mg, 522 mg Tablets(B): 75 mg, 100 mg Sustained-release tablets(C): 100 mg, 150 mg, 200 mg(B) Extended-release tablets: 150 mg, 300 mg, 450 mg(B)

* Refer to Health Canada's Drug Product Database or the FDA's Drugs@FDA for the most current availability information   * Developed by a taskforce consisting of representatives from the American College of Neuropsychopharmacology (ACNP), the Asian College of Neuropsychopharmacology (AsCNP), the European College of Neuropsychopharmacology (ECNP), the International College of Neuropsychopharmacology (CINP), and the International Union of Basic and Clinical Pharmacology (IUPHAR) (see https://nbn2r.com), (A) Generic preparations may be available,   (B) Not marketed in Canada,   (C) Not marketed in the USA,   (D) Marketed as aid in smoking cessation (as 150 mg)

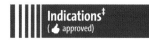 **Indications‡** (👍 approved)

- 👍 Major depressive disorder (MDD)
- 👍 Seasonal affective disorder (SAD)
- 👍 Smoking cessation
- Dysthymia and chronic fatigue syndrome – efficacy reported
- MDD, recurrent: Prophylaxis
- Bipolar disorder: Depressed phase (use with an antimanic agent)
- Social phobia – case reports of efficacy
- ADHD – controlled studies suggest benefit in adults and children; primarily in individuals with simple ADHD or with comorbid depression, cigarette smoking or active substance use disorder
- Sexual dysfunction (e.g., reduced sexual desire, anorgasmia, erectile problems) induced by SSRIs and SNRIs; promising role in mitigating sexual dysfunction in opioid substitution therapy
- Neuropathic pain – randomized control studies suggest benefit
- Trichotillomania – case reports of benefit
- Addictive disorders (e.g., cocaine, alcohol[15], marijuana)
- Internet gaming disorder
- Weight loss in patients taking naltrexone

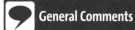 **General Comments**

- May have a lower switch rate (to hypomania or mania) than other antidepressants, although a recent meta-analysis found a similar phase shifting rate
- May enhance energy and motivation early in treatment due to effects on norepinephrine and dopamine; reported to improve neurocognitive function in patients with depression
- Compared to IR, SR preparation appears to be better tolerated and is associated with a decreased risk of seizures and lower risk of sexual dysfunction
- Monitor patients for worsening of depression and suicidal thinking
- Monitor patients taking bupropion for smoking cessation as serious neuropsychiatric events have occurred in this population
- Superior to placebo for smoking cessation at 3 months and 12 months. Abstinence rates at 12 months: Bupropion 19% (vs. 9% on placebo)
- Least likely of all antidepressants to impair sexual functioning
- Case reports of recreational abuse with bupropion via oral, intranasal, and intravenous administration

‡ Indications listed here do not necessarily apply to all NDRIs or all countries. Please refer to a country's regulatory database (e.g., US Food and Drug Administration, Health Canada Drug Product Database) for the most current availability information and indications

Norepinephrine Dopamine Reuptake Inhibitor (NDRI) (cont.)

Pharmacology	• Inhibits the reuptake of primarily norepinephrine (and dopamine to a lesser extent) into presynaptic neurons • Its major metabolite (hydroxybupropion), which in humans is present at blood levels 10- to 20-fold higher than bupropion, blocks only norepinephrine reuptake
Dosing	• See p. 94 • Regular immediate-release bupropion and SR preparation should be prescribed in divided doses (preferably 8 h or more apart), with a maximum of 150 mg per IR dose and 200 mg per SR dose; XL preparation formulated for once daily dosing • Initiate doses for depression at 100–150 mg daily. Dose may be increased to 300 mg/day in patients who do not respond to 150 mg/day; if tolerated, may be further titrated as necessary to a maximum of 200 mg bid for SR and 450 mg XL for major depressive disorder (doses beyond 300 mg/day not studied in seasonal affective disorder) • Forfivo XL for treatment of depression may only be used after initial titration with other bupropion products; patients receiving 300 mg daily of bupropion HCL (as immediate-release, SR or XL) for at least 2 weeks and requiring a dose increase, or patients already taking 450 mg daily of bupropion HCL may switch to Forfivo XL 450 mg daily • Aplenzin (bupropion hydrobromide): Initial dosing of 174 mg daily and may increase on day 4 (for treatment of depression) or on day 7 (for treatment of SAD) to 348 mg daily; maximum dose is 522 mg daily; Bupropion HCL (as immediate-release, SR or XL): 150 mg, 300 mg, 450 mg is equivalent to 174 mg, 348 mg, 522 mg bupropion hydrobromide, respectively • For smoking cessation: Initial dosing of 150 mg daily for 3 days, then 150 mg twice daily. Treatment should continue for 1 week before target quit date and continue for 7-12 weeks • In adults with ADHD, begin at 150 mg/day and titrate dose gradually to a maximum of 450 mg/day in divided doses; up to 4 weeks may be required for maximum drug effect • In renal impairment, reduce dose and frequency and monitor for adverse effects such as insomnia, dry mouth, or seizures that could indicate higher than normal levels; Forfivo XL not recommended in renal impairment • In mild to moderate hepatic impairment (Child-Pugh Grade A or B), initiate treatment at the lowest recommended dose. Use with extreme caution in patients with severe hepatic impairment. Forfivo XL not recommended
Pharmacokinetics	• Rapid absorption with peak concentration occurring within 2 h after administration of immediate-release tablets, 3 h after administration of sustained-release tablets, 5 h after administration of extended-release tablets; peak plasma concentration of sustained-release preparation is 50–85% that of the immediate-release tablets after single dosing, and 25% after chronic dosing • Protein binding 80–85% • Metabolized predominantly by the liver, primarily via CYP2B6 and to a lesser extent by other isoenzymes – 6 metabolites; 3 are active • Bupropion and hydroxybupropion exhibit dose-dependent inhibition of CYP2D6 isoenzyme • Elimination half-life: 11–14 h; with chronic dosing: 21 h (mean); increased half-life of bupropion and its metabolites and decreased clearance reported in the elderly
Onset & Duration of Action	• Therapeutic effect typically seen after 28 days (though effects may be sooner in some patients)
Adverse Effects	• See chart on p. 91 for incidence of adverse effects
CNS Effects	• A result of effects on dopamine and norepinephrine • Insomnia – IR or SR formulations may be associated with significantly more insomnia compared with XL formulation; vivid dreams and nightmares reported; decreased REM latency and increased REM sleep • Agitation, anxiety, irritability, dysphoria, aggression, hostility, depersonalization, coupled with urges of self-harm or harm to others

- Traditionally, precipitation of hypomania or mania felt to be less likely than with other cyclic antidepressants
- Can exacerbate psychotic symptoms
- Very high doses can result in CNS toxicity including delirium, confusion, impaired concentration, hallucinations, delusions, EPS, and seizures
- Reported to exacerbate symptoms of OCD
- Short-term memory loss reported
- Risk of seizures with SR formulation at doses of 100–300 mg/day = 0.1% and at doses of 400 mg/day = 0.4%. With immediate-release formulation, seizure incidence of 0.4% with dosing of 300-450 mg/day, risk increases almost tenfold with dosing of 450-600 mg/day; in clinical trials for XL formulation, overall seizure incidence was 0.1% – in those treated with 450 mg, incidence with higher dose was 0.39%; however, seizures have been observed across all doses and formulations in the post-marketing setting
- Disturbance in gait, fine tremor, myoclonus
- Reversible dyskinesia reported; may aggravate neuroleptic-induced tardive dyskinesia
- Headache, arthralgia (4%), neuralgias (5%), myalgia [Management: Analgesics prn]
- Tinnitus reported

Anticholinergic Effects	

- No appreciable affinity for cholinergic receptors
- Occur rarely
- Mydriasis
- Dry mouth
- Constipation

Cardiovascular Effects	

- Modest sustained increases in blood pressure reported in adults and children (more likely in patients with pre-existing hypertension and in those receiving nicotine replacement therapy) – caution in patients with ischemic heart disease
- Orthostatic hypotension, dizziness occurs occasionally, especially when bupropion added to SSRI – caution in the elderly
- Palpitations
- Case of transient ischemic attacks reported
- Rare cases of myocarditis, myocardial infarction, and cardiac death

Endocrine & Metabolic Effects	

- Menstrual irregularities reported (up to 9% risk)
- Cases of hypoglycemia, hyperglycemia, SIADH

Other Adverse Effects	

- Urticarial or pruritic rashes have been reported; rare cases of erythema multiforme and Stevens-Johnson syndrome
- Anaphylactoid reactions with pruritus, urticaria, angioedema, and dyspnea (up to 0.3%)
- Delayed hypersensitivity reactions with arthralgia, myalgia, fever, and rash. The symptoms may resemble serum sickness. Post-marketing reports of hypersensitivity reactions in those who consumed alcohol
- Rarely hepatotoxicity with hepatocellular and/or cholestatic pattern of damage; predominantly immune-mediated, typically accompanied by hypersensitivity reactions; onset is highly variable but appears to occur more consistently in the first 2 months
- Dose-dependent urinary frequency and diurnal enuresis reported
- Nausea, anorexia, and weight loss with acute and long-term treatment
- Rarely febrile neutropenia
- Alopecia
- Sweating (also due to NE-reuptake inhibition)
- Rare cases of stuttering and exacerbation of tics
- Case reports of premature ejaculation, spontaneous ejaculation, and spontaneous orgasm

D/C Discontinuation Syndrome	

- Abrupt discontinuation may cause a syndrome consisting of dizziness, lethargy, nausea, vomiting, diarrhea, headache, fever, sweating, chills, malaise, incoordination, insomnia, vivid dreams, myalgia, paresthesias, dyskinesias, "electric-shock-like" sensations, visual discoordination, anxiety, irritability, confusion, slowed thinking, disorientation; rarely aggression, impulsivity, hypomania, and depersonalization
- Brain "zaps" (or electric-shock-like sensations), often associated with lateral eye movements, hearing static sounds, and feelings of dizziness/wooziness; usually transitory but may last for months
- Case of mania reported 2 weeks after abrupt discontinuation of bupropion 300 mg/day taken for 5 weeks to aid in smoking cessation

Norepinephrine Dopamine Reuptake Inhibitor (NDRI) (cont.)

- Rare cases of acute dystonia following abrupt discontinuation
- Most likely to occur within 1–7 days after drug stopped or dose drastically reduced, and typically disappears within 3 weeks

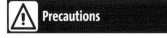
Precautions

- Monitor all patients for worsening depression and suicidal thoughts, especially at the start of therapy and following an increase or decrease in dose
- May lower the seizure threshold; therefore administer cautiously to patients with organic brain disease and when combining with other drugs that may lower the seizure threshold; contraindicated in patients with a history of or current seizure disorder. To minimize seizures with regular-release bupropion, do not exceed a dose increase of 100 mg in a 3-day period. No single dose should exceed 150 mg for the immediate-release or the sustained-release preparation
- Contraindicated in patients with a history of anorexia or bulimia, undergoing alcohol or benzodiazepine withdrawal or with other conditions predisposing to seizures
- Use with caution (i.e., use lower dose and monitor regularly) in patients with hepatic impairment
- Zyban, marketed for smoking cessation, contains bupropion – DO NOT COMBINE with other bupropion products
- Caution in patients with narrow-angle glaucoma

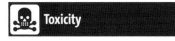
Toxicity

- Commonly causes agitation, drowsiness, seizures (delayed in onset 18 h), and sinus tachycardia; rarely causes hypotension, bradycardia, serious cardiac dysrhythmia, hyperreflexia, elevated transaminases
- High risk of QTc interval prolongation following overdose
- Rare reports of death following massive overdose, preceded by uncontrolled seizures, bradycardia, cardiac failure, and cardiac arrest

Management

- Single dose of activated charcoal if patient presents within 1 h of ingestion
- Supportive treatment
- Monitor ECG and vital signs for 18 h as well as EEG
- Benzodiazepines are first-line therapy for seizures

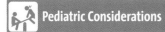
Pediatric Considerations

- For detailed information on the use of bupropion in this population, please see the *Clinical Handbook of Psychotropic Drugs for Children and Adolescents*[8]
- No approved indications in children and adolescents
- In ADHD, controlled studies suggest benefit in children, primarily in individuals with simple ADHD or with comorbid depression
- May exacerbate tics in patients with ADHD and evoke tics in patients with Tourette's syndrome
- Dosage in children: Initiate at 1 mg/kg/day (in divided doses) and increase gradually to a maximum of 6 mg/kg/day (in divided doses)
- Rash reported in up to 17% of youths

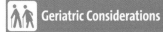
Geriatric Considerations

- The elderly are at risk for accumulation of bupropion and its metabolites due to decreased clearance
- Initiate at the lowest recommended dose
- Orthostatic hypotension or dizziness reported; may predispose to falls
- Extrapyramidal effects have been reported; they are not dose related and can develop with short-term or long-term use
- Prior to prescribing bupropion, screen for factors that may predispose an elderly patient to seizures

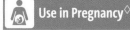
Use in Pregnancy◊

- Data from the international Bupropion Pregnancy Registry (675 first trimester exposures) and a retrospective cohort study using the United Healthcare database (1,213 first trimester exposures) did not show an increased risk of malformations overall
- No increased risk of cardiovascular malformations overall has been observed after bupropion exposure during the first trimester
- No harm to fetus reported in animal studies; no teratogenic effects reported in humans following use of bupropion in the first trimester
- Higher umbilical cord concentration of metabolites suggest a higher fetal exposure vs. parent drug – consequences of exposure yet to be determined

◊ See p. 473 for further information on drug use in pregnancy and effects on breast milk

- There appears to be no clinically meaningful difference in the stereoselective disposition of the parent drug (or its metabolite) during pregnancy, suggesting that dose adjustment during pregnancy may not be necessary

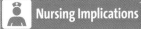

Breast Milk

- Bupropion and metabolites are secreted in breast milk; infant can receive up to 2.7% of maternal dose
- Seizures and sleep disturbances reported in breastfed infants following bupropion exposure via breast milk
- Infants of mothers using psychotropic medications should be monitored daily for changes in sleep, feeding patterns, and behavior as well as infant growth and neurodevelopment
- If a patient is breastfeeding and requires the addition of an antidepressant, other agents may be preferable as first-line options; however, maternal use of bupropion is not considered a reason to discontinue breastfeeding

Nursing Implications

- Risk of seizures increases if any single dose exceeds 150 mg (immediate-release or sustained-release) or if total daily dose exceeds 300 mg; doses above 150 mg daily should be given in divided doses, preferably 8 h or more apart
- Crushing or chewing the sustained or extended-release preparation destroys the slow-release activity of the product; cutting or splitting the SR preparation in half will increase the rate of drug release in the first 15 min. If the tablet is split, the unused half should be discarded unless used within 24 h
- Do not crush, split or chew Forfivo tablets
- Can be administered with or without food
- Bupropion degrades rapidly on exposure to moisture, therefore tablets should not be stored in an area of high humidity
- Monitor therapy by watching for adverse effects and mood and activity level changes including worsening depression and suicidal thoughts, especially at the start of therapy or following an increase or decrease in dose
- If the patient has difficulty sleeping, ensure that the last dose of bupropion is no later than 1500 h
- Ensure the patient is not currently being treated for smoking cessation with Zyban (also contains bupropion)

Patient Instructions

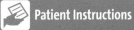

- For detailed patient instructions on bupropion, see the Patient Information Sheet (details on p. 474)

Drug Interactions

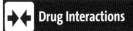

- Clinically significant interactions are listed below
- For more interaction information on any given combination, also see the corresponding chapter for the second agent

Class of Drug	Example	Interaction Effects
Antiparkinsonian	Amantadine, L-dopa	Caution with concurrent use with amantadine or L-dopa; increased side effects, including excitement, restlessness, and tremor due to increased dopamine availability Case reports of neurotoxicity in elderly patients; delirium
Antiarrhythmic (Type 1c)	Flecainide, propafenone	Increased plasma level of antiarrhythmic due to inhibited metabolism via CYP2D6
Antibiotic	Ciprofloxacin, linezolid	Seizure threshold may be reduced Case report of severe intraoperative hypertension in combination with linezolid via MAO inhibition
Anticholinergic	Orphenadrine	Altered levels of either drug due to competition for metabolism via CYP2B6
Anticonvulsant	Carbamazepine, phenobarbital, phenytoin	Decreased plasma level of bupropion and increased level of its metabolite hydroxybupropion due to increased metabolism by the anticonvulsant
	Valproate	Increased level of hydroxybupropion due to inhibited metabolism; level of bupropion not affected
Antidepressant SSRI	Fluoxetine	Case of delirium, anxiety, panic, and myoclonus with fluoxetine due to inhibited metabolism of bupropion and/or fluoxetine (via CYP2D6), competition for protein binding, and additive pharmacological effects Additive antidepressant effect in treatment-refractory patients; bupropion may mitigate SSRI-induced sexual dysfunction
SNRI	Venlafaxine	3-fold increase in venlafaxine level due to inhibited metabolism via CYP2D6, and reduction of level of OD-metabolite Potentiation of noradrenergic effects

Norepinephrine Dopamine Reuptake Inhibitor (NDRI) (cont.)

Class of Drug	Example	Interaction Effects
SMS	Vortioxetine	May increase vortioxetine levels significantly. Recommend reducing dose by 50% when combining
Nonselective cyclic	Desipramine, imipramine, nortriptyline	Elevated imipramine level (by 57%) and nortriptyline level (by 200%) with combination; desipramine peak plasma level and half-life increased 2-fold due to decreased metabolism (via CYP2D6) Seizure threshold may be reduced
Irreversible MAOI	Phenelzine	DO NOT COMBINE – dopamine metabolism inhibited Washout of 14 days recommended between drugs
Antimalarial	Chloroquine, mefloquine	Seizure threshold may be reduced
Antiplatelet	Clopidogrel	May inhibit CYP2B6-catalysed bupropion hydroxylation; increased plasma bupropion concentration and reduced hydroxybupropion concentration. May affect efficacy of bupropion and increase risk of seizures
Antipsychotic		
First generation	Chlorpromazine	Seizure threshold may be reduced
	Thioridazine	Increased plasma level of thioridazine due to decreased metabolism via CYP2D6; increased risk of thioridazine-related ventricular arrhythmias and sudden death. DO NOT COMBINE. Washout of 14 days recommended between drugs
Second generation	Risperidone	Inhibits CYP2D6, leading to decreased metabolism of antipsychotic and/or bupropion – risk of delirium
Antiretroviral		
Non-nucleoside reverse transcriptase inhibitor (NNRTI)	Efavirenz, nevirapine	Decreased AUC of bupropion by 55% via CYP2B6 induction of efavirenz and nevirapine; an increase in bupropion dose may be required, but do not exceed maximum daily bupropion dose
Protease inhibitor	Nelfinavir, ritonavir	CYP2B6 inducers may decrease bupropion AUC by 22–67%, extent seems to vary based on dose, at least with ritonavir; in contrast, a short 2-day course of ritonavir (200 mg bid) had minimal effects on bupropion kinetics, suggesting a slightly delayed onset. Note that ritonavir-boosted nirmatrelvir may be co-administered without dose adjustment
Antitubercular	Rifampin	Decreased bupropion AUC by 67% reported via CYP2B6 induction; potential reduced efficacy of bupropion
β-blocker	Metoprolol	Increased plasma level of β-blocker possible due to inhibited metabolism via CYP2D6
Benzodiazepine	Diazepam	Bupropion may antagonize the functional impairment and drowsiness associated with diazepam; bupropion is contraindicated during abrupt withdrawal of benzodiazepines due to an additive decrease in seizure threshold
CNS depressant	Alcohol	Post-marketing reports of adverse neuropsychiatric events/reduced alcohol tolerance and hypersensitivity reactions. Avoid alcohol while taking bupropion
Corticosteroid (systemic)		Seizure threshold may be reduced
Ginkgo biloba		Seizure threshold may be reduced
Hormone	Estrogen/progesterone	Decreased metabolism (hydroxylation) of bupropion via CYP2B6; interaction with combined oral contraceptive is unlikely to be clinically significant
Hypnotic/sedative	Zolpidem	Case reports of visual hallucinations with combination
Methylene blue		Due to risk of hypertensive reaction through inhibition of MAO by methylene blue, the concurrent use of IV methylene blue and bupropion is contraindicated
Nicotine transdermal		Combination reported to promote higher rates of smoking cessation than either drug alone Increased risk of hypertension with combination
Nitrogen mustard analog	Cyclophosphamide, ifosfamide	Altered levels of either drug due to competition for metabolism via CYP2B6

Class of Drug	Example	Interaction Effects
Opioid	Tramadol	Increased risk of seizures Possible decreased analgesic effect due to decreased conversion to the active M1 metabolite
Selective norepinephrine reuptake inhibitor	Atomoxetine	Increased plasma level and half-life of atomoxetine due to inhibited metabolism via CYP2D6 5-fold increase in atomoxetine exposure
St. John's wort		Case report of orofacial dystonia due to additive effect on serotonin reuptake
Sympathomimetic	Methylphenidate Pseudoephedrine	Case reports of grand mal seizures and myocardial infarction associated with concurrent use with methylphenidate Report of manic-like reaction with pseudoephedrine Seizure threshold may be reduced
Tamoxifen		Combination appears to reduce the conversion of tamoxifen to its active metabolite (endoxifen) and may decrease the therapeutic efficacy of this drug
Theophylline		Seizure threshold may be reduced

Serotonin Norepinephrine Reuptake Inhibitors (SNRIs)

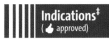 **Product Availability***

Generic Name	Chemical Class	Neuroscience-based Nomenclature* (Pharmacological Target/Mode of Action)	Trade Name[A]	Dosage Forms and Strengths
Desvenlafaxine	Bicyclic (phenethylamine)	Serotonin, norepinephrine/Reuptake inhibitor	Khedezla[B], Pristiq	Extended-release tablets: 25 mg[B], 50 mg, 100 mg
Duloxetine	Bicyclic (phenethylamine)	Serotonin, norepinephrine/Reuptake inhibitor	Cymbalta, Irenka[B]	Capsules, delayed-release pellets: 20 mg[B], 30 mg, 40 mg[B], 60 mg
Levomilnacipran	Bicyclic (phenethylamine)	Norepinephrine, serotonin/Reuptake inhibitor	Fetzima Fetzima Titration	Extended-release capsules: 20 mg, 40 mg, 80 mg, 120 mg Extended-release capsules (28 pack): 20 mg, 40 mg
Venlafaxine	Bicyclic (phenethylamine)	Serotonin, norepinephrine/Reuptake inhibitor	Effexor Effexor XR	Tablets[B]: 25 mg, 37.5 mg, 50 mg, 75 mg, 100 mg Extended-release tablets: 37.5 mg[B], 50 mg[C], 75 mg[B], 100 mg[C], 150 mg[B], 225 mg[B] Extended-release capsules: 37.5 mg, 75 mg, 150 mg

* Refer to Health Canada's Drug Product Database or the FDA's Drugs@FDA for the most current availability information. * Developed by a taskforce consisting of representatives from the American College of Neuropsychopharmacology (ACNP), the Asian College of Neuropsychopharmacology (AsCNP), the European College of Neuropsychopharmacology (ECNP), the International College of Neuropsychopharmacology (CINP), and the International Union of Basic and Clinical Pharmacology (IUPHAR) (see https://nbn2r.com), [A] Generic preparations may be available, [B] Not marketed in Canada, [C] Not marketed in the USA,

Indications‡
(👍 approved)

- 💊 Major depressive disorder (MDD) – all
- 💊 Generalized anxiety disorder (GAD) (venlafaxine and duloxetine)
- 💊 Social anxiety disorder (venlafaxine)
- 💊 Panic disorder with or without agoraphobia (venlafaxine)
- 💊 Pain due to diabetic peripheral neuropathy (duloxetine)
- 💊 Pain due to fibromyalgia (duloxetine)

‡ Indications listed here do not necessarily apply to all SNRIs or all countries. Please refer to a country's regulatory database (e.g., US Food and Drug Administration, Health Canada Drug Product Database) for the most current availability information and indications

Serotonin Norepinephrine Reuptake Inhibitors (SNRIs) (cont.)

- 🔥 Chronic musculoskeletal pain: low back pain and pain due to osteoarthritis of the knee (duloxetine)
- Bipolar disorder: Depressed phase (venlafaxine)
- Treatment-resistant depression, dysthymia, postpartum depression, and melancholic depression
- OCD – higher doses of venlafaxine
- PTSD (venlafaxine, duloxetine)
- Premenstrual dysphoric disorder (small studies showed benefit with venlafaxine)
- ADHD in children and adults – potential for benefit with venlafaxine and duloxetine (evidence is weak for these indications)
- Hot flashes in menopausal women – double-blind studies have shown reduction by venlafaxine (for women with natural or surgical menopause as well as a history of breast cancer), desvenlafaxine (natural or surgical menopause), and open label study by duloxetine (for those with concurrent depression)
- Migraine and tension headaches (preliminary data suggest venlafaxine may be superior to amitriptyline in migraine prophylaxis)
- Urinary incontinence, stress induced (duloxetine)
- Vasomotor symptoms (moderate to severe) and neuropathic pain – desvenlafaxine has shown effect but for the latter possibly at doses higher than for depression
- Binge eating (duloxetine, venlafaxine) – preliminary data

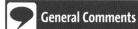

General Comments

- SNRIs are associated with increased suicidal ideation, hostility, and psychomotor agitation in clinical trials involving children and adolescents. Monitor all patients for worsening depression and suicidal thinking
- Trials and post-marketing reports suggest that SNRIs can also be associated with severe agitation-type adverse events that include aggression, agitation, akathisia, depersonalization, disinhibition, emotional lability, and hostility in both pediatric and adult patients
- Meta-analysis of trials with venlafaxine versus SSRI for depression showed superiority in achieving remission and response but with higher rates of discontinuation due to adverse effects. Results not reproduced in other meta-analyses[16]
- Desvenlafaxine is the major active metabolite of venlafaxine and does not undergo metabolism via CYP2D6. This may result in a reduced risk of drug interactions and susceptibility to genetic polymorphism
- In the updated French guidelines for neuropathic pain, first-line treatments include duloxetine, venlafaxine, gabapentin, and TCAs
- Using the WHO Pharmacovigilance database, the risk of antidepressant-associated withdrawal syndrome was highest with paroxetine, desvenlafaxine, venlafaxine, and duloxetine
- Levomilnacipran is the more active enantiomer of milnacipran. A network meta-analysis of 24 studies does not indicate greater benefits or less harm from levomilnacipran compared with other second-generation antidepressants

Pharmacology

- Potent uptake inhibitors of serotonin and norepinephrine; venlafaxine reliably inhibits NE reuptake at 225 mg, while duloxetine and desvenlafaxine have equal affinity to both NE and serotonin transporter "reuptake" proteins; inhibition of dopamine reuptake occurs at high doses
- Levomilnacipran has approximately 2-fold greater potency for inhibition of norepinephrine relative to serotonin reuptake. Compared with desvenlafaxine, duloxetine, and venlafaxine, levomilnacipran has more than 10-fold higher selectivity for norepinephrine relative to serotonin reuptake inhibition
- The higher selectivity of levomilnacipran for norepinephrine occurs at lowest effective dose; as dose is titrated upwards, levomilnacipran has equipotent effects on 5HT and NE transporters and no effects on dopamine transporters

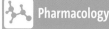

Dosing

- See p. 95
- Desvenlafaxine: Initiate drug at 50 mg once daily – usual maintenance dose; dose may be increased to 100 mg/day if needed. In patients with renal insufficiency (CrCl 30–50 mL/min), use maximum of 50 mg/day; if less than 30 mL/min, use 50 mg every other day. A meta-analysis of registration trials showed no increased efficacy with doses greater than 50 mg/day; however, adverse effects and discontinuations increase with dose
- Duloxetine: Initiate drug at 30–60 mg daily; 30 mg daily may be considered to improve tolerability (e.g. lower incidence of nausea), with a target dose of 60 mg daily within 1–2 weeks. Although 120 mg is effective, there is no evidence that it confers additional benefit. AVOID in severe renal insufficiency as AUC increased 100% and metabolites increase up to 9-fold; in hepatic disorders, AUC increased 5-fold and half-life increased 3-fold

- Levomilnacipran: Initiate drug at 20 mg once daily for 2 days, increase to 40 mg once daily, may then be increased in increments of 40 mg at intervals of 2 or more days; maintenance: 40–120 mg once daily; maximum: 120 mg/day. In patients with renal insufficiency (CrCl 30–59 mL/min), use maximum of 80 mg/day; if CrCl 15–29 mL/min, use maximum of 40 mg/day. Use not recommended in end-stage renal disease (ESRD). No adjustments necessary for any hepatic impairment or in the elderly
- Venlafaxine: Initiate drug at 37.5–75 mg (once daily for XR preparation, twice daily for regular preparation) and increase after 1 week in increments no greater than 75 mg q 4 days, up to 225 mg/day for moderately depressed patients. There is very limited experience at higher doses (375 mg/day) in severely depressed inpatients. Decrease dose by 50% in hepatic disease, by 25–50% in renal disease, and by 50% if undergoing hemodialysis. For panic disorder, start at 37.5 mg/day. For social anxiety disorder, there is no evidence that doses above 75 mg/day confer any additional benefit

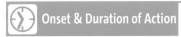 **Pharmacokinetics**	

- See p. 95
- Desvenlafaxine: Well absorbed from GI tract; food has no effect on absorption; peak plasma concentration reached in about 7.5 h and mean half-life is about 11 h. Metabolized primarily in the liver by UGT conjugation and, to a lesser extent, by CYP3A4; potentially lower risk for significant drug interactions and susceptibility to genetic polymorphism. May be a better choice of agent for MDD compared with venlafaxine in patients with decreased CYP2D6 activity. Steady state achieved in 4 days
- Duloxetine: Can be given with or without meals, although food delays T_{max} by 6–10 h. Bioavailability is reduced by about 30% in smokers. Duloxetine is metabolized by CYP1A2 and 2D6 and is an inhibitor of CYP2D6; potential risk for drug interactions and susceptibility to genetic polymorphism; elimination half-life increased from 12 h (mean) to 47.8 h (mean) in patients with liver impairment
- Levomilnacipran: Can be given with or without food; bioavailability is 92%. Peak plasma concentration C_{max} is reached in 6–8 h and mean half-life is about 12 h. Metabolized in the liver primarily by CYP3A4, therefore if utilized with strong CYP3A4 inhibitor recommendations to not exceed 80 mg/day; with minor contributions by CYP2C8, CYP2C19, CYP2D6 to inactive metabolites. Levomilnacipran and its metabolites are eliminated primarily by renal excretion. Approximately 58% of dose is excreted in urine as unchanged levomilnacipran. N-desethyl levomilnacipran is the major metabolite excreted in urine and accounts for approximately 18% of the dose. The metabolites are inactive. Displays linear pharmacokinetics over the therapeutic dosage range (and up to 300 mg). No clinically relevant effects of gender, age, bodyweight or hepatic impairment on pharmacokinetics
- Venlafaxine: Well absorbed from GI tract, food has no effect on absorption; absorption of XR formulation is slow (15 ± 6 h); peak plasma level (C_{max}) reached by parent drug in 1–3 h and by active metabolite (O-desmethylvenlafaxine, ODV) in 2–6 h; with XR formulation, C_{max} reached by parent drug in 6 h and metabolite in 8.8 h (mean). Elimination half-life of oral tablet: Parent = 3–7 h and metabolite = 9–13 h; XR elimination half-life is dependent on absorption half-life (15 h mean). Steady state of parent and metabolite reached in about 3 days. Parent drug metabolized by CYP2D6 and is also a weak inhibitor of this enzyme; ODV metabolite is metabolized by CYP3A3/4; potential risk for drug interactions and susceptibility to genetic polymorphism

Onset & Duration of Action	

- Therapeutic effect on emotional/psychological symptoms can take up to 28 days or longer (though some patients may respond sooner) but physical symptoms may respond sooner (within 1-2 weeks)

Adverse Effects	

- Generally dose-related; see chart p. 91 for incidence of adverse effects

CNS Effects	

- Both sedation and insomnia reported; prolonged sleep onset latency, disruption of sleep cycle, decreased REM sleep, increased awakenings, reduced sleep efficiency, vivid nightmares
- Headache, dizziness common
- Nervousness, agitation, hostility, suicidal urges
- Asthenia, fatigue, difficulty concentrating, decreased memory – more likely with higher doses of venlafaxine
- 10–30% of patients on venlafaxine who improve initially can have breakthrough depression after several months ("poop-out syndrome") – an increase in dosage or augmentation therapy may be of benefit
- Seizures reported rarely (less than 2%) with venlafaxine, desvenlafaxine, levomilnacipran; dose related
- Case reports of restless leg syndrome, periodic limb movement, and myoclonus with venlafaxine
- Extrapyramidal symptoms reported with duloxetine and levomilnacipran

Serotonin Norepinephrine Reuptake Inhibitors (SNRIs) (cont.)

Anticholinergic Effects	• Dry mouth common • Urinary retention; cases of urinary frequency and incontinence in females on venlafaxine as well as reports of both retention and hesitancy with duloxetine; dose-related side effect of levomilnacipran, with case reports indicating successful treatment with tamsulosin • Constipation • Mydriasis; cases of elevated ocular pressure in patients with narrow-angle glaucoma (duloxetine and levomilnacipran contraindicated for those with uncontrolled narrow angle glaucoma)
Cardiovascular Effects	• Increased blood pressure: Venlafaxine: Modest, sustained increase in blood pressure can occur, usually within 2 months of dose stabilization; seen in over 3% of individuals on less than 100 mg/day of venlafaxine and up to 13% of individuals on doses above 300 mg/day of immediate-release drug, and 3–4% with sustained-release product. Duloxetine is associated with case reports of increase in blood pressure and, rarely, hypertensive crisis. Desvenlafaxine: 1.3% incidence of sustained hypertension with 50 mg, 0.7% with 100 mg, 1.1% with 200 mg, 2.3% with 400 mg • Levomilnacipran: As expected for the class, some individuals experienced increases in heart rate and blood pressure. Incidence of patients with sustained hypertension for all short-term clinical studies: systolic blood pressure $\geq$ 140 mmHG and $\geq$ 15 mmHG above baseline was 0.8% (levomilnacipran) vs. 0.2% (placebo), and diastolic blood pressure $\geq$ 90 mmHG and $\geq$ 10 mmHG above baseline was 1.4% (levomilnacipran) vs. 1.1% (placebo) • Tachycardia; increase by 4 beats/min – more likely in the elderly • Dizziness and orthostatic hypotension (OH) common – with venlafaxine, OH occurs more frequently vs. incident hypertension and is associated with increased risk of falls and associated injury • QTc prolongation: Venlafaxine at therapeutic doses may not have any clinically significant concern but can occur in situations of overdose and should be used cautiously in patients with risk factors including CHF, previous MI, congenital long QT syndrome, electrolyte imbalance, concomitant medications known to increase QT interval, and the elderly; desvenlafaxine and levomilnacipran do not seem to have any clinically relevant impact but data for both are limited; duloxetine has no effect on QTc interval • Takotsubo cardiomyopathy reported in postmarketing adverse effects for levomilnacipran
Endocrine & Metabolic Effects	• No weight gain reported; treatment-emergent anorexia and weight loss has been associated with venlafaxine for patients with depression and GAD, social anxiety disorder, and panic disorder (in placebo-controlled trials) • Minor changes in blood glucose and cholesterol are infrequently noted with all SNRIs; duloxetine capsules contain sucrose therefore should not be used in patients with fructose intolerance, glucose-galactose malabsorption, or sucrase-isomaltase insufficiency • Incidence of hyponatremia in some studies found to be comparable to SSRIs, higher risk if volume depleted or dehydrated (e.g., the elderly and with concurrent use of diuretics)
GI Effects	• Nausea and vomiting occur frequently at start of therapy and tends to decrease after 1–2 weeks; less frequent with XR formulation of venlafaxine but higher rates than with SSRIs and duloxetine; 37% incidence with IR venlafaxine, 31% with XR venlafaxine; 22–41% with desvenlafaxine – most common side effect (dose related); 17% incidence with levomilnacipran – most common side effect • Potential for gastrointestinal obstruction: desvenlafaxine is a nondeformable controlled-release product and should not be administered to patients with pre-existing GI narrowing conditions (e.g., small bowel inflammatory disease, "short gut" syndrome, history of peritonitis, cystic fibrosis) • Case report of glossodynia (burning mouth syndrome) in a female on venlafaxine • Flatulence (levomilnacipran)
Urogenital & Sexual Effects	• Sexual side effects reported include: Decreased libido, delayed orgasm/ejaculation, anorgasmia, no ejaculation, and erectile dysfunction (see SSRIs p. 8 for suggested treatments); reports of long-lasting sexual dysfunction despite discontinuation • Risk increased with increasing age, use of higher doses, and concomitant medication • No large studies comparing venlafaxine to SSRIs but one small study found that rates of sexual dysfunction for venlafaxine were between those for moclobemide and the SSRIs paroxetine and sertraline • Duloxetine and desvenlafaxine appear to have significantly fewer sexual dysfunction effects than the SSRIs[17] • Levomilnacipran may cause dose-related erectile dysfunction, ejaculatory disorder, and testicular pain; spontaneous reports of sexual dysfunction were greater than with placebo; urinary hesitancy (dose related), dysuria, pollakiuria, urinary retention

Other Adverse Effects	

- Sweating (in more than 10%)
- Risk of bone fractures: Caution in the elderly and those with low bone density
- Hepatotoxicity – duloxetine and venlafaxine: Cases of hepatitis accompanied by abdominal pain, hepatomegaly, and serum transaminase concentrations more than 20 times the upper limit of normal, with or without jaundice, have been reported during postmarketing surveillance. Elevation in serum transaminase concentrations has in some cases required the discontinuation of duloxetine. Laboratory findings suggestive of severe hepatic injury with evidence of cholestasis were reported in 3 patients who received duloxetine in clinical studies. Case reports of elevated hepatic enzyme levels, hepatitis, bilirubinemia, and jaundice with venlafaxine. Case reports of life-threatening toxicity requiring transplantation reported for both
- Epistaxis, bruising and abnormal bleeding with venlafaxine
- Venlafaxine: Case reports of breast engorgement and pain, SIADH with hyponatremia, Stevens-Johnson syndrome
- Duloxetine: Severe skin reactions, including erythema multiforme and Stevens-Johnson syndrome, can occur

 Discontinuation Syndrome

- Abrupt discontinuation may cause a syndrome consisting of dizziness, lethargy, nausea, vomiting, diarrhea, headache, fever, sweating, chills, malaise, incoordination, insomnia, vivid dreams, myalgia, paresthesias, dyskinesias, "electric-shock-like" sensations, tinnitus, visual discoordination, anxiety, irritability, confusion, slowed thinking, disorientation, rarely aggression, impulsivity, hypomania, and depersonalization
- Brain "zaps" (or electric-shock-like sensations), often associated with lateral eye movements, hearing static sounds, and feelings of dizziness/wooziness; occur most commonly with abrupt discontinuation of venlafaxine and duloxetine; usually transitory but may last for months
- Most likely to occur within 1–7 days after drug stopped or dose drastically reduced, and typically disappears within 3 weeks
- Cases of inter-dose withdrawal reported with regular-release tablet; withdrawal reactions also reported with XR product; withdrawal from venlafaxine can be problematic, with symptom severity occasionally preventing cessation of the medication even when a prolonged taper is used
- Case of mania reported following venlafaxine taper, despite adequate concomitant mood stabilizing treatment
- Although levomilnacipran studies reported comparable rates of discontinuation symptoms between active treatment and placebo, gradual titration still recommended
- ☞ THEREFORE THESE MEDICATIONS SHOULD BE WITHDRAWN GRADUALLY (OVER SEVERAL WEEKS) AFTER PROLONGED USE

Management	

- Suggested to taper slowly over a 2-week period (some suggest over 6 weeks)
- Substituting one dose of fluoxetine (10 or 20 mg) near the end of the taper may help in the withdrawal process
- To withdraw desvenlafaxine, increase the dosing interval by giving it every other day, then increase this interval gradually

⚠ Precautions

- Monitor all patients for worsening depression and suicidal thoughts, especially at start of therapy and following an increase or decrease in dose
- Risk of hypomania/mania estimated to be 0.5% with venlafaxine, 0.1% with desvenlafaxine in Phase 2 and 3 studies, 0.1% with duloxetine in placebo-controlled trials; caution in bipolar patients with comorbid substance abuse
- Serotonin syndrome may occur, particularly when used with other agents that affect the serotonin system
- Treatment with medications that inhibit the serotonin transporter may be associated with abnormal bleeding, particularly when combined with NSAIDs, acetylsalicylic acid, or other medications that affect coagulation
- AVOID duloxetine in patients with severe renal insufficiency (CrCl less than 30 mL/min)
- AVOID duloxetine in patients with underlying liver disease; DO NOT USE in patients with substantial alcohol use, chronic liver disease or hepatic insufficiency
- AVOID levomilnacipran in end-stage renal disease; should not use in patients with MI, history of cardiac intervention within the past 12 months, CHF, uncontrolled tachyarrhythmias, uncontrolled hypertension, or history of cerebrovascular accident
- Do not use in patients with uncontrolled hypertension, as SNRIs can cause modest, sustained increases in blood pressure [blood pressure monitoring recommended for all patients]

 Toxicity

- Fatality rates secondary to overdose were second to that of TCA
- Symptoms of toxicity include vomiting, excess adrenergic stimulation, mydriasis, tachycardia, hypotension, arrhythmias, increase in QTc interval, bowel dysmotility, decreased level of consciousness, seizures – increased risk of fatal outcomes following overdose
- Delayed onset rhabdomyolysis

Serotonin Norepinephrine Reuptake Inhibitors (SNRIs) (cont.)

- Fatal outcomes have been reported for acute overdoses, primarily with mixed overdoses, but also with duloxetine alone, at doses as low as 1000 mg. Signs and symptoms of overdose (duloxetine alone or with mixed drugs) included somnolence, serotonin syndrome, seizures, vomiting, and tachycardia
- There is limited clinical experience with desvenlafaxine overdosage in humans. No cases of fatal acute overdose reported in premarketing clinical trials. The most common symptoms associated with desvenlafaxine overdose are headache, vomiting, agitation, dizziness, nausea, constipation, diarrhea, dry mouth, paresthesia, and tachycardia. Desvenlafaxine is the major active metabolite of venlafaxine. Published retrospective studies report that venlafaxine overdosage may be associated with an increased risk of fatal outcomes compared to that observed with SSRI antidepressant products, but lower than that of tricyclic antidepressants
- Epidemiological studies have shown that venlafaxine-treated patients have a higher burden of suicide risk than SSRI patients; high risk of QTc prolongation in overdose
- Cardiac toxicity and serotonin syndrome reported in a woman who ingested 3 g of levomilnacipran

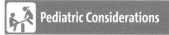 **Pediatric Considerations**

- For detailed information on the use of SNRIs in this population, please see the *Clinical Handbook of Psychotropic Drugs for Children and Adolescents*[8]
- CAUTION: No approved indications in children and adolescents due to lack of efficacy and concerns about increased hostility and suicidal ideation (rate 2% vs. placebo 1%)

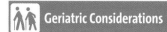 **Geriatric Considerations**

- Treatment of the acute phase of MDD with SNRIs, but not SSRIs, associated with a greater number of overall adverse events vs. placebo[18]
- Dosage adjustments in healthy elderly patients are not usually required; 14% increase in metabolite level and 24% increase in half-life reported with venlafaxine
- Can increase heart rate in frail elderly, related to its noradrenergic activity; increased cardiovascular and cerebrovascular adverse effects reported
- Hyponatremia reported in older aldults
- Clearance of desvenlafaxine decreased in the elderly; higher incidence of orthostatic hypotension
- Monitor for SIADH
- Extrapyramidal effects have been reported with duloxetine; they are not dose related and can develop with short-term or long-term use
- Four levomilnacipran studies included patients older than 65 years

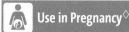 **Use in Pregnancy**◊

- Duloxetine and venlafaxine have been associated with increased risk of postpartum hemorrhage; venlafaxine has also been associated with an increased risk of hypertension during pregnancy
- In utero exposure to venlafaxine may be higher compared with other antidepressants; low absolute risk of cardiac malformations with venlafaxine and exposure may be a marker, for which fetal echocardiography may be considered; there may be a trend toward higher rates of spontaneous abortion. Use of duloxetine during pregnancy is associated with an increased risk of spontaneous abortion; one study suggests an absolute risk of 18% and another suggests a trebled relative risk
- Neonates exposed to venlafaxine and desvenlafaxine in third trimester have developed complications upon delivery including respiratory distress, temperature instability, feeding difficulties, agitation, irritability, changes in muscle tone, and seizures
- No developmental toxicity or other signs of toxicity were observed in an infant exposed to duloxetine during the second half of gestation and during breast-feeding in the first 32 days after birth
- There are no adequate well-controlled studies of levomilnacipran in pregnant women
- Special caution should be taken when prescribing SNRIs to women before 16th week of gestation because of risk of gestational hypertension and preeclampsia

Breast Milk

- The total dose of venlafaxine and its ODV metabolite ingested by a breastfed infant can be as high as 9.2% of the maternal dose
- An exclusively breastfed infant would receive an estimated 5.7–7.4% of the maternal weight-adjusted dose of desvenlafaxine

◊ See p. 473 for further information on drug use in pregnancy and effects on breast milk

- Infant exposure to duloxetine in breast milk is less than 1% of the maternal weight-adjusted dose, implying that a woman receiving duloxetine can probably safely breast feed her infant
- The effect of levomilnacipran on lactation and nursing in humans is unknown

 Nursing Implications

- A gradual titration of dosage at start of therapy will minimize nausea
- Psychotherapy and education are also important in the treatment of depression
- Monitor therapy by watching for adverse effects as well as mood and activity level changes including worsening of suicidal thoughts, especially at start of therapy or following an increase or decrease in dose; keep physician informed
- Be aware that the medication may increase psychomotor activity; this may create concern about suicidal behavior
- Excessive ingestion of caffeinated foods, drugs or beverages may increase anxiety and agitation and confuse the diagnosis
- Instruct patient not to chew or crush the venlafaxine XR tablets, the extended-release desvenlafaxine tablets, the extended-release levomilnacipran capsules, or the delayed-release duloxetine capsules, but to swallow these sustained-release products whole. Venlafaxine XR capsules may be opened and the contents sprinkled onto applesauce. This drug/food mixture should be swallowed immediately without chewing and followed with a glass of water
- If a dose is missed, do not attempt to make it up; continue with regular daily schedule (divided doses)
- SNRIs should not be stopped suddenly due to risk of precipitating a withdrawal reaction; desvenlafaxine can be withdrawn by gradually increasing the dosing interval
- Patients taking desvenlafaxine may see an "empty" tablet in their stool since the outer inert tablet does not dissolve

 Patient Instructions

- For detailed patient instructions on venlafaxine, see the Patient Information Sheet (details p. 474)

Drug Interactions

- Clinically significant interactions are listed below
- For more interaction information on any given combination, also see the corresponding chapter for the second agent
- Drug–lab interaction: Desvenlafaxine and venlafaxine may result in false positive urine result for PCP and amphetamine

Class of Drug	Example	Interaction Effects
α_2 agonist	Clonidine	Inhibition of antihypertensive effect of clonidine
Analgesic	Acetylsalicylic acid	Increased risk of upper GI bleeding with combined use
Antiarrhythmic	Flecainide, propafenone	Increased plasma level of venlafaxine and duloxetine due to inhibited metabolism via CYP2D6 Duloxetine may increase plasma levels of propafenone
	Quinidine	Increased plasma level of duloxetine due to inhibited metabolism
Antibiotic	Ciprofloxacin, enoxacin	Increased plasma level of duloxetine due to inhibition of metabolism via CYP1A2
	Clarithromycin, telithromycin	Increased plasma level of levomilnacipran due to inhibited metabolism vial CYP3A4. Do not exceed a maximum of 80 mg/day
	Linezolid	Due to linezolid's weak MAOI activity, monitor for increased serotonergic and noradrenergic effects
Anticholinergic	Antiparkinsonian agents, antipsychotics, etc.	Increased anticholinergic effects
Anticoagulant	Apixaban, dabigatran, rivaroxaban, warfarin	Increased risk of bleeding possible due to decreased platelet aggregation secondary to depletion of serotonin in platelets
Anticonvulsant	Stiripentol	Strong CYP3A4 inhibitors may increase levomilnacipran concentrations significantly. Do not exceed a maximum of 80 mg/day
Antidepressant SSRI	Paroxetine, fluoxetine	Reports that combination with SSRIs that inhibit CYP2D6 can result in increased levels of venlafaxine and duloxetine, with possible increases in blood pressure, anticholinergic effects, and serotonergic effects
	Fluvoxamine	6-fold increase in AUC, 2.5-fold increase in C_{max}, and 3-fold increase in half-life of duloxetine due to inhibited metabolism via CYP1A2 (AVOID concomitant use)

Serotonin Norepinephrine Reuptake Inhibitors (SNRIs) (cont.)

Class of Drug	Example	Interaction Effects
NDRI	Bupropion	3-fold increase in venlafaxine plasma level due to inhibited metabolism via CYP2D6 and reduction in level of ODV metabolite Potentiation of noradrenergic effects Bupropion may mitigate SNRI-induced sexual side effects
SARI	Nefazodone	May increase plasma level of levomilnacipran through inhibition of CYP3A4
	Trazodone	Case report of serotonin syndrome with venlafaxine
NaSSA	Mirtazapine	Case report of serotonin syndrome with venlafaxine
Nonselective cyclic	Desipramine	Desipramine (metabolite) clearance reduced by 20% with venlafaxine; desipramine level increased 3-fold with duloxetine Increased levels of cyclic antidepressants metabolized by CYP2D6 possible with duloxetine
	Imipramine	C_{max} and AUC of imipramine increased by 40% with venlafaxine
	Trimipramine	Case report of seizure in combination with venlafaxine – postulated to be a result of inhibited metabolism via CYP2D6
RIMA	Moclobemide	Enhanced effects of norepinephrine and serotonin; CAUTION – no data on safety with combined use
Irreversible MAOI	Phenelzine	AVOID; possible hypertensive crisis and serotonergic reaction
Antifungal	Fluconazole, itraconazole, ketoconazole	Strong CYP3A4 inhibitors may increase levomilnacipran concentrations significantly. Do not exceed a maximum of 80 mg/day Moderate CYP3A4 inhibitors may increase levomilnacipran levels
Antihistamine	Diphenhydramine	Decreased metabolism of venlafaxine via CYP2D6
Antihypertensive		Case reports of hypertension with use of SNRIs for patients previously well controlled with antihypertensives; reduction in SNRI dose or stopping SNRIs altogether may be required
Antiplatelet	Clopidogrel	Increased risk of upper GI bleeding with combined use
Antipsychotic	General	Increased levels of antipsychotics metabolized by CYP2D6 possible with duloxetine
First generation	Haloperidol	Increased C_{max} and AUC of haloperidol with venlafaxine; no change in half-life
	Thioridazine	Increased plasma level of venlafaxine and decreased concentration of ODV metabolite Increased plasma levels of thioridazine and other phenothiazines possible with duloxetine due to inhibition of CYP2D6 – AVOID duloxetine and CAUTION with other SNRIs due to possible additive prolongation of QTc interval
Second generation	Clozapine	Increased levels of both clozapine and venlafaxine possible due to competitive inhibition of CYP2D6 and/or CYP3A4. A study with venlafaxine doses of 150 mg/day or less suggests no clinically significant interaction. Case report of NMS/serotonin syndrome
	Risperidone	Increased AUC of risperidone by 32% and decreased renal clearance by 20% with venlafaxine
Third generation	Aripiprazole	Case report of parkinsonism with venlafaxine 225 mg/day and aripiprazole 15 mg/day
Antiretroviral		
Non-nucleoside reverse transcriptase inhibitor (NNRTI)	Delavirdine, efavirenz	Strong CYP3A4 inhibitors (cobicistat, delavirdine) may increase levomilnacipran concentrations significantly. Do not exceed a maximum of 80 mg/day Moderate CYP3A4 inhibitors (efavirenz) may increase levomilnacipran levels
Protease inhibitor	Indinavir	Both increases (by 13%) and decreases (by 60%) in total concentration (AUC) of indinavir reported with venlafaxine
	Ritonavir	Ritonavir moderately decreases clearance of venlafaxine
β-blocker	Propranolol	Increased plasma level of venlafaxine due to competition for metabolism via CYP2D6
Calcium channel blocker	Nicardipine	Strong CYP3A4 inhibitors may increase levomilnacipran concentrations significantly. Do not exceed a maximum of 80 mg/day
	Verapamil	Moderate CYP3A4 inhibitors may increase levomilnacipran levels

Class of Drug	Example	Interaction Effects
CNS depressant	Alcohol	Increased risk of psychomotor impairment and hepatotoxicity
Diuretic		Concurrent use of diuretics may increase risk of developing hyponatremia
H$_2$ antagonist	Cimetidine	Increased plasma level of venlafaxine due to decreased clearance (by 43%); peak concentration increased by 60% Increased plasma level of duloxetine due to inhibited metabolism
Hypnotic/sedative	Zolpidem	Case report of delirium and hallucinations with venlafaxine
Lithium		Case report of serotonin syndrome with venlafaxine (see p. 10)
Licorice		Increased serotonergic effects possible
Lomitapide		Moderate CYP3A4 inhibitors may increase levomilnacipran levels
L-tryptophan		Additive effects with duloxetine in treatment-resistant patients May potentiate the risk of serotonin syndrome. Monitor for increased serotonergic effects
MAO-B inhibitor	Selegiline (L-deprenyl)	Case reports of serotonergic reaction with venlafaxine
Methylene blue		Enhanced serotonergic effects through inhibition of MAO-A and B by methylene blue. Risk for serotonin syndrome (see Precautions p. 10)
Metoclopramide		Case report of extrapyramidal and serotonergic effects with venlafaxine
NSAID		Increased risk of upper GI bleed with combined use. CAUTION
Opioid	Meperidine	Increased risk of serotonin syndrome
	Tramadol	Increased risk of seizures and serotonin syndrome
Smoking (tobacco)		Can lower median serum duloxetine concentrations via induction of CYP1A2; higher doses may be required
St. John's wort		May augment serotonergic effects – increased risk of serotonin syndrome
Stimulant	Dextroamphetamine	Case report of serotonin syndrome with venlafaxine
	Methylphenidate	Potentiated effect in the treatment of depression and ADHD
Tolterodine		C_{max} and half-life of tolterodine increased; no effect on active metabolites
Triptan	Rizatriptan, sumatriptan	Inadequate data available to determine the risk of serotonin syndrome with the addition of a triptan to SNRIs. However, given the seriousness of serotonin syndrome, caution is warranted

Serotonin-2 Antagonists/Reuptake Inhibitors (SARIs)

℞ Product Availability*

Generic Name	Chemical Class	Neuroscience-based Nomenclature* (Pharmacological Target/Mode of Action)	Trade Name[A]	Dosage Forms and Strengths
Nefazodone[B]	Phenylpiperidine	Serotonin/Antagonist and agonist	Serzone	Tablets: 50 mg, 100 mg, 150 mg, 200 mg, 250 mg
Trazodone	Triazolopyridine	Multimodal	Desyrel Oleptro[C]	Tablets: 50 mg, 100 mg, 150 mg, 300 mg[B] Extended-release caplets: 150 mg, 300 mg

* Refer to Health Canada's Drug Product Database or the FDA's Drugs@FDA for the most current availability information. ● Developed by a taskforce consisting of representatives from the American College of Neuropsychopharmacology (ACNP), the Asian College of Neuropsychopharmacology (AsCNP), the European College of Neuropsychopharmacology (ECNP), the International College of Neuropsychopharmacology (CINP), and the International Union of Basic and Clinical Pharmacology (IUPHAR) (see https://nbn2r.com), [A] Generic preparations may be available, [B] Not marketed in Canada, [C] Not marketed in the USA

Serotonin-2 Antagonists/Reuptake Inhibitors (SARIs) (cont.)

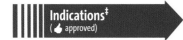

Indications‡
(👍 approved)

- 👍 Major depressive disorder (MDD)
- Secondary depression in other mental illnesses (e.g., schizophrenia, dementia)
- MDD, recurrent: Prophylaxis
- Agoraphobia associated with panic disorder
- Dysthymia
- Social phobia
- Posttraumatic stress disorder (PTSD)
- Insomnia
- Impotence, erectile dysfunction (trazodone), anorgasmia (nefazodone)
- Fibromyalgia, in open-label studies – monitor for tachycardia
- Diabetic neuropathy
- Antipsychotic-induced akathisia
- Bulimia
- Schizophrenia: Negative symptoms (trazodone)
- Neuroleptic-associated akathisia
- Barré-Lièou syndrome
- Obstructive sleep apnea in comorbid ischemic stroke (trazodone) – decreased severity without increasing nocturnal hypoxia

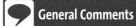 **General Comments**

- Nefazodone was withdrawn in Canada in November 2003 due to risk of hepatotoxicity
- Trazodone is the best-known antidepressant for improving sleep. Has been shown to enhance slow-wave sleep and improve sleep quality. Has also been shown to improve the results of CBT in patients with primary insomnia
- Nefazodone is associated with enhanced REM sleep. Unlike trazodone, nefazodone appears to improve quality and quantity of sleep with minimal daytime somnolence
- Monitor all patients for worsening depression and/or suicidal thoughts

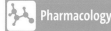 **Pharmacology**

- Exact mechanism of action unknown; equilibrate the effects of biogenic amines through various mechanisms; cause downregulation of β-adrenergic receptors
- Trazodone: Potent antagonist of the 5-HT$_{2A}$ receptor as well as a dose-dependent blockade of serotonin transporter; also blocks 5-HT$_{2C}$, α_1, and H$_1$ receptors; antidepressant effects thought to occur when both 5-HT$_{2A}$ and serotonin transporters are antagonized at doses of 150–600 mg; hypnotic effects occur at lower doses of 25–100 mg due to antagonizing 5-HT$_{2A}$, H$_1$, and α_1 receptors
- Nefazodone: Inhibits neuronal reuptake of serotonin and norepinephrine; also blocks 5-HT$_{2A/C}$ receptors and α_1 receptors; has no significant affinity for α_2, β-adrenergic, 5-HT$_{1A}$, cholinergic, dopaminergic, or benzodiazepine receptors

 Dosing

- See p. 95
- Initiate drug at a low dose and increase dose every 3–5 days to a maximum tolerated dose based on side effects; there is a wide variation in dosage requirements; prophylaxis is most effective if therapeutic dose is maintained
- For treatment of depression with trazodone regular-release formulation: start with 150-200 mg/day in 2 or 3 divided doses; usual maximum is 300 mg/day in divided doses
- Doses of trazodone up to 400 mg and, rarely, 600 mg have been used in hospitalized patients
- Trazodone should be taken on an empty stomach when used for sedation, as food delays absorption, but otherwise should be taken after a light meal or snack to reduce side effects

‡ Indications listed here do not necessarily apply to all SARIs or all countries. Please refer to a country's regulatory database (e.g., US Food and Drug Administration, Health Canada Drug Product Database) for the most current availability information and indications

- XR formulation (Oleptro) dosing: 150–375 mg daily, should be given on an empty stomach in the late evening, caplets can be halved along score line but should not be crushed or chewed
- For treatment of depression with nefazodone, start with 50 mg daily and increase by 50–100 mg at 1-week intervals as necessary. Usual daily dose range is 150–300 mg
- Trazodone doses of 25–100 mg at bedtime used in chronic sleep disorders

 Pharmacokinetics

- See p. 95
- Completely absorbed from the GI tract; food significantly delays (from 1 to several h) and decreases peak plasma effect of regular-release trazodone; peak plasma level of XR formulation not affected by food
- Nefazodone bioavailability only 20% due to high first-pass metabolism; can be given without regard to meals
- Highly bound to plasma protein (trazodone 85–95%; nefazodone more than 99%)
- Metabolized primarily by the liver; half-life of nefazodone is dose dependent, varying from 2 h at 100 mg/day to 4–5 h at 600 mg/day; half-life and AUC of nefazodone and hydroxy metabolite doubled in patients with severe liver impairment
- Trazodone metabolized by CYP3A4 to active metabolite m-chlorophenylpiperazine (mCPP); elimination half-life 4–9 h in adults and 11.6 h (mean) in the elderly; steady state reached in about 3 days
- Nefazodone is a potent inhibitor of CYP3A4 and may decrease the metabolism of drugs metabolized by this isoenzyme (see Drug Interactions, pp. 38–39)
- Regular ingestion of grapefruit juice while on nefazodone may affect the antidepressant plasma level (see Drug Interactions, p. 39)

Onset & Duration of Action

- Therapeutic effect is typically seen after 28 days (though some patients may respond sooner)
- Sedative effects are seen within a few hours of oral administration; decreased sleep disturbance reported after a few days

Adverse Effects

- The pharmacological and side effect profile of SARI antidepressants is dependent on their affinity for and activity on neurotransmitters/receptors (see table p. 89)
- See chart p. 91 for incidence of adverse effects at therapeutic doses; incidence of adverse effects may be greater in early days of treatment; patients adapt to many side effects over time

CNS Effects

- A result of antagonism at histamine H_1 receptors and α_1 adrenoreceptors
- Drowsiness (most common adverse effect; reported in 20–50%) [Management: Prescribe bulk of dose at bedtime]
- Weakness, lethargy, fatigue
- Conversely, excitement, agitation, and restlessness have occurred
- Confusion, disturbed concentration, and disorientation
- Nefazodone increases REM sleep and sleep quality
- Improved psychomotor and complex memory performance reported with nefazodone after single doses; dose-related impairment noted after repeated doses
- Precipitation of hypomania or mania, increased risk in bipolar patients with comorbid substance abuse
- Psychosis, panic reactions, anxiety or euphoria may occur
- Fine tremor
- Akathisia (rare – check serum iron for deficiency)
- Seizures can occur rarely following abrupt drug increase or after drug withdrawal; risk increases with high plasma levels
- Myoclonus; includes muscle jerks of lower extremities, jaw, and arms, and nocturnal myoclonus – may be severe in up to 9% of patients [If severe, clonazepam, valproate or carbamazepine may be of benefit]
- Dysphasia, stuttering
- Disturbance in gait, parkinsonism, dystonia
- Restless legs syndrome
- Headache; worsening of migraine reported with trazodone and nefazodone

Anticholinergic Effects

- A result of antagonism at muscarinic receptors
- Include dry eyes, blurred vision, constipation, dry mouth [see p. 57 for treatment suggestions]

Serotonin-2 Antagonists/Reuptake Inhibitors (SARIs) (cont.)

Cardiovascular Effects	• A result of antagonism at α_1 adrenoreceptors, muscarinic, 5-HT$_{2A/C}$, and H$_1$ receptors, and inhibition of sodium fast channels • More common in the elderly • Risk increases with high plasma levels • Bradycardia seen with nefazodone • Dizziness (10–30%), orthostatic hypotension, and syncope • Trazodone can exacerbate ischemic attacks; arrhythmias reported (with doses above 200 mg/day) including torsades de pointes • Cases of prolonged conduction time with trazodone and nefazodone (by inhibiting hERG potassium ion channels); contraindicated in heart block or post-myocardial infarction
Endocrine & Metabolic Effects	• Decreases in blood sugar levels reported (nefazodone) • Can induce SIADH with hyponatremia; risk increased with age • Weight gain reported with trazodone; rare with nefazodone
GI Effects	• A result of inhibition of 5-HT uptake and M$_1$ receptor antagonism • Peculiar taste, "black tongue," glossitis • Nausea, vomiting • Reports of upper GI bleeding; one study showed risk with trazodone may be higher than with citalopram
Urogenital & Sexual Effects	• A result of altered dopamine (D$_2$) activity, 5-HT$_{2A}$ blockade, inhibition of 5-HT reuptake, α_1 blockade, and M$_1$ blockade • Occur rarely • Testicular swelling, painful ejaculation, retrograde ejaculation, increased libido; spontaneous orgasm with yawning (trazodone) • Priapism with trazodone and nefazodone due to prominent α_1 blockade in the absence of anticholinergic activity
Hypersensitivity Reactions	• Rare • Rash, urticaria, pruritus, edema, blood dyscrasias
Other Adverse Effects	• Jaundice, hepatitis, hepatic necrosis and hepatic failure reported with therapeutic doses of nefazodone (laboratory evidence includes: Increased levels of ALT, AST, GGT, and bilirubin and increased prothrombin time) – cases of liver failure and death reported. Recommend baseline and periodic liver function tests with nefazodone. Monitor for signs of hepatotoxicity • Cases of palinopsia with both trazodone and nefazodone and scotoma with nefazodone – may be dose related • Rare reports of alopecia with nefazodone • Case reports of burning sensations in various parts of the body with nefazodone
D/C **Discontinuation Syndrome**	• Abrupt discontinuation may cause a syndrome consisting of dizziness, lethargy, nausea, vomiting, diarrhea, headache, fever, sweating, chills, malaise, incoordination, insomnia, vivid dreams, myalgia, paresthesias, dyskinesias, "electric-shock-like" sensations, visual discoordination, anxiety, irritability, confusion, slowed thinking, disorientation; rarely aggression, impulsivity, hypomania, and depersonalization • Brain "zaps" (or electric-shock-like sensations), often associated with lateral eye movements, hearing static sounds, and feelings of dizziness/wooziness; usually transitory but may last for months • Most likely to occur within 1–7 days after drug stopped or dose drastically reduced, and typically disappears within 3 weeks • Paradoxical mood changes reported on abrupt withdrawal, including hypomania or mania ☞ **THEREFORE THESE MEDICATIONS SHOULD BE WITHDRAWN GRADUALLY AFTER PROLONGED USE**
Management	• Reinstitute the drug at a lower dose and taper gradually over several days
⚠ **Precautions**	• May induce manic reactions in patients with bipolar disorder and, rarely, in unipolar depression; because of risk of increased cycling, bipolar disorder is a relative contraindication • May impair the mental and physical ability to perform hazardous tasks (e.g., driving a car or operating machinery); will potentiate the effects of alcohol

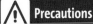

- Trazodone is a substrate for CYP3A4 and its metabolism can be inhibited by CYP3A4 inhibitors; nefazodone is a potent inhibitor of CYP3A4 (see Drug Interactions, pp. 38–39)
- Use caution in combination with drugs that prolong the QT interval (see Drug Interactions p. 38)
- Combination with SSRIs can lead to increased plasma level of trazodone. Combination therapy has been used in the treatment of resistant patients; use caution and monitor for serotonin syndrome
- Treatment with medications that inhibit the serotonin transporter may be associated with abnormal bleeding, particularly when combined with NSAIDs, acetylsalicylic acid or other medications that affect coagulation (see p. 38)
- May lower the seizure threshold; therefore, administer cautiously to patients with a history of convulsive disorders, organic brain disease or a predisposition to convulsions (e.g., alcohol withdrawal)
- May be arrhythmogenic in patients with a history of cardiac disease
- Priapism has occurred with trazodone requiring surgical intervention in one third of cases; use with caution in men with sickle cell anemia, multiple myeloma, leukemia, autonomic dysfunction, hypercoagulable state, and penile anatomic variation
- Use nefazodone cautiously in patients in whom excess anticholinergic activity could be harmful (e.g., prostatic hypertrophy, urinary retention, narrow-angle glaucoma)
- Use nefazodone with caution in patients with respiratory difficulties, since antidepressants with anticholinergic properties can dry up bronchial secretions and make breathing more difficult
- Use caution in prescribing nefazodone for patients with a history of alcoholism or liver disorder. Monitor liver function tests at baseline and periodically during treatment, and at first symptom or clinical sign of liver dysfunction
- Use caution when switching from trazodone to fluoxetine and vice versa (see Drug Interactions, pp. 38–39, and Switching Antidepressants p. 97)

| 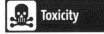 **Toxicity** | • Acute poisoning results in drowsiness, ataxia, nausea, vomiting; deep coma as well as arrhythmias (including torsades de pointes) and AV block reported; no seizures reported |

| 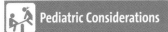 **Pediatric Considerations** | • For detailed information on the use of trazodone in this population, please see the *Clinical Handbook of Psychotropic Drugs for Children and Adolescents*[8]
• No approved indications in children and adolescents
• Trazodone used in acute and chronic treatment of insomnia and night terrors, and in MDD and behavior disturbances in children (agitation, aggression)
• Start drug at a low dose (10–25 mg) and increase gradually by 10–25 mg every 5 days to a maximum tolerated dose based on side effects |

| 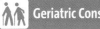 **Geriatric Considerations** | • Trazodone is used (off-label) in the treatment of insomnia and also agitation accociated with insomnia in dementia
• Initiate dose lower and more slowly than in younger patients; elderly patients may take longer to respond and may require trials of up to 12 weeks before response is noted
• AUC increased in the elderly; highest in elderly females
• Monitor for excessive CNS and anticholinergic effects
• Caution when combining with other drugs with CNS and anticholinergic properties; additive effects can result in confusion, disorientation, and delirium; the elderly are sensitive to anticholinergic effects
• Caution regarding cardiovascular side effects: Orthostatic hypotension (can lead to falls). Can potentiate effects of antihypertensive drugs
• Cognitive impairment can occur |

| 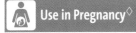 **Use in Pregnancy**◊ | • Trazodone in high doses was found to be teratogenic and toxic to the fetus in some animal species; trazodone and nefazodone found not to increase rates of malformations in humans above the baseline of 1–3%
• If possible, avoid during first trimester |
| Breast Milk | • SARI antidepressants are secreted into breast milk
• The American Academy of Pediatrics classifies SARI antidepressants as drugs "whose effects on nursing infants are unknown but may be of concern" |

◊ See p. 473 for further information on drug use in pregnancy and effects on breast milk

Serotonin-2 Antagonists/Reuptake Inhibitors (SARIs) (cont.)

 Nursing Implications

- Psychotherapy and education are also important in the treatment of depression
- Monitor therapy by watching for adverse side effects and mood and activity level changes, including worsening of suicidal thoughts; keep physician informed
- Be aware that as the medication reduces the degree of depression it may increase psychomotor activity; this may create concern about suicidal behavior
- Expect a lag time of up to 28 days before antidepressant effects will be noticed
- Reassure patient that drowsiness and dizziness usually subside after first few weeks; if dizzy, patient should get up from lying or sitting position slowly, and dangle legs over edge of bed before getting up
- Excessive consumption of caffeine may increase anxiety and agitation and confuse the diagnosis
- These drugs should not be stopped suddenly due to risk of precipitating withdrawal reactions
- Because these drugs can cause drowsiness, caution patient that activities requiring mental alertness should not be performed until response to the drug has been determined
- With nefazodone, monitor for signs of hepatotoxicity, including nausea, vomiting, fatigue, pruritus, jaundice, and dark urine
- Trazodone should be taken on an empty stomach when used for sedation, as food delays absorption, but otherwise should be taken after a light meal or snack to reduce side effects
- Ingestion of grapefruit juice while taking nefazodone should be avoided as the blood level of the antidepressant may increase

 Patient Instructions

- For detailed patient instructions on SARI antidepressants, see the Patient Information Sheet (details p. 474)

 Drug Interactions

- Clinically significant interactions are listed below
- For more interaction information on any given combination, also see the corresponding chapter for the second agent

Class of Drug	Example	Interaction Effects
Antibiotic	Linezolid	Monitor for increased serotonergic effects due to weak MAOI activity of linezolid
	Macrolide (clarithromycin, erythromycin)	Increased plasma level and decreased clearance of trazodone reported via potent CYP3A4 inhibition by clarithromycin; reduction in trazodone dose may be necessary when used concurrently with macrolides
Anticholinergic	Antihistamines, antiparkinsonian agents	Increased anticholinergic effect; may increase risk of hyperthermia, confusion, urinary retention, etc.
Anticoagulant	Apixaban, dabigatran, rivaroxaban, warfarin	Increased risk of bleeding possible due to decreased platelet aggregation secondary to depletion of serotonin in platelets
Anticonvulsant	Barbiturates, carbamazepine, phenytoin	Decreased plasma level of trazodone and its mCPP metabolite (by 76% and 60%, respectively, with carbamazepine) and of nefazodone, due to enzyme induction via CYP3A4
	Carbamazepine, phenytoin	Increased plasma level of carbamazepine or phenytoin, possibly due to competitive inhibition of metabolism via CYP3A4 with trazodone Increased plasma level of carbamazepine with nefazodone due to inhibited metabolism via CYP3A4
Antidepressant SSRI	Fluoxetine, fluvoxamine, paroxetine, sertraline	Elevated SSRI plasma level (due to inhibition of oxidative metabolism); monitor plasma level and for signs of toxicity Nefazodone metabolite (mCPP) level increased 4-fold with fluoxetine; case report of serotonin syndrome with combination
SNRI	Venlafaxine	Combined use may increase risk of serotonin syndrome
	Levomilnacipran	Nefazodone may increase plasma level of levomilnacipran through inhibition of CYP3A4
RIMA	Moclobemide	Monitor for serotonergic effects

Class of Drug	Example	Interaction Effects
Irreversible MAOI	Phenelzine, tranylcypromine	Low doses of trazodone (25–50 mg) used to treat antidepressant-induced insomnia Monitor for serotonergic effects
Antifungal	Ketoconazole	Increased plasma level of trazodone due to inhibited metabolism via CYP3A4
Antihypertensive	Acetazolamide, thiazide diuretics	Hypotension augmented
	Clonidine	Additive hypotension and sedation
	Guanethidine, methyldopa	Decreased antihypertensive effect due to inhibition of α-adrenergic receptors
Antipsychotic First generation	Chlorpromazine, haloperidol, perphenazine	Potential for additive adverse effects (e.g., sedation, orthostatic hypotension)
	Pimozide	Elevated pimozide levels and cardiac arrhythmias may occur with combination
Second generation	Clozapine, olanzapine, quetiapine, risperidone	Increased plasma levels of clozapine (case report) and quetiapine (in vitro data), possibly due to inhibited metabolism via CYP3A4 and associated adverse effects (e.g., dizziness, hypotension) Case report of NMS with nefazodone and olanzapine Case report of serotonin syndrome with trazodone, sertraline, and risperidone
	Lurasidone	Contraindicated with concomitant use of potent CYP3A4 inhibitors such as nefazodone
Antiretroviral Non-nucleoside reverse transcriptase inhibitor (NNRTI)	Delavirdine	Potential increased concentration of trazodone via CYP3A4 inhibition; monitor for increased adverse effects
Protease inhibitor	Indinavir, ritonavir	Increased plasma levels of trazodone and nefazodone due to decreased metabolism (with ritonavir, trazodone clearance decreased 52%)
Anxiolytic	Alprazolam, triazolam	Increased plasma levels of alprazolam (by 200%) and triazolam (by 500%), due to inhibited metabolism via CYP3A4 by nefazodone
	Buspirone	Concomitant use increases the risk of serotonin syndrome
Calcium channel blocker	Amlodipine	Elevated amlodipine level due to inhibited metabolism via CYP3A4 with nefazodone
Cardiac glycoside	Digoxin	Increased digoxin plasma level, with possible toxicity
CNS depressant	Alcohol	Short-term or acute use reduces first-pass metabolism of antidepressant and increases its plasma level; chronic use induces metabolizing enzymes and decreases its plasma level
	Antihistamines, benzodiazepines	Increased sedation, CNS depression
Cholestyramine		Decreased absorption of antidepressant, if given together
Ginkgo biloba		Case report of coma with trazodone (postulated to be due to excess stimulation of GABA receptors)
Grapefruit juice		Decreased metabolism of trazodone and nefazodone via CYP3A4
L-Tryptophan		Additive antidepressant effect; monitor for serotonergic effects
MAO-B inhibitor	Selegiline (L-deprenyl)	Reports of serotonergic reactions
Methylene blue		Enhanced serotonergic effects through inhibition of MAO-A and B by methylene blue. Risk for serotonin syndrome (see Precautions p. 10)
Opioid	Tramadol	Increased risk of seizures and serotonin syndrome
Phosphodiesterase type 5 (PDE5) inhibitor	Sildenafil	Possible enhanced hypotension due to inhibited metabolism of sildenafil via CYP3A4 with nefazodone
Statins	Atorvastatin, pravastatin, simvastatin	Inhibited metabolism of statins by nefazodone (via CYP3A4); increased plasma level and adverse effects – myositis and rhabdomyolysis reported
St. John's wort		May augment serotonergic effects – case reports of serotonergic reactions
Sulfonylurea	Tolbutamide	Increased hypoglycemia

Serotonin-1A Partial Agonist/Serotonin Reuptake Inhibitor (SPARI)

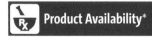 **Product Availability***

Generic Name	Chemical Class	Neuroscience-based Nomenclature* (Pharmacological Target/Mode of Action)	Trade Name	Dosage Forms and Strengths
Vilazodone	Indolalkylamine	Serotonin/Multimodal	Viibryd	Tablets: 10 mg, 20 mg, 40 mg

* Refer to Health Canada's Drug Product Database or the FDA's Drugs@FDA for the most current availability information · Developed by a taskforce consisting of representatives from the American College of Neuropsychopharmacology (ACNP), the Asian College of Neuropsychopharmacology (AsCNP), the European College of Neuropsychopharmacology (ECNP), the International College of Neuropsychopharmacology (CINP), and the International Union of Basic and Clinical Pharmacology (IUPHAR) (see https://nbn2r.com),

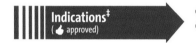 **Indications‡**
(👍 approved)

- 👍 Major depressive disorder (MDD)
- 👍 Generalized anxiety disorder (GAD)

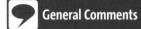 **General Comments**

- Clinical profile similar to SARIs and SSRIs. A network meta-analysis of 24 studies does not indicate greater benefits or fewer harms of vilazodone, compared with other second-generation antidepressants
- In a double-blind study, nonresponders to citalopram 20 mg/day showed improvement if dose was increased to 40 mg/day or switched to vilazodone
- The efficacy of vilazodone (over placebo) was established in four 8- to 10-week, randomized, double-blind, controlled trials in adult patients with a diagnosis of MDD; 41–58% of patients on vilazodone had a response compared to 31–47% of patients who received placebo
- The efficacy of vilazodone (over placebo) for generalized anxiety disorder was studied in two 10-week, randomized, double-blind, controlled trials in adults; 46–55% of patients on vilazodone had a response compared to 42–48% of patients who received placebo
- In a 28-week randomized double-blind, fixed-dose (vilazodone 20 mg/day, vilazodone 40 mg/day, or placebo) trial, the time to relapse with vilazodone was not statistically different from placebo

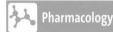 **Pharmacology**

- Dual 5-HT_{1A} receptor partial agonist and 5-HT reuptake inhibitor. Vilazodone binds with high affinity to the serotonin reuptake site ($K_i = 0.1$ nM) and potently and selectively inhibits reuptake of serotonin ($IC_{50} = 1.6$ nM); also binds selectively with high affinity to 5-HT_{1A} receptors ($IC_{50} = 2.1$ nM)
- 5-HT_{1A} agonism produces a more rapid desensitization of presynaptic 5-HT_{1A} autoreceptors

 Dosing

- See p. 95
- Initial dose of 10 mg once daily with food for 7 days, followed by 20 mg once daily for an additional 7 days, and then increase to 40 mg once daily; slower dose titration helps to minimize GI side effects
- Some patients were unable to reach 40 mg in clinical trials due to lack of tolerability
- No dosage adjustment required in renal insufficiency or moderate liver impairment
- Give with food as absorption decreased by up to 50% in fasting state

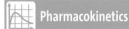 **Pharmacokinetics**

- See p. 95
- The pharmacokinetics of vilazodone (5–80 mg) are dose proportional. Vilazodone concentrations peak at a median of 4–5 h (T_{max}) after administration and decline with a terminal half-life of approximately 25 h
- The bioavailability is 72% with food. Administration with food (high-fat or light meal) increases oral bioavailability (C_{max} increased by approximately 147–160%, and AUC increased by approximately 64–85%)
- Distribution: Vilazodone is widely distributed and approximately 96–99% protein bound

‡ Indications listed here do not necessarily apply to all countries. Please refer to a country's regulatory database (e.g., US Food and Drug Administration, Health Canada Drug Product Database) for the most current availability information and indications

- Metabolism and elimination: Elimination of vilazodone is primarily by hepatic metabolism through CYP and non-CYP pathways (possibly by carboxylesterase), with only 1% of the dose recovered in urine and 2% of the dose recovered in feces as unchanged vilazodone. CYP3A4 is primarily responsible for its metabolism, with minor contributions from CYP2C19 and CYP2D6. It has no active metabolites

 Adverse Effects

- See chart p. 92 for incidence of adverse effects at therapeutic doses

CNS Effects

- Headache was a common side effect (over 10%) but this was no different to placebo or citalopram
- In pooled analysis of pivotal trials, dizziness was also a common side effect (16.5% vs. 3.3% placebo), as were insomnia (11.1% vs. 5.4%), fatigue (8.7% vs. 3%), and lethargy (6.8% vs. 0.5%)
- Restlessness and abnormal dreams, nightmares reported in initial trials
- Effects on sleep were specifically investigated in a randomized crossover study with 10 healthy young men (20 mg single dose); slow-wave sleep increased in the first and third one-third of the night, whereas wakefulness was enhanced in the second and third one-third of the night; rapid eye movement almost totally disappeared in patients receiving vilazodone

Cardiovascular Effects

- A thorough ECG study in healthy volunteers found that vilazodone had no clinically significant effect on heart rate, PR interval, or corrected QT interval, indicating a low potential for it to induce cardiac arrhythmias

Endocrine & Metabolic Effects

- No statistically significant weight gain in the two pivotal trials; mean weight increase in the long-term study was 1.7 kg
- Increased appetite reported, but incidence was low and not significantly different to placebo
- Case report of hyperglycemia in diabetic patient
- In one GAD trial, a higher percentage of vilazodone-treated patients compared to placebo-treated patients shifted from normal baseline values to high values at the end of treatment for total cholesterol (18% vs. 11%), glucose (10% vs. 4%), and triglycerides (19% vs. 12%)

GI Effects

- Diarrhea (> 25%) and nausea (> 20%) were the most common side effects
- Vomiting, dyspepsia, abdominal pain, dry mouth, and flatulence also reported

Urogenital & Sexual Effects

- Spontaneously-reported sexual side effects were generally more frequent with vilazodone than placebo in 8- or 10-week trials, decreased libido being most common (4% vs. less than 1% in men and 2% vs. less than 1% in women for vilazodone 40 mg once daily); in open-label treatment with vilazodone for 1 year, the most frequent sexual function-related adverse effects were decreased libido (4.2%), erectile dysfunction (4.2%), delayed ejaculation (3.1%), and abnormal orgasm (2.3%)
- In 3 trials prospectively evaluating sexual dysfunction using validated scales, over half of the participants had baseline sexual dysfunction; scores for those whose MADRS score was reduced by ≥ 50% improved in all treatment groups with a small numerical (but not statistically significant) difference between vilazodone (20 mg/40 mg) and placebo relative to citalopram 40 mg

Other Adverse Effects

- Hyperhidrosis, night sweats, blurred vision, arthralgia, tremor, dry mouth, and dry eyes

 Discontinuation Syndrome

- Abrupt discontinuation may cause a syndrome consisting of dizziness, lethargy, nausea, vomiting, diarrhea, headache, fever, sweating, chills, malaise, incoordination, insomnia, vivid dreams, myalgia, paresthesias, dyskinesias, "electric-shock-like" sensations, visual discoordination, anxiety, irritability, confusion, slowed thinking, disorientation; rarely aggression, impulsivity, hypomania, and depersonalization
- Brain "zaps" (or electric-shock-like sensations), often associated with lateral eye movements, hearing static sounds, and feelings of dizziness/wooziness; usually transitory but may last for months
- Most likely to occur within 1–7 days after drug stopped or dose drastically reduced, and typically disappears within 3 weeks
- Paradoxical mood changes reported on abrupt withdrawal, including hypomania or mania
- ☞ **THEREFORE THIS MEDICATION SHOULD BE WITHDRAWN GRADUALLY AFTER PROLONGED USE**

Management

- Reinstitute the drug at a lower dose and taper gradually over several days

 Precautions

- Strong CYP3A4 inhibitors can result in elevated plasma levels of vilazodone, recommended dose reduction to 20 mg/day; alternatively, potent inducers of CYP3A4 can lower plasma levels of the drug and decrease its effectiveness

Serotonin-1A Partial Agonist/Serotonin Reuptake Inhibitor (SPARI) (cont.)

- Black-box warning regarding increased risk of suicidal thinking and behavior in children, adolescents, and young adults taking antidepressants for MDD and other psychiatric disorders
- Similar to other antidepressants, vilazodone labeling carries warnings about serotonin syndrome, seizures, abnormal bleeding, activation of mania/hypomania (reported in 0.1% of patients in clinical trials), and hyponatremia
- If urgent treatment with linezolid or IV methylene blue is required in a patient already receiving vilazodone and potential benefits outweigh potential risks, discontinue vilazodone promptly and administer linezolid or IV methylene blue. Monitor for serotonin syndrome for 2 weeks or until 24 h after the last dose of linezolid or IV methylene blue, whichever comes first. May resume vilazodone 24 h after the last dose of linezolid or IV methylene blue
- Dose tapering is recommended when the drug is discontinued

Toxicity

- There is limited clinical experience regarding human overdose; 4 patients and 1 patient's child experienced an overdose and all recovered
- Case report of a 23-month-old, 11 kg child ingesting 60 mg vilazodone (unwitnessed) who developed recurrent seizure activity along with lethargy, fever, and hyperreflexia; managed with supportive care, benzodiazepines, and phenobarbital – patient recovered 24 h following ingestion. No serum analysis was performed to confirm exposure or establish pharmacokinetic parameters
- The adverse reactions associated with overdose at doses of 200–280 mg as observed in clinical trials included serotonin syndrome, lethargy, restlessness, hallucinations, and disorientation

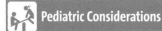
Pediatric Considerations

- For detailed information on the use of vilazodone in this population, please see the *Clinical Handbook of Psychotropic Drugs for Children and Adolescents*[8]
- Efficacy of vilazodone for MDD in adolescents (ages 12–17) could not be confirmed in an 8-week, double-blind, randomized, placebo-controlled, fixed dose study (vilazodone 15 mg/day [175 participants], vilazodone 30 mg/day [180 participants], placebo [174 participants])
- No approved indications in children and adolescents
- The safety and efficacy of vilazodone in children and adolescents has not been adequately studied

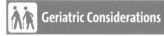
Geriatric Considerations

- No dosage adjustments recommended on the basis of age, renal or mild liver impairment although there is no published data evaluating use in geriatric depression
- GAD trials included patients up to 70 years of age

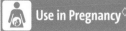
Use in Pregnancy◊

- There are no adequate, well-controlled studies of vilazodone in pregnant women and no human data regarding vilazodone concentrations in breast milk
- One published case report of vilazodone used in pregnancy: 32-year-old woman unexpectedly became pregnant while on 40 mg/day, continued medication and gave birth to a healthy child. The child experienced transient neonatal jaundice but none of the irritability or feeding or respiratory difficulties reported with other serotonergic antidepressants

Breast Milk

- No human data regarding vilazodone concentrations in breast milk

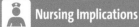
Nursing Implications

- Psychotherapy and education are also important in the treatment of depression
- Expect a lag time of up to 28 days before antidepressant effects will be noticed, significant improvement may not be seen before 6 weeks
- Monitor therapy by watching for adverse side effects and mood and activity level changes, including worsening of suicidal thoughts; keep physician informed
- Reassure patient that most early side effects usually subside after the first few weeks; if dizzy, patient should get up from lying or sitting position slowly and dangle legs over edge of bed before getting up
- Vilazodone may cause drowsiness; caution patient that activities requiring mental alertness should not be performed until response to the drug has been determined

◊ See p. 473 for further information on drug use in pregnancy and effects on breast milk

- MUST give with a meal for full absorption
- Instruct patient to avoid ingestion of grapefruit juice, as otherwise the blood level of vilazodone may increase
- Avoid excessive use of caffeinated foods, drugs, or beverages as these may increase anxiety and agitation that can occur during initial titration
- Be aware that as the medication reduces the degree of depression it may increase psychomotor activity; this may create concern about suicidal behavior
- Should not be stopped suddenly due to risk of precipitating withdrawal reactions

 Patient Instructions

- For detailed patient instructions on vilazodone, see the Patient Information Sheet (details p. 474)

 Drug Interactions

- Clinically significant interactions are listed below
- For more interaction information on any given combination, also see the corresponding chapter for the second agent

Class of Drug	Example	Interaction Effects
Analgesic	Acetylsalicylic acid	May impair platelet aggregation, resulting in increased risk of bleeding events
Antibiotic	Clarithromycin, erythromycin	Increased plasma level of vilazodone due to inhibition of metabolism via CYP3A4; reduce dose to maximum of 20 mg
	Linezolid	May enhance serotonergic effect. May increase risk for serotonin syndrome (see Precautions p. 10)
Anticoagulant	Apixaban, dabigatran, rivaroxaban, warfarin	Increased risk of bleeding possible due to decreased platelet aggregation secondary to depletion of serotonin in platelets
Antidepressant		
SSRI, SNRI		SSRIs and SNRIs may enhance serotonergic effects. May increase risk for serotonin syndrome
MAOI	Moclobemide, phenelzine, tranylcypromine	Risk of serotonin syndrome. Contraindicated if used concurrently or within 14 days of stopping
Antiemetic	Metoclopramide	May enhance serotonergic effect. May increase risk for serotonin syndrome
Antifungal	Ketoconazole	Increased plasma level of vilazodone due to inhibition of metabolism via CYP3A4; reduce dose to maximum of 20 mg
Antipsychotic	Pimozide	May enhance antipsychotic side effects due to inhibition of metabolism via CYP3A4
Antiretroviral		
Protease inhibitor	Ritonavir	Increased plasma level of vilazodone due to inhibition of metabolism via CYP3A4; reduce dose to maximum of 20 mg
Anxiolytic	Buspirone	May enhance serotonergic effect. May increase risk for serotonin syndrome
Calcium channel blocker	Verapamil	Increased plasma level of vilazodone due to inhibition of metabolism via CYP3A4; reduce dose to maximum of 20 mg
Cardiac glycoside	Digoxin	C_{max} of digoxin increased significantly when co-administered with vilazodone, monitoring of digoxin plasma concentrations and possible digoxin dosage reduction may be required
CYP450 inducers	Carbamazepine, cimetidine, phenytoin, rifampin	May induce the metabolism of vilazodone due to induction of metabolism via CYP3A4
Diuretic	Hydrochlorothiazide	May increase risk for hyponatremia
Grapefruit juice		Increased plasma level of vilazodone possible due to inhibition of metabolism via CYP3A4
Herbal preparation/supplement	Alfalfa, anise, ginger, glucosamine, omega-3 fatty acids	Enhanced antiplatelet properties that can result in increased risk of bleeding events
	St. John's wort	May enhance serotonergic effect. May increase risk for serotonin syndrome
Methylene blue		Enhanced serotonergic effects through inhibition of MAO-A and B by methylene blue. Risk for serotonin syndrome (see Precautions p. 10)
NSAID	Acetylsalicylic acid, ibuprofen, naproxen	May impair platelet aggregation, resulting in increased risk of bleeding events

Serotonin-1A Partial Agonist/Serotonin Reuptake Inhibitor (SPARI) (cont.)

Class of Drug	Example	Interaction Effects
Opioid	Meperidine, pentazocine	May enhance serotonergic effect. May increase risk for serotonin syndrome
	Tramadol	May also increase risk of seizure
Stimulant	Methylphenidate	May enhance serotonergic effect. May increase risk for serotonin syndrome
Triptan	Rizatriptan, sumatriptan, zolmitriptan	May enhance serotonergic effect. May increase risk for serotonin syndrome

Serotonin Modulator and Stimulator (SMS)

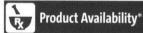 **Product Availability***

Generic Name	Chemical Class	Neuroscience-based Nomenclature* (Pharmacological Target/Mode of Action)	Trade Name	Dosage Forms and Strengths
Vortioxetine	Bisarylsulfanyl amine	Serotonin/Multimodal	Trintellix	Tablets: 5 mg, 10 mg, 15 mg, 20 mg

* Refer to Health Canada's Drug Product Database or the FDA's Drugs@FDA for the most current availability information   * Developed by a taskforce consisting of representatives from the American College of Neuropsychopharmacology (ACNP), the Asian College of Neuropsychopharmacology (AsCNP), the European College of Neuropsychopharmacology (ECNP), the International College of Neuropsychopharmacology (CINP), and the International Union of Basic and Clinical Pharmacology (IUPHAR) (see https://nbn2r.com),

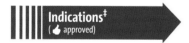 **Indications‡**
(👍 approved)

- 👍 Major depressive disorder (MDD)
- Generalized anxiety disorder (GAD)
- Alcohol use disorder (AUD) comorbid with major depressive disorder (MDD) – preliminary evidence suggests this may be a rational treatment consideration, even in cases of subclinical depression but clinically significant anhedonia

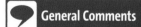 **General Comments**

- Structurally related to buspirone, citalopram, and ondansetron, each of which shares some mechanisms of action with vortioxetine
- Non-US-based trials demonstrated efficacy for MDD at lower doses (5 mg) compared to US trials
- A network meta-analysis of 24 studies does not indicate greater benefits or fewer harms of vortioxetine compared with other second-generation antidepressants
- Post-hoc analyses of short-term trials to assess safety of vortioxetine in later life depression (defined as 55 years or older with a majority having stable chronic physical diseases for these analyses) suggest no differences in this population
- Beneficial cognitive effects were initially demonstrated as a secondary outcome in the late-life depression trial; effects confirmed in a short-term prospective, active comparator (duloxetine) trial with non-elderly patients where cognitive effect was the primary outcome. This was determined to be a direct effect of treatment not simply an epiphenomenon of symptomatic improvement. Improvements in functionality, anxiety and quality of life seem to be more substantial in GAD subpopulations who are working or pursuing education
- A Canadian study demonstrated significant economic savings extending from improved workplace productivity following treatment with vortioxetine. Notably, there are no other antidepressant trials that monetized economic impact available for comparison; however, a previous US study that estimated the economic impact of lost productivity for the overall population of patients suffering from MDD had relatively similar findings

‡ Indications listed here do not necessarily apply to all countries. Please refer to a country's regulatory database (e.g., US Food and Drug Administration, Health Canada Drug Product Database) for the most current availability information and indications

- Some very limited data derived from post-hoc analyses demonstrate significant improvement in depression-related physical symptoms as well as sleep (quality/continuity) which, as residual issues, increase the risk of illness recurrence
- As with the other antidepressants, vortioxetine carries the warning regarding clinical worsening, suicidality, and unusual changes in behavior

 Pharmacology

- The mechanism of action of vortioxetine is thought to be related to its direct modulation of serotonergic receptor activity and inhibition of the serotonin (5-HT) transporter
- Based on PET data, the mean 5-HT transporter occupancy in the raphe nuclei was approximately 50% at 5 mg/day, 65% at 10 mg/day, and increased to above 80% at 20 mg/day
- Nonclinical data indicate that vortioxetine inhibits the serotonin transporter protein (K_i = 1.6) and, in decreasing order of affinity, acts as a 5-HT$_3$ antagonist (K_i = 3.7), 5-HT$_{1A}$ receptor agonist (K_i = 15), 5-HT$_7$ antagonist (K_i = 19), 5-HT$_{1B}$ receptor partial agonist (K_i = 33), and 5-HT$_{1D}$ receptor antagonist (K_i = 54). Based on rat studies only – clinical correlation is not yet clear – this leads to modulation of serotonin, norepinephrine, dopamine, acetylcholine, GABA, glutamate, and histamine in the medial prefrontal cortex and ventral hippocampus
- Often referred to as a multimodal antidepressant because it has partial agonist and antagonist effects, plus inhibits serotonin reuptake
- 5-HT$_{1A}$ agonism produces a more rapid desensitization of presynaptic 5-HT$_{1A}$ autoreceptors
- 5-HT$_3$ affinity for vortioxetine is greater than that of mirtazapine (K_i = 7–8) and olanzapine (K_i = 6) but it is lacking in H$_1$ affinity, which may explain the high rates of nausea despite strong 5-HT$_3$ antagonist activity. Further, its inhibitory activity at 5-HT$_3$ receptors differs from these other antagonists, possibly inducing a brief initial agonistic response
- Serotonergic modulation of glutamate neurotransmission via 5-HT$_{1A}$, 5-HT$_{1B}$, 5-HT$_3$, and 5-HT$_7$ receptors has been postulated as a potential mechanism of action for relief of depression-related cognitive dysfunction

 Dosing

- See p. 95
- Initial dose of 10 mg once daily without regard to meals; increase to 20 mg once daily after one week as tolerated because higher doses demonstrated better treatment effects in trials conducted in the USA; consider 5 mg once daily for patients who do not tolerate higher doses. Maintenance: 5–20 mg once daily. Limited evidence that 20 mg may yield a better outcome but dose adjustment should be individualized based on both efficacy and safety. The recommended maximum dose is 10 mg/day in known CYP2D6 poor metabolizers
- No dose adjustment necessary on the basis of age, renal function or mild–moderate hepatic impairment
- Not recommended in more severe hepatic impairment (Child-Pugh class C) because it has not been studied in patients with this degree of liver dysfunction
- Vortioxetine can be discontinued abruptly. However, it is recommended that doses of 15 mg/day or 20 mg/day be reduced to 10 mg/day for one week prior to full discontinuation, if possible

Pharmacokinetics

- See p. 95
- Displays linear pharmacokinetics (up to 60 mg after multiple doses); bioavailability (75%) is NOT affected by food
- Intrinsic factors such as ethnicity, age, sex, or body size have no clinically meaningful effects on drug exposure
- Vortioxetine concentrations peak in 7–11 h (T_{max}). Widely distributed and about 98% protein bound
- Elimination half-life is 57–66 h. Elimination is via hepatic metabolism, primarily through oxidation (CYP2D6 is the major isoenzyme responsible for metabolism) with subsequent glucuronic acid conjugation. The major metabolite has no clinical activity and a minor metabolite has the capacity to inhibit the serotonin transport protein, but it has limited ability to penetrate blood/brain barrier
- In obese individuals, half-life following cessation of the drug is significantly prolonged compared with normal-weight controls. Therefore, in cases of switching to a MAOI, it is suggested to extend the time between vortioxetine discontinuation and MAOI initiation beyond product monograph recommendation to reduce risk of serotonin syndrome
- In healthy patients, oral clearance was approximately 2-fold higher in extensive metabolizers compared to poor CYP2D6 metabolizers; no clinically relevant differences in overall incidence of adverse events in clinical trials. Routine CYP2D6 genotyping test not required before starting vortioxetine
- Vortioxetine or its metabolites have not shown any potential for clinically meaningful CYP450 inhibition or induction. It is also not considered a good P-glycoprotein substrate, nor does it have any P-glycoprotein inhibitory effects
- Steady state levels occur in about 14 days
- Excretion via urine (59%) and feces (26%). Negligible amounts of the unchanged drug remain in the urine

Serotonin Modulator and Stimulator (SMS) (cont.)

Adverse Effects

- See chart p. 92 for incidence of adverse effects at therapeutic doses

CNS Effects

- Fatigue, sedation or somnolence possible but not common
- During short-term clinical trials in patients with no history of seizure disorders, seizures were reported in less than 0.1% of patients receiving vortioxetine
- Headaches common in maintenance trials
- One industry-sponsored RCT suggests vortioxetine (at 10 mg/day over a 15-day period) has no significant impact on cognitive and psychomotor performance in the context of driving
- Although symptoms of mania/hypomania were seen in less than 0.1% of patients treated with vortioxetine in pre-marketing trials, caution is still warranted in using vortioxetine in patients with a personal or family history of bipolar disorder, mania or hypomanic symptoms
- Rare reports of restless legs syndrome

Cardiovascular Effects

- No significant effects on blood pressure, heart rate, and ECG parameters were seen in premarketing trials at doses up to 40 mg/day

Endocrine & Metabolic Effects

- No significant effect on body weight as measured by the mean change from baseline (5.8% of patients in one long-term trial reported a mean weight increase of 1 kg)
- Rare reports of amenorrhea with or without hyperprolactinemia

GI Effects

- Nausea was the most common adverse effect (20.9–30.2%); generally dose related (seems to plateau at 15 mg) and usually transient, with a median duration of 10–16 days. Some suggest splitting daily dose or even combining low-dose mirtazapine in the short term to prevent onset of nausea
- Diarrhea common, also dry mouth, constipation, vomiting, abdominal discomfort, dyspepsia, and flatulence
- Liver test abnormalities in a small proportion of patients (less than 1%) on long-term vorioxetine therapy, but elevations are usually mild, asymptomatic, and transient, reversing even with continuation of medication. No instances of acute liver injury with jaundice attributable to vortioxetine reported, but the total experience with its use has been limited

Urogenital & Sexual Effects

- Impact on sexual function appears to be dose related; limited comparative evidence suggests rates are likely lower relative to SSRIs or SNRIs when using 5–10 mg/day
- When trials used ASEX to evaluate sexual dysfunction in patients without baseline sexual dysfunction, rates were higher: Incidence of treatment-related sexual dysfunction (TRSD) across the dosing range was 22–34% for women and 16–29% for men

Hypersensitivity Reactions

- Rash and urticaria reported infrequently
- Rare post-marketing reports of angioedema and allergic dermatitis

Other Adverse Effects

- Generalized pruritus, hyperhidrosis, nasopharyngitis, and arthralgia relatively common

D/C Discontinuation Syndrome

- In clinical trials, vortioxetine doses of 10 mg, 15 mg, and 20 mg daily were abruptly discontinued, with non-significant differences in the Discontinuation–Emergent Signs and Symptoms checklist total scores vs. placebo (likely explained by long serum half-life)
- However, because of individual variation and sensitivity, some may still experience withdrawal symptoms. Most likely to occur within first weeks after drug stopped or dose drastically reduced, and typically disappear within 1 week
- ☞ **THEREFORE THIS MEDICATION SHOULD BE WITHDRAWN GRADUALLY AFTER PROLONGED USE**

Management

- Reinstitute the drug at a lower dose and taper more gradually

⚠ Precautions

- Strong CYP2D6 inhibitors can result in elevated plasma levels of vortioxetine. Vortioxetine should be reduced by 50% in the presence of strong inhibitors such as bupropion

- Although CYP3A4 is not a primary metabolic pathway, the product label recommends increasing the dose of vortioxetine when a strong CYP3A4 inducer such as carbamazepine, phenytoin or rifampin is co-administered for more than 14 days. The maximum recommended dose should not exceed 3 times the original dose
- Contraindicated in patients taking MAOIs or in patients who have taken MAOIs within the preceding 14 days. Using MAOIs within 21 days of stopping treatment with vortioxetine is also contraindicated
- As with other serotonergic antidepressants, serotonin syndrome may occur with vortioxetine, both when taken alone and especially when co-administered with other serotonergic agents. If such symptoms occur, discontinue the medications and initiate supportive treatment. If concomitant use of vortioxetine with other serotonergic drugs is clinically warranted (note that linezolid or intravenous methylene blue use is specifically mentioned as a contraindication), patients should be made aware of a potential increased risk for serotonin syndrome, particularly during treatment initiation and dose increases
- As with other antidepressants, vortioxetine should be introduced cautiously in patients who have a history of seizures or in patients with unstable epilepsy
- Treatment with medications that inhibit the serotonin transporter may be associated with abnormal bleeding, particularly when combined with NSAIDs, acetylsalicylic acid, or other medications that affect coagulation

 Toxicity

- Ingestion of vortioxetine in the dose range of 40–75 mg has caused an aggravation of the following adverse reactions: nausea, postural dizziness, diarrhea, abdominal discomfort, generalized pruritus, somnolence, and flushing. Management of overdose should consist of treating clinical symptoms and relevant monitoring

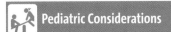 **Pediatric Considerations**

- For detailed information on the use of vortioxetine in this population, please see the *Clinical Handbook of Psychotropic Drugs for Children and Adolescents*[8]
- No approved indications in children and adolescents
- The safety and efficacy of vortioxetine in children and adolescents has not been adequately studied. Limited to a single open-label exploratory study

Geriatric Considerations

- No dosage adjustments recommended on the basis of age, renal or mild hepatic impairment
- Elderly patients, especially those taking diuretics, are at higher risk of developing hyponatremia

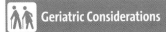 **Use in Pregnancy**◇

- Very limited human data; in a single case report, a healthy baby was delivered following 1 month of exposure to vortioxetine 5 mg
- Adverse events such as decreased fetal weight and delayed ossification observed in animal reproduction studies. Non-teratogenic effects in the newborn following serotonergic exposure late in the third trimester include respiratory distress, cyanosis, apnea, seizures, temperature instability, feeding difficulty, vomiting, hypoglycemia, hypo- or hypertonia, hyperreflexia, jitteriness, irritability, constant crying, and tremor. In the majority of instances, such complications began immediately or soon (less than 24 h) after delivery. Symptoms may be due to the toxicity of serotonergic antidepressants or a discontinuation syndrome – although no specific reports of such exist to date related specifically to vortioxetine exposure, it may be a possibility
- Epidemiological data suggest that the use of SSRIs in pregnancy, particularly in late pregnancy, may increase the risk of persistent pulmonary hypertension (PPHN) in the newborn. Although no studies have investigated the association of PPHN with vortioxetine treatment, this potential risk cannot be ruled out, taking into account the related mechanism of action (increase in serotonin concentrations)

Breast Milk

- No evidence in humans at this time. Available data in animals have shown excretion of vortioxetine and metabolites in milk. It is expected that vortioxetine is excreted into human milk. A risk to the nursing child cannot be excluded. A decision must be made whether to discontinue breastfeeding or to discontinue/abstain from vortioxetine, taking into account the benefit of breastfeeding for the child and the benefit of therapy for the woman

 Nursing Implications

- Psychotherapy and education are also important in the treatment of depression
- Monitor therapy by watching for adverse side effects and mood and activity level changes, including worsening of suicidal thoughts; keep physician informed

◇ See p. 473 for further information on drug use in pregnancy and effects on breast milk

Serotonin Modulator and Stimulator (SMS) (cont.)

- Be aware that as the medication reduces the degree of depression it may increase psychomotor activity; this may create concern about suicidal behavior
- Expect a lag time of up to 28 days before antidepressant effects are noticed
- Reassure patient that most early side effects usually subside after the first few weeks; if dizzy, patient should get up from lying or sitting position slowly and dangle legs over edge of bed before getting up
- Excessive use of caffeinated foods, drugs, or beverages may increase anxiety and agitation and confuse the diagnosis
- Should not be stopped suddenly due to risk of precipitating withdrawal reactions

 Patient Instructions

- For detailed patient instructions on vortioxetine, see the Patient Information Sheet (details p. 474)

 Drug Interactions

- Clinically significant interactions are listed below
- For more interaction information on any given combination, also see the corresponding chapter for the second agent

Class of Drug	Example	Interaction Effects
Analgesic	Acetylsalicylic acid	Increased risk of abnormal bleeding
Antibiotic	Linezolid	May enhance serotonergic effect. May increase risk for serotonin syndrome (see Precautions p. 10)
Anticoagulant	Apixaban, dabigatran, rivaroxaban, warfarin	Increased risk of bleeding possible due to decreased platelet aggregation secondary to depletion of serotonin in platelets
Antidepressant		
SSRI	Fluoxetine, paroxetine	May increase vortioxetine levels significantly. Recommend reducing dose by 50% when combining with these significant CYP2D6 inhibitors
NDRI	Bupropion	May increase vortioxetine levels significantly. Recommend reducing dose by 50% when combining
Antifungal	Fluconazole, ketoconazole	Moderate to strong CYP2C9/2C19/3A4 inhibitors can increase AUC and C_{max} of vortioxetine only modestly (15–46%), therefore no dosage adjustment is recommended but monitoring may be warranted
CYP450 inducers	Carbamazepine, phenytoin, rifampin	May reduce vortioxetine levels due to CYP3A4 induction Broad CYP inducer rifampin decreased the exposure of vortioxetine by 72%
CYP450 inhibitor	Protease inhibitors, quinidine	Strong CYP2D6 inhibitors can increase vortioxetine levels significantly. May require reducing vortioxetine dose by 50% with such combinations
Desmopressin		Increased risk of hyponatremia if combined with vortioxetine, particularly in the elderly
Diuretic	Hydrochlorothiazide	Increased risk of hyponatremia if combined with vortioxetine, particularly in the elderly
Methylene blue		Enhanced serotonergic effects through inhibition of MAO-A and B by methylene blue. Risk for serotonin syndrome (see Precautions p. 10)
NSAID		Increased risk of abnormal bleeding
Opioid	Meperidine	Increased risk of serotonin syndrome

Noradrenergic/Specific Serotonergic Antidepressant (NaSSA)

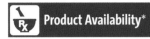 **Product Availability***

Generic Name	Chemical Class	Neuroscience-based Nomenclature* (Pharmacological Target/Mode of Action)	Trade Name(A)	Dosage Forms and Strengths
Mirtazapine	Tetracyclic agent	Norepinephrine, serotonin/Multimodal	Remeron Remeron RD(C), Remeron SolTab(B)	Tablets: 7.5 mg(B), 15 mg, 30 mg, 45 mg Oral disintegrating tablets: 15 mg, 30 mg, 45 mg

* Refer to Health Canada's Drug Product Database or the FDA's Drugs@FDA for the most current availability information. * Developed by a taskforce consisting of representatives from the American College of Neuropsychopharmacology (ACNP), the Asian College of Neuropsychopharmacology (AsCNP), the European College of Neuropsychopharmacology (ECNP), the International College of Neuropsychopharmacology (CINP), and the International Union of Basic and Clinical Pharmacology (IUPHAR) (see https://nbn2r.com), (A) Generic preparation may be available, (B) Not marketed in Canada, (C) Not marketed in the USA

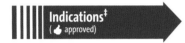 **Indications‡**
(👍 approved)

- 👍 Major depressive disorder (MDD) (with or without comorbid anxiety)
- Sexual dysfunction, SSRI-induced, and "poop-out" syndrome (see p. 3): May be mitigated by mirtazapine
- Panic disorder, generalized anxiety disorder, social anxiety disorder, somatoform disorder, OCD, PTSD, dysthymia, and premenstrual dysphoric disorder – preliminary reports of efficacy[19]
- Pervasive developmental disorders (autism) – improvement in symptoms of aggression, self-injury, irritability, hyperactivity, anxiety, depression, insomnia, and inappropriate sexual behaviors
- Schizophrenia and psychotic depression – mirtazapine may benefit negative symptoms
- Akathisia – some early evidence demonstrating that low doses (7.5-15 mg) may reduce incidence, particularly that related to aripiprazole
- Chronic pain (e.g., tension headache, fibromyalgia); effect size compared to placebo in recent fibromyalgia (without comorbid depression) trial was similar to placebo-controlled trials with duloxetine and pregabalin
- Alcohol withdrawal – has been found helpful; may help maintain abstinence
- Substance use: Methamphetamine – addition of mirtazapine to substance use counseling decreased methamphetamine use among active users and was associated with decreases in sexual risk despite low to moderate medication adherence
- Nausea/vomiting in a variety of clinical scenarios including cyclical vomiting syndrome; longer half-life and decreased cost relative to traditional 5-HT$_3$ antagonists but formal comparative trials are lacking
- Headaches and nausea induced by ECT – case series suggests benefit
- Appetite stimulation
- Functional dyspepsia (FD) – short-term evidence (pilot trial) suggests that, of the various symptoms encountered in FD, issues with early satiety may respond best to mirtazapine
- Refractory gastroparesis – possibly independent of antidepressant effect
- Insomnia – although both sleep latency and sleep quantity may be improved, additional promotion of slow-wave sleep may benefit sleep quality
- Malignancy-related pruritus unresponsive to standard treatment

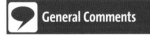 **General Comments**

- Reduces sleep latency and prolongs sleep duration due to H$_1$ and 5-HT$_{2A/C}$ blockade – may be helpful in treating depression with prominent insomnia or agitation
- Has mild anxiolytic effects at lower doses
- A Cochrane review found mirtazapine was more effective at 2 weeks and at the end of acute-phase treatment than SSRIs and venlafaxine and was more likely to cause weight gain or increased appetite and somnolence than SSRIs but less likely to cause nausea or vomiting and sexual dysfunction
- Monitor all patients for worsening depression and suicidal thinking

‡ Indications listed here do not necessarily apply to all countries. Please refer to a country's regulatory database (e.g., US Food and Drug Administration, Health Canada Drug Product Database) for the most current availability information and indications

Noradrenergic/Specific Serotonergic Antidepressant (NaSSA) (cont.)

- A randomized, double-blind, placebo-controlled trial in participants with probable or possible Alzheimer's disease and agitation unresponsive to non-drug treatment reported no benefit of mirtazapine 45 mg/day compared with placebo. The authors observed a potentially higher mortality rate with use of mirtazapine[20]

 Pharmacology

- Presynaptic α_2-adrenergic antagonist effects, which result in increased release of norepinephrine and serotonin. It is also a potent antagonist of 5-HT$_{2A}$, 5-HT$_{2C}$, 5-HT$_3$, and H$_1$ receptors and a moderate peripheral α_1-adrenergic and muscarinic antagonist; it does not inhibit the reuptake of norepinephrine or serotonin

 Dosing

- See p. 95
- Initiate at 15 mg daily for a minimum of one week before considering further dose increases since mirtazapine has a half-life of 20–40 h. The optimal dose balancing efficacy for depression and tolerability is at the lower end of the licensed dosing range (15–30 mg) for a majority; however, dosing should be individualized, as there are limitations to the available evidence and significant heterogeneity amongst individuals with depression. Patients who do not respond may benefit from increases up to 45 mg daily
- Lower dosage range suggested if specifically targeting sleep (7.5–15 mg)
- The dose is best administered in the evening prior to sleep

 Pharmacokinetics

- Bioavailability is approximately 50% due to gut wall and hepatic first-pass metabolism; food slightly decreases absorption rate
- Remeron SolTabs dissolve on the tongue within 30 seconds; can be swallowed with or without water, chewed, or allowed to dissolve
- Peak plasma level achieved in 2 h
- Protein binding of 85%
- Females and the elderly show higher plasma concentrations than males and young adults
- Extensively metabolized via CYP1A2, 2D6, and 3A4; desmethyl metabolite has some clinical activity
- Half-life 20–40 h – significantly longer in females than in males
- Hepatic clearance decreased by 40% in patients with cirrhosis
- Clearance reduced by 30–50% in patients with renal impairment

 Onset & Duration of Action

- Therapeutic effect is typically seen after 28 days (though some effects may be seen sooner), especially on symptoms related to sleep and appetite
- Meta-analysis of double-blind trials in patients with depression suggests an earlier onset of efficacy with mirtazapine than with SSRIs although no difference in number of responders at study end

 Adverse Effects

- See p. 92
- Somnolence, hyperphagia, and weight gain are the most commonly reported side effects[19]

CNS Effects

- Fatigue, sedation in over 30% of patients; may have less sedation at doses above 15 mg due to increased effect on α_2 receptors and increased release of NE (based on relatively limited evidence)
- Shown to impair driving performance and decreased psychomotor functioning during the acute treatment phase although a prospective randomized study in depressed patients using a simulator showed a significant improvement in performance and decrease in crash rates
- Insomnia, agitation, hostility, depersonalization, restlessness, and nervousness reported occasionally, coupled with urges of self-harm or harm to others
- Increases slow-wave sleep and decreases stage 1 sleep. Reported to shorten sleep onset latency, improve sleep efficiency and increase total sleep time; vivid dreams reported – does not appear to be dose related; case reports of REM sleep behavior disorder with hallucinations and confusion; case report of somnambulism on dose increase
- Case report of panic attack during dose escalation
- Rarely delirium, hallucinations, psychosis

- Cases of altered visual perception and visual hallucinations reported in elderly patients
- Seizures (very rare – 0.04%)

Anticholinergic Effects	• Dry mouth frequent; thirst, constipation [for treatment suggestions see Nonselective Cyclic Antidepressants, p. 57] • Blurred vision, and urinary retention reported rarely
Cardiovascular Effects	• Hypotension, hypertension, vertigo, tachycardia, and palpitations reported rarely • Edema 1–2% • Risk of QTc prolongation and torsades de pointes
Endocrine & Metabolic Effects	• Carbohydrate craving, increased appetite and leptin concentrations, and weight gain (of over 4 kg) reported in over 16% of patients (due to potent antihistaminic properties); occur primarily in the first 4 weeks of treatment and may be dose related – may be of benefit in depressed patients with marked anorexia. Weight gain may appear more slowly in elderly patients, especially octogenarians, relative to younger individuals • May be less likely than SSRIs to cause hyponatremia • Increases in plasma cholesterol, to over 20% above the upper limit of normal, seen in 15% of patients; increases in nonfasting triglyceride levels (7%)
GI Effects	• Rare reports of bitter taste, dyspepsia, nausea, vomiting, and diarrhea • Decreased appetite and weight loss occasionally reported
Other Adverse Effects	• Sexual dysfunction occurs occasionally; risk increased with age, use of higher doses, and concomitant medication • Case reports of erotic dream-related ejaculation in elderly patients • Rates of sexual dysfunction in a naturalistic study were citalopram 60%, venlafaxine 54.5%, paroxetine 54.2%, fluoxetine 46.2%, and mirtazapine 18.2% • Increased sweating • Rare reports of tremor, hot flashes • Transient elevation of ALT reported in about 2% of patients; cases of hepatitis • Febrile neutropenia (1.5% risk) and agranulocytosis (0.1%) reported; monitor WBC if patient develops signs of infection [some recommend doing baseline and annual CBC] • Cases of joint pain or worsening of arthritis reported • Myalgia and flu-like symptoms in 2–5% of patients • Case of palinopsia reported • Cases of pancreatitis and of gall-bladder disorder • Cases of rhabdomyolysis reported with mirtazapine used alone, in combination with risperidone, and in overdose • Reports of venous thromboembolism including deep vein thrombosis • Cases of paradoxical tremors, akathisia, dystonia, and dyskinesias reported – these hyperkinetic reactions may be more likely in older individuals or with higher doses

D/C Discontinuation Syndrome	• Abrupt discontinuation may cause a syndrome consisting of dizziness, lethargy, nausea, vomiting, diarrhea, headache, fever, sweating, chills, malaise, incoordination, insomnia, vivid dreams, myalgia, paresthesias, dyskinesias, "electric-shock-like" sensations, visual discoordination, anxiety, irritability, confusion, slowed thinking, disorientation; rarely aggression, impulsivity, hypomania, and depersonalization • Most likely to occur within 1–7 days after drug stopped or dose drastically reduced, and typically disappears within 3 weeks • Case reports of hypomania, akathisia, panic attack, and pruritis (without rash or urticarial) following abrupt cessation of treatment ☞ **THEREFORE THIS MEDICATION SHOULD BE WITHDRAWN GRADUALLY AFTER PROLONGED USE**
Management	• Reinstitute drug at a lower dose and taper gradually over several days

⚠ Precautions	• Monitor all patients for worsening depression and suicidal thoughts, especially at start of therapy or following an increase or decrease in dose; see Pediatric Considerations (p. 52) • Cases of QT prolongation and torsades de pointes; caution in patients with risk factors such as known cardiovascular disease, family history of QT prolongation, and concomitant use of QT-prolonging medications

Noradrenergic/Specific Serotonergic Antidepressant (NaSSA) (cont.)

- Caution in patients with compromised liver function or renal impairment
- Monitor WBC if patient develops signs of infection; a low WBC requires discontinuation of therapy
- May induce manic reactions in patients with BD and rarely in unipolar depression
- Treatment with medications that inhibit the serotonin transporter may be associated with abnormal bleeding, particularly when combined with NSAIDs, acetylsalicylic acid or other medications that affect coagulation

 Toxicity

- Low liability for toxicity in overdose if taken alone; depression of CNS with disorientation and prolongation of sedation, with tachycardia and mild hyper or hypotension
- Cases of QT prolongation and torsades de pointes
- Post-marketing case reports of fatalities; none during clinical trials except in mixed overdose

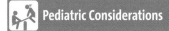 **Pediatric Considerations**

- For detailed information on the use of mirtazapine in this population, please see the *Clinical Handbook of Psychotropic Drugs for Children and Adolescents*[8]
- No approved indications in children and adolescents. There are limited well-conducted randomized controlled trials of mirtazapine in pediatric patients for any indication
- CAUTION: Episodes of self-harm and potential suicidal behaviors reported with certain serotonergic antidepressants in patients under age 18

 Geriatric Considerations

- Clearance reduced in elderly males by up to 40%, and in elderly females by up to 10%
- Dosing: Start at 7.5 mg at bedtime and increase to 15 mg after 1–2 weeks, depending on response and side effects; monitor for sedation, hypotension, and anticholinergic effects
- Used to counteract or stabilize weight loss in patients with dementia
- Hyponatremia reported in older adults

 Use in Pregnancy◊

- Limited data suggests no major teratogenic effects in humans
- Although some evidence suggests higher rate of spontaneous abortions, preterm births, and low birth weight, no correction has been made for depressive symptoms, a known risk factor
- No long-term outcome data or evidence available on neonatal abstinence syndrome

Breast Milk

- Mirtazapine and its metabolite are secreted into breast milk in low concentrations (e.g., undetectably low to 2.86% of the maternal weight-adjusted dose)
- Very limited information regarding outcomes – no apparent short-term adverse effects but small sample size (less than 50 published cases) makes overall safety index unknown
- If a patient is breastfeeding and requires the addition of an antidepressant, other agents may be preferable as first-line options; however, maternal use of mirtazapine is not considered a reason to discontinue breastfeeding

 Nursing Implications

- Psychotherapy and education are also important in the treatment of depression
- Monitor therapy by watching for adverse effects and mood and activity level changes, including worsening of suicidal thoughts
- Signs and symptoms of infections (e.g., sore throat, fever, mouth sores, elevated temperature) should be reported to the physician as soon as possible
- Because mirtazapine can cause drowsiness, caution patient not to perform activities requiring mental alertness until response to this drug has been determined
- Mirtazapine should not be stopped suddenly due to risk of precipitating a withdrawal reaction

◊ See p. 473 for further information on drug use in pregnancy and effects on breast milk

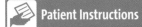 **Patient Instructions**

- For detailed patient instructions on mirtazapine, see the Patient Information Sheet (details on p. 474)

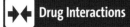 **Drug Interactions**

- Clinically significant interactions are listed below
- For more interaction information on any given combination, also see the corresponding chapter for the second agent

Class of Drug	Example	Interaction Effects
Antibiotic	Linezolid	Monitor for increased serotonergic and noradrenergic effects due to linezolid's weak MAO inhibition
Anticoagulant	Warfarin	May increase INR; monitor
Anticonvulsant	Carbamazepine, phenytoin	Decreased plasma level of mirtazapine by 60% with carbamazepine and 46% with phenytoin due to induction of metabolism via CYP3A4
Antidepressant		
SSRI	Fluoxetine, sertraline	Combination reported to alleviate insomnia and augment antidepressant response; may have activating effects
		May mitigate SSRI-induced sexual dysfunction and "poop-out" syndrome
	Fluvoxamine	Increased serotonergic effects possible; case reports of increased mirtazapine concentrations (3–4 fold)
		Increased sedation and weight gain reported with combination
SNRI	Venlafaxine	Increased plasma level of mirtazapine (3- to 4-fold) due to inhibited metabolism
		Case report of serotonin syndrome (see p. 10)
Irreversible MAOI	Phenelzine, tranylcypromine	Possible serotonergic reaction; DO NOT COMBINE
Irreversible MAO-B inhibitor	Rasagiline, selegiline	Possible serotonergic reaction
Antiemetic (5-HT$_3$ antagonist)	Dolasetron, granisetron, ondansetron	Case reports of serotonin syndrome
Antifungal	Ketoconazole	Increased peak plasma levels of mirtazapine (by about 40%)
Antihypertensive	Clonidine, guanabenz, guanfacine	Antihypertensive effect may be antagonized by mirtazapine
Antiplatelet	Clopidogrel	Increased risk of bleeding possible
Antipsychotic	Olanzapine	Case report of status epilepticus with mirtazapine and olanzapine; and of serotonin syndrome with mirtazapine, tramadol, and olanzapine
		Potential for additive metabolic adverse effects (e.g., increased cholesterol, sedation) and increased appetite
CNS depressant	Alcohol, benzodiazepines, opioid analgesics etc.	Impaired cognition and motor performance
H$_2$ antagonist	Cimetidine	Increased serum levels of mirtazapine (by 61%), dose adjustments of mirtazapine may be required
Methylene blue		Enhanced serotonergic effects through inhibition of MAO-A and B by methylene blue. Risk for serotonin syndrome (see Precautions p. 10)
Opioid	Tramadol	Case of lethargy, hypotension, and hypoxia in elderly patient
		Increased risk of seizures and serotonin syndrome
Smoking (tobacco)		Significantly decreased levels of mirtazapine
Stimulant	Dextroamphetamine, methylphenidate, phentermine	May increase agitation and risk of mania, especially in patients with bipolar disorder

Nonselective Cyclic Antidepressants

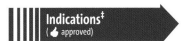 **Product Availability***

Generic Name	Chemical Class	Neuroscience-based Nomenclature* (Pharmacological Target/Mode of Action)	Trade Name[A]	Dosage Forms and Strengths
Amitriptyline[E]	Tricyclic antidepressant (TCA)	Serotonin, norepinephrine/Multimodal	Elavil, Levate[C]	Tablets: 10 mg, 25 mg, 50 mg, 75 mg, 100 mg[B], 150 mg[B]
Amoxapine[B]	Dibenzoxazepine	Norepinephrine, serotonin/Reuptake inhibitor	Asendin	Tablets: 25 mg, 50 mg, 100 mg, 150 mg
Clomipramine[D]	TCA	Serotonin, norepinephrine/Reuptake inhibitor (SERT, NET (metabolite))	Anafranil	Tablets[C]: 10 mg, 25 mg, 50 mg Capsules[B]: 25 mg, 50 mg, 75 mg
Desipramine	TCA	Norepinephrine/Reuptake inhibitor	Norpramin	Tablets: 10 mg, 25 mg, 50 mg, 75 mg, 100 mg, 150 mg[B]
Doxepin	TCA	Norepinephrine, serotonin/Multimodal	Adapin[B], Sinequan Silenor Zonalon	Capsules: 10 mg, 25 mg, 50 mg, 75 mg, 100 mg, 150 mg Oral solution[B]: 10 mg/mL Tablets: 3 mg, 6 mg 5% topical cream
Imipramine HCl	TCA	Serotonin, norepinephrine/Reuptake inhibitor	Tofranil	Tablets: 10 mg, 12.5 mg[C], 25 mg, 50 mg, 75 mg[C]
Imipramine pamoate[B]	TCA	Serotonin, norepinephrine/Reuptake inhibitor	Tofranil PM	Capsules: 75 mg, 100 mg, 125 mg, 150 mg
Maprotiline	Tetracyclic	Norepinephrine/Reuptake inhibitor	Ludiomil	Tablets: 10 mg, 25 mg, 50 mg, 75 mg
Nortriptyline	TCA	Norepinephrine/Reuptake inhibitor	Aventyl[C]	Capsules: 10 mg, 25 mg, 50 mg[B], 75 mg[B]
Protriptyline[B]	TCA	Norepinephrine/Reuptake inhibitor	Vivactil	Tablets: 5 mg, 10 mg
Trimipramine	TCA	Serotonin, dopamine/Antagonist	Surmontil	Tablets[C]: 12.5 mg, 25 mg, 50 mg, 75 mg[B], 100 mg Capsules: 25 mg[B], 50 mg[B], 75 mg[C], 100 mg[B]

* Refer to Health Canada's Drug Product Database or the FDA's Drugs@FDA for the most current availability information.   * Developed by a taskforce consisting of representatives from the American College of Neuropsychopharmacology (ACNP), the Asian College of Neuropsychopharmacology (AsCNP), the European College of Neuropsychopharmacology (ECNP), the International College of Neuropsychopharmacology (CINP), and the International Union of Basic and Clinical Pharmacology (IUPHAR) (see https://nbn2r.com), [A] Generic preparations may be available,   [B] Not marketed in Canada,   [C] Not marketed in the USA,   [D] Not approved for depression in the USA,   [E] Available in combination with perphenazine and also in combination with chlordiazepoxide in the USA

Indications‡
(👍 approved)

- 👍 Major depressive disorder (MDD): Acute treatment and maintenance
- 👍 Secondary depression in other mental illnesses (e.g., schizophrenia, dementia)
- 👍 Bipolar disorder: Depressed phase
- 👍 Obsessive-compulsive disorder (OCD) (clomipramine)
- 👍 Childhood enuresis (imipramine)
- 👍 Depression and/or anxiety associated with alcoholism or organic disease (doxepin)
- 👍 Psychoneuroses with MDD (doxepin)
- 👍 Insomnia (doxepin 3 and 6 mg at bedtime, for difficulty with sleep maintenance)
- Panic disorder (imipramine, clomipramine)
- Agoraphobia associated with panic disorder
- Dysthymia – efficacy reported (imipramine, desipramine)
- Depression, poststroke (nortriptyline)
- Posttraumatic stress disorder (PTSD) – efficacy against intrusive symptoms reported
- Generalized anxiety disorder (GAD) (imipramine)

‡ Indications listed here do not necessarily apply to all nonselective cyclic antidepressants or all countries. Please refer to a country's regulatory database (e.g., US Food and Drug Administration, Health Canada Drug Product Database) for the most current availability information and indications

- Temporomandibular joint disorders
- Attention-deficit/hyperactivity disorder (ADHD) not responsive to other agents (desipramine, nortriptyline)
- Premenstrual dysphoric disorder (clomipramine, nortriptyline)
- Premature ejaculation (clomipramine)
- Sialorrhea induced by clozapine (amitriptyline)
- Pain management, including migraine headache, diabetic neuropathy, postherpetic neuralgia, irritable bowel syndrome, chronic oral-facial pain, chronic pelvic pain, interstitial cystitis, and adjuvant analgesic; may help with sleep problems associated with fibromyalgia and other pain syndromes (i.e., amitriptyline, maprotiline, nortriptyline)
- Smoking cessation (nortriptyline), alone or in combination with nicotine patch. Nortriptyline (25–75 mg/day) appears as effective as bupropion for smoking cessation and has been recommended as second-line therapy for treating smoking dependence
- Chronic idiopathic urticaria (doxepin)
- Overactive bladder (imipramine, doxepin)
- Behavioral and psychological symptoms of dementia (BPSD)
- Neurogenic cough (nortriptyline)

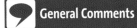 **General Comments**

- Antidepressants are associated with a small (2–3%) risk of hostility or suicidal ideation and associated behaviors in children, adolescents, and young adults (aged up to 24 years). Risk for suicide should be assessed and closely monitored during the initial weeks of antidepressant therapy
- In patients presenting with depression and a high risk of suicide, treatment selection should consider safety in overdose (i.e., consider using newer antidepressant agents rather than nonselective cyclic and MAOI antidepressants). Prescription quantities should be consistent with safe patient care
- Prior to using, consider a thorough cardiac evaluation that includes: known/existing heart disease (e.g., congenital or acquired prolonged QT syndrome), family history of heart disease (sudden death, cardiac dysrhythmias, cardiac conduction disturbances); baseline ECG for patients over 40 years old
- The presence of hallucinations or delusions is a negative predictor of response to tricyclic antidepressants (TCAs)
- Men may respond better to TCAs and less well to SSRIs than women
- Studies suggest improved outcomes in panic disorder with combination of imipramine and psychotherapy

 Pharmacology

- Exact mechanism of action unknown
- TCAs equilibrate the effects of biogenic amines through various mechanisms (i.e., reuptake blockade, downregulation of β-adrenergic receptors); tertiary amine agents (amitriptyline, clomipramine, doxepin, imipramine, trimipramine) have greater affinity for serotonin blockade; secondary amine agents (desipramine, nortriptyline, protriptyline) have greater affinity for norepinephrine blockade
- TCAs may facilitate management of enuresis; anticholinergic effects inhibit urination and CNS stimulation encourages easier arousal when stimulated by a full bladder
- The analgesic effects observed with TCAs may be due to sodium channel blockade
- Low-dose doxepin's histamine (H_1) blockade enables its use as a sedative and in urticaria (affinity for H_1 receptor greater than that of diphenhydramine)

 Dosing

- There is wide variation in dosage requirements between individuals; dosage should be individualized
- Monitoring serum drug levels may support dosage adjustment (most evidence for nortriptyline)
- Initiate at a low dose and increase dosage every 3–5 days to a maximum tolerated dose based on side effects. TCAs demonstrate a clear dose-response relationship
- Once steady state is achieved, medications can be provided as a single bedtime dose; this facilitates compliance, helps with sleep, and reduces daytime sedation. Exception: protriptyline, which is usually given in the morning
- Dosages can be divided or the entire dose given in the morning if the patient develops nightmares or experiences insomnia or stimulation
- Adolescent and geriatric patients generally require lower doses
- Prophylaxis is most effective if the therapeutic dose is maintained

Nonselective Cyclic Antidepressants (cont.)

- Hepatic disease: CAUTION may require a lower dosage
- Renal disease: CAUTION may require a lower dosage

Pharmacokinetics	

- See p. 95
- Completely absorbed from the GI tract
- Large percentage metabolized by first-pass effect
- Highly lipophilic; primarily concentrated in myocardial and cerebral tissue
- Highly bound to plasma and tissue proteins
- Metabolized by the liver; poor metabolizers (e.g., CYP2D6) may experience an up to 8-fold increase in plasma concentrations, resulting in increased adverse effects (e.g., cardiac toxicity, etc.)
- Most TCAs demonstrate linear pharmacokinetics (except desipramine), a change in dose results in a proportional change in the plasma concentration
- Pharmacokinetics may vary between males and females; data suggest that plasma levels of TCAs may decrease in female patients prior to menstruation
- Primary route of elimination is urinary excretion
- Elimination half-life: see p. 95; steady state reached in about 5 half-lives or 5 days
- Concurrent ingestion of TCAs with high-fiber foods or laxatives (e.g., bran, psyllium) can result in decreased absorption of the antidepressant

 Onset & Duration of Action

- TCAs and related drugs are long acting and can be provided as a single daily dose
- Onset of antidepressant effect typically occurs after 28 days although some patients may respond sooner, analgesic effects can take up to 3 weeks
- Sedative effects occur within a few hours of oral administration; sleep disturbance is reduced after a few days
- Patients may report a loss of antidepressant response or "poop-out syndrome" [Management: Check compliance; optimize dose, plasma levels may be helpful; consider switching antidepressants or augmenting therapy]

 Adverse Effects

- The pharmacological and side effect profile of TCAs is dependent on their affinity for and activity on neurotransmitters/receptors (see table p. 89)
- See chart p. 91 for the incidence of common adverse effects at therapeutic doses
- Adverse effects may be more problematic early in treatment; patients may adapt to side effects over time, e.g., anticholinergic effects, hypotension, sedation, etc. [Management: Initiate at low doses, gradually increase dose]

CNS Effects

- Occur due to antagonism at histamine H_1 receptors and α_1 adrenoreceptors
- CNS and neuromuscular effects occur frequently
- Drowsiness is the most common adverse effect; weakness, lethargy, and fatigue also occur. Conversely, excitement, agitation, restlessness, and insomnia have been reported
- Secondary amines reduce sleep efficiency and increase wake time after sleep onset; tertiary amines improve sleep continuity; decrease REM sleep (exception: trimipramine); vivid dreaming or nightmares can occur, especially if all the medication is given at bedtime
- Confusion, disturbed concentration, delusions, disorientation, and hallucinations can occur; more common in geriatric patients
- Precipitation of hypomania or mania (patients with a history of bipolar disorder – less frequent in patients on a mood stabilizer) and episode acceleration (occurs in up to 67% of patients)
- Anxiety, euphoria, panic reactions, and hostility may occur
- Fine tremor; dose dependent; observed in young and old patients
- Disturbance in gait, parkinsonism, and dystonia; geriatric patients are more likely to experience parkinsonism at high doses
- Akathisia can occur following abrupt drug withdrawal; reported with amoxapine, imipramine, and desipramine
- Paresthesias, numbing and tingling; approximate risk 4%
- Myoclonus, including muscle jerks of lower extremities, jaw, and arms, and nocturnal myoclonus; more likely with serotonergic agents; severe symptoms occur in up to 9% of patients [Management: If severe, clonazepam, valproate or carbamazepine may be of benefit]

- Dysphasia, stuttering
- Tardive dyskinesia; reported with amoxapine but also seen with other antidepressants on rare occasions
- Tinnitus – more likely with serotonergic agents
- Seizures; see Precautions p. 58; can occur following an abrupt increase in the drug dosage or after drug withdrawal; risk both dose and concentration dependent

Anticholinergic Effects

- Occur due to antagonism at muscarinic receptors
- Most common side effects associated with TCAs: increased frequency noted in elderly patients
- Dry mucous membranes predispose patient to monilial infections and dental caries [Management: Review oral hygiene, sugar-free gum or candy, oral lubricants (e.g., Moi-Stir, OraCare D), pilocarpine tablets or mouthwash (tablets 10–15 mg/day, mouthwash 4% solution 4–12 drops in water swished in mouth and spat out), bethanechol]
- Blurred vision, increased intraocular pressure
- Dry eyes; may be a problem in the elderly or those wearing contact lenses [Management: Patients who wear contact lenses should use their usual wetting solutions or comfort drops, others may use artificial tears]
- TCAs can induce or exacerbate existing hiatus hernia; TCAs should be discontinued if esophageal reflux develops
- Constipation; frequent side effect in children on therapy for enuresis [Management: Increase dietary bulk and fluid intake, fecal softener, bulk-forming laxative]
- Urinary retention, delayed micturition [Management: Bethanechol 10–30 mg tid]
- Confusion, disorientation, delirium, delusions, and hallucinations (more common in the elderly, especially with higher doses)
- Hyperthermia; increased risk when combined with other agents with anticholinergic activity or those that affect thermoregulation

Cardiovascular Effects

- Occur due to antagonism at α_1 adrenoreceptors, muscarinic, 5-HT$_2$, and H$_1$ receptors and inhibition of sodium fast channels
- Risk increases with high plasma levels
- Orthostatic hypotension common; additional risk factors include pre-existing postural hypotension and concurrent use of antihypertensive medications [Management: Sodium chloride tablets, caffeine, fludrocortisone (0.1–0.2 mg/day), midodrine (2.5–10 mg tid), support stockings]
- Hypertensive episodes reported in patient on TCAs receiving surgery [Management: Whenever possible, discontinue TCAs several days prior to surgery]
- Prolonged conduction time by delaying the inward sodium current into cardiomyocytes, slowing cardiac depolarization and lengthening the QTc interval; see Precautions p. 58; risk factors for ventricular arrhythmias can include combination with other antidepressant medications, underlying bundle branch block, preexisting conduction delays, higher doses of TCA, baseline QTc interval of $\geq$ 450 ms
- QTc prolongation; nortriptyline at therapeutic doses does not affect QTc interval
- Tachycardia; may be more pronounced in younger patients
- Syncope, thrombosis, thrombophlebitis, stroke, and congestive heart failure have been reported on occasion

Endocrine & Metabolic Effects

- Both increased and decreased blood sugar levels reported
- Weight gain reported in up to 30% of patients with chronic use; average gain of up to 7 kg; weight gain is linear over time and often accompanied by a craving for sweets [Management: Nutritional counseling, exercise, dose reduction, consider switching antidepressants]
- Menstrual irregularities, amenorrhea, and galactorrhea in females, breast enlargement in males
- Can induce SIADH with hyponatremia; risk increases with age

GI Effects

- Occur due to inhibition of 5-HT uptake and ACh antagonism
- Anorexia, nausea, vomiting, diarrhea, and abdominal cramps
- Increased pancreatic enzymes
- Constipation (see Anticholinergic Effects, p. 57)
- Peculiar taste, "black tongue," glossitis

Urogenital & Sexual Effects

- Occur due to altered dopamine activity, 5-HT$_{2A}$ blockade, inhibition of 5-HT reuptake, α_1 blockade, and ACh antagonism
- Decreased libido, impotence [Management: Amantadine (100–400 mg prn), bethanechol (10 mg tid or 10–25 mg prn), neostigmine (7.5–15 mg prn), cyproheptadine (4–16 mg prn), yohimbine (5.4–16.2 mg prn)]
- Anorgasmia or marked delay in up to 90% of clomipramine-treated patients [Management: Amantadine (100–400 mg prn), cyproheptadine (4–16 mg prn), yohimbine (5.4–10.8 mg od or prn), ginseng, ginkgo biloba (180–900 mg)]

Nonselective Cyclic Antidepressants (cont.)

- Testicular swelling, painful ejaculation, retrograde ejaculation, increased libido, and priapism; spontaneous orgasm with yawning reported with clomipramine
- Amitriptyline may have lower frequency of sexual dysfunction

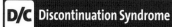

Hypersensitivity Reactions
- Rare
- Drug fever, edema, erythema, petechiae, pruritus, rash, and urticaria
- Photosensitivity, skin hyperpigmentation; 13 case reports with imipramine, also reported with desipramine
- Rarely agranulocytosis, eosinophilia, leukopenia, purpura, and thrombocytopenia

Other Adverse Effects
- Asymptomatic increases in aminotransferase levels
- Jaundice, hepatitis; reversible on discontinuation of TCA [Management: Monitor LFTs, discontinue if levels continue to increase]
- Excessive sweating [Management: Daily showering, talcum powder; in severe cases: Drysol solution, terazosin 1–10 mg daily, oxybutynin up to 5 mg bid, clonidine 0.1 mg bid; consider switching antidepressant]
- Rare reports of alopecia with TCAs

D/C Discontinuation Syndrome
☞ **THESE MEDICATIONS SHOULD BE WITHDRAWN GRADUALLY AFTER PROLONGED USE**
- Most frequent with clomipramine; likely due to cholinergic and adrenergic rebound
- Abrupt withdrawal from high doses may cause a "flu-like" syndrome consisting of fever, fatigue, sweating, coryza, malaise, myalgia, headache. Anxiety, agitation, hypomania or mania, insomnia, vivid dreams, as well as dizziness, nausea, vomiting; akathisia and dyskinesia also reported
- Symptoms are most likely to occur 24–48 h after withdrawal, or a large dosage decrease
- Paradoxical mood changes reported on abrupt withdrawal, including hypomania or mania

Management
- Re-institute drug, consider a slightly lower dose, and gradually taper the dose over several days
- Alternatively, can treat specific withdrawal symptoms:
  - Cholinergic rebound (e.g., nausea, vomiting, sweating) – ginger, benztropine 0.5–4 mg prn, atropine 1–4 mg tid to qid
  - Anxiety, agitation, insomnia – benzodiazepine (e.g., lorazepam 0.5–2 mg prn)
  - Neurological symptoms: Akathisia (propranolol 10–20 mg tid to qid), dyskinesia (clonazepam 0.5–2 mg prn), dystonia (benztropine 0.5–4 mg prn)

⚠ Precautions
- TCAs have a low therapeutic margin (lethal dose is about 3 times the maximum therapeutic dose); monitor during initiation of therapy and during dose increases. Prescribe limited quantities
- **Contraindicated**
  - in the acute recovery phase following a myocardial infarction and in heart block; caution in patients with pre-existing cardiovascular disease
  - if hypersensitive to tricyclics
  - within 14 days of stopping a MAOI
- May lower the seizure threshold; administer cautiously to patients with a history of convulsive disorders, organic brain disease or a predisposition to convulsions (e.g., alcohol withdrawal), patients with eating disorder
- Patients with existing cardiovascular disease may be sensitive to the cardiac adverse effects associated with TCAs; particularly those who have an eating disorder, are underweight, malnourished, or elderly
- Patients in whom excess anticholinergic activity could be harmful (e.g., increased intraocular pressure, narrow-angle glaucoma, prostatic hypertrophy, urinary retention), reduced GI motility, paralytic ileus
- Patients with respiratory difficulties as anticholinergic properties can dry up bronchial secretions, making breathing more difficult
- May induce manic reactions in up to 50% of patients with bipolar disorder; risk of increased cycling, bipolar disorder is a relative contraindication; screen for bipolar depression before the initiation of therapy
- May impair the mental and physical ability to perform hazardous tasks (e.g., driving a car or operating machinery); will potentiate the effects of alcohol

- Combining TCAs with SSRIs can result in increased plasma level of the TCA. Combination therapy has been used in the treatment of resistant patients; see Drug Interactions p. 60
- Combining serotonergic TCAs with SSRIs can cause a serotonin syndrome (see p. 10)

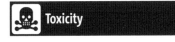 **Toxicity**

- Symptoms of toxicity are extensions of the common adverse effects; anticholinergic effects, CNS stimulation followed by CNS depression, myoclonus, hallucinations, respiratory depression, and seizures (can develop rapidly after overdose)
- Symptoms of CNS stimulation include agitation, confusion, delirium, irritability, hallucinations, and hyperpyrexia
- Increased risk of seizures in children
- CNS depression follows stimulation and may present with drowsiness, depressed level of consciousness, cyanosis, hypotension, hypothermia, respiratory depression, and coma
- Cardiac irregularities are extremely dangerous and common; duration of QRS complex on the electrocardiogram (ECG) reflects the severity of the overdose; a QRS equaling or exceeding 0.12 sec should be considered a danger sign (normal 0.08–0.11 sec)
- Patients with cardiac disease, eating disorders or renal disease, as well as the elderly and children are more susceptible to TCA cardiotoxicity
- Acid-base imbalances can occur

Management

- Hospitalize; monitor and provide supportive treatment
- Activated charcoal (25-100 g if patient presents within an hour of ingestion); forced diuresis and dialysis are of little benefit
- DO NOT GIVE IPECAC due to possibility of rapid neurological deterioration and high incidence of seizures
- Seizures: Recommend benzodiazepines, diazepam IV is the drug of choice. **Caution** – CNS and respiratory depression may occur

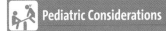 **Pediatric Considerations**

- For detailed information on the use of nonselective cyclic antidepressants in this population, please see the *Clinical Handbook of Psychotropic Drugs for Children and Adolescents*[8]
- Approved for OCD in children above age 10 (clomipramine) and for enuresis in children above age 5 (imipramine)
- Tricyclics have been tried in pediatric patients with variable success in treating ADHD, MDD, OCD, panic disorder, separation anxiety disorder, bulimia nervosa, and Tourette's disorder (clomipramine)
- Prior to treatment, consider a baseline ECG. A steady state serum level and ECG should be obtained when an effective daily dose is reached. Follow-up ECGs should be obtained at any dose change. Plasma levels should be obtained every few months
- The U.S. FDA defines the following ECG and examination values as unsafe in children treated with tricyclics: (a) PR interval > 200 ms, (b) QRS interval > 30% above a baseline (or > 120 ms), (c) BP > 140 mmHg systolic or 90 mmHg diastolic, (d) Heart rate > 130 beats/min at rest
- Sudden death has been reported rarely with desipramine, despite therapeutic plasma levels; plasma levels may be higher by 42% in children than adults, at the same dose
- Start TCAs at a low dose (10–25 mg) and increase gradually by 10–25 mg every 4–5 days to a maximum dose of 3–5 mg/kg

 Geriatric Considerations

- Safety and efficacy of TCAs in elderly patients has not been systematically studied
- Monitor for excessive CNS and anticholinergic effects; select an antidepressant least likely to cause these effects (e.g., nortriptyline, desipramine)
- Caution when combining with other medications with CNS and anticholinergic properties; additive effects can result in confusion, disorientation, and delirium; the elderly are sensitive to anticholinergic effects
- Cognitive impairment can occur, including decreased word recall and facial recognition
- Caution regarding cardiovascular side effects: Orthostatic hypotension (can lead to falls), tachycardia, and conduction slowing
- Initiate at low doses and increase the dosage more slowly than in younger patients; elderly patients may take longer to respond and may require trials of up to 12 weeks before response is noted

 Use in Pregnancy◇

- Clomipramine, nortriptyline, and possibly others cross the placenta
- Fetal malformations and developmental delay have been reported in children of mothers who received TCAs during pregnancy
- CNS effects, urinary retention, and withdrawal symptoms have also been reported
- Avoid TCAs during first trimester if possible
- The dosage required to achieve therapeutic plasma levels may increase during the third trimester, particularly for trimipramine and nortriptyline

◇ See p. 473 for further information on drug use in pregnancy and effects on breast milk

Nonselective Cyclic Antidepressants (cont.)

Breast Milk	

- The American Academy of Pediatrics classifies antidepressants as drugs "whose effects on nursing infants are unknown but may be of concern"
- TCAs are secreted into breast milk; estimates indicate that the baby will receive up to 4% of the mother's dose
- The half-life of antidepressants in the neonate is increased 3- to 4-fold
- Reports indicate that the doxepin metabolite concentration reaches similar plasma levels in mothers and infants; one case report of respiratory depression; doxepin is contraindicated in breastfeeding
- Recommend to either discontinue medication or bottle feed

Nursing Implications

- Be aware that although antidepressants reduce symptoms of depression they may increase psychomotor activity, thus increasing concern about suicidal behavior
- Monitor therapy by observing for changes in mood and activity and the emergence of adverse side effects; keep physician informed
- Although antidepressant effect can be seen within 2 weeks in some individuals, response may take as long as 6–8 weeks
- Psychotherapy and education are important in the treatment of MDD
- Antidepressants can cause sedation, caution patient not to perform activities requiring alertness until response to the drug has been determined
- Reassure patient that drowsiness and dizziness usually subside after the first few weeks; if dizzy, patient should get up from lying or sitting position slowly, and dangle legs over edge of bed before getting up
- Excessive use of caffeinated foods, drugs or beverages may increase anxiety and agitation, confusing the diagnosis
- Artificial tears may be useful for patients who complain of dry eyes; suggest using wetting solutions for those wearing contact lenses
- Expect a dry mouth; suggest rinsing the mouth frequently with water and using sour or sugarless hard candy or gum
- Check for constipation; recommend increasing fluid and dietary fiber intake but avoid ingesting high-fiber foods or laxatives (e.g., bran) concurrently with medication, as this may interfere with absorption, reducing antidepressant levels
- Check for urinary retention; if required, the physician may order bethanechol orally or by subcutaneous injection
- Caution patient to avoid suddenly stopping the antidepressant due to risk of precipitating a withdrawal reaction

Patient Instructions

- For detailed patient instructions on cyclic antidepressants, see the Patient Information Sheet (details p. 474)

Drug Interactions

- Clinically significant interactions are listed below
- For more interaction information on any given combination, also see the corresponding chapter for the second agent

Class of Drug	Example	Interaction Effects
ACE inhibitor	Enalapril	Increased plasma level of clomipramine due to decreased metabolism
Anesthetic	Enflurane	Report of seizures with amitriptyline
Antiarrhythmic	Procainamide, propafenone, quinidine	Increased plasma level due to CYP2D6 inhibition; risk for increased side effects)
Antibiotic	Azithromycin, clarithromycin, erythromycin	Additive QTc prolongation, arrhythmia
	Ciprofloxacin, ofloxacin	Decreased clearance due to CYP1A2 inhibition; risk of increased side effects
	Linezolid	Monitor for increased serotonergic and noradrenergic effects due to linezolid's weak MAO inhibition
Anticholinergic	Antihistamines, antiparkinsonian agents, antipsychotics	Increased anticholinergic effect; may increase risk of hyperthermia, confusion, urinary retention, etc.
Anticoagulant	Apixaban, dabigatran, rivaroxaban, warfarin	Increased risk of bleeding possible due to decreased platelet aggregation secondary to depletion of serotonin in platelets

Class of Drug	Example	Interaction Effects
Anticonvulsant	Barbiturates, carbamazepine, phenytoin	Decreased plasma level of TCAs due to enzyme induction; increased levels of carbamazepine
	Divalproex, valproate, valproic acid	Increased plasma level of TCAs
	Phenobarbital	Increased plasma level of phenobarbital with clomipramine
Antidepressant		
SSRI	Fluoxetine, fluvoxamine, paroxetine, sertraline (less likely with citalopram or escitalopram)	Elevated TCA plasma level (due to inhibition of oxidative metabolism); monitor plasma level and for signs of toxicity, also for additive QTc prolongation effects
NDRI	Bupropion	Elevated imipramine level (by 57%), desipramine level (by 82%), and nortriptyline level (by 200%) with combination
NDRI	Venlafaxine	Cases of serotonin syndrome, increased antimuscarinic adverse effects (dry mouth, urinary retention, constipation), movement disorders, and seizures reported with concurrent use of venlafaxine and tricyclic antidepressants
Irreversible MAOI	Isocarboxazid, phenelzine, tranylcypromine	If used together, do not add TCAs to MAOI: Start TCAs first or simultaneously with MAOI; for patients already on MAOI, discontinue MAOI 10–14 days before starting combination therapy Combined TCA and MAOI therapy has additive antidepressant effects in treatment-resistant patients Serotonin syndrome and deaths have been reported
Antifungal	Fluconazole, itraconazole, ketoconazole, miconazole	Increased plasma level of antidepressant due to inhibited metabolism (89% with amitriptyline; 70% with nortriptyline); 20% increase with imipramine and no increase with desipramine
	Terbinafine	Prolonged increase in plasma level of amitriptyline and its metabolite nortriptyline, due to inhibited metabolism via CYP2D6
Antihistamine	Diphenhydramine	Increased plasma level of antidepressants metabolized via CYP2D6 is possible (e.g., amitriptyline, desipramine, clomipramine, imipramine) due to inhibited metabolism Additive CNS and anticholinergic effects
Antihypertensive	Acetazolamide, thiazide diuretics	Hypotension augmented
	Clonidine, guanethidine, methyldopa, reserpine	Decreased antihypertensive effect due to inhibition of α-adrenergic receptors Abrupt discontinuation of clonidine may precipitate hypertensive crisis
	Labetalol	Increased plasma level of imipramine (by 54%) and desipramine
Antipsychotic		
First generation	Chlorpromazine, fluphenazine, haloperidol, perphenazine, pimozide, thioridazine	Haloperidol and phenothiazines may increase the plasma level of TCAs. TCAs may increase the plasma level of chlorpromazine. Clinical significance unknown DO NOT COMBINE pimozide or thioridazine with TCAs; NOT recommended with phenothiazines or zuclopenthixol. CAUTION with all other FGAs. Possible additive prolongation of QT interval and associated life-threatening cardiac arrhythmias Additive sedation, hypotension, and anticholinergic effects
Second generation	Clozapine	Possible serotonin syndrome reported in a patient taking clomipramine following the withdrawal of clozapine
Antiretroviral		
Combination	Stribild (elvitegravir + cobicistat + emtricitabine + tenofovir)	Increased plasma level of desipramine (AUC by 65%, C_{max} by 24%) via CYP2D6 inhibition
Protease inhibitor	Ritonavir	Dose-dependent increase in plasma levels of tricyclic antidepressant due to decreased metabolism (AUC of desipramine increased by 145% and peak plasma level increased by 22% with ritonavir 500 mg bid, while ritonavir 100 mg bid has no significant effects on desipramine pharmacokinetics)

Nonselective Cyclic Antidepressants (cont.)

Class of Drug	Example	Interaction Effects
Anxiolytic	Alprazolam	Increased plasma levels of desipramine and imipramine with alprazolam (by 20% and 31%, respectively)
	Buspirone	Concomitant use of serotonergic agents (clomipramine, amitriptyline) increases the risk of serotonin syndrome
	Triazolam	Desipramine and triazolam: Report of hypothermia (neither drug causes this effect alone); triazolam potentiates anorexic effect of desipramine
Calcium channel blocker	Diltiazem, verapamil	Increased imipramine plasma level (by 30% and 15%, respectively); increased level of trimipramine
	Nifedipine	May antagonize the efficacy of antidepressant drugs
Cannabis/marijuana		Case reports of tachycardia, lightheadedness, confusion, mood lability, and delirium with nortriptyline and desipramine; may evoke cardiac complications in youth
CNS depressant	Alcohol	Short-term or acute use reduces first-pass metabolism of TCAs, increasing plasma levels; chronic use induces metabolizing enzymes, decreasing plasma levels Additive effects on sedation and CNS depression
	Antihistamines, benzodiazepines, hypnotics	Increased sedation, CNS depression
Cholestyramine		Decreased absorption of antidepressant due to binding by cholestyramine, if given together
Evening primrose oil		May lower the seizure threshold
Grapefruit juice		Decreased conversion of clomipramine to metabolite due to inhibition of CYP3A4
H_2 antagonist	Cimetidine	Increased plasma level of antidepressant; for desipramine, inhibition of hydroxylation only occurs in patients who are rapid metabolizers
Hormone	Estrogen/progesterone oral contraceptive	Increased plasma level of antidepressant due to decreased metabolism Reduced clearance of combined oral contraceptive possible with amitriptyline due to inhibited metabolism
Insulin		Decreased insulin sensitivity reported with amitriptyline
Lithium		May increase risk of neurotoxicity
L-tryptophan		May potentiate the risk of serotonin syndrome. Monitor for increased serotonergic effects
MAO-B inhibitor	Selegiline (L-deprenyl)	Reports of serotonergic reactions
Muscle relaxant	Baclofen	Warning of tricyclic antidepressants potentiating the effects of baclofen, resulting in pronounced muscular hypotonia; case report of a patient taking baclofen being unable to walk after taking nortriptyline and imipramine (reversed after discontinuing tricyclics)
Opioid	Codeine	Marked inhibition of conversion of codeine to morphine (active moiety) with amitriptyline, clomipramine, desipramine, imipramine, and nortriptyline
	Methadone	Increased plasma level of desipramine (by about 108%)
	Morphine	Enhanced analgesic effect
	Tramadol	Increased risk of seizures and serotonin syndrome
Oxybutynin		Increased metabolism of clomipramine (may be due to induction of CYP3A4) and additive anticholinergic effects
Proton pump inhibitor	Omeprazole	Increased plasma level of antidepressant due to inhibited metabolism
Rifampin		Decreased plasma level of antidepressant due to increased metabolism

Class of Drug	Example	Interaction Effects
Stimulant	Methylphenidate	Plasma level of antidepressant may be increased
		Used together to augment antidepressant effect and response to symptoms of ADHD
		Cardiovascular effects increased with combination, in children – monitor
		Case reports of neurotoxic effects with imipramine, considered rare – monitor
		Decreased seizure threshold
		Elevated heart rate and diastolic pressure (by 20–30%); increased risk of arrhythmia
St. John's wort		Decreased amitriptyline concentration
		Additive serotonergic effects
Sulfonylurea	Tolbutamide	Increased hypoglycemia
Sympathomimetic	Epinephrine, norepinephrine (levarterenol), phenylephrine	Enhanced pressor response from 2- to 8-fold; benefit may outweigh risks in anaphylaxis
		Avoid concurrent use of parenteral epinephrine, norepinephrine, phenylephrine, or other direct-acting sympathomimetic amines due to increased risk of hypertension and cardiac arrhythmias
	Isoproterenol	May increase likelihood of arrhythmias
Tamoxifen		Decreased plasma level of doxepin (by 25%) due to induced metabolism via CYP3A4
Triptan	Sumatriptan, zolmitriptan	Possible serotonergic reaction when combined with antidepressants with serotonergic activity (e.g., clomipramine)
Zolpidem		Case report of visual hallucinations in combination with desipramine
		In one study, 5 of 8 patients on imipramine experienced anterograde amnesia

Monoamine Oxidase Inhibitors

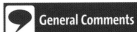 **General Comments**

- Monoamine oxidase inhibitors are classified as follows:

Chemical Class	Agent	Page
Reversible Inhibitor of MAO-A (RIMA)	Moclobemide[C]	See p. 64
Irreversible MAO (A&B) Inhibitors (MAOIs)	Isocarboxazid[B]	See p. 67
	Phenelzine	See p. 67
	Tranylcypromine	See p. 67
Irreversible MAO-B Inhibitor	Selegiline (L-deprenyl)[B]	See p. 74

[B] Not marketed in Canada,   [C] Not marketed in the USA

Reversible Inhibitor of MAO-A (RIMA)

 Product Availability*

Generic Name	Neuroscience-based Nomenclature* (Pharmacological Target/Mode of Action)	Trade Name[(A)]	Dosage Forms and Strengths
Moclobemide[(C)]	Serotonin, norepinephrine, dopamine/Enzyme inhibitor	Manerix	Tablets: 100 mg, 150 mg, 300 mg

* Refer to Health Canada's Drug Product Database or the FDA's Drugs@FDA for the most current availability information.   * Developed by a taskforce consisting of representatives from the American College of Neuropsychopharmacology (ACNP), the Asian College of Neuropsychopharmacology (AsCNP), the European College of Neuropsychopharmacology (ECNP), the International College of Neuropsychopharmacology (CINP), and the International Union of Basic and Clinical Pharmacology (IUPHAR) (see https://nbn2r.com), [(A)] Generic preparations may be available,   [(C)] Not marketed in the USA

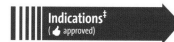 **Indications‡**
(👍 approved)

- 👍 Major depressive disorder (MDD)
- 👍 Dysthymia, chronic
- Seasonal affective disorder (SAD), chronic fatigue syndrome, and obsessive-compulsive disorder (OCD) – weak evidence suggests efficacy
- Borderline personality disorder – suggested to modulate impulsivity/aggression and affective instability
- Social anxiety disorder

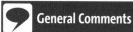 **General Comments**

- In patients presenting with depression and a high risk of suicide, treatment selection should consider safety in overdose (i.e., consider using newer antidepressant agents rather than nonselective cyclic and MAOI antidepressants). Prescription quantities should be consistent with safe patient care
- Increases REM sleep

 Pharmacology

- Short-acting reversible inhibitor of the enzyme MAO-A; inhibits the metabolism of serotonin, norepinephrine, and dopamine
- Chronic dosing over 400 mg daily will inhibit 20–30% of MAO-B in platelets
- Inhibition reverses within 24 h
- Combining moclobemide with TCAs or lithium may increase antidepressant effect

 Dosing

- Starting dose: 300 mg daily in divided doses; further dose increases should wait at least 1 week; bioavailability increases over the first week. Usual dose range: 300–600 mg daily; some patients respond to 150 mg daily, but most require doses above 450 mg/day
- Moclobemide should be taken after meals to minimize tyramine-related effects (e.g., headache)
- Preliminary data suggests that once daily dosing is as effective as divided dosing
- Dosing is not affected by age
- Hepatic disease: Decreases clearance [Management: Decrease dose by one third to one half in patients with severe hepatic impairment]
- Renal disease: Use with caution, does not affect dosing

 Pharmacokinetics

- See p. 96
- Rapidly absorbed from the gut with a high first-pass effect; absorption increases from 50% with first dose to approximately 90% after 2 weeks
- Relatively lipophilic, but highly water soluble at low pH
- Low plasma-protein binding, approximately 50%, primarily albumin
- Peak effect occurs between 0.7 and 1.1 h in the absence and presence of food, respectively
- Plasma levels increase in proportion to dose; blockade of MAO-A correlates with plasma concentrations
- Extensively metabolized by oxidation; partial metabolism primarily via CYP2C19 and 2D6

‡ Indications listed here do not necessarily apply to all countries. Please refer to a country's regulatory database (e.g., US Food and Drug Administration, Health Canada Drug Product Database) for the most current availability information and indications

- Clearance decreases as dosage increases because of auto-inhibition or metabolite-induced inhibition
- Elimination half-life 1–3 h; 4.6 h in the elderly

 Onset & Duration of Action
- Therapeutic effects are typically observed by 28 days

 Adverse Effects
- See table p. 93

CNS Effects
- Most common: Insomnia, sedation, agitation, nervousness, anxiety, headache, and dizziness
- Dose-related stimulant effects include restlessness, anxiety, agitation, and aggression
- Tremor
- Hypomania reported, especially in patients with bipolar disorder

Anticholinergic Effects
- Dry mouth, blurred vision

Cardiovascular Effects
- Tachycardia, hypotension

Endocrine & Metabolic Effects
- Reports of galactorrhea in females
- Both weight loss and weight gain

GI Effects
- Constipation, nausea, vomiting, diarrhea, abdominal pain

Urogenital & Sexual Effects
- Low incidence of sexual dysfunction; 24% compared to 62% for SSRIs

 Discontinuation Syndrome
- Case report of moclobemide discontinuation syndrome presenting with influenza-like symptoms (muscular cramps, shivering, neck pain, headache, nausea, hot flush without fever)

 Precautions
- Patients prescribed doses above 600 mg/day should minimize consumption of tyramine-rich foods
- Hypertensive patients should avoid ingesting large quantities of tyramine-rich foods
- Hypertensive reactions may occur in patients with thyrotoxicosis or pheochromocytoma
- Use caution when combining with serotonergic drugs as serotonin syndrome has been reported (see p. 10) with CNS irritability, increased muscle tone, myoclonus, diaphoresis, and elevated temperature (see Drug Interactions, p. 66)
- Reduce dose by one third to one half in patients with severe liver impairment

 Toxicity
- Symptoms of toxicity are the same as side effects but intensified: drowsiness, disorientation, stupor, hypotension, tachycardia, hyperreflexia, grimacing, sweating, agitation, and hallucinations; serotonin syndrome has been reported, convulsions
- Fatalities have occurred when combined with citalopram or clomipramine in overdose

Management
- Gastric lavage, emesis, activated charcoal may be of benefit
- Monitor vital functions, supportive treatment

 Pediatric Considerations
- For detailed information on the use of moclobemide in this population, please see the *Clinical Handbook of Psychotropic Drugs for Children and Adolescents*[8]

Geriatric Considerations
- Dosing is not affected by age or renal function
- Improvement in cognitive functioning in elderly depressed patients has been noted

Reversible Inhibitor of MAO-A (RIMA) (cont.)

Use in Pregnancy◊	• Data on safety in pregnancy is lacking • Animal studies have not shown any particular adverse effects on reproduction
Breast Milk	• Moclobemide is secreted into breast milk at about 1% of maternal dose
Nursing Implications	• Monitor for signs of suicidal ideation • Monitor blood pressure • Warn patient not to self-medicate with over-the-counter drugs or herbal preparations; consult physician or pharmacist to prevent drug-drug interactions • It is not necessary to maintain a special diet when moclobemide is prescribed in low to moderate doses; excessive amounts of foods with high tyramine content can lead to headache • Patients should be instructed to recognize signs of hypertensive crisis (e.g., headache, neck stiffness, palpitations, etc.) • Administer moclobemide after food to minimize side effects; avoid big meals after taking moclobemide • If patient has difficulty sleeping, ensure that the last dose of moclobemide is no later than 1700 h
Patient Instructions	• For detailed patient instructions on moclobemide, see the Patient Information Sheet (details p. 474)
Food Interactions	• No particular precautions are required; avoid excessive consumption of tyramine-containing food to minimize the risk of hypertension
Drug Interactions	• Clinically significant interactions are listed below • For more interaction information on any given combination, also see the corresponding chapter for the second agent

Class of Drug	Example	Interaction Effects
Anesthetic, general		Stop antidepressant two days prior
Antibiotic	Linezolid	MAOIs increase the adverse effects of linezolid; AVOID concomitant use
Anticholinergic	Antiparkinsonian drugs	Enhanced anticholinergic adverse effects
Antidepressant		MAOIs may enhance the adverse effects of other antidepressants
SSRI	Citalopram, escitalopram, fluoxetine, fluvoxamine	Use cautiously and monitor for serotonergic adverse effects (e.g., serotonin syndrome), especially with citalopram and escitalopram Higher incidence of insomnia may occur; increased headache reported with fluvoxamine Fluoxetine and fluvoxamine can inhibit the metabolism of moclobemide
NDRI	Bupropion	Enhanced neurotoxic effects; MAOIs may increase the antihypertensive effects of bupropion; AVOID
SNRI	Venlafaxine	Enhanced effects of serotonin and/or norepinephrine; no data on safety with combination; AVOID
SARI	Nefazodone	Enhanced effects of serotonin and/or norepinephrine; no data on safety with combination; AVOID
Nonselective cyclic	Desipramine, nortriptyline	Potentiation of weight gain, hypotension, and anticholinergic effects; use cautiously and monitor for serotonergic adverse effects (e.g., serotonin syndrome)
	Clomipramine	Enhanced serotonergic effects; AVOID
MAOI		Concurrent use contraindicated

◊ See p. 473 for further information on drug use in pregnancy and effects on breast milk

Class of Drug	Example	Interaction Effects
Antipsychotic	General	May enhance dopamine blockade; antipsychotic agents may enhance serotonergic effects resulting in serotonin syndrome Additive hypotension, particularly with low-potency FGAs such as chlorpromazine
Anxiolytic	Buspirone	Buspirone may increase the adverse effects of MAOIs (e.g., increased blood pressure); AVOID MAOIs may potentiate the activity of buspirone via inhibition of serotonin metabolism; serotonergic reaction possible
H₂ antagonist	Cimetidine	May decrease metabolism of moclobemide; plasma level may double
L-ryptophan		May enhance adverse effects of moclobemide. Serotonin syndrome possible; AVOID
MAO-B inhibitor	Selegiline (L-deprenyl)	CAUTION with combination; dietary restrictions recommended as both A + B MAO enzymes will be inhibited
Methylene blue		Enhanced serotonergic effects through inhibition of MAO-A and B by methylene blue. Risk for serotonin syndrome (see Precautions p. 10)
Opioids and related drugs	Dextromethorphan, meperidine, pentazocine	MAOIs will enhance the serotonergic effects; may cause serotonin syndrome; increased restlessness; death reported with meperidine – AVOID COMBINATION Vertigo, tremor, nausea, and vomiting reported; increased risk of serotonin syndrome; AVOID COMBINATION
	Tramadol	May enhance neuroexcitatory effects, increasing the risk of seizures and serotonin syndrome
Selective norepinephrine reuptake inhibitor	Atomoxetine	MAOIs may enhance the neurotoxic effects of atomoxetine; AVOID
Stimulant	Amphetamine, methylphenidate	MAOIs enhance the antihypertensive effects; AVOID
St. John's wort		May augment serotonergic effects and cause serotonin syndrome. AVOID combination
Sympathomimetic	*Indirect-acting:* Amphetamine, ephedrine, L-dopa, methylphenidate, etc.	Increased blood pressure and enhanced effects if used over prolonged periods or at high doses; AVOID
	Direct-acting: Epinephrine, salbutamol, etc.	Increased blood pressure and enhanced effects if used over prolonged periods or at high doses; AVOID
Triptan	Rizatriptan	Decreased metabolism of rizatriptan; AUC and peak plasma level increased by 119% and 41%, respectively, and AUC of metabolite increased by 400%
	Sumatriptan, zolmitriptan	Possible increased serotonergic effects

Irreversible Monoamine Oxidase (A&B) Inhibitors (MAOIs)

℞ Product Availability*

Generic Name	Chemical Class	Neuroscience-based Nomenclature˙ (Pharmacological Target/Mode of Action)	Trade Name[A]	Dosage Forms and Strengths
Isocarboxazid[B]	Hydrazine derivative	Serotonin, norepinephrine, dopamine/Enzyme inhibitor	Marplan	Tablets: 10 mg
Phenelzine	Hydrazine derivative	Serotonin, norepinephrine, dopamine/Enzyme inhibitor	Nardil	Tablets: 15 mg
Tranylcypromine	Non-hydrazine derivative	Serotonin, norepinephrine, dopamine/Enzyme inhibitor	Parnate	Tablets: 10 mg

* Refer to Health Canada's Drug Product Database or the FDA's Drugs@FDA for the most current availability information.   ˙ Developed by a taskforce consisting of representatives from the American College of Neuropsychopharmacology (ACNP), the Asian College of Neuropsychopharmacology (AsCNP), the European College of Neuropsychopharmacology (ECNP), the International College of Neuropsychopharmacology (CINP), and the International Union of Basic and Clinical Pharmacology (IUPHAR) (see https://nbn2r.com), [A] Generic preparations may be available,   [B] Not marketed in Canada

Irreversible Monoamine Oxidase (A&B) Inhibitors (MAOIs) (cont.)

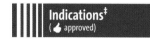

Indications‡
(👍 approved)

- 👍 Depression, atypical
- 👍 Major depressive disorder (MDD) unresponsive to other antidepressants (phenelzine, tranylcypromine)
- Bipolar depression, atypical (anergic)
- Phobia: Phobic anxiety states or social phobia
- Panic disorder: Prophylaxis
- Obsessive-compulsive disorder (OCD)
- MDD in patients with borderline personality disorder
- Dysthymia, chronic
- Posttraumatic stress disorder (PTSD) – efficacy reported
- Schizophrenia, chronic: May improve negative symptoms
- Herpes: Possible antiherpetic effect

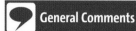

General Comments

- In patients presenting with depression and a high risk of suicide, treatment selection should consider safety in overdose (i.e., consider using newer antidepressant agents rather than nonselective cyclic and MAOI antidepressants). Prescription quantities should be consistent with safe patient care
- Ability of patient to adhere to dietary and drug restrictions should be assessed before prescribing
- Use with caution in elderly, debilitated patients and those with hypertension, cardiovascular or cerebrovascular disease due to increased risk for hypertensive crisis or hyperthermia
- Monitor BP and heart rate
- Premenopausal women may respond better to MAOIs than to TCAs
- A network meta-analysis of 52 RCTs involving 6462 subjects found MAOIs were similar to TCAs and SSRIs with respect to efficacy (response rate) and acceptability (all-cause dropout)

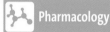

Pharmacology

- Nonselectively inhibit MAO-A and B enzymes; involved in oxidative deamination of serotonin, norepinephrine, and dopamine; down-regulate β adrenoceptors
- Inhibition is irreversible and lasts about 10 days

Dosing

- See p. 96
- Bid or more frequent dosing required due to short half-life (see individual agents); give doses in the morning and mid-day to avoid overstimulation and insomnia; sedation can occur occasionally
- Delay in therapeutic response; allow sufficient time between dose increases (e.g., 1–2 weeks)
- Gradual dose increases are recommended in debilitated, emaciated or geriatric patients
- Hepatic disease: AVOID
- Renal disease: CAUTION, may have to decrease the dose

Pharmacokinetics

- See p. 96
- Rapidly absorbed from the GI tract, metabolized by the liver and excreted almost entirely in the urine
- Peak plasma level of tranylcypromine occurs in 1–2 h, of phenelzine in up to 1 h and correlates with elevations in supine blood pressure, orthostatic drop in systolic blood pressure, and rise in pulse rate. Blood pressure elevation correlates with dose
- Irreversible MAOIs can impair their own metabolism with long-term use, resulting in nonlinear pharmacokinetics and the potential for drug accumulation

‡ Indications listed here do not necessarily apply to all MAOIs or all countries. Please refer to a country's regulatory database (e.g., US Food and Drug Administration, Health Canada Drug Product Database) for the most current availability information and indications

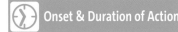 **Onset & Duration of Action**
- The energizing effect often observed within a few days
- May require up to 2 weeks to reach maximum MAO inhibition
- Duration of MAO inhibition can be up to 2 weeks after discontinuation of phenelzine; 10 days for tranylcypromine
- Tolerance to anti-panic effects reported

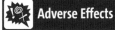 **Adverse Effects**
- See p. 93

CNS Effects
- Most common effects; dizziness, drowsiness (phenelzine most sedating), fatigue, headache (without increased blood pressure), hyperreflexia, and sleep disturbance that can occur early on [Management: slowing dosage titration, divided dosing, bedtime dosing]
- Other symptoms include akinesia, confusion, disorientation, euphoria, memory loss, and nystagmus
- Stimulant effects include agitation, anxiety, hyperexcitability, manic symptoms, precipitation of psychosis, and restlessness (may be more prevalent with higher doses of tranylcypromine)
- Hypomania and mania: reported in patients with bipolar disorder (risk up to 35%; lower risk with concomitant use of a mood stabilizer); in MDD, risk about 4%
- Increased sleep onset latency and reduced sleep efficiency; REM sleep decreased and may be eliminated at start of therapy, rebound REM of up to 250% above baseline reported on drug withdrawal
- Paresthesias or "electric-shock-like" sensations and carpal tunnel syndrome (numbness) reported; may be due to vitamin B6 deficiency [Management: Pyridoxine 50–150 mg/day]
- Myoclonic movements (especially during sleep, 10–15%), muscle cramps, tension, tremor and twitching, and dose-related akathisia [Management: Cyproheptadine may be helpful for cramps or jerks; clonazepam or valproate for nocturnal myoclonus]

Anticholinergic Effects
- Constipation common [Management: Increase bulk and fluid intake, fecal softener, bulk-forming laxative]
- Dry mouth
- Urinary retention

Cardiovascular Effects
- Dizziness, weakness, orthostatic hypotension (can be early or late effect); usually temporary but if symptoms persist the drug may need to be discontinued [Management: slower dosage titration, divided dosing, increased fluid intake, fludrocortisone 0.1–0.2 mg/day]
- Occasionally, hypertensive patients may experience a rise in blood pressure (prevalence may be higher with tranylcypromine)
- Edema in lower extremities (more common with tranylcypromine) [Management: Restrict sodium; support hose; amiloride 5–10 mg/day up to bid, monitor frequently for hypotension]

Hematological Effects
- Normocytic, normochromic anemia, agranulocytosis, and neutropenia reported
- Case reports of thrombocytopenia

Endocrine & Metabolic Effects
- Hyponatremia and SIADH reported
- Increased appetite and weight gain
- Hypoglycemia reported

GI Effects
- Most common are anorexia, nausea, and vomiting

Urogenital & Sexual Effects
- Urinary frequency, incontinence, and retention reported
- Decreased libido, impotence, anorgasmia, and ejaculation difficulties [Management: See SSRIs p. 8]
- May diminish sperm count
- Rarely priapism

Other Adverse Effects
- The most common adverse effect is elevated transaminase levels; rare reports of liver toxicity
- Rare reports of hair loss with tranylcypromine

Hypertensive Crisis
- Can occur with irreversible MAOIs due to ingestion of incompatible foods (containing substantial levels of tyramine) or drugs (see lists pp. 71–72)
- Not related to drug dosage
- Other risk factors can include: elderly, debilitated patients, pre-existing hypertension, cardiovascular or cerebrovascular disease

Irreversible Monoamine Oxidase (A&B) Inhibitors (MAOIs) (cont.)

Signs and Symptoms	• Occipital headache, neck stiffness or soreness, nausea, vomiting, sweating (sometimes with fever and sometimes with cold, clammy skin), dilated pupils and photophobia, sudden nosebleed, tachycardia, bradycardia, and constricting chest pain • Headache is usually the first symptom • Warn patients to discontinue the medication immediately if they experience any of the above symptoms
Management	• Withhold medication and notify physician immediately • Monitor blood pressure and clinical status • Monitor vital signs, ECG • Sublingual captopril 25 mg may decrease blood pressure (occasionally drastically – monitor) • Phentolamine is an alternative parenteral treatment • Patient should stand and walk, rather than lie down, during a hypertensive reaction; BP will drop somewhat

 D/C Discontinuation Syndrome

- Can occur 1–4 days after abrupt withdrawal of medications
- Reports of muscle weakness, agitation, vivid nightmares, headache, palpitations, nausea, sweating, irritability, and myoclonic jerking; acute organic psychosis with hallucinations also reported
- REM rebound (up to 250% above baseline)
- Important to maintain dietary and drug restrictions for at least 10 days after stopping MAOI

 Precautions

- Monitor for worsening of depression or suicidal ideation, especially during initiation of therapy or with dose changes
- CONTRAINDICATED in patients with a history of liver disease or abnormal liver function tests
- Should not be administered to patients with cerebrovascular disease, cardiovascular disease, or a history of hypertension
- Use with caution in patients with hyperthyroidism, Parkinsonian syndrome, impaired renal function or a history of seizures
- Should not be used alone in patients with marked psychomotor agitation
- Need 10–14 days washout before an incompatible drug or food is given; hypertensive crisis can occur if given concurrently with certain drugs or foods (see lists pp. 71–72)
- When changing from one MAOI to another, or to a TCA, allow a minimum of 10 medication-free days
- Discontinue at least 7–14 days before elective surgery (tranylcypromine: 7 days; phenelzine, isocarboxazid: 10 days); may want to discontinue use prior to ECT
- Use caution when combining with serotonergic drugs; serotonin syndrome has been reported (see p. 10)

 Toxicity

- Symptoms same as side effects but intensified
- Severe cases progress to extreme dizziness and shock due to effects on cardiac conduction
- Overdose, whether accidental or intentional, can be fatal; patient may appear symptom-free up to 6 h, then progress to restlessness-coma-death; close medical supervision is indicated for 48 h following an overdose

 Pediatric Considerations

- Ideally should not be used in this patient population. For detailed information on the use of MAOIs in this population, please see the *Clinical Handbook of Psychotropic Drugs for Children and Adolescents*[8]

Geriatric Considerations

- Suggested that MAOIs may have particular efficacy in the elderly, as monoamine oxidase activity in the brain increases with age
- The elderly are also more susceptible to adverse effects associated with MAOI use and these effects are associated with an increased mortality
- Initiate at low doses and monitor
- Orthostatic hypotension may be problematic, use divided doses [Management: Support stockings, sodium chloride tablets, fludrocortisone]

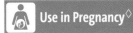

Use in Pregnancy◇	• Experience is too limited to adequately assess risk; increased incidence of malformations associated with use in first trimester
Breast Milk	• Limited data on tranylcypromine, phenelzine, or isocarboxazid; molecular weight is low enough to expect excretion into breast milk • Use with caution in nursing women

| Nursing Implications | • Advise patient to inform physicians and dentists that they are taking a MAOI
• Educate patient regarding which foods and drugs to avoid; a diet sheet should be provided for each patient
• Warn patient to avoid self-medicating with over-the-counter drugs or herbal preparations; always consult a physician or pharmacist to prevent drug-drug interactions
• Monitor BP and heart rate and report increases to physician immediately
• Advise patient to immediately report severe headache, neck stiffness, palpitations or other atypical or unusual symptoms not previously experienced
• The incidence of orthostatic hypotension is high, especially in the elderly and at the start of treatment [Management: Advise patient to get up and out of bed slowly]
• If patient has difficulty sleeping, ensure that the last dose of MAOI is taken no later than 3 p.m. |

| Patient Instructions | • For detailed patient instructions on MAOIs, see the Patient Information Sheet (details on p. 474) |

| **Food Interactions** | There are many serious food and drug interactions that can precipitate a hypertensive crisis; maintain dietary and drug restrictions for at least 10 days after stopping MAOI
☞ **MAKE SURE ALL FOOD IS FRESH, STORED PROPERLY, AND EATEN SOON AFTER BEING PURCHASED – refrigerated products will show an increase in tyramine content after several days**
• Never consume food that is fermented or possibly "off"
• Avoid restaurant sauces, gravy, and soup
Foods to avoid (high tyramine content):
• All matured or aged cheeses (e.g., cheddar, brie, blue, Stilton, Roquefort, camembert)
• Broad bean pods (e.g., Fava) – contain dopamine
• Concentrated yeast extracts (e.g., Marmite)
• Dried salted fish, pickled herring
• Packet soup, especially miso
• Sauerkraut
• Aged/smoked meats (especially salami, mortadella, pastrami, summer sausage), sausage, other unrefrigerated fermented meats, game meat that has been hung, liver
• Soy sauce or soybean condiments, tofu
• Tap (draft) beer, alcohol-free beer
• Improperly stored or spoiled meats, poultry or fish
SAFE to use in moderate amounts but only if fresh:
• Cottage cheese, cream cheese, farmer's cheese, processed cheese, Cheez Whiz, ricotta, Havarti, Boursin, brie without rind, gorgonzola
• Liver (as long as it is fresh), fresh or processed meats, poultry or fish (e.g., hot dogs, bologna)
• Spirits (in moderation)
• Sour cream
• Soy milk
• Salad dressings
• Worcestershire sauce |

◇ See p. 473 for further information on drug use in pregnancy and effects on breast milk

Irreversible Monoamine Oxidase (A&B) Inhibitors (MAOIs) (cont.)

- Yeast-leavened bread

Reactions have been reported with the following (moderate tyramine content) – use moderately with caution:
- Smoked fish, caviar, snails, tinned fish, shrimp paste
- Yogurt
- Meat tenderizers
- Homemade red wine, Chianti, canned/bottled beer, sherry, champagne
- Cheeses (e.g., Parmesan, muenster, Swiss, gruyere, mozzarella, feta)
- Pepperoni
- Overripe fruit: bananas, avocados, raspberries, plums, tomatoes, canned figs or raisins, orange pulp
- Meat extract (e.g., Bovril, Oxo)
- Asian foods
- Spinach, eggplant

Over-the-counter drugs – DO NOT USE without prior consultation with doctor or pharmacist:
- Cold remedies, decongestants (including nasal sprays and drops), some antihistamines and cough medicines
- Opioid painkillers (e.g., products containing codeine)
- All stimulants including pep-pills (Wake-ups, Nodoz)
- All appetite suppressants
- Anti-asthma drugs (Primatine P)
- Sleep aids and sedatives (Sominex, Nytol)
- Yeast, dietary supplements (e.g., Ultrafast, Optifast)

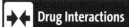 **Drug Interactions**

- Clinically significant interactions are listed below
- For more interaction information on any given combination, also see the corresponding chapter for the second agent

Class of Drug	Example	Interaction Effects
Anesthetic, general		MAOIs may exaggerate the hypotension and CNS effects of anesthetics; discontinue 10 days prior to elective surgery
Antibiotic	Linezolid	Monitor for increased serotonergic and noradrenergic effects due to linezolid's weak MAO inhibition
Anticholinergic	Antihistamines, antiparkinsonian agents	Severe reactions reported, including prolonging and intensifying some anticholinergic effects Increased atropine-like effects
Anticonvulsant	Carbamazepine	Possible decrease in metabolism and increased plasma level of carbamazepine with phenelzine
Antidepressant		
SSRI	Citalopram, fluoxetine, fluvoxamine, paroxetine, sertraline	Serotonin syndrome and death reported with serotonergic antidepressants; AVOID; do not use within 5 weeks of fluoxetine and 2 weeks of other SSRIs
NDRI	Bupropion	MAOIs enhance toxic effects of bupropion; AVOID
SNRI	Venlafaxine	Metabolism of serotonin and norepinephrine inhibited; AVOID
SARI	Trazodone	Low doses of trazodone (25–50 mg) used to treat antidepressant-induced insomnia Monitor for serotonergic adverse effects
NaSSA	Mirtazapine	Possible serotonergic reaction; AVOID

Class of Drug	Example	Interaction Effects
Nonselective cyclic	Amitriptyline, desipramine	If used together, do not add cyclic antidepressant to MAOI. Start cyclic antidepressant first or simultaneously with MAOI. For patients already on MAOI, discontinue the MAOI for 10–14 days before starting combination therapy Combined cyclic and MAOI therapy has increased antidepressant effects and will potentiate weight gain, hypotension, and anticholinergic effects Serotonin syndrome and deaths have been reported
	Clomipramine	Serotonin syndrome (see p. 10) reported; AVOID
Antihypertensive	α-blockers, β-blockers, ACE inhibitors	MAOIs should not be administered with hypotensive agents as marked hypotension may occur
	Guanethidine	Severe pressor response can occur due to catecholamine release; AVOID
Antipsychotic	General	Additive hypotension and anticholinergic effects
Second generation	Quetiapine	Case report of serotonin syndrome with quetiapine and phenelzine
	Ziprasidone	Case report of serotonin syndrome with tranylcypromine
Anxiolytic	Buspirone	Several cases of increased blood pressure reported; AVOID; discontinue MAOIs at least 10 days before initiation of buspirone
Atropine		Prolonged action of atropine
Bromocriptine		Increased serotonergic effects
CNS depressant	Alcohol, barbiturates, sedatives	May enhance CNS depression
Diuretic		MAOIs should not be administered with hypotensive agents as marked hypotension may occur
Ginseng		May cause headache, tremulousness or hypomania; case report of irritability and visual hallucinations with combination
Insulin		Enhanced hypoglycemic response through stimulation of insulin secretion and inhibition of gluconeogenesis
L-dopa		Increase in storage and release of dopamine and/or norepinephrine Headache, hyperexcitability, hypertension, and related symptoms reported
Licorice		Increased serotonergic effects possible
Lithium		Increased serotonergic effects
L-tryptophan		Reports of serotonin syndrome (see p. 10) with hyperreflexia, tremor, myoclonic jerks, and ocular oscillations; AVOID
MAO-B inhibitor	Selegiline (L-deprenyl)	Increased serotonergic effects
Methylene blue		Enhanced serotonergic effects through inhibition of MAO-A and B by methylene blue. Risk for serotonin syndrome (see Precautions p. 10)
Muscle relaxant	Succinylcholine	Phenelzine may prolong muscle relaxation by inhibiting metabolism
Nicotine		Low doses of tranylcypromine reported to inhibit nicotine metabolism by competitive inhibition via CYP2A6
Opioids and related drugs	Dextromethorphan	Reports of bizarre behavior and psychosis. Case reports of serotonin syndrome; AVOID
	Dextromethorphan, diphenoxylate, meperidine, tramadol	Excitation, sweating, and hypotension reported; may lead to development of encephalopathy, convulsions, coma, respiratory depression, and serotonin syndrome. If an opioid is required, meperidine should not be used; institute other opioids cautiously
	Tramadol	Increased risk of seizures and serotonin syndrome
Reserpine		Central excitatory syndrome and hypertension reported due to central and peripheral release of catecholamines
Stimulants	MDA, MDMA ("Ecstasy")	Case reports of serotonin syndrome (see p. 10) and hypertensive crisis
St. John's wort		Increased serotonergic effects possible
Sulfonylurea	Tolbutamide	Enhanced hypoglycemic response

Irreversible Monoamine Oxidase (A&B) Inhibitors (MAOIs) (cont.)

Class of Drug	Example	Interaction Effects
Sympathomimetic	*Indirect-acting:* Amphetamine, dopamine, ephedrine, methylphenidate, pseudoephedrine, tyramine	Release of large amounts of norepinephrine with hypertensive reaction; AVOID
	Direct-acting: Epinephrine, isoproterenol, norepinephrine (levarterenol), salbutamol	No interaction
	Phenylephrine	Increased pressor response
Tetrabenazine		Central excitatory syndrome and hypertension reported due to central and peripheral release of catecholamines
Triptan	Rizatriptan, sumatriptan, zolmitriptan	Serotonin syndrome (see p. 10); AVOID; recommended that 2 weeks elapse after discontinuing an irreversible MAOI before using sumatriptan

Irreversible MAO-B Inhibitor

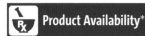 **Product Availability***

Generic Name	Chemical Class	Neuroscience-based Nomenclature* (Pharmacological Target/Mode of Action)	Trade Name	Dosage Forms and Strengths
Selegiline (L-deprenyl)	Levo-acetylenic derivative of phenethylamine	Dopamine, norepinephrine, serotonin/Enzyme inhibitor	EMSAM(B)	Transdermal system: 20 mg/20 cm², 30 mg/30 cm², 40 mg/40 cm² that deliver on average 6 mg/24 h, 9 mg/24 h, 12 mg/24 h, respectively
			Zelapar(B)	Orally disintegrating tablet: 1.25 mg

* Refer to Health Canada's Drug Product Database or the FDA's Drugs@FDA for the most current availability information. * Developed by a taskforce consisting of representatives from the American College of Neuropsychopharmacology (ACNP), the Asian College of Neuropsychopharmacology (AsCNP), the European College of Neuropsychopharmacology (ECNP), the International College of Neuropsychopharmacology (CINP), and the International Union of Basic and Clinical Pharmacology (IUPHAR) (see https://nbn2r.com), (B) Not marketed in Canada

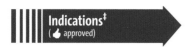 **Indications‡** (👍 approved)

- 👍 Major depressive disorder (MDD) in adults (US only)
- Cocaine use: Selegiline may reduce physiological and subjective effects

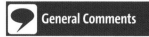 **General Comments**

- In patients presenting with depression and a high risk of suicide, treatment selection should consider safety in overdose (i.e., consider using newer antidepressant agents rather than nonselective cyclic and MAOI antidepressants). Prescription quantities should be consistent with safe patient care
- Oral formulation approved in low doses for the treatment of Parkinson's disease; higher doses required for treatment of MDD
- Transdermal patches contain 1 mg of selegiline per cm² and deliver approximately 0.3 mg of selegiline per cm² over 24 h

‡ Indications listed here do not necessarily apply to all countries. Please refer to a country's regulatory database (e.g., US Food and Drug Administration, Health Canada Drug Product Database) for the most current availability information and indications

- A case series of 6 patients with treatment-resistant depression failing both ECT and oral antidepressants found IV ketamine with simultaneous administration of selegiline transdermal system to resolve suicidality and increase food intake in all patients. Five patients showed sustained improvement with the selegiline transdermal system
- Dietary restrictions are not required at lowest doses; use caution at higher doses as selegiline loses its selectivity for MAO-B inhibition
- May produce false-positive drug screen (L-amphetamine metabolites)

 Pharmacology

- Transdermal selegiline provides sustained plasma concentrations of the parent compound, increasing the amount of drug delivered to the brain and decreasing metabolite production
- At low doses, selegiline irreversibly inhibits MAO-B, which is involved in oxidative deamination of dopamine in the brain and also inhibits the uptake of dopamine
- At higher doses, selegiline inhibits both MAO-A and B, which are involved in the catabolism of norepinephrine, dopamine, and serotonin. In vivo animal models using the transdermal patch suggest that both MAO-A and MAO-B inhibition is required for antidepressant effects
- The transdermal formulation allows for targeted inhibition of central nervous system MAO-A and MAO-B with minimal effects on MAO-A in the GI (gut wall) and hepatic systems, avoiding first-pass effect, reducing the risk of interactions with tyramine-rich foods
- Induces antioxidant enzymes and decreases the formation of oxygen radicals; it interferes with early apoptotic signaling events induced by various kinds of insults in cell cultures, protecting cells from apoptotic death

 Dosing

- See p. 96
- EMSAM should be applied to dry, intact skin on the upper torso (below the neck and above the waist), upper thigh or the outer surface of the upper arm once every 24 h. Avoid using the same site on consecutive days
- The 6 mg/24 h patch is the recommended starting and target dose. If dose increases are indicated for individual patients, they should occur in dose increments of 3 mg/24 h (up to a maximum dose of 12 mg/24 h) at intervals of no less than 2 weeks
- No adjustment in dosage necessary in moderate hepatic or renal insufficiency

Pharmacokinetics

- See p. 96
- On average, 25–30% of the selegiline content is systemically delivered over 24 h (range ~ 10–40%) following dermal application
- Absorption of selegiline is similar when transdermal selegiline is applied to the upper torso or upper thigh; the drug is not metabolized in human skin
- Transdermal selegiline bypasses the GI tract, thus avoids inhibiting MAO-A in the GI tract; patient sensitivity to dietary tyramine is more than 20 times less than with oral tranylcypromine, the effect of avoiding excessive amounts of tyramine entering the bloodstream
- Transdermal dosing avoids extensive first-pass metabolism, resulting in substantially higher selegiline exposure and lower exposure to metabolites compared to oral dosing
- Selegiline is approximately 90% bound to plasma protein
- Steady-state selegiline plasma concentrations are achieved within 5 days of daily dosing
- Extensively metabolized by CYP450 enzymes including CYP2B6, CYP2C9, and CYP3A4/5 and CYP2A6
- Selegiline is initially metabolized via N-dealkylation or N-depropargylation to form N-desmethylselegiline or R(–)-methamphetamine, respectively. Both of these metabolites can be further metabolized to R(–)-amphetamine
- Selegiline and N-desmethylselegiline produce a concentration-dependent inhibition of CYP2D6 at 10–250 μM and CYP3A4/5 at 25–250 μM; CYP2C19 and CYP2B6 were also inhibited at concentrations ≥ 100 μM. All inhibitory effects of selegiline and N-desmethylselegiline occurred at concentrations that were several orders of magnitude higher than clinical concentrations
- Mean half-lives of selegiline and its three metabolites, R(–)-N-desmethylselegiline, R(–)-amphetamine, and R(–)-methamphetamine, range from 18 to 25 h

 Onset & Duration of Action

- Therapeutic effects are typically seen within 28 days; a lack of an antidepressant response within 6–8 weeks may require a dosage increase or selegiline may not work at all

 Adverse Effects

- See p. 93
- Insomnia is common [Management: Take the patch off before bedtime]

Irreversible MAO-B Inhibitor (cont.)

- Dermatological reactions are common at the site of application; usually erythema (24%) [Management: Rotate application sites]
- Diarrhea, pharyngitis, dizziness, lightheadedness, headache (18%); hypotension (10%); dry mouth
- Increased blood pressure at doses above 6 mg/24 h possible
- Increased anxiety, agitation, irritability, increase in suicidal thoughts; activation of mania/hypomania (0.4%)
- Weight loss of more than 5% of body weight (5% incidence)

 Contraindications

- Simultaneous administration of drugs with serotonergic properties (see Interactions, p. 77)
- Combination with sympathomimetic amines, amphetamines, cold products, and weight-reducing preparations that contain vasoconstrictors or local vasoconstrictors (i.e., cocaine or local anesthesia containing sympathomimetic vasoconstrictors)
- Carbamazepine, oxcarbazepine (see Drug Interactions, p. 77)

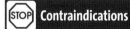 **Precautions**

- Both adults and children with depression (whether under treatment or not) may experience worsening of their MDD, unusual changes in their behavior, and/or the emergence of suicidal ideation and behavior (see Nursing Implications p. 77 for monitoring)
- Although dietary restrictions are not required for the 6 mg/24 h dose, higher doses can negate drug selectivity and a pressor response can occur on exposure to tyramine-rich foods. Patients should observe dietary and drug restrictions for doses over 6 mg (as per irreversible MAO inhibitors p. 71)
- A 14-day washout is required between termination of selegiline and initiating an antidepressant with serotonergic activity; prevents serotonin syndrome (see Drug Interactions, p. 17 and Switching Antidepressants pp. 97–99)
- Patients should be carefully evaluated for a history of drug abuse; patients should be closely observed for signs of transdermal selegiline misuse or abuse (e.g., development of tolerance, increases in dose, or drug-seeking behavior)

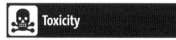 **Toxicity**

- No information available on overdose by selegiline patches. Overdose with MAOI agents is typically associated with CNS and cardiovascular toxicity
- Delays of up to 12 h between ingestion of drug and appearance of symptoms may occur; peak effects may not be observed for 24–48 h
- Death has been reported following overdosage with MAOI agents; hospitalization and close monitoring during this period are essential

Management

- Symptomatic and supportive

 Pediatric Considerations

- Not recommended

 Geriatric Considerations

- Recommended dose for elderly patients is 6 mg/24 h
- Observe closely for orthostatic BP changes during treatment
- Patients aged 50 and older appear to be at higher risk for rash (4.4% vs. 0% placebo) than younger patients

 Use in Pregnancy◇

- Very limited human data, avoid when possible

Breast Milk

- It is not known whether selegiline hydrochloride is excreted in human milk but low molecular weight suggests that it will be. Significant neurotoxicity observed in animals

 Nursing Implications

- Dietary restrictions are not necessary at a dose of 6 mg/24 h; however, patients should be informed about the signs and symptoms associated with MAOI-induced hypertensive crisis and urged to seek immediate medical attention if these symptoms occur
- Follow MAOI dietary restrictions for doses over 6 mg/24 h
- Patients should be advised to immediately report severe headache, neck stiffness, palpitations or other atypical or unusual symptoms not previously experienced

◇ See p. 473 for further information on drug use in pregnancy and effects on breast milk

- Advise patient to avoid exposing the application site of patches to external sources of direct heat, such as heating pads or electric blankets, heat lamps, saunas, hot tubs, heated water beds, and prolonged direct sunlight, as this may result in an increase in the amount of selegiline absorbed from the patch, producing elevated serum levels
- Theoretically, there is a 3-day reservoir of drug in each patch; discard patches in a manner that prevents accidental application or ingestion by children, pets, etc.
- All patients being treated with antidepressants should be observed closely for clinical worsening, suicidality, and unusual changes in behavior, especially during the initial few months of therapy or following an increase or decrease in dose

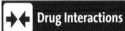 **Patient Instructions**

- For detailed patient instruction on transdermal selegiline, see the Patient Information Sheet (details p. 474)

Drug Interactions

- Clinically significant interactions are listed below
- For more interaction information on any given combination, also see the corresponding chapter for the second agent

Class of Drug	Example	Interaction Effects
Antibiotic	Linezolid	Monitor for increased serotonergic and noradrenergic effects due to linezolid's weak MAO inhibition
Anticonvulsant	Carbamazepine, oxcarbazepine	Increased level of selegiline and its metabolite (2-fold)
Antidepressant SSRI, SNRI, SARI, NaSSA, tricyclic, RIMA, MAOI		Increased serotonergic effects with possibility of serotonin syndrome
Anxiolytic	Buspirone	Several cases of elevated blood pressure have been reported
Opioid	Meperidine	Stupor, muscular rigidity, severe agitation, and elevated temperature reported in some patients receiving the combination of selegiline and meperidine
	Tramadol	Increased risk of seizures and serotonin syndrome
St. John's wort		Increased serotonergic effects with possibility of serotonin syndrome
Sympathomimetic	Amphetamines, dextromethorphan, ephedrine, phenylephrine, phenylpropanolamine, pseudoephedrine	Risk of hypertensive crisis

GABA$_A$ Receptor Positive Modulator

 Product Availability*

Generic Name	Neuroscience-based Nomenclature* (Pharmacological Target/Mode of Action)	Trade Name[A]	Dosage Forms and Strengths
Brexanolone	GABA/Positive allosteric modulator	Zulresso[B]	Injection: 100 mg/20 mL (5 mg/mL) single-dose vial

* Refer to Health Canada's Drug Product Database or the FDA's Drugs@FDA for the most current availability information. * Developed by a taskforce consisting of representatives from the American College of Neuropsychopharmacology (ACNP), the Asian College of Neuropsychopharmacology (AsCNP), the European College of Neuropsychopharmacology (ECNP), the International College of Neuropsychopharmacology (CINP), and the International Union of Basic and Clinical Pharmacology (IUPHAR) (see https://nbn2r.com), [A] Generic preparations may be available, [B] Not marketed in Canada

GABA$_A$ Receptor Positive Modulator (cont.)

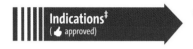 **Indications‡**
(👍 approved)

👍 Treatment of postpartum depression (PPD) in adults

 General Comments

- A healthcare provider must be available on site to continuously monitor the patient, and intervene as necessary, for the duration of the infusion
- Initiate brexanolone treatment early enough in the day to allow for recognition of excessive sedation
- Because of the risk of serious harm resulting from excessive sedation or sudden loss of consciousness, brexanolone is available only through a restricted program under a Risk Evaluation and Mitigation Strategy (REMS) called the ZULRESSO REM
- A meta-analysis of 3 RCTs reported that a single brexanolone infusion appears to have ultra-rapid antidepressant effect for PPD, lasting for up to 1 week[21]

 Pharmacology

- Mechanism of action in the treatment of PPD in adults is not fully understood; thought to be related to positive allosteric modulation of GABA$_A$ receptors

 Dosing

- See p. 96
- Administered as a continuous IV infusion over 60 hours (2.5 days) as follows:
  - 0–4 h: Initiate with a dosage of 30 micrograms/kg/h
  - 4–24 h: Increase dosage to 60 micrograms/kg/h
  - 24–52 h: Increase dosage to 90 micrograms/kg/h (alternatively, consider a dosage of 60 micrograms/kg/hr for those who do not tolerate 90 micrograms/kg/h)
  - 52–56 h: Decrease dosage to 60 micrograms/kg/h
  - 56–60 h: Decrease dosage to 30 micrograms/kg/h

Renal Impairment

- No dosage adjustment recommended in patients with mild (eGFR 60–89 mL/min/1.73 m^2), moderate (eGFR 30–59 mL/min/1.73 m^2), or severe (eGFR 15–29 mL/min/1.73 m^2) renal impairment

Hepatic Impairment

- No dosage adjustment necessary

 Pharmacokinetics

- Brexanolone exhibits dose-proportional pharmacokinetics over a dosage range of 30–270 micrograms/kg/h
- Mean steady state exposure at 60 and 90 micrograms/kg/h was around 52 and 79 nanograms/mL, respectively
- Volume of distribution: 3 L/kg, suggesting extensive distribution into tissues
- Plasma protein binding: >99%, is independent of plasma concentration
- Terminal half-life: approximately 9 h
- Clearance: approximately 1 L/h/kg
- Metabolism: extensively metabolized by non-CYP-based pathways via three main routes – keto reduction, glucuronidation, and sulfation. There are 3 inactive major metabolites
- Excretion: 47% recovered in feces (primarily as metabolites) and 42% in urine (with less than 1% as unchanged brexanolone)

 Adverse Effects

- See chart p. 93
- Data presented below reflect exposure of brexanolone in 140 patients with PPD; titration to a target dose of 90 or 60 micrograms/kg/h was evaluated in 102 and 38 patients, respectively (placebo control group: 107 patients). Patients were followed for 4 weeks

CNS Effects

- Headache: 14% (placebo); 18% (60 micrograms/kg/h); 15% (90 micrograms/kg/h)
- Dizziness, presyncope, vertigo: 7% (placebo); 13% (60 micrograms/kg/h); 12% (90 micrograms/kg/h)

‡ Indications listed here do not necessarily apply to all countries. Please refer to a country's regulatory database (e.g., US Food and Drug Administration, Health Canada Drug Product Database) for the most current availability information and indications

- Loss of consciousness: none with placebo; 5% (60 micrograms/kg/h); 3% (90 micrograms/kg/h)
- Sedation, somnolence: 6% (placebo); 21% (60 micrograms/kg/h); 13% (90 micrograms/kg/h)

Anticholinergic Effects	- Dry mouth: 1% (placebo); 11% (60 micrograms/kg/h); 3% (90 micrograms/kg/h)
Cardiovascular Effects	- Tachycardia: none with placebo and 60 micrograms/kg/h; 3% (90 micrograms/kg/h)
GI Effects	- Diarrhea: 1% (placebo); 3% (60 micrograms/kg/h); 2% (90 micrograms/kg/h) - Dyspepsia: none with placebo and 60 micrograms/kg/h; 2% (90 micrograms/kg/h) - Oropharyngeal pain: non with placebo; 3% (60 micrograms/kg/h); 2% (90 micrograms/kg/h)
Other Adverse Effects	- Flushing, hot flush: none with placebo; 5% (60 micrograms/kg/h); 2% (90 micrograms/kg/h) - Rash: 4% (placebo); 3% (60 micrograms/kg/h); 1% (90 micrograms/kg/h)

 D/C Discontinuation Syndrome
- In the PPD clinical studies conducted, end of treatment occurred through tapering. Thus, not possible to assess whether abrupt discontinuation of brexanolone produced withdrawal symptoms indicative of physical dependence
- Recommended that brexanolone be tapered according to the dosage recommendations, unless symptoms warrant immediate discontinuation

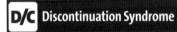 **Contraindications**
- Avoid in patients with end stage renal disease with eGFR of less than 15 mL/min/1.73 m^2 because of potential accumulation of the solubilizing agent, betadex sulfobutyl ether sodium

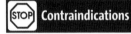 **Precautions**
- Suicidal thoughts and behaviors: Consider changing therapeutic regimen, including discontinuing brexanolone, in patients whose PPD worsens or who experience emergent suicidal thoughts and behaviors
- Excessive sedation: In clinical studies, brexanolone caused sedation and somnolence that required dose interruption or reduction (5% with brexanolone compared to none with placebo). Assess for excessive sedation every 2 h during non-sleep periods. If excessive sedation occurs at any time during infusion, immediately stop infusion until symptoms resolve. Infusion may be resumed at the same or lower dose as clinically appropriate
- Sudden loss of consciousness or altered states of consciousness during infusion reported in some patients (4% with brexanolone compared to none with placebo). Time to full recovery, after dose interruption, ranged from 15 to 60 min. All patients recovered with dose interruption
- Hypoxia: Monitor patients for hypoxia using continuous pulse oximetry equipped with an alarm. Immediately stop infusion if pulse oximetry reveals hypoxia. Infusion should not be resumed
- Concomitant use of opioids, antidepressants, or other CNS depressants such as benzodiazepines or alcohol may increase likelihood or severity of adverse reactions related to sedation

 Pediatric Considerations
- Not approved for use in pediatric patients
- Safety and effectiveness of brexanolone in pediatric patients have not been established

 Geriatric Considerations
- PPD is a condition associated with pregnancy; there is no geriatric experience with brexanolone

 Use in Pregnancy◇
- Based on animal studies of other drugs that enhance GABA-ergic inhibition, brexanolone may cause fetal harm
- No available data on brexanolone use in pregnant women to determine drug-associated risk of major birth defects, miscarriage, or adverse maternal or fetal outcomes

Breast Milk
- Brexanolone is present in human milk; however, relative infant dose is low, 1–2% of maternal weight-adjusted dose. Also, as brexanolone has low (less than 5%) oral bioavailability in adults, infant exposure is expected to be low
- The developmental and health benefits of breastfeeding should be considered along with the mother's clinical need for brexanolone

 Nursing Implications
- Initiate brexanolone treatment early enough in the day to allow for recognition of excessive sedation
- Brexanolone is supplied as a concentrated solution that requires dilution prior to administration

◇ See p. 473 for further information on drug use in pregnancy and effects on breast milk

GABA$_A$ Receptor Positive Modulator (cont.)

- After dilution, product can be stored in infusion bags under refrigerated conditions for up to 96 h
- As diluted product can be used at room temperature for only 12 h, each 60 h infusion will require preparation of at least 5 infusion bags
- Administer brexanolone via a dedicated line. Do not inject other medications into the infusion bag or mix with brexanolone
- Monitor patients for hypoxia using continuous pulse oximetry equipped with an alarm. Immediately stop infusion if pulse oximetry reveals hypoxia. Infusion should not be resumed
- Assess for excessive sedation every 2 h during non-sleep periods. If excessive sedation occurs at any time during infusion, immediately stop infusion until symptoms resolve. Infusion may be resumed at the same or lower dose as clinically appropriate
- Patients must be accompanied during interactions with their child(ren) while receiving the infusion because of potential for excessive sedation and sudden loss of consciousness
- Psychotherapy and education are also important in the treatment of depression
- Monitor therapy by watching for adverse side effects and mood and activity level changes, including worsening of suicidal thoughts

 Drug Interactions

- Clinically significant interactions are listed below
- For more interaction information on any given combination, also see the corresponding chapter for the second agent

Class of Drug	Example	Interaction Effects
Antidepressant		In placebo-controlled studies, a higher percentage of brexanolone-treated patients who used concomitant antidepressants reported sedation-related events
CNS depressant	Benzodiazepines, opioids	May increase likelihood or severity of adverse reactions related to sedation

NMDA Receptor Antagonist

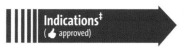 **Product Availability***

Generic Name	Chemical Class	Neuroscience-based Nomenclature* (Pharmacological Target/Mode of Action)	Trade Name	Dosage Forms and Strengths
Esketamine	NMDA receptor antagonist	Glutamate/Antagonist	Spravato	Nasal spray: 28 mg of esketamine per device Each spray device delivers two sprays containing a total of 28 mg

* Refer to Health Canada's Drug Product Database or the FDA's Drugs@FDA for the most current availability information ˙ Developed by a taskforce consisting of representatives from the American College of Neuropsychopharmacology (ACNP), the Asian College of Neuropsychopharmacology (AsCNP), the European College of Neuropsychopharmacology (ECNP), the International College of Neuropsychopharmacology (CINP), and the International Union of Basic and Clinical Pharmacology (IUPHAR) (see https://nbn2r.com),

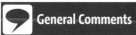 **Indications‡** (👍 approved)

- 👍 Treatment-resistant depression (in conjunction with an oral antidepressant)

💬 **General Comments**

- Must be administered under the direct supervision of a healthcare provider. A treatment session consists of nasal administration of esketamine and post-administration observation under supervision for at least 2 h

‡ Indications listed here do not necessarily apply to all countries. Please refer to a country's regulatory database (e.g., US Food and Drug Administration, Health Canada Drug Product Database) for the most current availability information and indications

- Because of the risk of serious adverse outcomes resulting from sedation and dissociation caused by esketamine administration, and the potential for abuse and misuse of the drug, it is only available through a restricted distribution system, under a Risk Evaluation and Mitigation Strategy (REMS)
- Monitor all patients for worsening depression and suicidal thinking
- A meta-analysis of 5 trials involving 774 patients reported that intranasal esketamine appears to be an effective treatment strategy for patients with MDD who are either treatment resistant or acutely suicidal[22]
- A disproportionality analysis of spontaneous reports was performed using the FDA Adverse Event Reporting System (FAERS) database (March 2019 to March 2020) and found esketamine-related adverse events (962 cases) that included: dissociation (ROR = 1,612.64), sedation (ROR = 238.46), feeling drunk (ROR = 96.17), suicidal ideation (ROR = 24.03), and completed suicide (ROR = 5.75). Signals for suicidal and self-injurious ideation, but not suicide attempt and completed suicide, remained when comparing esketamine to venlafaxine

 Pharmacology

- Esketamine, the S-enantiomer of racemic ketamine, is a non-selective, non-competitive antagonist of the N-methyl-D-aspartate (NMDA) receptor, an ionotropic glutamate receptor
- The mechanism by which esketamine exerts its antidepressant effect is unknown
- The major circulating metabolite of esketamine (noresketamine) demonstrated activity at the same receptor with lower affinity

 Dosing

- See p. 96
- Assess blood pressure prior to dosing. If baseline BP is elevated (e.g., higher than 140 mmHg systolic, higher than 90 mmHg diastolic), consider the risk of short-term increases in BP and benefit of esketamine. Do not administer esketamine if an increase in BP or intracranial pressure poses a serious risk. After dosing, reassess BP at approximately 40 min (corresponds to C_{max}) and subsequently as clinically warranted
- Dosage adjustments should be made based on efficacy and tolerability
- Evidence of therapeutic benefit should be evaluated at the end of the induction phase to determine need for continued treatment
- Induction phase (weeks 1–4, administer twice per week): Day 1 starting dose 56 mg; subsequent doses 56 mg or 84 mg
- Maintenance phase (weeks 5–8, administer once weekly): 56 mg or 84 mg
- Maintenance phase (week 9 and after, administer every 2 weeks or once weekly): 56 mg or 84 mg. Dosing frequency should be individualized to the least frequent dosing to maintain remission/response
- Esketamine is for nasal use only. The nasal spray device delivers a total of 28 mg of esketamine. To prevent loss of medication, do not prime the device before use. Use 2 devices (for a 56 mg dose) or 3 devices (for an 84 mg dose), with a 5-minute rest between use of each device
- If a patient misses treatment sessions and there is worsening of depression symptoms, consider returning to the patient's previous dosing schedule

 Pharmacokinetics

- The mean absolute bioavailability is approximately 48% following nasal spray administration
- Time to reach maximum esketamine plasma concentration is 20–40 min after the last nasal spray of a treatment session
- C_{max} (inter-subject variability) ranges from 27% to 66%; C_{max} (intra-subject variability) is approximately 15%
- AUC (inter-subject variability) ranges from 18% to 45%; AUC (intra-subject variability) is approximately 10%
- Mean steady-state volume of distribution is 709 L
- Protein binding is approximately 43–45%
- Brain-to-plasma ratio of noresketamine is 4–6 times lower than that of esketamine
- Half-life ranges from 7 to 12 h
- AUC and half-life higher in patients with moderate hepatic impairment
- Clearance is approximately 89 L/h following IV administration
- Primarily metabolized to noresketamine via CYP2B6 and CYP3A4 and to a lesser extent via CYP2C9 and CYP2C19
- Noresketamine is metabolized via CYP-dependent pathways and certain subsequent metabolites undergo glucuronidation

 Onset & Duration of Action

- In a 4-week study comparing esketamine (plus oral antidepressant) vs. intranasal placebo (plus oral antidepressant), a significant improvement in MADRS score was observed at 4 h with esketamine compared to placebo with the greatest treatment difference observed at 24 h
- Patients in stable remission who continued treatment with esketamine (plus oral antidepressant) experienced a statistically significantly longer time to relapse of depressive symptoms than did patients on intranasal placebo (plus oral antidepressant)

NMDA Receptor Antagonist (cont.)

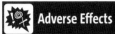 **Adverse Effects**

- See chart p. 92 for incidence of adverse effects at therapeutic doses
- Dissociation, dizziness, nausea, sedation, vertigo, hypoesthesia, anxiety, lethargy, blood pressure increase, vomiting, and feeling drunk are the most commonly reported side effects (incidence ≥ 5% and at least twice that of placebo plus oral antidepressant)
- Approximately 5% of patients will discontinue treatment due to adverse effects

CNS Effects

- Sedation in 49–61% of patients
- Dissociative or perceptual changes (including distortion of time/space and illusions), derealization, and depersonalization in 61–75% of patients
- Anxiety 13% in patients treated with esketamine (plus oral antidepressant) vs. 6% in placebo (plus oral antidepressant)
- Dizziness 29%, lethargy 11%, and feeling drunk 5% in patients treated with esketamine (plus an oral antidepressant) vs. 8%, 5%, and 0.5%, respectively, with placebo (plus oral antidepressant)
- Hypoesthesia 18% in patients treated with esketamine (plus oral antidepressant) vs. 2% with placebo (plus oral antidepressant)
- Two placebo-controlled studies found comparable driving performance between patients treated with esketamine (84 mg) and placebo at 6 h and 18 h post dose (except two esketamine-treated patients who discontinued the driving test at 8 h post dose due to esketamine-related adverse reactions)
- May impair short-term cognitive performance (no effect on cognitive performance in a one-year open-label safety study, but unknown beyond one year)

Anticholinergic Effects

- Not significant

Cardiovascular Effects

- Increase of 40 mmHg in systolic blood pressure (BP) and/or 25 mmHg in diastolic BP in 8–17% of esketamine-treated patients vs. 1–3% of placebo-treated patients in the first 1.5 h during the first 4 weeks of treatment
- Increase in BP peaks approximately 40 min after administration

Endocrine & Metabolic Effects

- Not significant

GI Effects

- Nausea 28% in patients treated with esketamine (plus oral antidepressant) vs. 9% with placebo (plus oral antidepressant)
- Vomiting 9% in patients treated with esketamine (plus oral antidepressant) vs. 2% with placebo (plus oral antidepressant)

Other Adverse Effects

- Vertigo 23% in patients treated with esketamine (plus oral antidepressant) vs. 3% with placebo (plus oral antidepressant)
- Higher rate of lower urinary tract symptoms (pollakiuria, dysuria, micturition urgency, nocturia, and cystitis) in esketamine-treated patients than with placebo

D/C Discontinuation Syndrome

- No discontinuation syndrome noted up to 4 weeks after esketamine cessation
- Withdrawal symptoms have been reported after discontinuation of frequently used (more than weekly) large doses of ketamine for long periods of time. Such withdrawal symptoms are likely to occur if esketamine were similarly abused. Symptoms may include craving, fatigue, poor appetite, and anxiety
- ☞ **THEREFORE THIS MEDICATION SHOULD BE WITHDRAWN GRADUALLY AFTER PROLONGED USE**

STOP Contraindications

- Contraindicated in patients with: Aneurysmal vascular disease or arteriovenous malformation, history of intracerebral hemorrhage, or hypersensitivity to esketamine, ketamine, or any of the excipients
- Esketamine should not be used in patients with severe hepatic impairment (Child-Pugh class C) due to lack of studies in this population

⚠ Precautions

- Assess blood pressure prior to dosing. If baseline BP is elevated (e.g., > 140 mmHg systolic, > 90 mmHg diastolic), consider the risks of short-term increases in BP and benefit of esketamine. Do not administer esketamine if an increase in BP or intracranial pressure poses a serious risk. After dosing, reassess BP at approximately 40 min (corresponds to C_{max}) and subsequently as clinically warranted
- Monitor for sedation during concomitant treatment with esketamine and CNS depressants

- Due to risks of sedation and dissociation, patient must be monitored for at least 2 h after each treatment session, followed by an assessment to determine when the patient is considered clinically stable and ready to leave the healthcare setting
- Assess each patient's risk for abuse or misuse prior to prescribing esketamine and monitor for the development of these behaviors or conditions, including drug-seeking behavior, while on therapy
- Monitor all patients for worsening depression and suicidal thoughts, especially during the initial few months of drug therapy and at times of dosage changes

 Pediatric Considerations

- Esketamine is not approved for use in pediatric patients
- The safety and effectiveness of esketamine in pediatric patients have not been established

 Geriatric Considerations

- Mean esketamine C_{max} and AUC higher in elderly patients
- Efficacy was assessed in a 4-week RCT comparing esketamine (plus an oral antidepressant) to intranasal placebo (plus an oral antidepressant) in patients aged 65 years and older. Esketamine was initiated at 28 mg twice weekly and titrated to 56 mg or 84 mg administered twice-weekly. At the end of the 4 weeks, there was no statistically significant difference between the groups on the primary efficacy endpoint of change from baseline to week 4 using MADRS

 Use in Pregnancy◊

- Not recommended during pregnancy
- Embryo-fetal toxicity; may cause fetal harm
- Insufficient data to draw conclusions about risk of major birth defects, miscarriage, or adverse maternal or fetal outcomes
- If a woman becomes pregnant while being treated with esketamine, treatment should be discontinued and the patient counseled about the potential risk to the fetus

Breast Milk

- Esketamine is present in human milk
- Potential for neurotoxicity in breastfed infants

 Nursing Implications

- Esketamine is for nasal use only
- Prior to esketamine administration, instruct patients not to engage in potentially hazardous activities, such as driving a motor vehicle or operating machinery, until the next day after a restful sleep
- Advise pregnant women of the potential risk of fetal harm
- To prevent loss of medication, do not prime the device before use
- If more than one spray device is used, allow a 5-minute rest period between use of devices
- Assess blood pressure prior to and 40 min (C_{max}) after esketamine administration
- Monitor for urinary tract and bladder symptoms during the course of esketamine treatment
- Psychotherapy and education are also important in the treatment of depression
- Monitor therapy by watching for adverse side effects and mood and activity level changes, including worsening of suicidal thoughts

 Patient Instructions

- For detailed patient instructions on esketamine, see the Patient Information Sheet (details p. 474)

 Drug Interactions

- Clinically significant interactions are listed below
- For more interaction information on any given combination, also see the corresponding chapter for the second agent

Class of Drug	Example	Interaction Effects
Antidepressant		
Irreversible MAOI	Phenelzine, tranylcypromine	May increase blood pressure
CNS depressant	Alcohol, benzodiazepines, opioids	May increase sedation
Psychostimulant	Amphetamines, armodafinil, methyphenidate, modafinil	May increase blood pressure

◊ See p. 473 for further information on drug use in pregnancy and effects on breast milk

NMDA Receptor Antagonist/CYP2D6 Inhibitor

 Product Availability*

Generic Name	Chemical Class	Neuroscience-based Nomenclature* (Pharmacological Target/Mode of Action)	Trade Name	Dosage Forms and Strengths
Dextromethorphan/bupropion combination	NMDA receptor antagonist/CYP2D6 inhibitor	Dextromethorphan: Glutamate/Antagonist Bupropion: Norepinephrine, dopamine/Reuptake inhibitor (NET, DAT), releaser (NE, DA)	Auvelity(B)	Extended-release tablets: 45 mg dextromethorphan hydrobromide/105 mg bupropion hydrochloride

* Refer to Health Canada's Drug Product Database or the FDA's Drugs@FDA for the most current availability information   * Developed by a taskforce consisting of representatives from the American College of Neuropsychopharmacology (ACNP), the Asian College of Neuropsychopharmacology (AsCNP), the European College of Neuropsychopharmacology (ECNP), the International College of Neuropsychopharmacology (CINP), and the International Union of Basic and Clinical Pharmacology (IUPHAR) (see https://nbn2r.com), (B) Not marketed in Canada

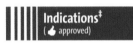 **Indications‡** (👍 approved)

👆 Major depressive disorder (MDD) in adults

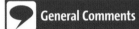 **General Comments**

- In a randomized, double-blind, phase 3 trial of dextromethorphan/bupropion (45 mg/105 mg extended-release tablet) vs. placebo (once daily for days 1–3, twice daily thereafter) for 6 weeks, significant improvements in depressive symptoms (i.e., change in MADRS total score from baseline) were noted in patients treated with dextromethorphan/bupropion compared to placebo starting 1 week after treatment initiation
- A randomized, double-blind trial evaluated dextromethorphan/bupropion (45 mg/105 mg extended-release tablet) vs. the active comparator sustained-release bupropion (105 mg) (once daily for days 1–3, twice daily thereafter) for 6 weeks in patients 18–65 years of age. MADRS score change and remission rates with dextromethorphan/bupropion were significantly greater than with bupropion at week 2 and every time point thereafter

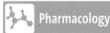 **Pharmacology**

- Dextromethorphan is an uncompetitive antagonist of the NMDA receptor (an ionotropic glutamate receptor) and a σ-1 receptor agonist
- Bupropion increases plasma levels of dextromethorphan by competitively inhibiting CYP2D6, a major metabolic pathway for dextromethorphan
- Bupropion is a relatively weak inhibitor of norepinephrine and dopamine reuptake into presynaptic neurons

 Dosing

- See p. 96
- Recommended starting dose (45 mg of dextromethorphan hydrobromide and 105 mg of bupropion hydrochloride) is one tablet once daily in the morning. After 3 days, increase to maximum recommended dose of one tablet twice daily, given at least 8 h apart
- Dose adjustment recommended in patients known to be poor CYP2D6 metabolizers as they have higher dextromethorphan concentrations than extensive/intermediate CYP2D6 metabolizers; recommended dose for such patients is one tablet once daily in the morning
- Recommended dose for patients with moderate renal impairment (eGFR 30–59 mL/min/1.73 m^2) is one tablet once daily in the morning. Not recommended in patients with severe renal impairment (eGFR 15–29 mL/min/1.73 m^2)
- Recommended dose when co-administered with strong CYP2D6 inhibitors is one tablet once daily in the morning

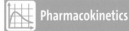 **Pharmacokinetics**

- Dextromethorphan is primarily metabolized by CYP2D6, bupropion inhibits the metabolism of dextromethorphan via CYP2D6
- Steady-state plasma concentrations of dextromethorphan and bupropion when given as dextromethorphan/bupropion combination are achieved within 8 days
- Median Tmax of dextromethorphan and bupropion when given as dextromethorphan/bupropion combination was 3 h and 2 h, respectively

‡ Indications listed here do not necessarily apply to all countries. Please refer to a country's regulatory database (e.g., US Food and Drug Administration, Health Canada Drug Product Database) for the most current availability information and indications

- C_{max} of hydroxybupropion metabolite occurred approximately 3 h post dose and was approximately 14 times the peak level of bupropion, and its AUC_{0-12} was about 19 times that of bupropion
- When dextromethorphan/bupropion combination was administered with food, dextromethorphan C_{max} was unchanged and AUC_{0-12} was decreased by 14%, and bupropion C_{max} and AUC_{0-12} were increased by 3% and 6%, respectively
- Plasma protein binding of dextromethorphan is approximately 60–70% and that of bupropion is 84%. The protein binding of the hydroxybupropion metabolite is similar to that of bupropion
- Mean elimination half-life of dextromethorphan and bupropion was 22 h and 15 h, respectively
- Bupropion is extensively metabolized with three active metabolites: hydroxybupropion (via CYP2B6), threohydroxybupropion, and erythrohydroxybupropion
- In CYP2D6 extensive metabolizers, approximately 37–52% of orally administered dose of dextromethorphan is recovered in the urine; approximately 45–83% in CYP2D6 poor metabolizers

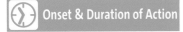 **Onset & Duration of Action**

- In a randomized, double-blind, phase 3 trial of dextromethorphan/bupropion (45 mg/105 mg extended-release tablet) vs. placebo (once daily for days 1–3, twice daily thereafter) for 6 weeks, significant improvements in depressive symptoms (i.e., change in MADRS total score from baseline) were noted in patients treated with dextromethorphan/bupropion compared to placebo starting 1 week after treatment initiation

Adverse Effects

- See p. 93
- In a 6-week placebo-controlled study, 6.2% of patients randomized to dextromethorphan/bupropion combination and 0.6% of patients randomized to placebo discontinued participation due to adverse reactions. The adverse reaction that led to study discontinuation in $\geq 1\%$ of patients was anxiety (2%)
- Most common adverse reactions in a 6-week placebo-controlled study (incidence $\geq 5\%$ with dextromethorphan/bupropion combination and more than twice as frequent as with placebo) were dizziness (16%), headache (8%), diarrhea (7%), somnolence (7%), dry mouth (6%), sexual dysfunction (6%), and hyperhidrosis (5%)
- Postmarketing experience with the individual components of the dextromethorphan/bupropion combination showed side effects for dextromethorphan as drowsiness, dizziness, nervousness or restlessness, nausea, vomiting, and stomach pain; for bupropion, arthralgia, myalgia, and fever with rash and other symptoms suggestive of delayed hypersensitivity (these symptoms may resemble serum sickness)

CNS Effects

- Abnormal electroencephalogram (EEG), aggression, agitation, akinesia, aphasia, coma, completed suicide, delirium, delusions, depression, dysarthria, euphoria, extrapyramidal syndrome (dyskinesia, dystonia, hypokinesia, parkinsonism), hallucinations, homicidal ideation, hostility, increased libido, manic reaction, neuralgia, neuropathy, panic, paranoid ideation, psychosis, restlessness, suicidal ideation, suicide attempt, and unmasked tardive dyskinesia

Cardiovascular Effects

- Complete atrioventricular block, extrasystoles, hypotension, hypertension (in some cases severe), phlebitis, and pulmonary embolism

Endocrine & Metabolic Effects

- Hyperglycemia, hypoglycemia, hyponatremia, syndrome of inappropriate antidiuretic hormone secretion, glycosuria

GI Effects

- Colitis, esophagitis, gastrointestinal hemorrhage, gum hemorrhage, hepatitis, intestinal perforation, pancreatitis, stomach ulcer

Urogenital & Sexual Effects

- Abnormal ejaculation, cystitis, dyspareunia, dysuria, gynecomastia, menopause, painful erection, salpingitis, urinary incontinence, urinary retention, and vaginitis

Hematological Effects

- Anemia, leukocytosis, leukopenia, pancytopenia, and thrombocytopenia. Altered PT and/or INR, infrequently associated with hemorrhagic or thrombotic complications, observed when bupropion co-administered with warfarin

Other Adverse Effects

- Lymphadenopathy
- Muscle rigidity/fever/rhabdomyolysis and muscle weakness
- Pneumonia
- Alopecia, angioedema, exfoliative dermatitis, hirsutism, Stevens-Johnson syndrome

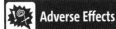 **Discontinuation Syndrome**

- No information is currently available regarding symptoms associated with the discontinuation of the dextromethorphan/bupropion combination product. The following is regarding the individual agents:

NMDA Receptor Antagonist/CYP2D6 Inhibitor (cont.)

- Dextromethorphan: Abrupt discontinuation may cause a syndrome consisting of restlessness, insomnia, cold flashes, diarrhea, and vomiting
- Bupropion:
  - Abrupt discontinuation may cause a syndrome consisting of dizziness, lethargy, nausea, vomiting, diarrhea, headache, fever, sweating, chills, malaise, incoordination, insomnia, vivid dreams, myalgia, paresthesias, dyskinesias, "electric-shock-like" sensations, visual discoordination, anxiety, irritability, confusion, slowed thinking, disorientation; rarely aggression, impulsivity, hypomania, and depersonalization
  - Brain "zaps" (or electric-shock-like sensations), often associated with lateral eye movements, hearing static sounds, and feelings of dizziness/wooziness; usually transitory but may last for months
  - Most likely to occur within 1–7 days after drug stopped or dose drastically reduced, and typically disappears within 3 weeks

 Contraindications

- Patient with seizure disorder
- Patient with current or prior diagnosis of bulimia or anorexia nervosa as a higher incidence of seizures was observed in such patients treated with the immediate-release formulation of bupropion
- Patient undergoing abrupt discontinuation of alcohol, benzodiazepines, barbiturates, or antiepileptic drugs
- Patient taking, or within 14 days of stopping, MAOIs due to the risk of serious and possibly fatal drug interactions including hypertensive crisis and serotonin syndrome
- Avoid use in patients with untreated narrow-angle glaucoma

 Precautions

- Assess blood pressure and monitor periodically during treatment
- Screen patients for personal or family history of bipolar disorder, mania, or hypomania
- Screen patients to determine if patient is receiving any other medications that contain bupropion or dextromethorphan

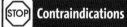 **Toxicity**

- Dextromethorphan: nausea, vomiting, stupor, coma, respiratory depression, seizures, tachycardia, hyperexcitability, toxic psychosis. Other adverse effects include ataxia, nystagmus, dystonia, blurred vision, and changes in muscle reflexes. Dextromethorphan may cause serotonin syndrome, and this risk is increased by overdose, particularly if taken with other serotonergic agents, including SSRIs or tricyclic antidepressants
- Bupropion:
  - Serious reactions reported with overdoses of bupropion alone included seizures, hallucinations, loss of consciousness, mental status changes, sinus tachycardia, ECG changes such as conduction disturbances (including QRS prolongation) or arrhythmias, clonus, myoclonus, and hyperreflexia. Fever, muscle rigidity, rhabdomyolysis, hypotension, stupor, coma, and respiratory failure have been reported mainly when bupropion was part of multiple drug overdoses
  - Rare reports of death following massive overdose, preceded by uncontrolled seizures, bradycardia, cardiac failure, and cardiac arrest

Management

- Single dose of activated charcoal if patient presents within 1 h of ingestion
- Supportive treatment
- Monitor ECG and vital signs for 18 h as well as EEG
- Benzodiazepines are first-line therapy for seizures

 Pediatric Considerations

- Not approved for use in pediatric patients
- The safety and effectiveness of the dextromethorphan/bupropion combination in pediatric patients has not been established

 Geriatric Considerations

- Clinical studies of the dextromethorphan/bupropion combination did not include patients aged 65 years and older to determine whether they respond differently than younger adult patients
- Bupropion:
  - The elderly are at risk for accumulation of bupropion and its metabolites due to decreased clearance
  - Orthostatic hypotension or dizziness reported; may predispose to falls
  - Extrapyramidal effects reported; not dose related and can develop with short-term or long-term use

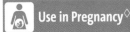

Use in Pregnancy◇

- Based on animal studies, the dextromethorphan/bupropion combination may cause fetal harm when administered during pregnancy. Discontinue treatment in pregnant females and advise patient about potential risk to fetus
- Insufficient clinical data for the dextromethorphan/bupropion combination during pregnancy to evaluate a drug-associated risk of major birth malformations, miscarriage, or other adverse maternal or fetal outcomes
- Available data on bupropion:
  - Epidemiological studies of pregnant women exposed to bupropion in the first trimester have not identified an increased risk of congenital malformations overall
  - Data from the international Bupropion Pregnancy Registry (675 first-trimester exposures) and a retrospective cohort study using the United Healthcare database (1,213 first-trimester exposures) did not show an increased risk of malformations overall
  - No increased risk for cardiovascular malformations overall observed after first-trimester exposure to bupropion
  - No harm to fetus reported in animal studies; no teratogenic effects reported in humans following bupropion use in first trimester
  - Higher umbilical cord concentration of metabolites suggests a higher fetal exposure vs. parent drug – consequences yet to be determined
  - Small prospective pharmacokinetic study concluded that although maternal exposure to bupropion may be slightly reduced over the course of pregnancy, exposure to the pharmacologically active metabolite appears similar to non-pregnant state

Breast Milk

- Bupropion and metabolites are secreted in breast milk; infant can receive up to 2% of maternal weight-adjusted dose
- Seizures and sleep disturbances reported in breastfed infants following bupropion exposure via breast milk
- Unknown whether dextromethorphan is present in human milk. No data on the effects of dextromethorphan in breastfed infants or the effects on milk production. Because of potential for neurotoxicity, advise patients that breastfeeding is not recommended during treatment with dextromethorphan/bupropion combination and for 5 days following final dose
- Infants of mothers using psychotropic medications should be monitored daily for changes in sleep, feeding patterns, and behavior as well as infant growth and neurodevelopment

 Nursing Implications

- Can be administered with or without food
- Tablets are to be swallowed whole and not crushed, divided, or chewed
- Crushing or chewing the extended-release tablets destroys the slow-release activity of the product
- Monitor therapy by watching for adverse effects and changes in mood and activity levels, including worsening depression and suicidal thoughts, especially at the start of therapy or following an increase or decrease in dose
- Can cause seizures; excessive use or abrupt discontinuation of alcohol, benzodiazepines, antiepileptic drugs, or sedative/hypnotics can increase the risk
- Assess blood pressure and monitor periodically

 Patient Instructions

- For detailed patient instructions on esketamine, see the Patient Information Sheet (details p. 474)

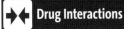 **Drug Interactions**

- Clinically significant interactions are listed below
- Also, see drug interactions for bupropion p. 23
- For more interaction information on any given combination, also see the corresponding chapter for the second agent

◇ See p. 473 for further information on drug use in pregnancy and effects on breast milk

NMDA Receptor Antagonist/CYP2D6 Inhibitor (cont.)

Class of Drug	Example	Interaction Effects
Cardiac glycoside	Digoxin	CNS toxicity reported with bupropion. Adverse reactions include restlessness, agitation, tremor, ataxia, gait disturbance, vertigo, and dizziness
CNS depressant	Alcohol	Bupropion can increase adverse neuropsychiatric events or reduce alcohol tolerance. Consumption of alcohol should be minimized or avoided during treatment with dextromethorphan/bupropion combination
CYP2B6 inducer (strong)	Carbamazepine, efavirenz, phenytoin	Decreased plasma concentrations of dextromethorphan and bupropion and may decrease efficacy of dextromethorphan/bupropion combination. Avoid co-administration of dextromethorphan/bupropion combination with strong inducers of CYP2B6
CYP2D6 inhibitor (strong)	Fluoxetine, paroxetine, quinidine, ritonavir	Increased plasma level of dextromethorphan. Dose adjustment necessary. Monitor for adverse reactions potentially attributable to dextromethorphan, such as somnolence and dizziness
CYP2D6 substrate	Atomoxetine, haloperidol, metoprolol, venlafaxine	Increased plasma level of dextromethorphan. Dose adjustment necessary. Monitor for adverse reactions potentially attributable to dextromethorphan, such as somnolence and dizziness.
Dopaminergic agent	Amantadine, levodopa	Decreased plasma level of bupropion and increased level of its metabolite hydroxybupropion due to increased metabolism by the anticonvulsant

Effects of Antidepressants on Neurotransmitters/Receptors*

	SSRIs						NDRI	SNRIs			SARIs		SPARI	SMS
	Citalo-pram	Escitalo-pram	Fluoxe-tine	Fluvoxa-mine	Paroxe-tine	Sertraline	Bupro-pion	Duloxetine	Levomil-nacipran	Venlafax-ine[(*)]	Nefazo-done	Trazodone	Vilazo-done	Vortioxe-tine
NE reuptake block	+	+	++	++	+++	++	+	++++	+++	+	++	−	+++	++
5-HT reuptake block	++++	++++	++++	++++	+++++	+++++	−	++++	+++	+++	++	++	+++++	++++
DA reuptake block	−	−	+	−	++	+++	++	++	−	+	++	−	+++	+
5-HT$_{1A}$ blockade	−	?	−	−	−	−	−	+	−	−	+++	+++	++++[(**)]	+++[(***)]
5-HT$_{2A}$ blockade	+	?	++	−	−	+	−	++	−	−	+++	+++	++	−
M$_1$(ACh) blockade	+	+	++	−	++	+	−	+	−	−	−	−	+	−
H$_1$ blockade	++	+	+	−	−	−	+	+	−	−	−	++	++	−
α$_1$ blockade	+	+	+	+	+	++	−	+	−	−	+++	+++	++	−
α$_2$ blockade	−	?	+	+	+	+	−	+	−	−	++	++	+	−
D$_2$ blockade	−	?	−	−	−	−	−	−	−	−	++	+	++	−
Selectivity	NE < 5-HT	NE < 5-HT	NE < 5-HT	NE < 5-HT	NE < 5-HT	NE < 5-HT	NE > 5-HT	NE < 5-HT	NE > 5-HT	NE < 5-HT	NE < 5-HT	NE < 5-HT	NE < 5-HT	NE < 5-HT

[(*)] Desvenlafaxine has similar effects on neurotransmitters as venlafaxine   [(**)] Vilazodone is a partial agonist at the 5-HT$_{1A}$ receptor,   [(***)] Vortioxetine is an agonist at the 5-HT$_{1A}$ receptor

	NaSSA	Nonselective Cyclics											GABA$_A$ Receptor Positive Modulator	NMDA Receptor Antagonist	NMDA Receptor Antagonist/ CYP2D6 Inhibitor
	Mirtaza-pine	Amitrip-tyline	Amoxa-pine	Clomipra-mine	Desipra-mine	Doxepin	Imipra-mine	Maproti-line	Nortrip-tyline	Protripty-line	Trimipra-mine	Brexano-lone	Esketa-mine	Dextro-methorphan/ Bupropion
NE reuptake block	+	+++	++++	+++	+++++	+++	+++	++++	++++	+++++	++	−	−	+
5-HT reuptake block	−	+++	++	++++	++	++	+++	+	++	++	+	−	−	−
DA reuptake block	−	+	+	+	+	+	+	+	+	+	+	−	−	++
5-HT$_{1A}$ blockade	+++	++	++	+	+	++	+	−	++	+	+	−	−	−
5-HT$_{2A}$ blockade	+++	+++	+++++	+++	++	+++	+++	++	+++	+++	+++	−	−	−
M$_1$(ACh) blockade	++	+++	++	+++	++	+++	+++	++	++	+++	+++	−	−	−
H$_1$ blockade	++++	++++	+++	+++	++	+++++	+++	++++	+++	+++	+++++	−	−	+
α$_1$ blockade	++	+++	+++	+++	++	+++	+++	+++	+++	++	+++	−	−	+
α$_2$ blockade	+++	++	+	+	+	+	+	+	+	+	++	−	−	−
D$_2$ blockade	+	+	++	++	+	+	+	++	+	+	++	−	−	−
Selectivity	NE = 5-HT	NE > 5-HT	NE > 5-HT	NE < 5-HT	NE > 5-HT	NE > 5-HT	NE > 5-HT	NE > 5-HT	NE > 5-HT	NE > 5-HT	NE > 5-HT	n/a	n/a	DA > NE

Key: K_i (nM) > 10,000 = −; 1000–10,000 = +; 100–1000 = ++; 10–100 = +++; 1–10 = ++++; 0.1–1 = +++++; ? = unknown

See also the National Institute of Mental Health's Psychoactive Drugs Screening Program. Available at http://pdsp.med.unc.edu

* The ratio of K_i values (inhibition constant) between various neurotransmitters/receptors determines the pharmacological profile for any one drug

Pharmacological Effects of Antidepressants on Neurotransmitters/Receptors

NE Reuptake Blockade
- Antidepressant effect
- Side effects: Tremors, tachycardia, hypertension, sweating, insomnia, erectile and ejaculation problems
- Potentiation of pressor effects of NE (e.g., sympathomimetic amines)
- Interaction with guanethidine (blockade of antihypertensive effect)

5-HT Reuptake Blockade
- Antidepressant, anti-anxiety, anti-panic, anti-obsessional effect
- Can increase or decrease anxiety, depending on dose
- Side effects: Dyspepsia, nausea, headache, nervousness, akathisia, extrapyramidal effects, anorexia, sexual side effects
- Potentiation of drugs with serotonergic properties (e.g., L-tryptophan); caution regarding serotonin syndrome

DA Reuptake Blockade
- Antidepressant, antiparkinsonian effect; may enhance motivation and cognition and mitigate against prolactin elevation
- Side effects: Psychomotor activation, aggravation of psychosis

5-HT$_{1A}$ Agonism
- Postulated to be associated with procognitive, anxiolytic, and antidepressant effects
- Enhances dopamine release in prefrontal cortex

5-HT$_{2A}$ Antagonism
- Sedation, prodopaminergic action may ameliorate EPS, and postulated to improve (not worsen) negative, cognitive, and mood symptoms
- Enhances dopamine release in prefrontal cortex

5-HT$_{2C}$ Antagonism
- Increased appetite, weight gain
- Postulated to be associated with procognitive and antidepressant effects
- Inhibits dopamine and norepinephrine release in prefrontal cortex

M$_1$ Antagonism
- Second most potent action of cyclic antidepressants
- Side effects: Dry mouth, blurred vision, constipation, urinary retention, sinus tachycardia, QRS changes, memory disturbances, sedation, exacerbation/attack of narrow-angle glaucoma
- Potentiation of effects of drugs with anticholinergic properties

H$_1$ Antagonism
- Anti-emetic effect, anxiolytic effects
- Side effects: Sedation, postural hypotension, weight gain

α_1 Antagonism
- Side effects: Postural hypotension, dizziness, reflex tachycardia, sedation
- Potentiation of antihypertensives acting via α_1 blockade (e.g., prazosin, doxazosin, labetalol)

α_2 Antagonism
- May improve cognitive deficits and have antidepressant effects
- Antagonism of presynaptic α_2-adrenergic receptors enhances serotonin and norepinephrine neurotransmission
- Side effect: Sexual dysfunction, priapism

D$_2$ Antagonism
- Antipsychotic effect
- In mesolimbic tract – reduction in positive symptoms (note: TGAs are partial agonists at D$_2$ receptors, partial agonism of this receptor may also reduce positive symptoms; partial agonist behaves like an antagonist in cases where a hyperdopaminergic state exists)
- In nigrostriatal tract – EPS (e.g., dystonias, pseudoparkinsonism, akathisia, tardive movement disorders, etc.)
- In tuberoinfundibular tract – prolactin elevation (e.g., galactorrhea, sexual dysfunction, etc.)
- In mesocortical tract – may exacerbate negative symptoms

Frequency of Adverse Reactions to Antidepressants at Therapeutic Doses

Reaction	SSRIs						NDRI	SNRIs				SARIs	
	Citalo-pram	Escitalo-pram	Fluoxe-tine	Fluvox-amine	Paroxe-tine	Sertraline	Bupro-pion	Desvenla-faxine	Duloxe-tine	Levomil-nacipran	Venla-faxine	Nefazo-done	Trazodone
CNS Effects ⁻													
Drowsiness, sedation	> 10%	> 2%	> 10%	> 10%	> 10%	> 10%	> 2%	> 10%	> 10%	–	> 10%	> 30%	> 30%
Insomnia	> 10%	> 10%	> 10%(a)	> 10%	> 10%	> 10%	> 10%	> 10%	> 10%	> 5%	> 10%(a)	> 2%	> 2%
Excitement, hypomania*	> 2%	< 2%	> 2%	> 10%	> 2%	> 10%	> 10%(b)	> 3%	> 2%	–	> 10%(b)	> 2%	–(b)
Disorientation/confusion	< 2%	< 2%	> 10%	> 2%	< 2%	< 2%	< 2%	< 2%	–	–	> 2%	> 10%	< 2%
Headache	> 10%	< 2%	> 10%	> 10%	> 10%	> 10%	> 10%	> 3%	> 10%	> 10%	> 10%	> 30%	> 2%
Asthenia, fatigue	> 10%	> 2%	> 10%	> 10%	> 10%	> 2%	> 2%	> 10%	> 10%	–	> 10%	> 10%	> 10%
Anticholinergic Effects													
Dry mouth	> 10%	> 10%	> 10%	> 10%	> 10%	> 10%	> 10%	> 10%	> 5%	> 10%	> 10%	> 10%	> 10%
Blurred vision	> 2%	< 2%	> 2%	> 2%	> 2%	> 2%	> 10%	> 3%	> 2%	< 2%	> 2%	> 10%	> 2%(c)
Constipation	> 2%	> 2%	> 2%	> 10%	> 10%	> 10%	> 10%	> 10%	> 10%	< 10%	> 10%	> 10%	> 2%
Sweating	> 10%	> 2%	> 2%	> 10%	> 10%	> 2%	> 10%	> 10%	> 10%	< 10%	> 10%	> 2%	–
Delayed micturition**	> 2%	–	> 2%	> 2%	> 2%	< 2%	> 2%	< 2%	< 2%	> 2%(d)	< 2%	< 2%	< 2%
Extrapyramidal Effects													
Unspecified	> 2%	< 2%	< 2%	> 2%(e)	> 2%	> 2%	< 2%	?	< 2%	< 2%	> 2%	< 2%	> 2%(e)
Tremor	> 2%	< 2%	> 10%	> 10%	> 10%	> 10%	> 10%	> 2%	> 2%	< 2%	> 2%	< 2%	> 2%
Cardiovascular Effects													
Orthostatic hypotension/dizziness	> 2%	> 2%	> 10%	> 2%	> 10%	> 10%	> 2%(f)	> 10%(f)	> 10%(f)	> 10%	> 10%(f)	> 10%	> 10%(g)
Tachycardia, palpitations	> 2%(h)	> 2%(h)	< 2%(h)	< 2%(h)	> 2%(h)	> 2%(h)	> 2%	> 3%	> 2%	> 2%	> 2%(i)	< 2%(h)	> 2%
ECG changes***	< 2%	< 2%	< 2%	< 2%	< 2%	< 2%	< 2%	< 2%	–	< 2%	< 2%(i)	< 2%	> 2%
Cardiac arrhythmia	< 2%	< 2%	< 2%(k)	< 2%	< 2%	< 2%	< 2%	< 2%	–	< 2%	< 2%	< 2%	> 2%(l)
GI distress	> 10%	> 10%	> 10%	> 30%	> 10%	> 30%	> 10%	> 30%	> 10%	> 20%	> 30%	> 10%	> 10%
Dermatitis, rash	< 2%	< 2%	> 2%	> 2%	< 2%	> 2%	> 2%	< 2%	> 2%	< 2%	> 2%	< 2%	< 2%
Weight gain (over 6 kg) #	> 2%	< 2%	> 2%(m)	> 2%(m)	> 10%(m)	≥ 2%(m)	< 2%(m)	?	> 2%	–	> 2%(m)	> 2%	> 2%
Sexual disturbances	> 30%	> 10%	> 30%(n)	> 30%	> 30%(n)	> 30%(n)	< 2%(n)(o)	> 3%	> 30%	< 10%	> 30%(n)	> 2%	< 2%(n)
Seizures ##	< 2%	< 2%	< 2%	< 2%	< 2%	< 2%	< 2%(p)	< 2%	< 2%	< 1%	< 2%	< 2%	< 2%

⁻ None reported in literature perused, * More likely in bipolar patients, ** Primarily in the elderly, *** ECG abnormalities usually without cardiac injury, # With chronic treatment, ## In nonepileptic patients; risk increased with elevated plasma levels (a) Especially if given in the evening, (b) Less likely to precipitate mania, (c) Found to lower intraocular pressure, (d) Dose-related (e) Tardive dyskinesia reported (rarely), (f) Hypertension reported; may be more common in patients with pre-existing hypertension, (g) Less frequent if drugs given after meals, (h) Decreased heart rate reported, (i) Increased risk with higher doses, (k) Slowing of sinus node and atrial dysrhythmia, (l) Patients with pre-existing cardiac disease have a 10% incidence of premature ventricular contractions, (m) Weight loss reported initially, (n) Priapism reported, (o) Improved sexual functioning, (p) Higher incidence if doses used above 450 mg/day of bupropion or in patients with bulimia

Frequency of Adverse Reactions to Antidepressants at Therapeutic Doses (cont.)

Reaction	SPARI Vilazodone	SMS Vortioxetine	NaSSA Mirtazapine	Nonselective Cyclics Amitriptyline	Amoxapine	Clomipramine	Desipramine	Doxepin	Imipramine	Maprotiline	Nortriptyline	Protriptyline	Trimipramine
CNS Effects ⁻													
Drowsiness, sedation	< 2%	< 2%	> 30%(q)	> 30%	> 10%	> 2%	> 2%	> 30%	> 10%	> 10%	> 2%	< 2%	> 30%
Insomnia	< 2%	–	> 2%	> 2%	> 10%	> 10%	> 2%	> 2%	> 10%	< 2%	< 2%	> 10%	> 2%(r)
Excitement, hypomania*	< 2%	< 0.1%	> 2%	< 2%	> 2%	< 2%	> 2%	< 2%	> 10%	> 2%	> 2%	> 10%	< 2%
Disorientation/confusion	< 2%	–	> 2%	> 10%	> 2%	> 2%	–	< 2%	> 2%	> 2%	> 10%	–	> 10%
Headache	< 2%	> 5%	> 2%	> 2%	> 2%	> 2%	< 2%	< 2%	> 10%	< 2%	< 2%	–	> 2%
Asthenia, fatigue	< 2%	> 2%	> 10%	> 10%	> 2%	> 2%	> 2%	> 2%	> 10%	> 2%	> 10%	> 10%	> 2%
Anticholinergic Effects													
Dry mouth	< 2%	> 5%	> 30%	> 30%	> 30%	> 30%	> 10%	> 30%	> 30%	> 30%	> 10%	> 10%	> 10%
Blurred vision	< 2%	–	> 10%	> 10%	> 2%	> 10%	> 2%	> 10%	> 10%	> 10%	> 2%	> 10%	> 2%
Constipation	< 2%	> 5%	> 10%	> 10%	> 30%	> 10%	> 2%	> 10%	> 10%	> 10%	> 10%	> 10%	> 10%
Sweating	< 2%	> 5%	> 2%	> 10%	> 2%	> 10%	> 2%	> 2%	> 10%	> 2%	< 2%	> 10%	> 2%
Delayed micturition**	> 2%	< 2%	> 2%	> 2%	> 10%	> 2%	–	< 2%	> 10%		< 2%	< 2%	< 2%
Extrapyramidal Effects													
Unspecified	< 2%	–	> 2%	> 2%(e)	> 2%(e)	< 2%(e)	< 2%	> 2%(e)	< 2%	> 2%	–	–	< 2%
Tremor	< 2%	–	> 2%	> 10%	> 2%	> 10%	> 2%	> 2%	> 10%	> 10%	> 10%	> 2%	> 10%
Cardiovascular Effects													
Orthostatic hypotension/dizziness	< 2%	< 10%	> 2%	> 10%	> 10%	> 10%	> 2%	> 10%	> 30%	> 2%	> 2%	> 10%	> 10%
Tachycardia, palpitations	< 2%	–	> 2%	> 10%	> 10%	> 10%	> 10%	> 2%	> 10%	> 2%	> 2%	> 2%	> 2%
ECG changes***	< 2%	–	< 2%	> 10%(s)	< 2%(s)	> 10%(s)	> 2%(s)	> 2%(s)	> 10%(s)	< 2%(s)	> 2%(s)	> 10%(s)	> 10%(s)
Cardiac arrhythmia	< 2%	–	< 2%	> 2%	< 2%	> 2%	> 2%	> 2%	> 2%	< 2%	> 2%	> 2%	> 2%
GI distress	> 2%	> 30%	> 2%	> 2%	> 2%	> 10%	> 2%	< 2%	> 10%	> 2%	< 2%	–	< 2%
Dermatitis, rash	< 2%	> 2%	< 2%	> 2%	> 10%	> 2%	> 2%	< 2%	> 2%	> 10%	< 2%	< 2%	< 2%
Weight gain (over 6 kg)	< 2%	–	> 30%	> 30%	< 2%	> 10%	> 2%	> 10%	> 10%	> 10%	> 2%	< 2%	> 10%
Sexual disturbances	< 2%	> 20%	> 2%	> 2%	> 2%	> 30%	> 2%	> 2%	> 30%	< 2%	< 2%	< 2%	< 2%
Seizures ##	< 2%	–	< 2%	< 2%	< 2%(t)	< 2%(t)	< 2%	< 2%	< 2%	< 2%(t)	< 2%	< 2%	< 2%

⁻ None reported in literature perused,   * More likely in bipolar patients,   ** Primarily in the elderly,   *** ECG abnormalities usually without cardiac injury,   ## In nonepileptic patients   (e) Tardive dyskinesia reported (rarely),   (q) Sedation decreased at higher doses (above 15 mg),   (r) No effect on REM sleep,   (s) Conduction delays: Increased PR, QRS or QTc interval,   (t) Higher incidence if dose above 250 mg daily clomipramine, 225 mg daily maprotiline, or 300 mg daily amoxapine

Reaction	MAOIs					GABA_A Receptor Positive Modulator	NMDA Receptor Antagonist	NMDA Receptor Antagonist/CYP2D6 Inhibitor
	Moclobemide	Isocarboxazid	Phenelzine	Tranylcypromine	Selegiline Transdermal	Brexanolone	Esketamine	Dextromethorphan/ Bupropion
CNS Effects [−]								
Drowsiness, sedation	> 2%	> 2%	> 10%	> 10%	< 2%	> 10%	> 10%	> 2%
Insomnia	> 10%[a]	> 2%[a]	> 10%[a]	> 10%[a]	> 10%	–	> 2%	> 2%
Excitement, hypomania[*]	> 10%	> 2%	> 10%	> 10%	> 2%	–	> 2%	–
Disorientation/confusion	> 2%	> 2%	> 2%	> 2%	< 2%	–	> 10%	–
Headache	> 10%	> 10%	> 2%	> 10%	> 10%	–	> 10%	> 2%
Asthenia, fatigue	< 2%	> 2%	< 2%	< 2%	< 2%	> 2%	> 2%	> 2%
Anticholinergic Effects								
Dry mouth	> 10%	> 10%	> 30%	> 10%	> 2%	> 2%	> 2%	> 2%
Blurred vision	> 10%	> 2%	> 10%	> 2%	< 2%	–	–	> 2%
Constipation	> 2%	> 2%	> 10%	> 2%	> 2%	–	> 2%	> 2%
Sweating	> 2%	< 2%	–	> 2%	> 2%	–	< 2%	< 2%
Delayed micturition[**]	< 2%	> 2%	> 2%	> 2%	< 2%	–	> 2%	–
Extrapyramidal Effects								
Unspecified	< 2%	> 2%	> 10%	< 2%	< 2%	–	–	–
Tremor	> 2%	> 10%	> 10%	> 2%	< 2%	–	> 2%	–
Cardiovascular Effects								
Orthostatic hypotension/dizziness	> 10%	> 10%	> 10%	> 10%	> 2%[g]	–	–	–
Tachycardia	> 2%	–	> 10%[h]	> 10%[h]	< 2%	> 2%	> 2%	–
ECG changes[***]	> 2%	> 2%	< 2%[u]	< 2%[u]	< 2%	–	–	–
Cardiac arrhythmia	> 2%	> 2%	< 2%	< 2%	< 2%	–	–	–
GI distress (nausea)	> 10%	> 10%	> 10%	> 2%	> 2%	> 2%	> 10%	> 10%
Dermatitis, rash	> 2%	> 2%	< 2%	> 2%	> 10%[w]	> 2%	–	–
Weight gain (over 6 kg)	< 2%	> 2%	> 10%	> 2%	> 2%[m]	–	–	–
Sexual disturbances	> 2%	> 2%	> 30%[n]	> 2%[n]	< 2%	–	–	–
Seizures [##]	< 2%	–	< 2%	–[x]	–	–	–	–

[−] None reported in literature perused,   [*] More likely in bipolar patients,   [**] Primarily in the elderly,   [***] ECG abnormalities usually without cardiac injury,   [##] In nonepileptic patients   [a] Especially if given in the evening,   [g] Hypertension reported,
[h] Decreased heart rate reported,   [m] Weight loss reported,   [n] Priapism reported,   [u] Shortened QTc interval,   [w] At site of patch application,   [x] May have anticonvulsant activity

Antidepressant Doses and Pharmacokinetics

Drug	Therapeutic Dose Range (mg)	Comparable Dose (mg)	Suggested Plasma Level (nmol/L)	Bioavai-lability (%)	Protein Binding (%)	Peak Plasma Level (h) (T_{max})	Elimination Half-life (h) ($T_{1/2}$)	Metabolizing Enzymes[*] (CYP450; other)	Enzyme Inhibition[**] (CYP450; other)
SSRIs									
Citalopram (Celexa)	10–40	10		80	80	4	23–45[b]	2D6[c][m], 2C19[m], 3A4[m]	2D6[w], 2C9[w], 2C19[w]
Escitalopram (Lexapro, Cipralex)	10–20	5		80	56	4–5 (metabolite = 14)	27–32[b] [d]	2D6[m], 3A4[m], 2C19[m]	2D6[w], 2C9[w], 2C19[w]
Fluoxetine (Prozac)	10–80[e]	10		72–85	94	6–8 (immediate release)	24–144 (parent)[b] 200–330 (metabolite)	1A2[w], 2B6[w], **2D6**[c] [p], 3A4[w], **2C9**[p], **2C19**[p], 2E1	1A2[m], 2B6[w], **2D6**[p], 3A4[c] [w], 2C9[w], 2C19[m]; P-gp
Fluoxetine delayed release (Prozac Weekly)	90 mg/week	10		72–85	94	6–8 (absorption delayed 1–2 h)	24–144 (parent)[b] 200–330 (metabolite)	1A2[w], 2B6[w], 2D6[c] [m], 3A4[w], **2C9**[p], **2C19**[p], 2E1	1A2[m], 2B6[w], **2D6**[p], 3A4[c] [w], 2C9[w], 2C19[m]; P-gp
Fluvoxamine (Luvox)	50–300[e]	35		60	77–80	1.5–8	9–28[b]	1A2[w], 2D6	**1A2**[p], 2B6[w], 2D6[m], 3A4[w], 2C9[m], **2C19**[p]; P-gp
Paroxetine (Paxil)	10–60[e]	10		> 90	95	5.2 (immediate release)	3–65[b] [d]	**2D6**[p]; P-gp	1A2[w], **2B6**[p], **2D6**[p], 3A4[w], 2C9[w], 2C19[m]; P-gp
Paroxetine CR (Paxil CR)	12.5–75	12.5		> 90	95	C_{max} = 6–10 (CR)	15–20	**2D6**[p]; P-gp	1A2[w], **2B6**[p], **2D6**[p], 3A4[w], 2C9[w], 2C19[m]; P-gp
Sertraline (Zoloft)	50–200[e]	25		70	98	6	22–36 (parent) [b] [d] 62–104 (metabolite)	2B6, 2D6, **3A4**[p], 2C9, 2C19[m]; UGT2B7	1A2[w], 2B6[m], 2D6[w], 3A4[w], 2C9[w], **2C19**[p]; P-gp
NDRI									
Bupropion (Wellbutrin)	225–450[f]	100[f]	75–350[a]	> 90	80–85	1.6 (immediate release)	10–14 (parent)[b]	1A2[w], **2B6**[p], 2D6[c], 3A4[w], 2C9[w], 2E1[m]	2D6[w]
Bupropion SR (Wellbutrin SR, Zyban)	150–300[f]	150[f]				3 (bupropion) 6 (metabolite) (SR)	20–27 (metabolites)		
Bupropion ER (Forfivo XL – only used after initial titration with other bupropion HCL products)	450	450				5 (fasting); delayed in fed state			
Bupropion ER (Aplenzin)	174–522	150–450				5			

Drug	Therapeutic Dose Range (mg)	Comparable Dose (mg)	Suggested Plasma Level (nmol/L)	Bioavai-lability (%)	Protein Binding (%)	Peak Plasma Level (h) (T_{max})	Elimination Half-life (h) ($T_{1/2}$)	Metabolizing Enzymes[*] (CYP450; other)	Enzyme Inhibition[**] (CYP450; other)
SNRIs									
Venlafaxine (Effexor)	75–375	40		13	27	2 (immediate release)	3–7 (parent)[b] [d] 9–13 (metabolite)	**2D6**[p], 3A4[c] [w], 2C9, 2C19	2D6[w], 3A4[w]
Venlafaxine XR (Effexor XR)						XR = 5.5	9–12 (absorption half-life)		
Desvenlafaxine (Pristiq)	50–100	40	–	80	30	7.5	11[d]	**UGT**[p], 3A4	2D6
Duloxetine (Cymbalta)	60–120	?		70	> 95	6	8–19[b] [d]	1A2, 2D6	2D6[m]
Levomilnacipran (Fetzima)	20–120	?	n/a	92	22	6–8	12	2C8, 2C19, **3A4**	
SARIs									
Nefazodone (Serzone)	100–600	130		99	15–23	2	2–5[h] (parent) 3–18 (metabolites)	2D6[c], **3A4**[p]	1A2[w], 2D6[w], **3A4**[p]; P-gp (acute dosing); inducer of P-gp
Trazodone (Desyrel)	150–600	100		70–90	93	2	4–9	2D6[c], **3A4**[p]	2D6[w]; inducer of P-gp
SPARI									
Vilazodone (Viibryd)	10–40	20	n/a	72 with food (50 fasting)	96–99	4–5	~25	1A2[w], 2D6[w], **3A4**[p]	2C8[w], 2D6[w]
SMS									
Vortioxetine (Brintellix)	5–20	?	n/a	75	98	7–11	57	2A6, 2B6, 2C8, 2C9, 2C19, **2D6**, 3A4/5	–
NaSSA									
Mirtazapine (Remeron)	15–60	12.5		50	85	2	20–40[b] [d]	**1A2**[p], 2D6[c] [p], **3A4**[p], 2C9	–
Nonselective cyclic agents									
Amitriptyline (Elavil)	75–300	30	250–825[a] [g]	43–48	92–96	2–8	10–46[b]	1A2[w], 2B6[w], 2D6[m], **3A4**[p], 2C9[w], **2C19**[p] 1A2[w], 2D6, 3A4[w], 2C9[w], 2C19[w]; P-gp	1A2, 2D6[m], 3A4, 2C9[w], 2C19[m], 2E1; P-gp; UGT
Amoxapine (Asendin)	100–600	100		46–82	?	1–2	8–14[b]	–	2D6
Clomipramine (Anafranil)	75–300	30	300–1000	98	98	2–6	17–37[b]	1A2, **2D6**[p]	2D6[m]; UGT
Desipramine (Norpramin)	75–300	50	400–1000[g]	73–92	73–92	2–6	12–76[b]	1A2, **2D6**[p], 3A4, 2C9[w], **2C19**[p]	2D6[m], 2C19[w], 2E1; P-gp
Doxepin (Sinequan, Triadapin)	75–300	35	500–950[a]	89	89	2–6	8–36[b]	1A2[w], 2B6[w], **2D6**[p], 3A4[m], 2C9[w], 2C19[m]; UGT1A3; UGT1A4	–
Imipramine (Tofranil)	75–300	35	500–800[a]	89	89	2–6	4–34[b]	**2D6**[p], 3A4[m], 2C9[w], 2C19[w]; UGT1A4	1A2, 2D6[m], 2C19[m], 2E1; P-gp; UGT1A3
Maprotiline (Ludiomil)	100–225	30	200–950[a]	66–100	88	9–16	27–58[b]	1A2, **2D6**[p]	2D6; P-gp

Drug	Therapeutic Dose Range (mg)	Comparable Dose (mg)	Suggested Plasma Level (nmol/L)	Bioavailability (%)	Protein Binding (%)	Peak Plasma Level (h) (T_{max})	Elimination Half-life (h) ($T_{1/2}$)	Metabolizing Enzymes* (CYP450; other)	Enzyme Inhibition** (CYP450; other)
Nortriptyline (Aventyl, Pamelor)	40–200	25	150–500(g)	89–92	89–92	2–6	13–88(b)	1A2, 2D6(m), 3A4(m), 2C19(w), P-gp	2D6, 2C19(w), 2E1
Protriptyline (Vivactil)	20–60	15	350–700	90–96	90–96	12	54–124(b)	?	?
Trimipramine (Surmontil)	75–300	50	500–800	95	95	2–6	7–30(b)	2D6, 2C9, 2C19	2D6; P-gp
RIMA									
Moclobemide (Manerix)	300–600	150	–	50–90 (after 2 weeks)	50	?	1–3(b)	2C19 (p)	1A2(m), 2D6(m), 2C9, 2C19(m)
MAOIs (irreversible)									
Isocarboxazid (Marplan)	30–50	10	?	?	?	?	2.5	–	–
Phenelzine (Nardil)	45–90	15	?	?	?	?	1.5–4	2E1	–
Tranylcypromine (Parnate)	20–60	10	–	?	?	?	2.4(b)	–	1A2(w), 2A6(p), 2D6(w), 2C9(w), 2C19(w), 3A4(w), 2E1(m)
MAO-B Inhibitor									
Selegiline Transdermal	6 mg/24 h to 12 mg/24 h	?	–	10–40	90	4	18–25	2A6, 2B6, 2C9, 3A4/5	2B6, 2D6, 3A4/5
GABA_A Receptor Positive Modulator									
Brexanolone (Zulresso)	30–90 micrograms/kg/h	n/a	n/a	100	> 99	–	6	AKRs, UGTs, SULTs	–
NMDA Receptor Antagonist									
Esketamine (Spravato)	56–84	n/a	n/a	48	43–45	.33–.66	7–12	2B6, 2C9, 2C19, 3A4	–
NMDA Receptor Antagonist/CYP2D6 Inhibitor									
Dextromethorphan/bupropion combination (Auvelity)	45/105 twice daily	n/a	n/a	?	Dextromethorphan: 60–70 Bupropion: 84	Dextromethorphan: 2 Bupropion: 3	Dextromethorphan: 22 Bupropion: 15	Dextromethorphan: 2D6 Bupropion: 1A2(w), **2B6**(p), 2C9(w), 2D6(c), 2E1(m), 3A4(w)	Bupropion: 2D6

* CYP450 isoenzymes involved in drug metabolism. ** CYP450 isoenzymes inhibited by the drug; magnitude may be influenced by drug dose and plasma concentration, and by genotype and basal metabolic capacity of each patient.

(a) Includes sum of drug and its metabolites. (b) Increased in liver disorders – consider dose adjustment. (c) Specific to metabolite. (d) Increased in moderate to severe renal impairment – consider dose adjustment. (e) SSRIs have a flat dose response curve. For depression most patients respond to the initial (low) dose. Higher doses are used in the treatment of OCD. (f) Give in divided doses (maximum of 150 mg per dose). (g) Established ranges for efficacy in major depressive disorder. (h) Dose-dependent. (m) Moderate activity. (p) Potent activity. (w) Weak activity.

P-gp = P-glycoprotein [a transporter of hydrophobic substances in or out of specific body organs (e.g., block absorption in the gut)]; UGT = uridine diphosphate glucuronosyl transferase [involved in Phase II reactions (conjugation)].

Clinical Handbook of Psychotropic Drugs, 25th edition, © 2023 Hogrefe Publishing

Switching Antidepressants

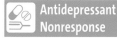

Antidepressant Nonresponse
- Ascertain that diagnosis is correct and that patient is compliant with therapy
- Ensure dosage prescribed is therapeutic; measure plasma level; ensure there has been an adequate trial period, i.e., up to 6 weeks at a reasonable dose
- Regular, systematic assessment of the patient's response to drug therapy, with the use of measurement tools for symptoms, adverse effects, and patient adherence is useful to guide future clinical decisions

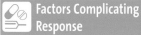

Factors Complicating Response
- Concurrent medical or psychiatric illness, e.g., hypothyroidism, OCD
- Personality disorders lead to poor outcome; however, depression may evoke personality problems that may disappear when the depression is alleviated
- Drug abuse may make management difficult (e.g., cocaine); see CANMAT recommendations
- Psychosocial factors may affect response
- Low folate levels associated with lack of remission, response and relapse
- Concurrent prescription drugs may interfere with efficacy (e.g., calcium channel blockers)
- Metabolic inducers (e.g., carbamazepine) or inhibitors (e.g., erythromycin) will affect plasma level of antidepressant
- Genetic variants

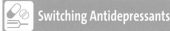

Switching Antidepressants
- Switching from one SSRI to another can enhance response in previously nonresponsive patients
- 20–25% remission rate when switching from SSRI to another class of antidepressant or a different SSRI after failure of first SSRI (STAR*D studies)
- Switching between tricyclic agents is of questionable benefit
- One study found significantly higher response rates when switching from imipramine to sertraline than vice versa and better tolerability
- Two studies have demonstrated that switching imipramine nonresponders to phenelzine was superior to switching phenelzine nonresponders to imipramine
- Use caution when switching to or from irreversible MAOIs (see Switching Antidepressants, pp. 97–99)

Advantages of Switching
- Minimizes polypharmacy
- Decreased risk of drug interactions
- Second agent may be better tolerated
- Improved compliance
- Less costly

Disadvantages of Switching
- Loss of partial efficacy of first agent
- Time required to taper first agent or need for a washout (risk of relapse)
- Delayed onset of action

Switching Strategies

Switching from		Switching to	Switching Method[a]
SSRI (not fluoxetine)	→	SSRI (including fluoxetine)	Direct switch, **OR** taper, stop, and switch
	→	NDRI, SPARI, clomipramine	Taper, stop, and switch
	→	SNRI	Taper, stop, and switch, **OR** cross-taper
	→	SARI, SMS, NaSSA, nonselective cyclics (not clomipramine)	Cross-taper
	→	RIMA, Irreversible MAOI, MAO-B	Taper, stop, washout (1 week), and switch

Switching Antidepressants (cont.)

Switching from		Switching to	Switching Method[a]
Fluoxetine	→	SSRI, NDRI, SPARI, SMS, nonselective cyclics (not clomipramine)	Taper, stop, washout (4–7 days), and switch
	→	SNRI	Taper, stop, and switch
	→	SARI	Cross-taper
	→	NaSSA	Taper, stop, washout (4–7 days), and switch **OR** cross-taper
	→	Clomipramine	Taper, stop, washout (2 weeks), and switch
	→	RIMA	Taper, stop, washout (5 weeks), and switch
	→	Irreversible MAOI, MAO-B	Taper, stop, washout (5–6 weeks), and switch
NDRI	→	SSRI (including fluoxetine), SNRI, SARI, SPARI, SMS, NaSSA, nonselective cyclics (including clomipramine)	Taper, stop and switch
	→	RIMA, Irreversible MAOI, MAO-B	Taper, stop, washout (1 week), and switch
SNRI	→	SSRI (not fluoxetine), SARI, SMS, NaSSA, nonselective cyclics (not clomipramine)	Cross-taper
	→	Fluoxetine, SPARI	Taper, stop and switch, **OR** cross-taper
	→	NDRI, SNRI, clomipramine	Taper, stop, and switch
	→	RIMA, Irreversible MAOI, MAO-B	Taper, stop, washout (1 week), and switch
SARI	→	SSRI (including fluoxetine), NDRI, SNRI, SPARI, SMS, NaSSA, nonselective cyclics (including clomipramine)	Cross-taper
	→	RIMA, Irreversible MAOI, MAO-B	Taper, stop, washout (1 week), and switch
SPARI[b]	→	SSRI (including fluoxetine), NDRI, SNRI, clomipramine	Taper, stop and switch
	→	SARI, SMS, NaSSA	Cross-taper
	→	Nonselective cyclics (not clomipramine)	Taper, stop, and switch **OR** cross-taper
	→	RIMA, Irreversible MAOI, MAO-B	Taper, stop, washout (2 weeks), and switch
SMS	→	SSRI (not fluoxetine)	Taper, stop, and switch **OR** cross-taper
	→	Fluoxetine, NDRI, clomipramine	Taper, stop and switch
	→	SNRI, SARI, SPARI, NaSSA, nonselective cyclics (not clomipramine)	Cross-taper
	→	RIMA, Irreversible MAOI, MAO-B	Taper, stop, washout (3 weeks), and switch
NaSSA	→	SSRI (including fluoxetine), SNRI, SPARI, nonselective cyclics (including clomipramine)	Taper, stop, and switch **OR** cross-taper
	→	NDRI	Taper, stop and switch
	→	SARI, SMS	Cross-taper
	→	RIMA	Taper, stop, washout (1 week), and switch
	→	Irreversible MAOI, MAO-B	Taper, stop, washout (2 weeks), and switch
Nonselective cyclic	→	SSRI (including fluoxetine), NDRI, SNRI, SARI, SPARI, SMS, nonselective cyclics (including clomipramine)	Cross-taper
	→	NaSSA	Taper, stop, and switch **OR** cross-taper
	→	RIMA	Taper, stop, washout (1 week), and switch
	→	Irreversible MAOI, MAO-B	Taper, stop, washout (2 weeks), and switch

Switching from		Switching to	Switching Method[a]
Clomipramine[c]	→	SSRI (not fluoxetine), SNRI, SPARI, SMS	Taper, stop and switch
	→	Fluoxetine	Taper, stop, washout (2–3 weeks), and switch
	→	NDRI, SARI, NaSSA, nonselective cyclics	Cross-taper
	→	RIMA	Taper, stop, washout (1 week), and switch
	→	Irreversible MAOIs, MAO-B	Taper, stop, washout (3 weeks), and switch
RIMA	→	SSRI (including fluoxetine), NDRI, SNRI, SARI, SMS, NaSSA, nonselective cyclics (including clomipramine), Irreversible MAOI, MAO-B	Taper, stop, washout (1 day), and switch
	→	SPARI	Taper, stop, washout (2 weeks), and switch
Irreversible MAOI[d]	→	SSRI (including fluoxetine), NDRI, SNRI, SARI, SPARI, SMS, NaSSA, nonselective cyclics (not clomipramine or imipramine), irrev. MAOI, MAO-B	Taper, stop, washout (2 weeks), and switch
	→	Clomipramine, imipramine	Taper, stop, washout (3 weeks), and switch
MAO-B	→	SSRI (including fluoxetine), NDRI, SNRI, SARI, SPARI, SMS, NaSSA, nonselective cyclics (not clomipramine or imipramine), irrev. MAOI, MAO-B	Taper, stop, washout (2 weeks), and switch
	→	Clomipramine, imipramine	Taper, stop, washout (3 weeks), and switch

[a] Switching Method:

Direct Switch: Stop the first antidepressant and start the new antidepressant the following day. Recommended if first antidepressant therapy duration is less than 6 weeks (interactions less likely) and/or switching to an antidepressant with similar mode of action (ameliorates withdrawal effects)

Taper, stop and switch: Gradually taper the first antidepressant and start the new antidepressant immediately after discontinuation. Recommended if first antidepressant therapy duration is more than 6 weeks

Taper, stop, washout, and switch: Gradually taper the first antidepressant and start the new antidepressant after a washout period

Cross-taper: Gradually taper down the first antidepressant and slowly simultaneously introduce and increase the dose of the new antidepressant

Speed of tapering and cross-taper is most commonly 1–2 weeks or longer and should be judged by monitoring tolerability of the individual patient, [b] Vilazodone is both an SSRI and a partial agonist of the 5-hydroxytryptamine 1A receptors. Caution is advised when switching to and from vilazodone due to limited relevant information from studies, [c] Clomipramine should not be co-administered with SSRIs, venlafaxine or duloxetine (except under specialist use) and cross-tapering is not recommended, [d] Should not be commenced before all other antidepressants have been trialed due to risk of hypertensive crisis and serotonin syndrome. Allow washout period and monitor patients individually

Antidepressant Augmentation Strategies

 Adjunctive Strategies | Largest evidence base for antidepressant nonresponders with MDD is the use of adjunctive atypical antipsychotics with at least 15 randomized double-blind studies to date

When to Consider an Adjunctive Medication
- Patient has already received at least 2 antidepressant trials
- Initial antidepressant is well tolerated
- Partial response (more than 25%) to initial agent
- Less time to wait for a response
- Patient prefers add-on

Advantages of Using an Adjunctive Medication
- May have rapid onset of response
- Response greater than 50% with most combinations
- No need to taper first agent or have a washout
- Avoids risk of withdrawal effects from first drug

Disadvantages of Using an Adjunctive Medication
- Increased potential for side effects
- Increased risk of drug interactions

Antidepressant Augmentation Strategies (cont.)

- Increased cost
- Decreased compliance possible due to need to take an increased number of tablets/capsules

Choosing Adjunctive Medications

- Adjunctive medication for nonresponse or partial response to antidepressant in MDD, according to the Canadian Network for Mood and Anxiety Treatments (CANMAT) 2016 clinical guidelines[23]

CANMAT Level of Evidence

- 1: Meta-analysis with narrow confidence intervals and/or 2 or more RCTs with adequate sample size, preferably placebo controlled
- 2: Meta-analysis with wide confidence intervals and/or 1 or more RCTs with adequate sample size
- 3: Small-sample RCTs or nonrandomized, controlled prospective studies or case series or high-quality retrospective studies
- 4: Expert opinion/consensus

CANMAT Line of Treatment

- First line: Level 1 or Level 2 evidence, plus clinical support
- Second line: Level 3 evidence or higher, plus clinical support
- Third line: Level 4 evidence or higher, plus clinical support

First-Line Adjunctive Medications

- Aripiprazole: Initial dose 2–5 mg/day; recommended dose 5–10 mg/day; maximum dose 15 mg/day
  - Level of evidence: 1
- Quetiapine: Initial dose 50 mg/day; recommended dose 150–300 mg/day; maximum dose 300 mg/day
  - Level of evidence: 1
- Risperidone: Initial dose 0.25 mg/day; recommended dose 1–3 mg/day
  - Level of evidence: 1
- Brexpiprazole: Initial dose 0.5–1 mg/day; recommended dose 1–3 mg/day
  - Level of evidence: 1

Second-Line Adjunctive Medications

- Bupropion: 150–300 mg/day
  - Level of evidence: 2
  - Of the 13 trials using bupropion as an adjunctive medication, 7 were open label
  - Of 5 studies with bupropion as an adjunctive to SSRIs, only one was a placebo-controlled, double-blind RCT. In a three-arm study (bupropion monotherapy vs. escitalopram monotherapy, vs. bupropion + escitalopram), the combination of bupropion + escitalopram was not significantly better than either medication used as monotherapy. There were more adverse events with the combination
  - There have been 2 studies using bupropion as an adjunctive to SNRIs. Positive results were found when bupropion was added to venlafaxine but not to when it was added to duloxetine
- Lithium: 600–1200 mg/day (use therapeutic serum levels to guide; 0.5–0.8 mmol/L)
  - Level of evidence: 2
  - Most lithium augmentation studies were with TCAs and had small sample sizes. Only three trials with lithium and SSRIs
  - Meta-analysis of 9 RCTs with 237 participants found overall comparison and the SSRI-only comparison to have significantly better efficacy than placebo. However, confidence intervals were wide, hence Level 2 evidence for efficacy
  - If no response within 7–10 days, consider alternative strategies
- Mirtazapine: 30–60 mg/day
  - Level of evidence: 2
  - A meta-analysis of 23 trials with 2435 participants, focusing on adverse events, found that an adjunctive antidepressant was associated with increased side effects compared to monotherapy, especially when adding mirtazapine or TCAs to SSRIs
- Modafinil: 100–400 mg/day
  - Level of evidence: 2
  - A meta-analysis of 4 trials involving 568 patients (of which only 2 with 211 patients were adjunctive trials) reported marginal evidence for efficacy in the modafinil-treated patients compared to placebo after an outlier was excluded

- Olanzapine: 2.5–10 mg/day
  - Level of evidence: 1
  - Considered second line due to unfavorable metabolic profile
- Triiodothyronine: 25–50 micrograms/day
  - Level of evidence: 2
  - There have only been 2 RCTs with lithium as an augmentation agent
  - Although not placebo controlled, triiodothyronine was also evaluated in the STAR*D study. No difference in remission rate compared to lithium, but triiodothyronine was better tolerated and had lower dropout rates
  - If no response within 3 weeks, consider alternative strategies

Third-Line Adjunctive Medications
- Other antidepressants
  - Level of evidence: 3
- Other stimulants (methylphenidate, lisdexamfetamine, etc.)
  - Level of evidence: 3
  - 2 RCTs of lisdexamfetamine showed efficacy as an adjunctive agent for partial responders to SSRIs. However, 2 unpublished phase III trials with 830 participants were negative
  - Other stimulants (e.g., methylphenidate) have negative studies
- TCAs (e.g., desipramine)
  - Level of evidence: 2
  - Considered third line due to higher side effect burden
- Ziprasidone
  - Level of evidence: 3

Brain Stimulation Strategies
- Repetitive transcranial magnetic stimulation (see pp. 117–120)
  - Typically used in medication-resistant patients, antidepressant effect reportedly greater in those with less chronic illness and fewer previous failed medication trials
- Electroconvulsive therapy (see pp. 104–110)
  - Concomitant treatment with an antidepressant can enhance the efficacy of ECT but may have variable effects on cognition

Complementary Adjunctive Medications
- Omega-3 fatty acids
  - Randomized double-blind placebo-controlled studies support the use of adjunctive omega-3 fatty acids (EPA and DHA) for patients with MDD who do not experience sufficient symptoms improvement following antidepressant therapy
  - Relatively well tolerated and accepted by patients
  - Conflicting results with dosing – one study found 2 g/day of ethyl-EPA to be superior to placebo as adjunctive therapy, a second found 1 g but not 2 g or 4 g to be superior to placebo, while a third found 660 mg/day of EPA-DHA mix to be superior to placebo
- S-Adenosyl-L-Methionine
  - Adjunctive treatment for use in mild to moderate MDD
  - Usual starting dose is 400 mg/day for the first 1-2 weeks, then increased by 200–400 mg/day every 5–7 days to a maximum dose of 800 mg bid
  - Variance in active ingredient(s) between manufacturers may limit efficacy
- Folate
  - Small overall benefits for unipolar depression; however, large doses (15 mg/day) of methylfolate as adjunctive therapy in MDD was found to have moderate-to-large benefits for depressive symptoms vs. placebo in a few small RCTs
  - Consider dietary enhancement first. Variance in active ingredient(s) between manufacturers may limit efficacy
  - Clinical utility of MTHFR genotyping unclear

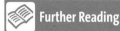 **Further Reading**

References

1. Cipriani A, Furukawa TA, Salanti G, et al. Comparative efficacy and acceptability of 21 antidepressant drugs for the acute treatment of adults with major depressive disorder: A systematic review and network meta-analysis. Lancet. 2018;391(10128):1357–1366. doi:10.1016/S0140-6736(17)32802-7

2. Hollander E, Soorya L, Chaplin W, et al. A double-blind placebo-controlled trial of fluoxetine for repetitive behaviors and global severity in adult autism spectrum disorders. Am J Psychiatry 2012;169(3):292–299. doi:10.1176/appi.ajp.2011.10050764

3. Singh, SP, Singh V, Kar N, et al. Efficacy of antidepressants in treating the negative symptoms of chronic schizophrenia: Meta-analysis. Br J Psychiatry. 2010;197(3):174–179. doi:10.1192/bjp.bp.109.067710

4. Albayrak Y, Hashimoto, K. Beneficial effects of the sigma-1 agonist fluvoxamine for tardive dyskinesia in patients with postpsychotic depressive disorder of schizophrenia: Report of 5 cases. Prim Care Companion CNS Disord. 2012;14(6):PCC.12br01401. doi:10.4088/PCC.12br01401

5. Jakubovski E, Johnson JA, Nasir M, et al. Systematic review and meta-analysis: Doses-response curve of SSRIs and SNRIs in anxiety disorders. Depress Anxiety. 2019;36(3):198–212. doi:10.1002/da.22854

6. Atmaca M. Selective serotonin reuptake inhibitor-induced sexual dysfunction: Current management perspectives. Neuropsychiatr Dis Treat. 2020;16:1043–1050. doi:10.2147/NDT.S185757

7. Jha MK, Rush AJ, Trivedi MH. When discontinuing SSRI antidepressants is a challenge: Management tips. Am J Psychiatry. 2018;175(12):1176–1184. doi:10.1176/appi.ajp.2018.18060692

8. Elbe D, Black TR, McGrane IR, et al. Clinical handbook of psychotropic drugs for children and adolescents. (4th ed.). Boston, MA: Hogrefe Publishing, 2019.

9. Seitz DP, Adunuri N, Gill SS, et al. Antidepressants for agitation and psychosis in dementia. Cochrane Database Syst Rev. 2011;2:CD008191. doi:10.1002/14651858.CD008191.pub2

10. Henry G, Williamson D, Tampi RR. Efficacy and tolerability of antidepressants in the treatment of behavioral and psychological symptoms of dementia, a literature review of evidence. Am J Alzheimers Dis Other Demen. 2011;26(3):169–183. doi:10.1177/1533317511402051

11. Sterke CS, Ziere G, van Beeck EF, et al. Dose-response relationship between selective serotonin re-uptake inhibitors and injurious falls: A study in nursing home residents with dementia. Br J Clin Pharmacol. 2012;73(5):812–820. doi:10.1111/j.1365-2125.2011.04124.x

12. Ames JL, Ladd-Acosta C, Fallin MD, et al. Maternal psychiatric conditions, treatment with selective serotonin reuptake inhibitors, and neurodevelopment disorders. Biol Psychiatry. 2021;90(4):253–262. doi:10.1016/j.biopsych.2021.04.002

13. Gao SY, Wu QJ, Sun C, et al. Selective serotonin reuptake inhibitor use during early pregnancy and congenital malformations: a systematic review and meta-analysis of cohort studies of more than 9 million births. BMC Medicine. 2018;16:205. doi:10.1186/s12916-018-1193-5

14. National Institutes of Health, COVID-19 Treatment Guidelines Panel. Coronavirus disease 2019 (COVID-19) treatment guidelines. https://www.covid19treatmentguidelines.nih.gov/

15. Karam-Hage M, Strobbe S, Robinson JD, et al. Bupropion-SR for smoking cessation in early recovery from alcohol dependence: A placebo-controlled, double-blind pilot study. Am J Drug Alcohol Abuse. 2011;37(6):487–490. doi:10.3109/00952990.2011.598591

16. de Silva VA, Hanwella R. Efficacy and tolerability of venlafaxine versus specific serotonin reuptake inhibitors in treatment of major depressive disorder: A meta-analysis of published studies. Int Clin Psychopharmacol. 2012;27(1):8–16. doi:10.1097/YIC.0b013e32834ce13f

17. Chokka PR, Hankey JR. Assessment and management of sexual dysfunction in the context of depression. Ther Adv Psychopharmco. 2018;8(1):13–23. doi:10.1177/2045125317720642

18. Sobieraj DM, Marinez BK, Hernandex AV, et al. Adverse effects of pharmacologic treatments of major depression in older adults. J Am Geriatr Soc 2019;67(8):1571–1581. doi:10.1111/jgs.15966

19. Benjamin S, Doraiswamy PM. Review of the use of mirtazapine in the treatment of depression. Expert Opin Pharmacother. 2011;12(10):1623–1632. doi:10.1517/14656566.2011.585459

20. Banerjee S, High J, Stirling S, et al. Study of mirtazapine for agitated behaviours in dementia (SYMBAD): A randomised, double-blind, placebo-controlled trial. Lancet. 2021;398(10310):1487–1497. doi:10.1016/S0140-6736(21)01210-1

21. Zheng W, Cia DB, Zheng W, et al. Brexanolone for postpartum depression: A meta-analysis of randomized controlled studies. Psychiatry Res. 2019;279:83–89. doi:10.1016/j.psychres.2019.07.006

22. Papakostas G, Salloum NC, Hock RS, et al. Efficacy of esketamine augmentation in major depressive disorder: A meta-analysis. J Clin Psychiatry. 2020;81(4):19r12889. doi:10.4088/jcp.19r12889

23. Kennedy SH, Lam RW, McIntyre RS, et al. Canadian Network for Mood and Anxiety Treatments (CANMAT) 2016 clinical guidelines for the management of adults with major depressive disorder: Section 3. Pharmacological treatments. Can J Psychiatry. 2016;61(9):540–560. doi:10.1177/0706743716659417

Additional Suggested Reading

- Caldiroli A, Capuzzi E, Tagliabue I, et al. Augmentative pharmacological strategies in treatment-resistant major depression: A comprehensive review. Int J Mol Sci. 2021;22(23):13070. doi:10.3390/ijms222313070

- Canuso CM, Singh JB, Fedgchin M, et al. Efficacy and safety of intranasal esketamine for the rapid reduction of symptoms of depression and suicidality in patients at imminent risk for suicide: Results of a double-blind, randomized, placebo-controlled study. Am J Psychiatry. 2018;175(7):620–630. doi:10.1176/appi.ajp.2018.17060720
- Citrome L. Vortioxetine for major depressive disorder: A systematic review of the efficacy and safety profile for this newly approved antidepressant – what is the number needed to treat, number needed to harm and likelihood to be helped or harmed? Int J Clin Pract. 2014;68(1):60–82. doi:10.1111/ijcp.12350
- Coupland C, Hill T, Morriss R, et al. Antidepressant use and risk of suicide and attempted suicide or self harm in people aged 20 to 64: Cohort study using a primary care database. BMJ. 2015;350:h517. doi:10.1136/bmj.h517
- Daly EJ, Singh JB, Fedgchin M, et al. Efficacy and safety of intranasal esketamine adjunctive to oral antidepressant therapy in treatment-resistant depression: A randomized clinical trial. JAMA Psychiatry. 2018;75(2):139–148. doi:10.1001/jamapsychiatry.2017.3739
- Fava GA, Cosci F. Understanding and managing withdrawal syndromes after discontinuation of antidepressant drugs. J Clin Psychiatry. 2019;80:19com12794. doi:10.4088/JCP.19com12794
- Hair P, Cameron F, Garnock-Jones KP. Levomilnacipran extended release: First global approval. Drugs. 2013;73(14):1639–1645. doi:10.1007/s40265-013-0116-1
- Henssler J, Alexander D, Schwarzer G, et al. Combining antidepressants vs antidepressant monotherapy for treatment of patients with acute depression: A systematic review and meta-analysis. JAMA Psychiatry. 2022;79(4):300–312. doi:10.1001/jamapsychiatry.2021.4313
- Jonkman K, Duma A, Olofsen E, et al. Pharmacokinetics and bioavailability of inhaled esketamine in healthy volunteers. Anesthesiology. 2017;127(4):675–683. doi:10.1097/ALN.0000000000001798
- Kato M, Hori H, Inoue T, et al. Discontinuation of antidepressants after remission with antidepressant medication in major depressive disorder: A systematic review and meta-analysis. Mol Psychiatry. 2021;26(1):118–133. doi:10.1038/s41380-020-0843-0
- Kennedy SH, Lam RW, McIntyre RS, et al. Canadian Network for Mood and Anxiety Treatments (CANMAT) 2016 clinical guidelines for the management of adults with major depressive disorder: Section 3. Pharmacological treatments. Can J Psychiatry. 2016;61(9):540–560. doi:10.1177/0706743716659417
- Mago R, Mahajan R, Thase ME. Levomilnacipran: A newly approved drug for treatment of major depressive disorder. Expert Rev Clin Pharmacol. 2014;7(2):137–145. doi:10.1586/17512433.2014.889563
- Malhi GS, Bassett D, Boyce P, et al. Royal Australian and New Zealand College of Psychiatrists clinical practice guidelines for mood disorders. Aust NZ J Psychiatr. 2015;49:1–185. doi:10.1177/0004867415617657
- Molero P, Ramos-Quiroga JA, Martin-Santos R, et al. Antidepressant efficacy and tolerability of ketamine and esketamine: A critical review. CNS Drugs. 2018;32(5):411–420. doi:10.1007/s40263-018-0519-3
- Ray S, Stowe Z. The use of antidepressant medication in pregnancy. Best Pract Res Clin Obstet Gynaecol. 2014;28(1):71–83. doi:10.1016/j.bpobgyn.2013.09.005
- van de Loo AJAE, Bervoets AC, Mooren L, et al. The effects of intranasal esketamine (84 mg) and oral mirtazapine (30 mg) on on-road driving performance: A double-blind, placebo-controlled study. Psychopharmacology (Berl). 2017;234(21):3175–3183. doi:10.1007/s00213-017-4706-6
- Van den Eynde V, Abdelmoemin WR, Abraham MM, et al. The prescriber's guide to classic MAO-inhibitors (phenelzine, tranylcypromine, isocarboxazid) for treatment-resistant depression. CNS Spectr. 2022;15:1–14. doi:10.1017/S1092852922000906
- Wajs E, Aluisio L, Holder R, et al. Esketamine nasal spray plus oral antidepressant in patients with treatment-resistant depression: Assessment of long-term safety in a phase 3, open-label study (SUSTAIN-2). J Clin Psychiatry. 2020;81:19m12891. doi:10.4088/JCP.19m12891
- Wang Y, Liu D, Li X, et al. Antidepressants use and the risk of type 2 diabetes mellitus: A systematic review and meta-analysis. J Affect Disord. 2021;287:41–53. doi:10.1016/j.jad.2021.03.023
- Zheng W, Sun H-L, Cai H, et al. Antidepressants for COVID-19: A systematic review. J Affect Disord. 2022;307:108–114. doi:10.1016/j.jad.2022.03.059

ELECTROCONVULSIVE THERAPY (ECT)

 Definition

- Noninvasive convulsive neurostimulation treatment whose therapeutic mechanism is mediated by a tonic-clonic generalized seizure induced by means of a brief current applied under general anesthesia, for the treatment of indicated psychiatric and neurological disorders (Note: Magnetic seizure therapy (MST) is a noninvasive convulsive therapy under investigation as an alternative means of seizure induction – electromagnetic induction)
- **Not** to be confused with the administration of sub-convulsive electric stimuli, referred to as cranial electrostimulation or electrosleep therapy; **nor** transcranial direct current stimulation (tDCS); **nor** the administration of aversive electric stimuli as a behavior modification protocol; **nor** repetitive transcranial magnetic stimulation (rTMS).

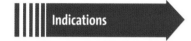 **Indications**

- Major depressive disorder (MDD); especially when associated with high suicide risk (rapid reduction in suicidal drive after 6–8 treatments), ina-nition/dehydration, severe agitation, depressive stupor, catatonia, delusions, nonresponse to one or more adequate trials of antidepressants or intolerance of therapeutic dosages[1, 2]
- MDD, recurrent: Prophylaxis or attenuation; i.e., "maintenance" ECT after response to an acute/index course of ECT, if previous antidepressants have not prevented recurrence[3]
- MDD: Prevention of relapse, i.e., "continuation" ECT for up to 6 months after response to an acute/index course of ECT, if previous antidepressants have not prevented rapid relapse; may provide better outcome than antidepressants alone following an acute/index course; ECT equivalent to most effective pharmacotherapy (nortriptyline or venlafaxine plus lithium) in preventing early relapse[4]
- Depression, atypical – a randomized trial found that patients with atypical depression were 2.6 times more likely to have remission with ECT than those with other types of depression
- Bipolar disorder: Prophylaxis of depressed and manic phases if mood stabilizers have been ineffective
- Bipolar disorder: Manic phase; adjunct to mood stabilizers and antipsychotics for severe mania (manic "delirium") and rapid-cycling illness
- Bipolar depression: A meta-analysis (19 studies) reported statistically higher response rates to ECT in bipolar depression compared to MDD; how-ever, remission rates were similar in patients with bipolar depression and those with MDD
- Mania, dysphoric ("mixed bipolar") or depressed phase
- Postpartum psychosis: Treatment of choice for some patients; secondary line of treatment after nonresponse to antidepressants and/or antipsy-chotics[5]
- Schizophrenia: Especially with concurrent catatonic and/or affective symptoms; adjunct to adequate dosage of antipsychotics for nonresponsive "positive" symptoms; clozapine-resistant schizophrenia[6]
- Schizoaffective disorder, first-episode psychosis: After nonresponse to one or more adequate drug trials
- Catatonia: Most dramatic improvement with ECT regardless of underlying condition[7]. Should be used if treatment with benzodiazepines does not elicit response or as first-line treatment. When catatonia is improved, ECT can be continued to treat underlying psychiatric disorder. Malignant forms of catatonia may respond dramatically to ECT (i.e., neuroleptic malignant syndrome or malignant catatonia)
- Parkinson's disease: ECT may be effective in treating mood, psychosis, and some motor symptoms ("on-off" phenomenon, dyskinesias)
- PTSD studied: Open trial suggests ECT may improve the core symptoms of treatment-refractory PTSD, independently of improvement in depres-sion[8]. Study results require replication and validation prior to using ECT for PTSD. Positive results reported in patients with comorbid MDD and PTSD
- Somatic symptoms and related disorders (SSDs): Case reports suggest ECT could be included for refractory SSD
- Treatment-refractory epilepsy (particularly non-focal) and status epilepticus (seizure threshold consistently increases over a course of ECT)

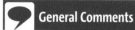 **General Comments**

- Consider ECT early in the treatment algorithm, in the presence of very severe illness (do not regard as treatment of last resort); may be first-line treatment for very severe depression or mania, active suicidality, psychotic depression in older adults (95% efficacy rates), or catatonic states[7]; however, very chronic episodes may reduce effectiveness

- High-dose, ultrabrief pulse width, right-sided unilateral ECT is considered to be equivalent in efficacy to moderate-dosage bilateral ECT and suggested to have advantages with respect to cognitive adverse effects, though reviews of studies still suggest right-sided unilateral ECT is somewhat less efficacious at improving depressive symptoms than bilateral ECT and there are small differences in cognition at 6 months post ECT[2, 9]
- Concomitant treatment with an antidepressant can enhance the efficacy of ECT, but may have variable effects on cognition
- Concomitant treatment with antipsychotic may result in faster and more pronounced symptom improvement but may cause more memory impairment – evidence is limited [7]
- Concomitant use of benzodiazepines and/or anticonvulsants has been associated with decreased efficacy. Consider temporarily stopping or reducing the dose of medications that interfere with seizure threshold
- Assess and document patient's capacity to consent to treatment; answer patient's questions about ECT; obtain signed and witnessed consent form (valid consent requires full disclosure to the patient of the nature of the procedure, all material risks and expected benefit of ECT and those of alternative available treatments, and the prognosis if no treatment is given); if patient incapable, obtain written consent from eligible substitute decision maker

Therapeutic Effects	<ul><li>ECT remains the most effective treatment for depression with overall response rates of 80%, and 60% remission rates. "Melancholic" and "psychotic" presentations respond best[10]</li><li>Vegetative symptoms of depression, such as insomnia and fatigue, and catatonic symptoms may respond initially; cognitive symptoms may improve with resolution of emotional symptoms, such as impaired self-esteem, helplessness, hopelessness, suicidal and delusional ideation</li><li>Manic symptoms which respond include agitation, euphoria, motor overactivity, and thought disorder</li><li>In psychosis, "positive" symptoms such as hallucinations and delusions may respond better than "negative" symptoms (e.g., abulia)</li></ul>
Mechanism of Action	<ul><li>Triggering controlled seizures is associated with an array of neurophysiological changes. The variety of neurophysiological effects may be related to the fact that ECT is effective in treating diverse neuropsychiatric conditions</li><li>Affects almost all neurotransmitters implicated in the pathogenesis of the mental disorders (norepinephrine, serotonin, acetylcholine, dopamine, GABA); dopamine potentiation may be especially relevant[11]</li><li>A meta-analysis of patients with depression treated with ECT using MRI (32 studies, involving 467 patients and 285 controls) failed to support the hypothesis that ECT causes brain damage; on the other hand, ECT induced volume increases in fronto-limbic areas</li><li>Neurophysiological effects include increased permeability of the blood-brain barrier, suppression of regional cerebral blood flow and neurometabolic activity; "anticonvulsant" effects may be related to outcome (inhibitory neurotransmitters are increased by ECT)</li><li>Affects neuroendocrine substances (CRF, ACTH, TRH, prolactin, vasopressin, met-enkephalins, β-endorphins)</li><li>A meta-analysis of patients with MDD (22 studies) reported that brain-derived neurotrophic factor (BDNF) level may increase afer ECT and may possibly be used as an indicator of treatment response after one or more weeks of ECT[12]</li><li>Suppression of REM sleep abnormalities[11]</li><li>COMT high/high genotype may be associated with better response</li></ul>
Dosage	<ul><li>In ECT, dose is measured in millicoulombs (mC), which is an absolute measure of electrons delivered. Dose is associated to the extent and intensity of the electric field elicited in the brain</li><li>Other variables that influence the distribution and intensity of the electric field elicited are electrode placement or resistance</li><li>A minimum of 15 seconds of seizure is considered necessary, shorter duration is considered an "aborted" seizure and an indication to re-stimulate. Barely supra-threshold seizures may be prolonged and are not associated with better outcome; augmenting agents (e.g., caffeine) are seldom used</li><li>Minimum stimulus energy/charge necessary to induce a convulsion is the "seizure threshold"; a multiple of this "threshold" stimulus is recommended for effective treatment (most accurate estimate of "threshold" is by "titration" dosing technique); threshold may be altered in patients who consume alcohol regularly or who are on medications that increase seizure threshold (e.g., benzodiazepines, anticonvulsants – avoid or reduce dose whenever possible)</li><li>Bilateral stimulus electrode placement (1.5 times "threshold" stimulus energy/charge) has been found more effective than unilateral placement; "high-energy" bilateral (2.5 times "threshold stimulus") may be effective for nonresponse to 1.5 times "threshold" bilateral treatment. No substantive difference in overall outcome or cognitive side effects between bitemporal and bifrontal placement[9]</li><li>Unilateral electrode placement can be as effective as bitemporal for many patients but, when used, the stimulus energy/charge should be substantially greater than the "threshold" stimulus (i.e., 4–6 times "threshold"); if no response after 6–8 treatments, recommend switch to bilateral</li></ul>

Electroconvulsive Therapy (ECT) (cont.)

- Ultrabrief stimulus pulse width may be effective with reduced cognitive side effects; efficacy of ultrabrief stimulus has been shown only in unilateral placement; generally lower seizure "threshold" on titration but may require more treatments
- Sex, age, and electrode placement affect seizure threshold: Males have higher thresholds than females, thresholds increase with age and are greater with bilateral than unilateral ECT
- Bifrontal placement may have advantages in selected indications (e.g., psychosis or Parkinson's disease)

Onset & Duration of Action

- An index course of ECT for depression usually involves 10–12 treatments; onset of therapeutic effect may be evident within 1–3 treatments in some cases. Index courses for schizophrenia tend to be more prolonged (15–20 treatments). If there is no benefit after 12–15 treatments, it is unlikely that ECT will be effective
- Relapse rate following discontinuation is high (30–70%) within 1 year, partly dependent on degree of medication resistance pre-ECT; prophylactic antidepressants should be administered in almost all cases; "continuation" ECT for up to 6 months (once per week for first 4–8 weeks, then one treatment every 2 weeks, then one treatment every 4 weeks) if antidepressant prophylaxis of rapid relapse is ineffective; lithium plus antidepressant may be the most effective medications to decrease relapse of major depression following ECT

Procedure

- Administer 3 times per week on alternate days, particularly for most severe cases. Twice a week has been associated with similar outcomes at the end of index course; twice-a-week treatments are also associated with less risk of cognitive side effects. Outpatient ECT is mostly delivered twice a week
- ECT must always be administered ("modified") under general anesthesia with partial neuromuscular blockade; "unmodified" ECT still used in developing countries with limited resources/personnel
- Induce light anesthesia with methohexital; little clinical advantage seen with newer agents such as propofol (results in briefer convulsions; may also raise the seizure threshold; reserve for patients with post-treatment delirium or severe nausea unresponsive to antinauseants, or very prolonged seizures)[13]; also consider propofol if patient is slow to recover from anesthesia[14]; if no seizures are elicited at maximum device output, etomidate or combination of methohexital/ketamine, methohexital/remifentanil may be used
- Induce neuromuscular blockade with succinylcholine or a short-acting non-depolarizing agent. Post-ECT myalgia may be due to insufficient relaxation or fasciculations (attenuate the latter if necessary with adjunctive non-depolarizing muscle relaxant – e.g., rocuronium – which necessitates a higher dosage of succinylcholine); if a reduction in the duration of neuromuscular blockade is necessary, a reversal agent can be used; rocuronium is indicated if there is cholinesterase deficiency or post-polio syndrome
- Pretreat with atropine or glycopyrrolate if excess oral secretions and/or significant bradycardia anticipated (i.e., during "threshold" titration, patient on a β-blocker); post-treat with atropine if bradycardia develops. It has also been used to reduce the parasympathetic effects of subconvulsive stimulation(s) (i.e., when more than one stimulation is required to elicit a seizure)
- Pretreat any concurrent physical illness which may complicate anesthesia (i.e., using antihypertensives, gastric acid/motility suppressants, hypoglycemics); special circumstances require anesthesia and/or internal medicine consultation
- If possible, discontinue or reduce dosage of all psychotropics with anticonvulsant properties (i.e., benzodiazepines, carbamazepine, valproate) during the course of treatment; use of anticonvulsant medication during a course of ECT has been associated with shorter seizure duration and higher dose required; if benzodiazepines cannot be discontinued, drugs with shorter half-life are recommended (lorazepam); pre-treat with flumazenil if necessary to reverse benzodiazepines (i.e., high dosage/dependent patient)
- Consider discontinuation of lithium or reduce dose during course of ECT due to increased risk of post-ECT delirium
- Continue all other psychotropics, except MAOIs (see Contraindications p. 108), when clinically necessary
- Outpatient treatment can be administered if warranted by the clinical circumstances, if there is no medical/anesthesia contraindication, and if the patient can comply with the pre- and posttreatment procedural requirements

Adverse Effects

- Anterograde amnesia occurs to some degree during most courses of ECT
  - Significant, patchy amnesia for the period during which ECT is administered; recall of period around time of ECT administration is usually vague
  - Retrograde episodic amnesia for some events up to a number of months pre-ECT; may be permanent; uncommonly, longer periods of retrograde amnesia

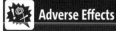

- Patchy anterograde amnesia for 3–6 months post-ECT
- Patients may rarely experience permanent anterograde memory impairment; unknown if this is a residual effect of the ECT or an effect of residual symptoms of the illness for which ECT was prescribed
- A number of pharmacological agents (i.e., liothyronine, cholinesterase inhibitors, thiamine), behavioral strategies (cognitive remediation), and treatment parameters (i.e., ultra-brief stimulus pulse width, right unilateral or more focal electrode placement) may attenuate some of the cognitive effects[15]

- Mortality rate 2 deaths per 100,000 treatments; higher risk in those with concurrent cardiovascular disease. Most recent evidence found no deaths over a course of 10 years and almost 80,000 treatments[16]
- Post-treatment delirium uncommon; usually of short duration
  - Reported in elderly patients; when more than one electric stimulus is used to induce a convulsion; after prolonged seizures
  - Due to concurrent drug toxicity (e.g., lithium carbonate, clozapine – see Drug Interactions p. 109)
  - May occur with too rapid pre-ECT discontinuation of some antidepressants
  - If occurs, consider propofol anesthesia for subsequent treatments
- Tachycardia and hypertension may be pronounced; duration several minutes post treatment; prevent with β-blocker if necessary
- Bradycardia (to the point of asystole) and hypotension may be pronounced, particularly if stimulus is subconvulsive or when right unilateral placement is used
  - Increased risk if patient on a β-blocker
  - Attenuated by the subsequent convulsion, atropine, and medication with anticholinergic effect
- Prolonged seizures and status epilepticus rare; monitor treatment with EEG until convulsion ends; seizures should be terminated after 3 min duration (with anesthetic dosage of propofol, repeated if necessary, or with a benzodiazepine – IV diazepam more rapidly effective than lorazepam)
- Limited evidence that etomidate may induce seizures during ECT; highest risk in patients with a history of epilepsy or cerebral cortical lesions
- Spontaneous seizures
  - Recent evidence suggests patients under age 40 who receive ECT might be at slightly increased risk of developing spontaneous seizures post-ECT, but patients older than 60 years may be at decreased risk of seizures after ECT
- Headache and muscle pain common but not usually severe
  - Try pre-treatment isometric exercises to prevent muscle pain
  - Pretreat with rocuronium bromide (approximately 3 mg) for severe muscle pain
- Temporomandibular joint pain; may be reduced with bifrontal electrode placement (compared to standard bitemporal placement)
  - All patients should have a bite block inserted in their mouth during the electric stimulus and seizure to minimize jaw pain and prevent dental injury, even if edentulous
- Temporary menstrual irregularity; possibly due to increased prolactin (transient). A meta-analysis investigating prolactin changes in ECT-treated patients (6 trials, 109 patients and 74 controls) reported significantly higher prolactin levels in ECT-treated patients compared to controls. Increases were large in methohexital-premedicated patients, women vs. men, and patients with bilateral vs. unilateral ECT
- Transient post-ictal paralysis (Todd's paralysis)

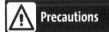 **Precautions**

- Obtain pretreatment anesthesia and/or internal medicine consultation for all patients with significant preexisting cardiovascular disease, potential gastro-esophageal reflux, compromised airway, and other circumstances which may complicate the procedure (i.e., personal or family history of significant adverse effects, or delay in recovery from general anesthesia); treat as indicated
- Monitor by ECG, pulse oximetry, and blood pressure, before, during, and after ECT; EEG during treatment
- Patients with insulin-dependent diabetes mellitus may have a reduced need for insulin after ECT, as ECT reduces blood glucose levels for several hours (may be related to pretreatment fasting)
- 10–30% of bipolar depressed patients can switch to hypomania or mania following ECT; important to continue antimanic medication if not unduly affecting the treatment procedure (i.e., increased seizure threshold)
- Modify electrode placement in patients with metallic face/skull implants or intracranial objects[17]
- ECT safely used with clozapine for treatment-refractory schizophrenia. May be associated with prolonged seizures or spontaneous tardive seizure

Electroconvulsive Therapy (ECT) (cont.)

Contraindications	**Note:** all contraindications should be regarded in the context of, and relative to, the risks of withholding ECT

- Rheumatoid arthritis complicated by erosion of the odontoid process
- Recent myocardial infarction, suggested wait is approximately 8 weeks
- Increased intracranial pressure
- Recent intracerebral hemorrhage/unstable aneurysm, recent ischemic stroke, suggested wait after event is approximately 8 weeks
- Extremely loose teeth which may be aspirated if dislodged
- Threatened retinal detachment
- Concurrent administration of an irreversible MAOI, which may interact with anesthetic agents (although most reports have implicated meperidine as the interacting drug). Severe impairment in cardiac output and hypotension during ECT may require resuscitation with a pressor agent; the choice may be limited in the presence of an irreversible MAOI. The literature therefore recommends that MAOIs be discontinued 14 days prior to elective anesthesia; if there are compelling reasons to continue the MAOI, or start ECT prior to this waiting period, obtain anesthesia consultation. The potential for a hypertensive response is much less in the presence of a selective, reversible MAOI (RIMA) such that their concurrent administration is acceptable
- Concurrent drug toxicity

 Lab Tests/Monitoring

- Full neuropsychological assessment may be needed if there is evidence of significant cognitive impairment; reassess if treatment-emergent loss is unduly severe. Otherwise, screening tools such as Montreal Cognitive Assessment of Mini Mental Status Examination before and after the course of ECT are sufficient
- Physical examination
- Hb, WBC, and differential for all patients over age 60 and when clinically indicated
- Electrolytes and creatinine for all patients on any diuretic, on lithium or with insulin-dependent diabetes, and as clinically indicated, including patients with a history or risk of water intoxication
- ECG for all patients over age 45, those being treated for hypertension, or with a history of cardiac disease and as clinically indicated
- Spinal x-rays for those patients with a history of compression fracture or other injury, significant back pain, and as clinically indicated; cervical spine x-rays for all patients with rheumatoid arthritis
- Sickle cell screening of all black patients of African descent
- Fasting blood glucose on day of each treatment for patients with diabetes mellitus or taking antidiabetic medication
- Prothrombin time and partial thromboplastin time for all patients on anticoagulants
- Serum lithium before and periodically during course of ECT

 Pediatric Considerations

- For detailed information on the use of ECT in this population, please see the *Clinical Handbook of Psychotropic Drugs for Children and Adolescents*[18]
- ECT may be used in most severe forms of psychosis, catatonia, or affective disorder with suicide risk in adolescence/childhood if medications are ineffective
- In pediatric population, ECT is also effective in treating severe self-injurious behavior
- Should never be prescribed without consultation by a specialist in child and adolescent psychiatry and a neurostimulation specialist
- ECT procedure in pediatric population is very similar to adult. Anesthetic medications need to be adjusted to weight. There is scarcity of data using any electrode placement other than bitemporal. Dose required to elicit seizures is significantly lower in this population as seizure threshold is lower than in adults

 Geriatric Considerations

- No specific risks, benefits or contraindications attributable to age
- Concurrent early dementia is not a contraindication; ECT may be administered for any concurrent diagnostic indication
- Evidence from randomized controlled trials is sparse; suggestions that response to ECT is at least equal to that in younger depressed patients. Evidence on use of ECT in the elderly suggests it is safe and effective at reducing symptoms of depression
- Lower speed of recovery after first and third treatment may predict worse outcome

Use in Pregnancy
- ECT may be used in all trimesters if a severe condition requires it; rates of fetal and maternal complications are not trivial; obtain obstetrical consultation, shared care is preferred
- Potential risk of adverse effects (to both mother and child) should be weighed against the benefits
- Should be administered by a highly skilled specialist team
- Fetal monitoring recommended
- Precaution: Increased risk of gastro-esophageal reflux; tilt position is recommended, especially in last trimester

Nursing Implications
- Patients must be kept NPO (especially for solid food) for approximately 8 h before treatment; continuous observation of potentially non-compliant patients may be required
- Dentures must be removed before treatment
- Observe and monitor vital signs until patient is recovered, oriented, and alert before discharge from recovery room; patient should be advised not to operate a motor vehicle or potentially dangerous equipment/machinery/tools until the day after each treatment. Outpatients should be escorted home after treatment
- When possible, avoid prn benzodiazepines and limit the use of sedatives and hypnotics the night prior to and the morning of treatment
- Lithium and anticonvulsants may be held the night prior to ECT as a way to decrease the risk of delirium (lithium) or increase seizure threshold (anticonvulsants)

Patient Instructions
- For detailed patient instructions on ECT, see the Patient Information Sheet (details p. 474)

Drug Interactions
- Clinically significant interactions are listed below
- For more interaction information on any given combination, also see the corresponding chapter for the interactant

Class of Drug	Example	Interaction Effects
Anesthetic	Propofol	Decreased seizure duration compared with methohexital (may be very substantial); may increase seizure threshold
	Thiopental	Increased time to recovery compared with propofol
Anticonvulsant	Carbamazepine, valproate	Increased seizure threshold with potential adverse effects of subconvulsive stimuli; carbamazepine interferes with muscle relaxants; valproate may prolong effects of thiopental
	Gabapentin, lamotrigine, topiramate	May have less of an effect on seizure threshold and duration
Antidepressant		
NDRI	Bupropion	Reported change to mania in two patients with recurrent depression, concomitant ECT and bupropion – limited evidence; lowers seizure threshold
SARI	Trazodone	Lower seizure threshold and prolonged seizures reported; clinical significance unknown. Rare case reports of cardiovascular complications in patients with and without cardiac disease – more likely to occur at high dosages (i.e., more than 300 mg/day)
Nonselective cyclic	Nortriptyline	Lowers seizure threshold; may increase the risk of cardiac arrhythmias (especially in the elderly and those with cardiovascular disease) In combination with sympathomimetic drugs, can cause hypertensive crisis
Irreversible MAOI	Phenelzine	Possible need for a pressor agent for resuscitation requires that this combination be avoided, if possible
Antihypertensive	β-blockers (e.g., propranolol)	May potentiate bradycardia and hypotension with subconvulsive stimuli Confusion reported with combined use
Antipsychotic	Clozapine	Increased seizure duration reported in 16.6% of patients; spontaneous (tardive) seizures reported following ECT Delirium reported with concurrent or shortly following clozapine treatment; however, there are many case reports of uncomplicated concurrent use, even with very high dosages. May be associated with increased tachycardia
	Risperidone	Minimal risk of convulsions compared to other antipsychotics; EEG abnormalities may occur
Benzodiazepine	Diazepam, lorazepam	Increased seizure threshold with potential adverse effects of subconvulsive stimuli or abbreviated seizure

Electroconvulsive Therapy (ECT) (cont.)

Class of Drug	Example	Interaction Effects
Caffeine		Increased seizure duration Reports of hypertension, tachycardia, and cardiac dysrhythmia
Hypnotic/sedative	Zopiclone	May reduce seizure duration (used the night before ECT)
Lithium		Lithium toxicity may occur, perhaps due to an increased permeability of the blood-brain barrier or release of lithium from cells by ECT resulting in systemic toxicity; prolongs seizure duration and succinylcholine action duration; may lower seizure threshold; decrease (aim for plasma level in the bottom range; ~0.6 mEq/L) or discontinue lithium and monitor patient. Concurrent administration not contraindicated if lithium level within the therapeutic range. Suggest hold dose night prior to ECT Ventricular tachycardia reported with the combination of lithium and duloxetine
L-tryptophan		Increased seizure duration
Theophylline		Increased seizure duration, status epilepticus. Concurrent administration not contraindicated if serum level within the therapeutic range

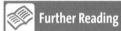 **Further Reading**

References

1 Fink M, Kellner CH, McDall WV. The role of ECT in suicide prevention. J ECT. 2014;30(1):5–9. doi:10.1097/YCT.0b013e3182a6ad0d

2 Fink M. What was learned: Studies by the consortium for research in ECT (CORE) 1997–2011. Acta Psychiatr Scand. 2014;129(6):417–426. doi:10.1111/acps.12251

3 Rabheru K. Maintenance electroconvulsive therapy (M-ECT) after acute response: Examining the evidence for who, what, when, and how? J ECT 2012;28(1):39–47. doi:10.1097/YCT.0b013e3182455758

4 Prudic J, Haskett RF, McCall WV, et al. Pharmacological strategies in the prevention of relapse after electroconvulsive therapy. J ECT. 2013;29(1):3–12. doi:10.1097/YCT.0b013e31826ea8c4

5 Focht A, Kellner CH. Electroconvulsive therapy (ECT) in the treatment of postpartum psychosis. J ECT. 2012;28(1):31–33. doi:10.1097/YCT.0b013e3182315aa8

6 Petrides G, Malur C, Braga RJ, et al. Electroconvulsive therapy augmentation in clozapine-resistant schizophrenia: A prospective, randomized study. Am J Psychiatry. 2015;172(1):52–58. doi:10.1176/appi.ajp.2014.13060787

7 Sienaert P. What we have learned about electroconvulsive therapy and its relevance for the practising psychiatrist. Can J Psychiatry. 2011;56(1):5–12. doi:10.1177/070674371105600103

8 Margoob MA, Ali Z, Andrade C. Efficacy of ECT in chronic, severe, antidepressant- and CBT-refractory PTSD: An open, prospective study. Brain Stimul. 2010;3(1):28–35. doi:10.1016/j.brs.2009.04.005

9 Kellner CH, Tobias KG, Wiegand J. Electrode placement in electroconvulsive therapy (ECT): A review of the literature. J ECT 2010;26(3):175–180. doi:10.1097/YCT.0b013e3181e48154

10 Rasmussen KG. Electroconvulsive therapy and melancholia: Review of the literature and suggestions for further study. J ECT. 2011;27(4):315–322. doi:10.1097/YCT.0b013e31820a9482

11 McCall WV, Andrade C, Sienaert P. Searching for the mechanism(s) of ECT's therapeutic effect. J ECT. 2014;30(2):87–89. doi:10.1097/YCT.0000000000000121

12 Luan S, Zhou B, Wu Q, et al. Brain-derived neurotrophic factor blood levels after electroconvulsive therapy in patients with major depressive disorder: A systematic review and meta-analysis. Asian J Psychiatr. 2020;51:101983. doi:10.1016/j.ajp.2020.101983

13 Vaidya PV, Anderson EL, Bobb A, et al. A within-subject comparison of propofol and methohexital anesthesia for electroconvulsive therapy. J ECT 2012;28(1):14–19. doi:10.1097/YCT.0b013e31823a4220

14 Lihua P, Su M, Ke W, et al. Different regimens of intravenous sedatives or hypnotics for electroconvulsive therapy (ECT) in adult patients with depression. Cochrane Database Syst Rev. 2014;4:CD009763. doi:10.1002/14651858.CD009763.pub2

15 Merk W, Kucia K. Combined use of ECT and psychotropic drugs. Psychiatr Pol. 2015;49(6):1241–1253. doi:10.12740/PP/37462

16 Watts B V, Groft A, Bagian JP, et al. An examination of mortality and other adverse events related to electroconvulsive therapy using a national adverse event report system. J ECT. 2011;27(2):105–108. doi:10.1097/YCT.0b013e3181f6d17f

17 Vila-Rodriguez F, McGirr A, Tham J, et al. Electroconvulsive therapy in patients with deep brain stimulators. J ECT. 2014;30(3):e16–e18. doi:10.1097/YCT.0000000000000074

18 Elbe D, Black TR, McGrane IR, et al. Clinical handbook of psychotropic drugs for children and adolescents. (5th ed.). Boston, MA: Hogrefe Publishing, 2023.

Additional Suggested Reading

• Amanullah S, Delva N, McRae H, et al. Electroconvulsive therapy in patients with skull defects or metallic implants: A review of the literature and case report. Prim Care Companion CNS Disord. 2012;14(2):[no pagination]. doi:10.4088/PCC.11r01228

- Cinderella MA, Nichols NA, Munjal S, et al. Antiepileptics in electroconvulsive therapy: A mechanism-based review of recent literature. J ECT. 2022;38(2):133–137. doi:10.1097/YCT.0000000000000805
- Elias A, Thomas N, Sackeim HA. Electroconvulsive therapy in mania: A review of 80 years of clinical experience. Am J Psychiatry. 2021;178(3):229–239. doi:10.1176/appi.ajp.2020.20030238
- Kellner CH, Obbels J, Sienaert P. When to consider electroconvulsive therapy (ECT). Acta Psychiatr Scand. 2020;141(4):304–315. doi:10.1111/acps.13134
- Kennedy SH, Lam RW, McIntyre RS, et al. Canadian network for mood and anxiety treatments (CANMAT) 2016 clinical guidelines for the management of adults with major depressive disorder: Section 3. Pharmacological treatments. Can J Psychiatry. 2016;61(9):540–560. doi:10.1177/0706743716659417
- Maguire S, Rea SM, Convery P. Electroconvulsive therapy – What do patients think of their treatment? Ulster Med J. 2016;85(3):182–186.
- Roumen VM, Giacobbe P, Kennedy SH, et al. Canadian network for mood and anxiety treatments (CANMAT) 2016 clinical guidelines for the management of adults with major depressive disorder: Section 4. Neurostimulation treatments. Can J Psychiatry. 2016;61(9):561–575. doi:10.1177/0706743716660033
- Versiani J, Cheniaux E, Landeira-Fernandez J. Efficacy and safety of electroconvulsive therapy in the treatment of bipolar disorder: A systematic review. J ECT 2011;27(2): 153–164. doi:10.1097/YCT.0b013e3181e6332e
- Ward HB, Fromson JA, Cooper JJ, et al. Recommendations for the use of ECT in pregnancy: Literature review and proposed clinical protocol. Arch Womens Ment Health. 2018;21(6):715–722. doi:10.1007/s00737-018-0851-0

BRIGHT LIGHT THERAPY (BLT)

Definition

- Regular daily exposure to ultraviolet-filtered visible light. For standard light boxes, this involves at least 5000 lux-hours (units of illumination per unit time) per day

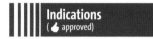

Indications
(👍 approved)

- 👍 Seasonal affective disorder (SAD)[1]
- Circadian rhythm sleep disorders (e.g., jet-lag, shift-work)
- Insomnia: A systematic review and meta-analysis reported that light therapy was found effective in the treatment of sleep problems in general (g = 0.39), and for circadian rhythm sleep disorders (g = 0.41), insomnia (g = 0.47), and sleep problems related to Alzheimer's disease/dementia (g = 0.30) specifically[2]
- Efficacy of light therapy for antepartum or postpartum depression reported in a few published studies that have produced mixed results[3]
- Nonseasonal depression: Randomized double-blind placebo-controlled studies showed that BLT, both as monotherapy and as adjunctive therapy, was efficacious and well tolerated in the treatment of adults with nonseasonal unipolar and bipolar depression; combination treatment had the most consistent effects.[4] BLT was more effective than placebo (sham treatment) in drug-resistant depression. Inconsistent results reported in a recent overview of systematic reviews of 18 RCTs.[5] A randomized double-blind study suggests that BLT may be promising in treating depression in patients with Type 2 diabetes with high insulin resistance
- Bipolar depression – BLT shown to be effective as adjunctive therapy in double-blind studies.[6, 7] Response reported within 48 h in conjunction with sleep deprivation and consecutive sleep phase advance; patients treated with bright white light experienced a significantly higher remission rate. Caution suggested regarding possible risk for mood shift. Meta-analyses of RCTs demonstrate efficacy of BLT in decreasing depressive severity in bipolar depression[8], however, no significant effect seen on remission rate[9]
- Parkinson's disease: Several studies have demonstrated a positive effect of BLT on quality of sleep; total salivary cortisol secretion was decreased; suggested to decrease daytime drowsiness[10]; variable effects seen on mood and motor function
- ADHD: Preliminary data suggest that morning BLT in combination with melatonin in the afternoon/evening effective in sleep-onset insomnia (delayed phase sleep disorder) in adolescents and adults. Pilot study in adults showed that BLT significantly advanced the phase of dim light melatonin onset and mid sleep time, which was correlated with decreased ADHD rating scale scores and hyperactive-impulsive sub scores; total sleep time, sleep efficiency, wake after sleep onset, or percent wake during sleep interval did not improve[11, 12]
- Dementia: Bright light is reported to improve circadian rhythms in patients with Alzheimer's dementia[13] and have a positive effect on sleep, mood, behavioral symptoms, and cognitive functioning. A systematic review and meta-analysis identified 7 multimodal intervention studies, all incorporating light exposure; 6 of these reported improved objective or subjective sleep[14]
- Fibromyalgia: A pilot study demonstrated that morning light treatment (3,000 lux for 1 h for 6 days) improved function and pain sensitivity in 10 female patients with fibromyalgia
- Delirium: A single-blind randomized controlled study of 62 postsurgical patients demonstrated that 3 days of BLT and supplemental oxygen protected 49 patients against delirium by targeting sleep-wake cycles and deficits in the bicarbonate buffer system; negative results reported in a randomized controlled study of ICU patients

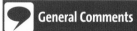

General Comments

- One explanation for inconsistent/mixed results of BLT for different disorders may be that current light therapy approaches are not standardized in terms of light intensity, wavelength spectrum, timing, distribution, duration, and individual circadian rhythms, leading, in some cases, to a weakening of the therapeutic effects of light
- Acceptable light boxes must filter out potentially harmful ultraviolet rays
- The wavelength of visible light used is not of great importance; the most consistent wavelength-specific effects have been found with short-wavelength light of 480 nm (blue light)[15]
- The magnitude of response increases with increased duration of exposure in a nonlinear fashion, as the majority of phase shift occurs at the beginning of the exposure
- Because they are used closer to the eyes, light visors produce much lower levels of light than do standard light boxes (which produce 2,500–10,000 lux). Brightness appears to be less important for visors than for light boxes

- Seasonal affective disorder: Hypersomnia appears to be most consistently associated with a good response to BLT; hyperphagia (especially carbo-hydrate craving) and a less severe symptom profile at baseline also predict response. Evidence is limited on light therapy as a preventive treatment for people with a history of SAD
- The efficacy of BLT is dependent on the time-of-day of the circadian cycle that the light is administered – see Dosing[2]
- Standard antidepressants may enhance the effects of BLT[16]
- Antidepressant effects of rTMS were enhanced and accelerated by its combination with BLT in treatment-resistant depression[17]

Therapeutic Effects	
	<ul><li>Eyes and retinas, not the skin, mediate the therapeutic effect of light. Notwithstanding, patients do not need to glance directly at the light source to experience a therapeutic effect</li><li>The specific mechanism of BLT remains unknown. While light suppresses melatonin, this may not be the primary mechanism of action. Modulation of serotonin and autonomic function have also been proposed[15]</li><li>Light induces gene expression in the adrenal gland via the suprachiasmatic nucleus (SCN)-sympathetic nervous system. This gene expression accompanies the surge of plasma and brain corticosterone levels without accompanying activation of the hypothalamo-adenohypophyseal axis; SCN activation is closely linked to the circadian clock. The magnitude of corticosterone response is dose-dependently correlated with the light intensity[15]</li><li>The ability of light to phase-advance delayed circadian rhythms may be important in some patients, particularly with sleep-wake disorders; manipulation of the circadian timing system via bright light (also sleep deprivation or pharmacological therapy) has been shown to alleviate depressive symptoms and suggests that circadian dysfunction may play a role in the pathophysiology of depression</li><li>Exposure to light in the late evening/early night causes phase delays, suppresses melatonin, and increases alertness; brief exposure may be more efficient than longer exposure</li><li>BLT usually works within several days; on discontinuation, benefits are lost after several days</li></ul>
Dosage	
	<ul><li>The standard "dose" of light is 5,000 lux-hours per day. The most popular method to achieve this is exposure for 30 min per day using a 10,000-lux light unit</li><li>One study suggests that 60 min of intermittent light (20 ms light flashes) may be more effective at eliciting circadian rhythm changes than continuous light exposure</li><li>Suggested guidelines for time of BLT for circadian rhythm sleep disorders[2]:<ul><li>Advanced sleep-phase syndrome (early sleep-wake times): BLT before bedtime and dim light after wake time</li><li>Delayed sleep-phase syndrome (late sleep-wake times, sleep-onset insomnia): BLT in the morning after awakening and dim light prior to bedtime</li><li>Shift work disorder (insomnia during daytime sleep, drowsiness/fatigue when awake): BLT in the evening/night, dim light after work, and strict adherence to regular sleep-wake times</li><li>Jet lag (eastward; sleep-onset insomnia, daytime drowsiness/fatigue): BLT in the morning after wake time (home time) and dim light prior to bedtime</li><li>Jet lag (westward; early morning awakening, daytime drowsiness/fatigue): BLT before bedtime (home time) and dim light after wake time</li><li>Non-24-hour sleep-wake disorder (no pattern to sleep-wake times): BLT in the morning after wake time if sleep episode occurs at night</li></ul></li><li>Nonseasonal depression: Augmentation with BLT administered at midday (e.g., between 12:00 p.m. and 2:30 p.m.) may be most efficacious and may minimize risk of manic switch. Suggested duration of treatment is 2–5 weeks</li><li>Bipolar depression: Review of BLT for bipolar depression recommends light intensity below 10,000 lux, depending on the duration of light exposure (e.g., 10,000 lux for 30 min per day or 5,000 lux for 1 h per day, or 2,500 lux for 2 h per day); they suggest a gradual increase in the duration of light exposure to prevent switching into mania, for instance, 5,000–7,000 lux with an increase of 15 min per week until 60 min per day reached</li><li>SAD: Several randomized trials indicate that BLT is more beneficial if administered early in the morning rather than later in the morning or in the evening. Treatment should be continued until the period of usual spontaneous remission in spring or summer</li></ul>
Adverse Effects	
	<ul><li>Cumulative exposure to light therapy over 6 years has shown no ocular damage. Notwithstanding, overuse of light may cause a decrease in sensitivity to light</li><li>Headache is most common (over 10%); nausea, diarrhea, nervousness/jitteriness, sleep disturbances, irritability, dizziness, and fatigue can occur</li><li>Case reports of suicidal ideation/attempts within days of starting treatment</li><li>Eye strain, blurred vision; eye irritation (itching, stinging) – gradually disappears with time (may need to sit further from the light source or initiate exposure gradually)</li></ul>

Bright Light Therapy (BLT) (cont.)

- Skin irritation – rare
- Hypomania or manic switch can occur (1–2.3% risk), particularly if light is overused or in patients with bipolar disorder[9]
- Paranoid delusions reported in patients with Alzheimer's disease; case report of induced psychotic episode in 38-year-old female
- Rarely, menstrual disturbances

 Precautions

- Patients with unidentified retinal conditions may be at risk; consult an ophthalmologist for such cases, if needed

 Contraindications

- Patients with glaucoma, cataracts, macular degeneration, retinal detachment, retinitis pigmentosa or retinopathy
- Light therapy is contraindicated in patients taking photosensitizing medications

 Pediatric Considerations

- Early data suggests benefit of BLT as monotherapy, and also as add-on therapy, in adolescents with nonseasonal depression; open label study of 39 inpatients aged 12–18, with moderate–severe depression, demonstrated that 4 weeks of BLT with light glasses, in addition to usual treatment, showed positive effects on depressive symptoms and sleep problems and significantly improved global clinical impression
- Used together with CBT in adolescents with delayed sleep phase disorder
- Randomized controlled study of adolescents with delayed sleep-phase disorder showed that BLT plus melatonin improved sleep onset and duration, and had continued benefit after 3 months

 Geriatric Considerations

- The elderly in their eighties and nineties retain only 10% of a 10-year-old child's circadian photoreception, mostly due to opacification of the lens, reductions in pupil diameter and loss of photoreceptor sensitivity, causing deficits in the absorption of 400–500 nm visible light, which is essential for circadian regulation. Suggested to use light between 500 and 10,000 lux, at eye level, to improve cognitive parameters, sleep quality, and circadian functions in the elderly
- Some of the factors influencing BLT effectiveness in the elderly are light intensity, spectral composition, duration, timing, exposure patterns, dementia type, sleep patterns, dementia severity, and acceptance of and adherence to the regimen
- Use of BLT in the morning had positive outcomes in elderly patients with sleep disturbances and non-seasonal mood disorders
- Meta-analysis of 8 studies reported that use of bright (white) light, or blue light, therapy resulted in significantly reduced severity of geriatric depression and was significantly more effective than comparative treatments, including placebo or dim light[18]
- Longer sleep times reported when BLT was used as part of a multicomponent delirium management program[19]

 Use in Pregnancy

- Open studies, case reports, and randomized studies suggest BLT is well tolerated during pregnancy and no adverse effects on the fetus have been reported

 Patient Instructions

- For detailed patient instructions on Bright Light Therapy, see the Patient Information Sheet (details p. 474)
- Prior to initiating BLT, consult with your physician and/or pharmacist to determine whether any drugs you are taking (including over-the-counter and herbal preparations) may interact with the therapy
- It is not necessary to glance directly at the light source

 Drug Interactions

- Clinically significant interactions are listed below
- For more interaction information on any given combination, also see the corresponding chapter for the interactant

Class of Drug	Example	Interaction Effects
Acne preparation	Benzoyl peroxide, retinoids (e.g., isotretinoin)	May cause photosensitivity reaction
Analgesic/anti-inflammatory	Naproxen, piroxicam	May cause photosensitivity reaction
Antiarrhythmic	Amiodarone	May cause photosensitivity reaction
Antibiotic	Doxycycline, nalidixic acid, tetracycline	May cause photosensitivity reaction
Antidepressant 　SSRI/SNRI 　MAOIs	 Citalopram, fluoxetine, paroxetine, sertraline, venlafaxine, etc. Tranylcypromine	 May augment the effects of bright light therapy Rarely used in SAD. May augment the effect of bright light therapy Standard MAOI precautions needed
Antifungal	Voriconazole	May cause photosensitivity reaction
Antipsychotic	Chlorpromazine, thioridazine	May cause photosensitivity reaction
Diuretic	Hydrochlorothiazide	May cause photosensitivity reaction
Hypoglycemic	Chlorpropamide	May cause photosensitivity reaction
L-tryptophan		May augment the effects of bright light therapy
St. John's wort		May cause photosensitivity reaction

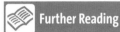 **Further Reading**

References
1. Pjrek E, Friedrich ME, Cambioli L, et al. The efficacy of light therapy in the treatment of seasonal affective disorder: A meta-analysis of randomized controlled trials. Psychother Psychosom. 2020;89(1):17–24. doi:10.1159/000502891
2. van Maanen A, Meijer AM, van der Heijden KB, et al. The effects of light therapy on sleep problems: A systematic review and meta-analysis. Sleep Med Rev. 2016;29:52–62. doi:10.1016/j.smrv.2015.08.009
3. Bais B, Kamperman AM, Bijma HH, et al. Effects of bright light therapy for depression during pregnancy: A randomised, double-blind controlled trial. BMJ Open. 2020;10(10):e038030. doi:10.1136/bmjopen-2020-038030
4. Lam RW, Levitt RJ, Levitan RD, et al. Efficacy of bright light treatment, fluoxetine, and the combination in patients with nonseasonal major depressive disorder: A randomized clinical trial. JAMA Psychiatry. 2016;73(1):56–63. doi:10.1001/jamapsychiatry.2015.2235
5. Haller H, Anheyer D, Cramer H, et al. Complementary therapies for clinical depression: An overview of systematic reviews. BMJ Open. 2019;9(8):e028527. doi:10.1136/bmjopen-2018-028527
6. Yorguner Kupeli N, Bulut NS, Carkaxhiu Bulut G, et al. Efficacy of bright light therapy in bipolar depression. Psychiatry Res. 2018;260:432–438. doi:10.1016/j.psychres.2017.12.020
7. Zhou TH, Dang WM, Ma YT, et al. Clinical efficacy, onset time and safety of bright light therapy in acute bipolar depression as an adjunctive therapy: A randomized controlled trial. J Affect Disord. 2018;227:90–96. doi:10.1016/j.jad.2017.09.038
8. Wang S, Zhang Z, Yao L, et al. Bright light therapy in the treatment of patients with bipolar disorder: A systematic review and meta-analysis. PLoS One. 2020;15(5):e0232798. doi:10.1371/journal.pone.0232798
9. Hirakawa H, Terao T, Muronaga M, et al. Adjunctive bright light therapy for treating bipolar depression: A systematic review and meta-analysis of randomized controlled trials. Brain Behav. 2020;10(12):e01876. doi:10.1002/brb3.1876
10. Videnovic A, Klerman EB, Wang W, et al. Timed light therapy for sleep and daytime sleepiness associated with Parkinson disease: A randomized clinical trial. JAMA Neurol. 2017;74(4):411–418. doi:10.1001/jamaneurol.2016.5192
11. Fargason RE, Fobian AD, Hablitz LM, et al. Correcting delayed circadian phase with bright light therapy predicts improvement in ADHD symptoms: A pilot study. J Psychiatr Res. 2017;91:105–110. doi:10.1016/j.jpsychires.2017.03.004
12. van Andel E, Bijlenga D, Vogel SWN, et al. Effects of chronotherapy on circadian rhythm and ADHD symptoms in adults with attention-deficit/hyperactivity disorder and delayed sleep phase syndrome: A randomized clinical trial. Chronobiol Int. 2021;38(2):260–269. doi:10.1080/07420528.2020.1835943
13. Roccaro I, Smirni D. Fiat lux: The light became therapy. An overview on the bright light therapy in Alzheimer's disease sleep disorders. J Alzheimers Dis. 2020;77(1):113–125. doi:10.3233/JAD-200478

Bright Light Therapy (BLT) (cont.)

14 O'Caoimh R, Mannion H, Sezgin D, et al. Non-pharmacological treatments for sleep disturbance in mild cognitive impairment and dementia: A systematic review and meta-analysis. Maturitas. 2019;127:82–94. doi:10.1016/j.maturitas.2019.06.0070

15 Oldham MA, Ciraulo DA. Bright light therapy for depression: A review of its effects on chronobiology and the autonomic nervous system. Chronobiol Int. 2014;31(3):305–319. doi: 10.3109/07420528.2013.833935

16 Geoffroy PA, Schroder CM, Reynaud E, et al. Efficacy of light therapy versus antidepressant drugs, and of the combination versus monotherapy, in major depressive episodes: A systematic review and meta-analysis. Sleep Med Rev. 2019;48:101213. doi:10.1016/j.smrv.2019.101213

17 Barbini B, Attanasio F, Manfredi E, et al. Bright light therapy accelerates the antidepressant effect of repetitive transcranial magnetic stimulation in treatment resistant depression: A pilot study. Int J Psychiatry Clin Pract. 2021;25(4):375–377. doi:10.1080/13651501.2021.1894579

18 Chang C, Liu C, Chen S, et al. Efficacy of light therapy on nonseasonal depression among elderly adults: A systematic review and meta-analysis. Neuropsychiatr Dis Treat. 2018;14:3091–3102. doi:10.2147/NDT.S180321

19 Chong MS, Tan KT, Tay L, et al. Bright light therapy as part of a multicomponent management program improves sleep and functional outcomes in delirious older hospitalized adults. Clin Interv Aging. 2013;8:565–572. doi:10.2147/CIA.S44926

Additional Suggested Reading

- Blakely KM, Drucker AM, Rosen CF. Drug-induced photosensitivity – An update: Culprit drugs, prevention and management. Drug Saf. 2019;42(7):827–847. doi:10.1007/s40264-019-00806-5
- Campbell PD, Miller AM, Woesner ME. Bright light therapy: Seasonal affective disorder and beyond. Einstein J Biol Med. 2017;32:E13–E25. https://www.ncbi.nlm.nih.gov/pmc/articles/PMC6746555/
- Cunningham JEA, Stamp JA, Shapiro CM. Sleep and major depressive disorder: A review of non-pharmacological chronotherapeutic treatments for unipolar depression. Sleep Med. 2019;61:6–18. doi:10.1016/j.sleep.2019.04.012
- Fifel K, Videnovic A. Light therapy in Parkinson's disease: Towards mechanism-based protocols. Trends Neurosci. 2018;41(5):252–254. doi:10.1016/j.tins.2018.03.00
- Figueiro MG. Light, sleep and circadian rhythms in older adults with Alzheimer's disease and related dementias. Neurodegener Dis Manag. 2017;7(2):119–145. doi:10.2217/nmt-2016-0060
- Spies M, James GM, Vraka C, et al. Brain monoamine oxidase A in seasonal affective disorder and treatment with bright light therapy. Transl Psychiatry. 2018;8:198. doi:10.1038/s41398-018-0227-2

REPETITIVE TRANSCRANIAL MAGNETIC STIMULATION (rTMS)

 Definition

- Repetitive transcranial magnetic stimulation (rTMS) is a noninvasive, non-convulsive, neuromodulation procedure that employs high-powered time-varying magnetic fields to alter cortical neuronal activity. rTMS is a first-line intervention for treatment-resistant depression[1] and has been approved for the treatment of depression in many countries, including the USA, three provinces in Canada, Great Britain, some European countries, Australia, Mexico, and Israel. Some private insurers cover the cost of treatment. Many double-blind, sham (i.e., simulated rTMS) controlled studies and several meta-analyses confirm the antidepressant efficacy of rTMS. The standard treatment involves delivering treatment to the left dorsolateral prefrontal cortex (DLPFC) with either high-frequency (10 Hz or 20 Hz) or intermittent theta-burst stimulation (iTBS) for 30 consecutive weekdays[2, 3]
- Pharmacoeconomic analysis suggests that, after two previously failed antidepressant drug trials, rTMS may be more cost-effective and lead to greater improvement of quality-adjusted life years (QALY) than a third antidepressant drug. The recent development of iTBS is associated with additional cost-effectiveness benefits[5]

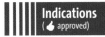 **Indications**
(👍 approved)

- 🔹 Medication-resistant major depressive disorder (MDD): Left high-frequency, iTBS, right low-frequency, or bilateral (left high- plus right low-frequency) rTMS are applied over the DLPFC to treat MDD. Sham-controlled studies and meta-analysis suggest rTMS can hasten the response to antidepressants
- 🔹 Obsessive compulsive disorder: Meta-analysis shows that low-frequency rTMS over the supplementary motor cortex or left orbitofrontal cortex or high-frequency deep transcranial magnetic stimulation (dTMS) over the medial frontal and anterior cingulate cortex may relieve some symptoms of OCD
- Maintenance treatment after remission of depression can prevent relapse after successful treatment with an acute series of rTMS[6]
- Schizophrenia: Left low-frequency temporoparietal rTMS in combination with antipsychotics may reduce auditory hallucinations; effects on other positive symptoms not established. Inconsistent results reported on efficacy for negative symptoms of schizophrenia
- Bipolar disorder: Meta-analysis suggests antidepressant effect but results are mixed for mania. RCT shows potential improvement of cognitive functioning. Case reports suggest that rTMS may precipitate mild hypomania in bipolar patients
- PTSD: Recent trials administering iTBS to right DLPFC have shown the highest level of efficacy.[7, 8] PTSD may respond less well to rTMS if major depression is absent. Pretreatment with rTMS may facilitate cognitive processing therapy for PTSD[9]
- Autism spectrum disorder: In a sham-controlled trial in 28 subjects with high-functioning autism or Asperger's, "social relating" impairment and socially-related anxiety were significantly reduced by bilateral rTMS
- Neurological disease: Meta-analysis shows that low-frequency rTMS can reduce seizure frequency in medication-resistant epilepsy. Patients with migraine and depression may experience improvement of both with rTMS. Both depression and damaged motor functioning after stroke may improve with rTMS.[10] Comparative study of rTMS and fluoxetine 20 mg/day showed similar response in depression in patients with Parkinson's disease, with additional improvement in motor function and cognition with rTMS. Meta-analysis suggests that rTMS may improve depressed mood and alleviate some motor symptoms in patients with Parkinson's disease. An RCT of sham vs. real high-frequency rTMS showed that 10 or more days of rTMS could improve cognitive functioning in patients with mild to moderate Alzheimer's disease. rTMS to the right hemisphere may improve verbal functioning in patients with aphasia and may reduce postconcussive symptoms after mild traumatic brain injury
- Addictions: Meta-analysis suggests that excitatory (high-frequency) rTMS to the left DLPFC or bilateral prefrontal cortex may reduce substance abuse cravings

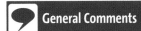 **General Comments**

- Noninvasive outpatient treatment that is only mildly uncomfortable and does not require anesthesia or sedation and is not associated with increased weight or sexual side effects
- iTBS treatment is administered over 3 min, 5 days/week, for up to 30 sessions per course of treatment
- Response to rTMS varies depending on individual patient pathophysiology, stimulus frequency and intensity, coil orientation, and brain region treated

Repetitive Transcranial Magnetic Stimulation (rTMS) (cont.)

Therapeutic Effect	• In the treatment of MDD, sham-controlled studies reported response rates of 18–58% and remission rates of 10–40% • Typically used in medication-resistant patients, antidepressant effect reportedly greater in those with less chronic illness and fewer previous failed medication trials • In a meta-analysis of 36 RCTs, antidepressant effect size was greater with rTMS treatment courses of 4 weeks compared to shorter ones, and greatest when the number of magnetic pulses delivered was 1200–1500 compared to higher or lower pulse numbers[11] • "Accelerated" rTMS with 2–3 sessions delivered each day may lead to slightly faster recovery of depression compared to standard once daily rTMS sessions[12] • rTMS may have an anti-suicide effect that is independent of the antidepressant effect[13, 14] • Depressive symptoms may continue to decrease following cessation of a course of rTMS treatment • Cognitive functioning may improve in depressed patients treated with rTMS • rTMS may be an alternative to ECT for some patients with MDD. Although early open-label trials suggest that ECT and rTMS are equivalent, larger open-label trials, meta-analysis, and clinical experience indicate that rTMS is less efficacious than ECT, particularly in psychotically depressed individuals[15] • After successful treatment of depression, relapse was observed in 14–40% after 3 months (depending on definition of relapse), even with use of prophylactic antidepressant medication[16] • Continuation or "maintenance": Open-label study suggests that single maintenance rTMS to the left prefrontal cortex, offered once weekly or at greater intervals, may reduce relapse rate in those successfully treated with either an acute course of rTMS or ECT • Robust antidepressant effects reported with combined ECT and rTMS, with fewer cognitive adverse effects than with ECT alone • Preliminary studies suggest that pre-treatment EEG may be used to predict antidepressant response to rTMS
Mechanism of Action	• The magnetic field penetrates the skull to enter brain tissue where, through the principle of Faraday induction, an electrical current is induced in those cortical neurons and glial cells beneath the coil. If the electric field generated is strong enough, it causes neurons to depolarize above the threshold to trigger action potentials. A recent concurrent TMS-fMRI study provided direct causal evidence that the pulses of TMS at the site of stimulation caused changes in functional connectivity in distal sites; these functional connectivity changes were associated with treatment response.[17] This may occur through trans-synaptic mechanisms • Low- and high-frequency rTMS may exert opposite neurophysiological effects. High-frequency pulses (more than 1 pulse/s) may increase cortical excitability while low-frequency pulses (1 pulse/s or less) may reduce cortical excitability by increasing cortical inhibition. These effects have been likened to the processes of "kindling" and "quenching" described in animals • The effects of rTMS appear to depend on the side of the brain treated (e.g., depression may respond to either high-frequency rTMS to the left dorsolateral prefrontal cortex (DLPFC) or to low-frequency rTMS to the right DLPFC); however, one study demonstrated that bilateral low-frequency rTMS may be an effective antidepressant. High-frequency rTMS to the right DLPFC may lessen mania while the same frequency to the left DLPFC may make it worse. PTSD symptoms are reported to respond more robustly to right high-frequency rTMS in some studies • As the neurophysiological effect of rTMS may depend on whether the subject is left or right handed, left-handed patients may theoretically respond better when treatment is given to the hemisphere opposite to that used for right handers • Though the neuronal depolarization and other changes in brain activity can be detected by electroencephalography and positron emission tomography (PET) imaging, the cellular and molecular mechanism of action of rTMS is not fully elucidated • Studies suggest that rTMS may downregulate α-adrenergic receptors, increase dopamine and serotonin levels in the striatum, frontal cortex, and hippocampus; increased prefrontal cortex metabolism and blood flow has been noted in patients responding to high-frequency rTMS. Glutamate levels may increase in brain regions below the coil. Theta burst rTMS over the prefrontal cortex appears to alter glucose utilization in the medial prefrontal, temporal, and anterior cingulate cortex

Dosing	• Dose is ascertained in each person by first determining their individual motor threshold, which is the minimum amount of energy that is required to elicit a motor-evoked potential when stimulating the primary motor cortex. Once the motor threshold has been established, dose is computed by multiplying the motor threshold 0.9 to 1.2 times. The total number of stimuli administered over a single treatment session can vary (e.g., 120–3,000 pulses)
	• The effects of rTMS on neuronal excitability is dependent on frequency
	• When used to treat depression, standard high-frequency rTMS is usually administered to the left DLPFC (in right handers) daily for 20–30 days. Duration of each treatment depends on treatment protocol (range 3 min for iTBS, 20 min for 10 Hz and 20 Hz dTMS)
	• An 8.5 min protocol using low-frequency rTMS to the right DLPFC was shown to be an effective antidepressant in a large multicenter controlled trial
Procedure	• A wire coil (encased in insulated plastic) is held over the skull and a very powerful electrical current is pulsed through the coil to generate a transient magnetic field of up to 2 Tesla in intensity. The patient is awake and alert throughout and may resume normal activity, including operating a motor vehicle, immediately after the rTMS session
	• The psychological effects, including those upon mood, depend on the pulse frequency and the region of the brain treated. Mood and anxiety seem to be most influenced when rTMS is administered over the DLPFC. PTSD may respond better to iTBS delivered to the right DLPFC.[7, 8] Pilot studies suggest that the antidepressant effect is greater with more lateral coil placement over the DLPFC
	• A spandex swim hat marked with cranial bony landmarks (nasion, inion, and tragus) can be used to record treatment site during the first session to assist with consistent coil placement over future sessions. Neuronavigation systems increase the accuracy and consistency of targeting. However, the use of these systems has not demonstrated to be associated with better clinical outcomes
	• A meta-analysis of bilateral vs. unilateral rTMS suggests no advantage for bilateral treatment
	• Different coil geometries (round, figure 8, H-coil) yield different patterns of induced electrical field in the brain. The H-coil (deep TMS or dTMS) generates a magnetic field that penetrates more deeply into the brain substance (6 cm vs. 2.5 cm for other coil geometries). Theoretically, deeper penetration with dTMS could be more effective than standard rTMS and some (but not all) meta-analyses of antidepressant effect size support this[19], although another failed to demonstrate superiority of dTMS over sham dTMS for depression[20]
Adverse Effects	• Usually very well tolerated; patients may feel discomfort or mild/moderate pain at the site of stimulation. The level of pain decreases over time after a few treatments
	• Discomfort in scalp most likely due to stimulation of pain receptors on the skin and bone
	• Headaches, usually with motor or premotor stimulation, commonly reported in rTMS studies; muscle tension headache can continue after the day's treatment session has ended [analgesics are of benefit]. Headache is less common as the course of rTMS proceeds and most patients no longer experience headache after the first 3–4 treatments
	• Some cases of nausea and tremor after rTMS have been reported but this is uncommon
	• The coil discharge noise artifact is loud and the coil is often placed very near the subject's ear, requiring use of foam ear plugs during treatment. This minimizes or eliminates the problem though transient increase in auditory thresholds has been described
	• Reports of mild neck pain, eye pain, toothache, likely due to stimulation of cranial nerves, and transient facial muscle twitches persisting after treatment session
	• Case reports of seizures with use of high-frequency rTMS; usually associated with sleep deprivation and/or substance use. There is no evidence showing increased risk of seizures with any particular antidepressant. Other sham-controlled trials report decreased seizure frequency in individuals with epilepsy treated with low-frequency rTMS
	• Case reports of switches to mania in patients with bipolar I and bipolar II disorders when treated with high-frequency rTMS of the left DLPFC; one case report with high-frequency treatment of the right DLPFC
	• Very rarely transient dysphasia may occur during stimulation (if coil placement is close to Broca's area in the inferior frontal cortex)
Contraindications	• Metallic implants in the head, cardiac pacemaker, personal history of seizures or history of seizures in first-degree relative
Pediatric Considerations	• rTMS has been used in children and adolescents for various diagnoses including ADHD, with and without Tourette's syndrome, and depression
	• A review study examining noninvasive brain stimulation techniques including rTMS in over 500 children and adolescents concluded that rTMS is safe

Repetitive Transcranial Magnetic Stimulation (rTMS) (cont.)

- One study reports response in 5 of 7 youths with depression treated with rTMS to the left DLPFC
- An open-label trial in 8 medication-resistant adolescents showed improvement of depression after 6–8 weeks of left high-frequency rTMS
- No significant adverse cognitive effects or seizures reported

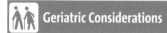 **Geriatric Considerations**

- A recent non-inferiority trial in older adults has shown that bilateral iTBS has similar effectiveness as bilateral high-frequency rTMS. Outcomes in this population were similar to those observed in adults[21]
- rTMS is considered safe and does not produce significant cognitive deficits, even among patients with clinical evidence of cerebrovascular disease. Improved cognitive functioning noted in some elderly subjects with cognitive impairment treated with rTMS[13]
- rTMS applied to the right DLPFC has been shown to improve motor performance in patients with Parkinson's disease
- Early data suggests response in late-onset vascular depression

 Use in Pregnancy

- Two case reports of successful treatment of females with depression; one in the second trimester, and the second through all 3 trimesters. No adverse effects were reported in mothers or infants (one of the babies was followed for 22 months)
- A case control study of infants of mothers with depression either untreated during pregnancy or treated with rTMS showed no abnormalities of cognitive functioning or motor development. Though the rTMS-treated mothers felt language development was delayed, this was similar to delays previously noted in children of mothers treated with SSRIs during pregnancy

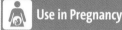 **Patient Instructions**

- For detailed patient instructions on rTMS , see the Patient Information Sheet (details p. 474)

Drug Interactions

- Clinically significant interactions are listed below
- For more interaction information on any given combination, also see the corresponding chapter for the interactant

Class of Drug	Example	Interaction Effects
Anticonvulsant	Clonazepam, valproate	Benzodiazepine use has been associated with poor outcomes in rTMS
	Gabapentin	One report suggests gabapentin may prolong duration of the antidepressant effect of rTMS

 Further Reading

References

1 Milev RV, Giacobbe P, Kennedy SH, et al. Canadian Network for Mood and Anxiety Treatments (CANMAT) 2016 clinical guidelines for the management of adults with major depressive disorder: Section 4. Neurostimulation treatments. Can J Psychiatry. 2016;61(9):561–575. doi:10.1177/0706743716660033

2 O'Reardon JP, Solvason HB, Janicak PG, et al. Efficacy and safety of transcranial magnetic stimulation in the acute treatment of major depression: A multisite randomized controlled trial. Biol Psychiatry. 2007;62(11):1208–1216. doi:10.1016/j.biopsych.2007.01.018

3 Blumberger DM, Vila-Rodriguez F, Thorpe KE, et al. Effectiveness of theta burst versus high-frequency repetitive transcranial magnetic stimulation in patients with depression (THREE-D): A randomised non-inferiority trial. Lancet. 2018;391(10131):1683–1692. doi:10.1016/S0140-6736(18)30295-2

4 Nguyen KH, Gordon LG. Cost-effectiveness of repetitive transcranial magnetic stimulation versus antidepressant therapy for treatment-resistant depression. Value Health. 2015;18(5):597–604. doi:10.1016/j.jval.2015.04.004

5 Mendlowitz AB, Shanbour A, Downar J, et al. Implementation of intermittent theta burst stimulation compared to conventional repetitive transcranial magnetic stimulation in patients with treatment resistant depression: A cost analysis. PLoS One. 2019;14(9):e0222546. doi:10.1371/journal.pone.0222546

6 Haesebaert F, Moirand R, Schott-Pethelaz AM, et al. Usefulness of repetitive transcranial magnetic stimulation as a maintenance treatment in patients with major depression. World J Biol Psychiatry. 2018;19(1):74–78. doi:10.1080/15622975.2016.1255353

7 Philip NS, Barredo J, Aiken E, et al. Theta-burst transcranial magnetic stimulation for posttraumatic stress disorder. Am J Psychiatry. 2019;176(11):939–948. doi:10.1176/appi.ajp.2019.18101160

8 Petrosino NJ, van't Wout-Frank M, Aiken E, et al. One-year clinical outcomes following theta burst stimulation for post-traumatic stress disorder. Neuropsychopharmacology. 2020;45(6): 940–946. doi:10.1038/s41386-019-0584-4

9 Kozel FA, Motes MA, Didehbani N, et al. Repetitive TMS to augment cognitive processing therapy in combat veterans of recent conflicts with PTSD: A randomized clinical trial. J Affect Disord. 2018;229:506–514. doi:10.1016/j.jad.2017.12.046

10 Shen X, Liu M, Cheng Y, et al. Repetitive transcranial magnetic stimulation for the treatment of post-stroke depression: A systematic review and meta-analysis of randomized controlled clinical trials. J Affect Disord. 2017;211:65–74. doi:10.1016/j.jad.2016.12.058

11 Teng S, Guo Z, Peng H, et al. High-frequency repetitive transcranial magnetic stimulation over the left DLPFC for major depression: Session-dependent efficacy: A meta-analysis. Eur Psychiatry. 2017;41:75–84. doi:10.1016/j.eurpsy.2016.11.002

12 Fitzgerald PB, Hoy KE, Elliot D, et al. Accelerated repetitive transcranial magnetic stimulation in the treatment of depression. Neuropsychopharmacology. 2018;43(7):1565–1572. doi: 10.1038/s41386-018-0009-9

13 Cheng CPW, Wong CSM, Lee KK, et al. Effects of repetitive transcranial magnetic stimulation on improvement of cognition in elderly patients with cognitive impairment: A systematic review and meta-analysis. Int J Geriatr Psychiatry. 2018;33(1):e1–e13. doi:10.1002/gps.4726

14 Weissman CR, Blumberger DM, Brown PE, et al. Bilateral repetitive transcranial magnetic stimulation decreases suicidal ideation in depression. J Clin Psychiatry. 2018;79(3). doi:10.4088/JCP.17m11692

15 Berlim MT, Van den Eynde F, Daskalakis ZJ. Efficacy and acceptability of high frequency repetitive transcranial magnetic stimulation (rTMS) versus electroconvulsive therapy (ECT) for major depression: A systematic review and meta-analysis of randomized trials. Depress Anxiety. 2013;30(7):614–623. doi:10.1002/da.22060

16 Mantovani A, Pavlicova M, Avery D, et al. Long-term efficacy of repeated daily prefrontal transcranial magnetic stimulation (TMS) in treatment-resistant depression. Depress Anxiety. 2012;29(10):883–890. doi:10.1002/da.21967

17 Ge R, Humaira A, Gregory E, et al. Predictive value of acute neuroplastic response to rtms in treatment outcome in depression: A concurrent TMS-fMRI trial. Am J Psychiatry. 2022;179(7):500–508. doi:10.1176/appi.ajp.21050541

18 Chen JJ, Liu Z, Zhu D, et al. Bilateral vs. unilateral repetitive transcranial magnetic stimulation in treating major depression: A meta-analysis of randomized controlled trials. Psychiatry Res. 2014;219(1):51–57. doi:10.1016/j.psychres.2014.05.010

19 Gellersen HM, Kedzior KK. Antidepressant outcomes of high-frequency repetitive transcranial magnetic stimulation (rTMS) with F8-coil and deep transcranial magnetic stimulation (DTMS) with H1-coil in major depression: A systematic review and meta-analysis. BMC Psychiatry. 2019;19:139. doi:10.1186/s12888-019-2106-7

20 Nordenskjold A, Martensson B, Pettersson A, et al. Effects of Hesel-coil deep transcranial magnetic stimulation for depression – A systematic review. Nord J Psychiatry. 2016;70(7):492–497. doi:10.3109/08039488.2016.1166263

21 Blumberger DM, Mulsant BH, Thorpe KE, et al. Effectiveness of standard sequential bilateral repetitive transcranial magnetic stimulation vs bilateral theta burst stimulation in older adults with depression: The FOUR-D randomized noninferiority clinical trial. JAMA Psychiatry. 2022;79(11):1065–1073. doi:10.1001/jamapsychiatry.2022.2862

Additional Suggested Reading

• Berlim MT, McGirr A, Beaulieu MM, et al. Are neuroticism and extraversion associated with the antidepressant effects of repetitive transcranial magnetic stimulation (rTMS)? An exploratory 4-week trial. Neurosci Lett. 2013;534:306–310. doi:10.1016/j.neulet.2012.12.029

• Connolly KR, Helmer A, Cristancho MA, et al. Effectiveness of transcranial magnetic stimulation in clinical practice post-FDA approval in the United States: Results observed with the first 100 consecutive cases of depression at an academic medical center. J Clin Psychiatry. 2012;73(4):e567–573. doi:10.4088/JCP.11m07413

• Cristancho MA, Helmer A, Connolly R, et al. Transcranial magnetic stimulation maintenance as a substitute for maintenance electroconvulsive therapy: A case series. J ECT. 2013;29(2):106–108. doi:10.1097/YCT.0b013e31827a70ba

• D'Agati D, Bloch Y, Levkovitz Y, et al. rTMS for adolescents: Safety and efficacy considerations. Psychiatry Res. 2010;177(3):280–285. doi:10.1016/j.psychres.2010.03.004

• Enticott PG, Fitzgibbon BM, Kennedy HA, et al. A double-blind, randomized trial of deep repetitive transcranial magnetic stimulation (rTMS) for autism spectrum disorder. Brain Stimul. 2014;7(2):206–211. doi:10.1016/j.brs.2013.10.004

• Galletta EE, Rao PR, Barrett AM. Transcranial magnetic stimulation (TMS): Potential progress for language improvement in aphasia. Top Stroke Rehabil. 2011;18(2):87–91. doi:10.1310/tsr1802-87

• Gaynes BN, Lloyd SW, Lux L, et al. Repetitive transcranial magnetic stimulation for treatment-resistant depression: A systematic review and meta-analysis. J Clin Psychiatry. 2014;75(5):477–489. doi:10.4088/JCP.13r08815

• Hebel T, Grözinger M, Landgrebe M, et al. Evidence and expert consensus based German guidelines for the use of repetitive transcranial magnetic stimulation in depression. World J Biol Psychiatry. 2022;23(5):327–348. doi:10.1080/15622975.2021.1995810

• Leggett LE, Soril LJ, Coward S, et al. Repetitive transcranial magnetic stimulation for treatment-resistant depression in adult and youth populations: A systematic literature review and meta-analysis. Prim Care Companion CNS Disord. 2015;17(6). doi:10.4088/PCC.15r01807

• Mayer G, Aviram S, Walter G, et al. (2012). Long-term follow-up of adolescents with resistant depression treated with repetitive transcranial magnetic stimulation. J ECT;28(2):84–86. doi:10.1097/YCT.0b013e318238f01a

Repetitive Transcranial Magnetic Stimulation (rTMS) (cont.)

- Nauczyciel C, Hellier P, Morandi X, et al. Assessment of standard coil positioning in transcranial magnetic stimulation in depression. Psychiatry Res. 2011;186(2–3):232–238. doi:10.1016/j.psychres.2010.06.012
- Parikh TK, Strawn JR, Walkup JT, et al. Repetitive transcranial magnetic stimulation for generalized anxiety disorder: A systematic literature review and meta-analysis. Int J Neuropsychopharmacol. 2022;25(2):144–146. doi:10.1093/ijnp/pyab077
- Slotema CW, Blom JD, Hoek HW, et al.: Should we expand the toolbox of psychiatric treatment methods to include repetitive transcranial magnetic stimulation (rTMS)? A meta-analysis of the efficacy of rTMS in psychiatric disorders. J Clin Psychiatry. 2010;71(7):873-884. doi:10.4088/JCP.08m04872gre
- Wall CA, Croarkin PA, Sim LA, et al. Adjunctive use of repetitive transcranial magnetic stimulation in depressed adolescents: A prospective, open pilot study. J Clin Psychiatry. 2011;72(9):1263–1269. doi:10.4088/JCP.11m07003

ANTIPSYCHOTICS

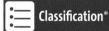 **Classification***

- Antipsychotics can be classified as follows:

Chemical Class	Agent	Page
First-Generation Antipsychotics (FGAs) [*]		See p. 128
Butyrophenone	Haloperidol	
Dibenzoxazepine	Loxapine	
Diphenylbutylpiperidine	Pimozide	
Phenothiazines		
– aliphatic	Example: Chlorpromazine	
– piperazine	Example: Perphenazine	
– piperidine	Example: Periciazine[C]	
Thioxanthenes	Example: Thiothixene	
Second-Generation Antipsychotics (SGAs) [**]		See p. 146
Benzisoxazole	Iloperidone[B], paliperidone, risperidone	
Benzisothiazol	Lurasidone	
Benzothiazolylpiperazine	Ziprasidone	
Butyrophenone	Lumateperone	
Dibenzodiazepine	Clozapine	
Dibenzo-oxepino pyrrole	Asenapine	
Dibenzothiazepine	Quetiapine	
Thienobenzodiazepine	Olanzapine	
Third-Generation Antipsychotics (TGAs)		See p. 177
Phenylpiperazine	Aripiprazole, Cariprazine	
N-arylpiperazine	Brexpiprazole	
5-HT$_{2A}$ Inverse Agonist Antipsychotic	Pimavanserin[B]	See p. 191

[*] Formerly called typical and conventional, [**] Formerly called atypical, which describes antipsychotics that have a decreased incidence of EPS at therapeutic doses; however, the boundaries between typical and atypical antipsychotics are not definitive. Atypical antipsychotics (1) may have low affinity for D$_2$ receptors and are readily displaced by endogenous dopamine in striatum (e.g., clozapine, quetiapine); (2) may have high D$_2$ blockade and high muscarinic blockade-anticholinergic activity; (3) block both D$_2$ and 5-HT$_2$ receptors (e.g., risperidone, clozapine, olanzapine, quetiapine); (4) may have high D$_4$ blockade (e.g., clozapine, olanzapine, loxapine); (5) may lack a sustained increased prolactin response (e.g., clozapine, quetiapine, olanzapine); (6) show mesolimbic selectivity (e.g., olanzapine, clozapine, quetiapine), [B] Not marketed in Canada. May be available through Health Canada's Special Access Programme, [C] Not marketed in the USA

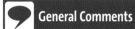 **General Comments**

- Antipsychotics are indicated in the treatment of a number of disorders, most notably schizophrenia and other related psychotic disorders and bipolar disorder. See the indications sections for FGAs (p. 129), SGAs (p. 147), and TGAs (p. 177) for detailed listings
- Despite the categorization of first, second, or third generation, these classes are heterogeneous and differences exist in the pharmacology and adverse effect profiles among them. These differences often help guide individualized treatment decisions. Non-industry-sponsored, randomized clinical trials comparing the effectiveness of a number of SGAs along with one FGA (i.e., perphenazine) suggest that some FGAs may be considered as appropriate first-line therapeutic alternatives. This has been reflected in a number of treatment guidelines that suggest selection of an antipsy-

* This classification system is under review.

Antipsychotics (cont.)

chotic agent should be tailored to best meet an individual's specific needs. Generally speaking, FGAs, especially high-potency agents, are associated with a higher incidence of extrapyramidal side effects (EPS) and tardive dyskinesia (TD). Haloperidol, in particular, appears to be associated with more EPS, even when lower doses are used. SGAs are less likely to result in EPS and TD but many are associated with a higher burden of metabolic adverse effects, most notably clozapine and olanzapine

- All classes have demonstrated efficacy in the treatment of positive symptoms of psychosis (e.g., hallucinations, delusions, hostility, and aggression) and relapse prevention
- Emerging data from cohort studies suggest that all classes of antipsychotics may decrease all-cause mortality in patients with schizophrenia[1], with some data suggesting nonsignificant, but modest between-class differences (long-acting injection vs. oral, FGA vs. SGA)[2]

 Pharmacology

- See p. 130, p. 149, and p. 179 for specific pharmacological statements relating to FGAs, SGAs, and TGAs, respectively, and the related charts listing effects on neurotransmitters/receptors (p. 194 and p. 195)

 Adverse Effects

- When individualizing therapy, the greater variation in adverse effect profiles observed among agents may play a more significant role in the selection of an antipsychotic than the smaller differences demonstrated in efficacy profiles
- See detailed discussion of adverse effects associated with SGAs (pp. 152–160), TGAs (p. 183), FGAs (pp. 131–136) and related charts (pp. 198–198)

Lab Tests/Monitoring

- Monitoring frequencies proposed below are guidelines only and should not replace good clinical judgment

Type	Details	Frequency
Initial history	Complete medical, substance use, smoking, and family history (including history of CVD, dyslipidemias, dementia, lung disease specifically for loxapine inhaler, and glucose dysregulation/diabetes in first-degree relatives)	Baseline
Physical assessment	Physical exam	Baseline and annually
	Waist circumference, weight, and BMI	Baseline and routinely thereafter (e.g., monthly for first 3 months, then every 3 months thereafter while on a stable antipsychotic dose)
	Blood pressure and pulse	Baseline and regularly thereafter (e.g., at 1 week, 1 month, 3 months, and every 6 months thereafter). More frequent assessments may be necessary during dosage titration with asenapine, chlorpromazine, clozapine, quetiapine, risperidone, thioridazine, and ziprasidone
	Temperature	When clinically indicated
Clinical assessment	Hyperprolactinemia	Screen for symptoms (e.g., decreased libido, erectile or ejaculatory dysfunction, menstrual changes, galactorrhea) at baseline and routinely thereafter (e.g., 1 month, 3 months, 6 months, and 12 months, then annually thereafter)
	EPS, TD, and other abnormal involuntary movements	Screen at baseline and routinely thereafter (e.g., at 2 weeks, monthly for 3 months, then every 6 months thereafter)
	Diabetes	Screen for symptoms (e.g., polydipsia, polyuria, polyphagia with weight loss, etc.) at baseline and routinely thereafter (e.g., baseline, at 6 months, 12 months, then annually thereafter)
	Sexual dysfunction	Screen at baseline and routinely (e.g., at 3 months, 6 months, and every 6 months thereafter)
	Sleep/sedation	Assess at baseline and routinely (e.g., at 2 weeks, 1 month, 2 months, 6 months, as clinically indicated thereafter)
	Anticholinergic effects	Screen for symptoms (e.g., confusion, constipation, dry eyes/mouth, blurred vision, urinary retention) at baseline and routinely as indicated (e.g., at 2 weeks, 1 month, 2 months, and as clinically indicated thereafter)

Type	Details	Frequency
Laboratory and other assessments	ECG	At baseline, along with serum potassium and magnesium levels in individuals with cardiac risk factors (e.g., heart disease – especially heart failure, recent MI, or preexisting conduction abnormalities; syncope; family history of early (before age 40) sudden cardiac death; or long QT syndrome) is recommended prior to prescribing antipsychotics with more definite associations/higher degrees of prolongation (e.g., chlorpromazine, haloperidol, pimozide)
	EEG	If seizures or myoclonus occur
	Fasting blood glucose	At baseline and routinely (e.g., at 6 months, 12 months, then annually thereafter). More frequent assessments may be required in patients with obesity, a family history of diabetes, or those who gain more than 5% of their body weight while on medication or experience a rapid increase in waist circumference
	A1c	If impaired fasting glucose or diabetes present
	Fasting lipid profile	At baseline and routinely (e.g., at 3 months, 12 months, and annually thereafter)
	Complete blood count	At baseline and as clinically indicated. Note: Specific hematological monitoring requirements exist for clozapine (see p. 162)
	Liver function tests	At baseline and at 1 month, then as clinically indicated thereafter
	Prolactin level	For prolactin-elevating antipsychotics: At baseline and at 3 months. If normal, no need for further testing. Also, as clinically indicated (e.g., signs of hyperprolactinemia on clinical assessment)

 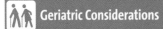 **Pediatric Considerations**

- For detailed information on the use of antipsychotics in this population, please see the *Clinical Handbook of Psychotropic Drugs for Children and Adolescents*[3]

Geriatric Considerations

- Pharmacokinetic and pharmacodynamic alterations associated with aging (decreased cardiac output, renal and hepatic blood flow, GFR, lean body mass, and hepatic metabolism – e.g., CYP3A4, etc.) may contribute to a marked sensitivity to the effects of antipsychotics
- Higher incidence of comorbid medical conditions often translates into use of multiple medications, thereby increasing the potential for adverse drug reactions, drug-drug interactions, and adherence issues
- Age-related sensory deficits and cognitive impairment may adversely impact adherence
- As a general rule, start with lower doses (e.g., 1/4–1/2 usual starting dose, and divide doses where possible) and titrate gradually. Assess tolerability following each dosage increase[4]
- Frequently reported adverse effects of antipsychotic medications in the elderly include neurological effects, orthostatic hypotension, sedation, and anticholinergic effects[4]
- **Neurological Effects**
  - The elderly are more sensitive to extrapyramidal reactions (e.g., akathisia, pseudoparkinsonism), which can be persistent and create difficulties in moving, eating, and sleeping and contribute to falls. These effects are typically dose related and are more common with high-potency FGAs. Exercise caution if opting to treat by adding anticholinergic agents or benzodiazepines, as these agents may exacerbate other conditions (e.g., constipation, memory impairment, falls, etc.) or precipitate a delirium
  - Consider comorbid medical conditions when choosing antipsychotic (e.g., Parkinson's disease, Lewy-body dementia)
  - The risk of TD increases with prolonged use and is higher with high-potency FGAs
- **Orthostatic Hypotension**
  - As most antipsychotics can cause orthostatic hypotension, use caution during dosage titration and when other hypotensive agents are prescribed – may result in falls and hip fracture. May be more common with low-potency FGAs, asenapine, clozapine, quetiapine, and risperidone
- **Sedation**
  - Tends to last longer in the elderly and can impair arousal levels during the day. May lead to confusion, disorientation, delirium, and increase risk of falls. Typically a dose related effect; more common with low-potency FGAs, asenapine, clozapine, olanzapine, and quetiapine. Caution when combining with other CNS depressants. If drug is prescribed in the morning or during the day, suggest moving it to evening or bedtime
- **Activation**
  - If activation or restlessness occurs, evaluate for drug-induced akathisia
  - If patient has problems sleeping, consider moving the dose to earlier in the day

Antipsychotics (cont.)

- **Anticholinergic Effects**
  - The elderly are more sensitive to anticholinergic effects; can result in physical as well as mental adverse effects (e.g., tachycardia, constipation, dry mouth and eyes, blurry vision, difficulty urinating, impairment in concentration and memory, delirium, worsening dementia, etc.). Most common with low-potency FGAs, clozapine, and olanzapine
- **Cognitive Effects**
  - Data contradictory as to cognitive decline secondary to use of antipsychotics for behavior disturbances in patients with Alzheimer's disease
- **Use in Dementia**
  - Individuals with dementia often develop neuropsychiatric symptoms such as agitation, aggression, and psychosis (e.g., delusions, hallucinations) over the course of illness. Many of these are challenging to control via nonpharmacological interventions and may result in the prescription of antipsychotic medication. SGAs and TGAs are preferred in this population (vs. FGAs), primarily as a consequence of their perceived improved tolerability (i.e., fewer EPS & other movement disorders)
  - A number of clinical trials evaluating these agents in the treatment of agitation and/or psychosis in dementia suggest minimal to modest clinical benefit, potentially negated in some cases by side effect burden. Recent meta-analysis describes nonsignificant improvement on standardized scale, but less discontinuation due to lack of efficacy with off-label use of olanzapine and aripiprazole
  - Recommendations for using antipsychotics to treat behavioral and psychological symptoms of dementia (BPSD) according to the Psychopharmacology Algorithm Project at the Harvard South Shore Program as follows: In an emergent setting – first-line recommendation is IM olanzapine. Second choice is IM haloperidol. In an urgent setting – first-line treatment would be oral aripiprazole or risperidone
  - Lack of efficacy of antipsychotics has been shown for numerous symptoms including: wandering, restless pacing, fidgeting/nervous twitching, repetitive vocalization, hoarding, inappropriate voiding, lack of social behavior skills, poor self-care practices, and indifference to surroundings
  - In 2005, both the FDA and Health Canada issued advisories concerning a small but significant increase in overall mortality in elderly patients with dementia-related psychosis treated with antipsychotic drugs. "Black box" warnings describing this risk were added to the labeling of these agents. The warnings were based on the analyses of 17 placebo-controlled trials (modal duration of 10 weeks), largely in patients taking atypical antipsychotics. The risk of death in drug-treated patients was 1.6–1.7 times the risk of death in placebo-treated patients. Over the course of a typical 10-week controlled trial, the rate of death in drug-treated patients was about 4.5%, compared to about 2.6% in the placebo group. Although causes of death varied, most deaths appeared to be either cardiovascular (e.g., heart failure, sudden death) or infectious (e.g., pneumonia) in nature. This "Black box" warning applies to all FGAs, SGAs, and TGAs
  - It is currently unknown if this risk extends beyond the early treatment period. Conversely, the benefits of long-term treatment with antipsychotics in this population are also uncertain
  - Consider individual's risk-benefit ratio when prescribing these agents in patients with dementia. It has been suggested to limit use to situations in which there is significant risk of harm to self or others, when hallucinations or delusions are problematic, or when symptoms are causing significant distress despite attempts to treat precipitating factors (e.g., infection, sleep deprivation, anticholinergic effects of medications) or implementation of alternative treatments, including nonpharmacological measures. Reassess the need for continued treatment regularly
  - Strategies for the use of antipsychotics in patients with dementia include slow dosage titration, using the lowest effective dose, avoiding agents with anticholinergic properties, avoiding using solely for indications of insomnia, depression, nonspecific agitation, and anxiety

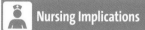 **Nursing Implications**

- Nurses may assist in baseline and routine assessment of mental status (to identify target symptoms & their subsequent response to drug therapy), physiological parameters (including weight, waist circumference, BP, heart rate, temperature, presence of abnormal movements), as well as documentation of any comorbidities, concomitant medications, and issues around medication adherence
- Excessive use of caffeine (e.g., colas, coffee, tea, chocolate) may worsen anxiety and agitation and counteract the beneficial effects of antipsychotics
- Adverse effects from therapy are a commonly cited reason for nonadherence
- Early onset (more common during the first 3 months of therapy) adverse effects include:
  - Anticholinergic effects – dry mouth, dry eyes, blurry vision, constipation, urinary retention, confusion/delirium, tachycardia
    - Frequent sips of water, chewing ice chips or sugarless gum, or artificial saliva products may relieve dry mouth. Artificial tears may relieve dry eyes. Blurred vision is usually transient; only near vision affected; if severe, pilocarpine eye drops may be prescribed
    - Anticholinergics reduce peristalsis and decrease intestinal secretions, leading to constipation; increasing fluids and bulk (e.g., bran, salads), as

well as fruit in the diet is beneficial; increasing exercise may help; if necessary, bulk laxatives (e.g., psyllium or polycarbophil), polyethylene glycol, or lactulose for chronic constipation
- Monitor patient's intake and output; urinary retention can occur, especially in the elderly and/or individuals with BPH; bethanechol (Urecholine) can reverse this
- Extrapyramidal side effects
  - Early-onset extrapyramidal side effects (EPS) (e.g., acute dystonias, akathisia, and pseudoparkinsonism); acute dystonias typically occur within the first few days and akathisia and pseudoparkinsonism within the first 6 weeks of treatment. These adverse effects are more commonly noted with FGAs, although they may occur with SGAs (most notably risperidone) and TGAs (e.g., aripiprazole and cariprazine). Anticholinergic agents (e.g., benztropine, procyclidine) may be used to prevent and/or treat some of these conditions (see p. 224 for details on treatment)
  - The use of prophylactic anticholinergic medications to prevent EPS is controversial as these agents can worsen anticholinergic adverse effects, including delirium. Young males on high-potency FGAs and individuals with a prior history of EPS may be at a higher risk for developing EPS and as such may be suitable candidates for prophylaxis. If an anticholinergic agent is prescribed to treat EPS, the need for its continued use should be reassessed periodically
  - Hold antipsychotic dose and notify physician if patient develops acute dystonia, severe persistent extrapyramidal reactions (longer than a few hours), or has symptoms of jaundice or blood dyscrasias (e.g., fever, sore throat, infection, cellulitis, weakness)
  - Be aware that akathisia can be misdiagnosed as anxiety or psychotic agitation and the incorrect treatment prescribed
- Postural hypotension, dizziness, and reflex tachycardia
  - Sitting on the side of the bed for a few minutes before rising or rising slowly from a seated position may help reduce falls
  - Hypotension may be compounded by concomitant administration of antihypertensives
- Somnolence, sedation
  - Caution patient not to perform activities requiring alertness until response to the drug has been determined
  - If drug is prescribed in the morning or during the day, suggest moving it to evening or bedtime
- Activation
  - If drug is suspected of causing activation or restlessness or if patient has problems sleeping, evaluate for drug-induced akathisia; moving the dose to earlier in the day may be helpful
- Weight gain
  - Weight gain may occur in patients receiving antipsychotics (especially SGAs); proper diet, exercise, and avoidance of calorie-laden beverages is important; monitor weight, waist circumference, and BMI during course of treatment
- Late-onset adverse effects include:
  - Metabolic effects – dyslipidemias, glucose intolerance, type 2 diabetes, weight gain
    - Baseline and periodic evaluation of weight, waist circumference, BP, and fasting blood glucose and lipid profiles recommended
  - Menstrual abnormalities, sexual dysfunction
    - Amenorrhea, sexual dysfunction including anorgasmia reported
  - Tardive movement disorders
    - Risk of developing TD believed to increase with duration of treatment and total dose
    - Use the lowest effective dose for the shortest possible duration to minimize risk of development
    - There is no effective treatment; consider discontinuing antipsychotic were feasible
- Other significant adverse effects (may not be time dependent) include:
  - Agranulocytosis/leukopenia/neutropenia
    - Patients with low neutrophil counts should be monitored closely for fever and other signs of infection and treated accordingly
    - Discontinue antipsychotic use if ANC counts less than 1500/µL 1.5 × 10^9/L
  - Diabetic Ketoacidosis
    - Has been noted to occur in individuals treated with antipsychotics despite no history of hyperglycemia
    - Signs/symptoms may include hypotension, tachycardia, fruity odor on breath, lethargy, shortness of breath, nausea, vomiting, abdominal pain, polyuria, polydipsia
  - Neuroleptic malignant syndrome (NMS)
    - Patients should avoid dehydration and exposure to extreme heat and humidity as antipsychotics affect the body's ability to regulate temperature
    - Signs of NMS may include autonomic instability, hyperpyrexia, altered mental status, rigidity, elevated creatine phosphokinase, elevated white blood cell count, and potentially renal failure
    - Antipsychotic should be discontinued immediately and supportive measures implemented

Antipsychotics (cont.)

- Seizures (typically dose related)
  - Use antipsychotics with caution in patients with seizure disorder, especially if poorly controlled
- QTc prolongation/arrhythmia
  - Monitor patients for symptoms that may be associated with QT prolongation (e.g., dizziness, fainting spells, palpitation, nausea, and vomiting). Symptomatic patients will require an ECG

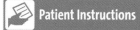 **Patient Instructions**

- For detailed patient instructions on antipsychotics, see the Patient Information Sheets (details on p. 474)

First-Generation Antipsychotics/FGAs

Product Availability*

Generic Name	Chemical Class	Neuroscience-based Nomenclature* (Pharmacological Target/ Mode of Action)	Trade Name[A]	Dosage Forms and Strengths
Chlorpromazine	Aliphatic phenothiazine	Dopamine, serotonin/Antagonist	Largactil[C]	Tablets: 10 mg[B], 25 mg, 50 mg, 100 mg, 200 mg[B] Short-acting injection: 25 mg/mL, 27.9 mg/mL[C]
Flupenthixol (Flupentixol)[C]	Thioxanthene	Dopamine, serotonin/Antagonist	Fluanxol Fluanxol Depot	Tablets[C]: 0.5 mg, 3 mg, 5 mg Long-acting IM injection (flupenthixol decanoate depot)[C]: 20 mg/mL, 100 mg/mL
Fluphenazine	Piperazine phenothiazine	Dopamine/Antagonist	Moditen[C], Prolixin[B] Modecate[C], Prolixin decanoate[B]	Tablets: 1 mg, 2 mg[C], 2.5 mg[B], 5 mg, 10 mg[B] Oral elixir[B]: 2.5 mg/5 mL Oral liquid concentrate[B]: 5 mg/mL Short-acting IM injection[B]: 2.5 mg/mL Long-acting IM injection (fluphenazine decanoate depot): 25 mg/mL, 100 mg/mL[C]
Haloperidol	Butyrophenone	Dopamine/Antagonist	Haldol Haldol Decanoate	Tablets: 0.5 mg, 1 mg, 2 mg, 5 mg, 10 mg, 20 mg Oral solution: 2 mg/mL Short-acting IM injection (haloperidol lactate): 5 mg/mL Long-acting IM injection (haloperidol decanoate depot): 50 mg/mL, 100 mg/mL
Loxapine	Dibenzoxazepine	Dopamine, serotonin/Antagonist	Loxapac[C], Loxitane[B] Adasuve[B]	Tablets[C]: 2.5 mg, 5 mg, 10 mg, 25 mg, 50 mg Capsules[B]: 5 mg, 10 mg, 25 mg, 50 mg Short-acting IM injection[C]: 50 mg/mL Inhalation powder: 10 mg in a single-use inhaler
Methotrimeprazine (Levomepromazine)[C]	Aliphatic phenothiazine	Not listed	Nozinan[C]	Tablets: 2 mg, 5 mg, 25 mg, 50 mg Short-acting IM injection: 25 mg/mL

Generic Name	Chemical Class	Neuroscience-based Nomenclature* (Pharmacological Target/ Mode of Action)	Trade Name(A)	Dosage Forms and Strengths
Periciazine(C)	Piperidine phenothiazine	Not listed	Neuleptil(C)	Capsules: 5 mg, 10 mg, 20 mg Oral drops: 10 mg/mL
Perphenazine	Piperazine phenothiazine	Dopamine/Antagonist	Trilafon Etrafon(B)	Tablets: 2 mg, 4 mg, 8 mg, 16 mg Tablets (perphenazine/amitriptyline): 2 mg/10 mg, 2 mg/24 mg, 4 mg/10 mg, 4 mg/25 mg, 4 mg/50 mg
Pimozide	Diphenylbutylpiperidine	Dopamine/Antagonist	Orap	Tablets: 1 mg(B), 2 mg, 4 mg(C), 10 mg(C)
Thioridazine(B), (D)	Piperidine phenothiazine	Dopamine, serotonin/Antagonist	Mellaril(B)	Tablets: 10 mg, 25 mg, 50 mg, 100 mg
Thiothixene(B)	Thioxanthene	Not listed	Navane(B)	Capsules: 1 mg, 2 mg, 5 mg, 10 mg
Trifluoperazine	Piperazine phenothiazine	Dopamine, serotonin/Antagonist	Stelazine	Tablets: 1 mg, 2 mg, 5 mg, 10 mg, 20 mg(C)
Zuclopenthixol(C)	Thioxanthene	Dopamine/Antagonist	Clopixol(C) Clopixol Acuphase(C) Clopixol Depot(C)	Tablets: 10 mg, 25 mg Short-acting IM injection (zuclopenthixol acetate depot): 50 mg/mL Long-acting IM injection (zuclopenthixol decanoate depot): 200 mg/mL

* Refer to Health Canada's Drug Product Database or the FDA's Drugs@FDA for the most current availability information   * Developed by a taskforce consisting of representatives from the American College of Neuropsychopharmacology (ACNP), the Asian College of Neuropsychopharmacology (AsCNP), the European College of Neuropsychopharmacology (ECNP), the International College of Neuropsychopharmacology (CINP), and the International Union of Basic and Clinical Pharmacology (IUPHAR) (see https://nbn2r.com), (A) Generic preparations may be available,   (B) Not marketed in Canada,   (C) Not marketed in the USA,   (D) Restricted to treatment-refractory schizophrenia in adults

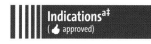

Indications[a][‡]
(👍 approved)

Schizophrenia and Psychotic Disorders

- 👍 Schizophrenia (chlorpromazine, fluphenazine, haloperidol, loxapine, perphenazine, thiothixene, trifluoperazine – Canada and USA; methotrimeprazine, thioproperazine, zuclopenthixol – Canada)
- 👍 Chronic schizophrenia (flupentixol, haloperidol, pimozide – Canada, in individuals whose main manifestations do not include excitement, agitation or hyperactivity; pipotiazine palmitate – Canada, in individuals who are non-agitated)
- 👍 Acute agitation associated with schizophrenia (loxapine inhalation powder – USA)
- 👍 Rapid control of acute manifestations of schizophrenia and acute psychotic episodes (haloperidol, zuclopenthixol acetate – Canada)
- 👍 Refractory schizophrenia (thioridazine – USA)
- 👍 Schizophrenia in patients with depressive symptoms (perphenazine + amitriptyline – USA)
- 👍 Psychotic disorders (chlorpromazine, fluphenazine, haloperidol – Canada and USA; methotrimeprazine, perphenazine, trifluoperazine – Canada)
- 👍 Adjunctive therapy in psychotic patients for control of residual prevailing hostility, impulsiveness, and aggressiveness (periciazine – Canada)
- • Psychotic depression (loxapine is metabolized to the antidepressant amoxapine)
- • Delusional disorder

Bipolar Disorder

- 👍 Manic phase of bipolar disorder/manic syndromes (chlorpromazine – Canada and USA; thioproperazine, trifluoperazine – Canada)
- 👍 Manic states: Rapid control of acute manifestations (haloperidol short-acting injection – Canada)
- 👍 Acute agitation associated with bipolar 1 disorder (loxapine inhalation powder – USA)
- 👍 Psychosis associated with manic-depressive syndromes (haloperidol, methotrimeprazine – Canada)

Acute Agitation, Delirium, and Dementia

- 👍 Chronic brain syndrome and mental retardation: Management of aggressive and agitated behavior (haloperidol – Canada)
- 👍 Senile psychoses (methotrimeprazine – Canada). In severe dementia, for the short-term symptomatic management of inappropriate behavior due to aggression and/or psychosis. The risks and benefits in this population should be considered

[a] Adult population unless otherwise stated   [‡] Indications listed here do not necessarily apply to all FGAs or all countries. Please refer to a country's regulatory database (e.g., US Federal Drug Administration, Health Canada Drug Product Database) for the most current availability information and indications

First-Generation Antipsychotics/FGAs (cont.)

- Delirium (chlorpromazine, haloperidol). A meta-analysis of 58 RCTs (1435 participants) demonstrated haloperidol plus lorazepam provided the best response rate for delirium treatment, compared with placebo/control. For delirium prevention, the dexmedetomidine hydrochloride, olanzapine, ramelteon, and risperidone groups had significantly lower delirium occurrence rates than placebo/control

Anxiety Disorders	

- ▲ Generalized nonpsychotic anxiety: Short-term management, no more than 6 mg/day or for longer than 12 weeks (trifluoperazine – USA)
- ▲ Depression/depressed mood with anxiety in association with chronic physical disease or with moderate to severe anxiety and/or agitation (perphenazine + amitriptyline – USA)
- ▲ Conditions associated with anxiety and tension: Autonomic disturbances, personality disturbances, emotional troubles secondary to such physical conditions as resistant pruritus (methotrimeprazine – Canada)
- ▲ Control of excessive anxiety, tension, and agitation seen in neuroses or associated with somatic conditions (trifluoperazine – Canada)

Movement Disorders	

- Dyskinesias: Management of various types, including Sydenham's chorea (haloperidol, risperidone)

Mental Health – Other	

- ▲ ADHD: Short-term treatment of hyperactive children who exhibit excessive motor activity that is manifested as impulsive behavior, difficulty sustaining attention, aggression, mood lability, and/or poor frustration tolerance (chlorpromazine, haloperidol – USA)
- ▲ Severe behavioral problems in children marked by combativeness and/or explosive hyperexcitable behavior that is not accounted for by immediate provocation with failure to respond to non-antipsychotic medication or psychotherapy (chlorpromazine, haloperidol – USA)
- ▲ Tourette's syndrome: Symptomatic control of tics and vocal utterances in adults and children (haloperidol – USA; pimozide – USA, in those who have failed standard treatment and daily life is severely compromised by motor and phonic tics)
- Trichotillomania

Other	

- ▲ Analgesia in pain due to cancer, zona (herpes zoster/shingles), trigeminal neuralgia, and neurocostal neuralgia, and in phantom limb pains and muscular discomforts (methotrimeprazine – Canada)
- ▲ Potentiator of anesthetics; in general anesthesia, can be used as both a pre- and post-sedative and analgesic (methotrimeprazine – Canada)
- ▲ Nausea and vomiting: Prevention and/or treatment (chlorpromazine, perphenazine – Canada and USA; methotrimeprazine, trifluoperazine – Canada; haloperidol – USA)
- ▲ Nausea, vomiting, and restlessness/anxiety associated with attacks of acute intermittent porphyria: Management (chlorpromazine – USA)
- ▲ Tetanus: Treatment adjunct (chlorpromazine – USA)
- Intractable hiccups (chlorpromazine, haloperidol – USA)

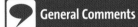

General Comments

- Low-potency FGAs are more likely to be associated with anticholinergic effects (e.g., constipation, dry mouth/eyes, blurred vision, urinary retention, confusion/delirium), antihistaminic effects (e.g., sedation, weight gain), and anti-adrenergic effects (e.g., orthostatic hypotension, dizziness, and reflex tachycardia). Significant metabolic effects appear to be less of a concern in comparison to some of the SGAs, although weight gain may occur, especially with the low-potency FGAs. Conduction abnormalities are a significant concern with some FGAs, notably pimozide and thioridazine
- For patients with schizophrenia, FGAs (e.g., chlorpromazine and haloperidol) are less effective in treating depressive symptoms than SGAs and TGAs[5]

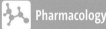

Pharmacology

- All first-generation (previously called typical or conventional) antipsychotics antagonize postsynaptic D_2 receptors as their main pharmacological activity. They may be further subclassified as low (e.g., chlorpromazine), moderate (e.g., perphenazine, loxapine, zuclopenthixol), or high (e.g., haloperidol) potency agents according to their affinity for the D_2 receptor
- Antagonism of D_2 receptors in the various dopaminergic pathways is thought responsible for the efficacy and also for some of the adverse effects associated with these agents. D_2 antagonism in the mesolimbic pathway relieves positive symptoms of psychosis; D_2 antagonism in the mesocortical pathway may worsen negative symptoms, mood, and cognition; D_2 antagonism in the nigrostriatal pathway may result in EPS (early onset) and TD (late onset); D_2 antagonism in the tuberoinfundibular tract may lead to hyperprolactinemia
- FGAs also have varying abilities to antagonize three other main receptors – α_1-adrenergic, H_1, and M_1 receptors. Generally, their affinities for these three receptors are the inverse of their affinities for the D_2 receptor

Dosing

- For dosing of individual oral and short-acting agents for schizophrenia and psychosis, see table pp. 200–202. For long-acting agents, see table p. 210
- For administration details, please see Nursing Implications pp. 138–139
- Current opinion suggests use of lower doses (i.e., haloperidol 2–10 mg daily, or equivalent); clinical efficacy of FGAs is correlated with D_2 binding above 60%, while hyperprolactinemia and EPS are associated with D_2 occupancies of 50–75% and 78%, respectively (see p. 131 and p. 133); outcome studies show that most patients respond similarly to low doses as to high doses, with decreased adverse effects
- Patients with acute symptoms may require slightly higher doses than chronic patients; manic patients may need even higher doses; maintenance doses for bipolar patients tend to be about half those used in schizophrenia
- Lower doses are used in first-episode patients, children, the elderly, and those with compromised liver and/or renal function

Pharmacokinetics

- See tables pp. 200–202 and p. 210 for kinetics of individual agents
- Hepatic primary route of metabolism: Chlorpromazine, haloperidol, loxapine, methotrimeprazine, perphenazine, pimozide, trifluoperazine
- Renal primary route of excretion: Chlorpromazine, pimozide, trifluoperazine

Oral

- Peak plasma levels of oral doses generally reached 1–4 h after administration
- Highly bound to plasma proteins
- Most phenothiazines and thioxanthenes have active metabolites
- Metabolized extensively by the liver; specific agents inhibit CYP450 metabolizing enzymes (see pp. 200–202)

Inhalation

- Peak plasma levels after inhalation (loxapine) achieved within 2 min
- Metabolized by the liver, with a similar half-life to oral administration

Short-acting IM

- Generally peak plasma level reached sooner than with oral preparation
- Bioavailability usually greater than with oral drug (loxapine excepted); dosage should be adjusted accordingly
- Loxapine single IM doses produce lower concentrations of active metabolite for first 12–16 h than oral therapy does – this may result in a different balance between D_2 and 5-HT$_2$ blockade
- Zuclopenthixol Acuphase: intermediate-acting depot injection (see p. 202) with a peak plasma level of 24–48 h and elimination half-life = 48–72 h

Long-acting IM

- See chart p. 210
- Bioavailability is greater than with oral agents (by a factor of at least 2); eliminates bioavailability problems related to absorption and first-pass metabolism and maintains stable plasma concentrations
- Presence of "free" fluphenazine in multi-dose vials of fluphenazine decanoate is responsible for high peak plasma level seen within 24 h of injection

Adverse Effects

- See charts p. 198 and p. 211 for incidence of adverse effects
- High-potency agents typically cause more D_2-related adverse effects (EPS and hyperprolactinemia), low-potency agents cause more α_1, H$_1$, and M$_1$-related adverse effects (e.g., postural hypotension, sedation, anticholinergic effects, respectively), and moderate-potency agents fall somewhere in the middle
- Some adverse effects may be preventable by employing simple strategies (e.g., slow upwards titration or dosing schedule manipulation – e.g., dosing a sedating drug at bedtime or dividing up the daily dose to minimize adverse effects related to higher peak levels)
- Many adverse effects may be transient in nature and require no intervention other than reassurance and follow-up to ensure they resolve

CNS Effects

- Confusion, disturbed concentration, disorientation (more common with high doses or in the elderly). Concomitant anticholinergic agents may exacerbate
- Extrapyramidal – acute onset: A result of antagonism at dopamine D_2 receptors (extrapyramidal reactions correlated with D_2 binding greater than approximately 80%)
  - Includes acute dystonia, akathisia, pseudoparkinsonism, Pisa syndrome, rabbit syndrome – see p. 224 for onset, symptoms, and treatment options and pp. 222–239 for detailed treatment options
  - More common with high-potency FGAs vs. moderate- to low-potency agents, also more common with FGAs vs. SGAs/TGAs – see pp. 224–227 to compare incidence of EPS associated with these agents
  - Most commonly occur within the first days to weeks of treatment and are dose related

First-Generation Antipsychotics/FGAs (cont.)

- Extrapyramidal – late onset or tardive movement disorders
  - Include tardive akathisia, tardive dyskinesia, and tardive dystonia – see p. 226 for onset, symptoms, and therapeutic management options. Valbenazine and deutetrabenazine are approved in the USA for treatment of tardive dyskinesia. They are VMAT2 inhibitors (vesicular monoamine transporter 2 inhibitors) and act to decrease dopamine release[6]
  - Late onset movement disorders usually develop after months or years of treatment
  - May be irreversible so prevention is key – use lowest doses for shortest possible time and assess for signs of movement disorders regularly. Symptoms are not alleviated and may be exacerbated by antiparkinsonian medications
  - Annual risk of TD with FGAs estimated to be 4–5% with a cumulative risk of up to 50%
- Neuroleptic malignant syndrome (NMS) – rare disorder characterized by autonomic dysfunction (e.g., tachycardia and hypertension), hyperthermia, altered consciousness, and muscle rigidity with an increase in creatine kinase and myoglobinuria. Can occur with any class of antipsychotic agent, at any dose, and at any time (although usually occurs early in the course of treatment). Risk factors may include dehydration, young age, male sex, organic brain syndromes, exhaustion, agitation, and rapid or parenteral antipsychotic administration
- Sedation – common, especially with low-potency agents, following treatment initiation, and with dosage increases. Usually transient, but some individuals may complain of persistent effects. [Management: Prescribe majority of daily dose at bedtime; minimize use of concomitant CNS depressants, if possible]
- Seizures – all FGAs may lower seizure threshold, resulting in seizures ranging from myoclonus to grand mal type. At usual dosage ranges, seizure rates are less than 1% for FGAs. Risk greater with low-potency agents and is dose related. May occur if dose increased rapidly or may also be secondary to hyponatremia associated with SIADH. Use with caution in patients with a history of seizures

Anticholinergic Effects

- See relative tolerability profiles table p. 196 for a comparison of the likelihood of anticholinergic effects among antipsychotics
- More common with low-potency FGAs
- Many of these adverse effects are often dose related and may also resolve over time without treatment. Treatment options may include reducing the dose of the FGA or switching to another antipsychotic with less potential to cause anticholinergic effects or employing a specific drug or non-drug strategy to treat the adverse effect (see below for suggestions)
- Blurred vision, dry eyes [Management: Use adequate lighting when reading; pilocarpine 0.5% eye drops]
- Constipation [Management/prevention: Increase dietary fiber and fluid intake, increase exercise, or use an osmotic agent (e.g., lactulose) or bulk laxative (e.g., psyllium)]
- Delirium – characterized by agitation, confusion, disorientation, visual hallucinations, tachycardia, etc. May result with use of high doses or combination anticholinergic medication. Drugs with high anticholinergic activity have also been associated with slowed cognition and selective impairments of memory and recall
- Dry eyes (Management: Artificial tears, wetting solutions)
- Dry mouth/mucous membranes – if severe or persistent, may predispose patient to candida infection [Management: Sugar-free gum and candy, oral lubricants (e.g., MoiStir, OraCare D), pilocarpine mouth wash – see p. 57]
- Urinary retention – may be more problematic for older patients, especially males with benign prostatic hypertrophy [Management: Bethanechol]

Cardiovascular Effects

- Arrhythmias and ECG changes (see p. 154):
  - Thioridazine has the most compelling evidence regarding QTc prolongation, with numerous reports of torsades de pointes and sudden cardiac death. There also appears to be an association for pimozide at higher doses. There have also been reports of torsades de pointes with chlorpromazine, droperidol and haloperidol. All the aforementioned agents are rated as "Risk of TdP – QT prolongation and clear association of risk of TdP even when used as directed" by CredibleMedsWorldwide[7]
  - See relative tolerability profiles table p. 196 for a comparison of the likelihood of QT prolongation among antipsychotics
  - The presence of other known risk factors for QT prolongation should be assessed and, to the extent possible, controlled (e.g., electrolyte imbalances corrected, interacting drugs or use of concomitant drugs that prolong QT avoided) before consideration is given to the initiation of treatment with a FGA. The effectiveness of baseline and follow-up ECGs as a monitoring tool has not been proven and may not be of value given the inherent variability within the QT interval (approximately 100 msec), though it has been recommended by some. See p. 154 for more information on QT/TdP

- Tachycardia may occur as a compensatory mechanism to orthostatic hypotension caused by α_1-adrenergic antagonism. Tachycardia due to anticholinergic effects in the absence of above conditions, may be treated with a low-dose peripherally-acting β-blocker
- Death/dementia – FGAs are associated with an increased risk of mortality in elderly patients treated for dementia-related psychosis with these agents, see p. 126
- Dyslipidemia (see p. 155)
- Orthostatic hypotension/compensatory tachycardia/dizziness/syncope – may occur as a result of α_1-adrenergic antagonism. More likely to occur with low-potency FGAs. DO NOT USE EPINEPHRINE, as it may further lower the blood pressure (see Drug Interactions p. 145). Elderly patients are susceptible to this adverse effect and syncopal episodes may result in falls and fractures. [Management: Rise slowly, divide the daily dose, consider a switch to another agent, increase fluid and salt intake, use support hose; treatment with fluid-retaining corticosteroid – fludrocortisone]
- Venous thrombosis – low-potency agents may be a risk factor for venous thrombosis in predisposed individuals, case reports of deep vein thrombosis in patients on chlorpromazine – usually occurs in first 3 months of therapy
- Cardiovascular disease (CVD) is the leading cause of death in individuals with schizophrenia. There may be a number of contributing factors to CVD in this population, including smoking, sedentary lifestyles, poverty, poor nutrition, reduced access to health care, and a number of metabolic abnormalities including weight gain, dyslipidemias, glucose intolerance, and hypertension. Please see p. 155 for more details on these endocrine and metabolic effects and their role in CVD

| Endocrine & Metabolic Effects |

- Antidiuretic hormone dysfunction:
  - Disturbances in antidiuretic hormone function: PIP (polydipsia, intermittent hyponatremia, and psychosis syndrome); prevalence in schizophrenia estimated at 6–20%, can range from mild cognitive deficits to seizures, coma, and death; increased risk in the elderly, smokers, and alcoholics. Monitor sodium levels in chronically treated patients to help identify risk for seizures [Management: Fluid restriction, demeclocycline up to 1200 mg/day, propranolol 30–120 mg/day; replace electrolytes, including salt tablets]
- Dyslipidemia:
  - See p. 124 for suggested monitoring guidelines
  - The comparative metabolic risks associated with various FGAs are less well studied, but in general these agents are associated with a lower metabolic risk (weight gain, glucose dysregulation, and lipid abnormalities) vs. many SGAs. In general, low-potency FGAs > moderate-potency FGAs > high-potency FGAs with respect to metabolic risk liability
  - Treatment options may include lifestyle and dietary modifications; switching to another antipsychotic associated with a lower potential for lipid dysregulation; adding cholesterol-lowering medication (e.g., statins, fibrates, salmon oil, etc.)
- Glucose intolerance, insulin resistance, hyperglycemia, type 2 diabetes, diabetic ketoacidosis:
  - Schizophrenia is a risk factor for the development of type 2 diabetes. Certain antipsychotic medications have also been associated with an increased risk for glucose intolerance/diabetes. While the risk appears highest with SGAs (most notably clozapine and olanzapine), there are also reports in the literature of glycosuria, glucose intolerance, hyperglycemia, and diabetes mellitus occurring in association with FGAs. Within FGAs, the risk may be greater with low-potency agents or phenothiazines
  - See p. 124 for suggested monitoring guidelines
  - Treatment options may include lifestyle and dietary modifications; switching to another antipsychotic associated with a lower potential for glucose dysregulation; adding hypoglycemic agent
- Hyperprolactinemia:
  - Prolactin level may be elevated up to 10-fold from baseline. Develops over first week of treatment and usually remains throughout treatment course
  - *Clinical consequences* of elevated prolactin levels may include short-term risks such as galactorrhea, gynecomastia, menstrual irregularities, and sexual dysfunction, and potential long-term risks such as osteoporosis (as a result of decreased bone density secondary to chronic hypogonadism), pituitary tumors, and breast cancer (data conflicting)
  - *Effects in women:* Breast engorgement and lactation (may be more common in women who have previously been pregnant), amenorrhea (with risk of infertility), menstrual irregularities, changes in libido, hirsutism (due to increased testosterone). Bone mineral density loss may be more intense in females than males and may vary by ethnic group; extent of loss may correlate with duration of hyperprolactinemia. Recommended women with hyperprolactinemia or amenorrhea for more than 12 months have a bone mineral density evaluation
  - *Risk of breast cancer:* A nationwide nested case-control study in Finland reported that exposure to prolactin-increasing antipsychotics for 5 or more years was significantly associated with increased odds of breast cancer in comparison with minimal exposure (less than 1 year). On the

other hand, exposure to prolactin-sparing antipsychotics (including clozapine, quetiapine, or aripiprazole) for 5 or more years was not associated with an increased risk of breast cancer in comparison with minimal exposure (less than 1 year)

- *Effects in men:* Gynecomastia, rarely galactorrhea, decreased libido, and erectile or ejaculatory dysfunction
- See relative tolerability profiles table p. 196 for a comparison of the likelihood of hyperprolactinemia among antipsychotics
- See p. 124 for suggested monitoring guidelines
- *Treatment options:* Assuming discontinuation of antipsychotic therapy is not an option, the preferred treatment is to switch to another antipsychotic agent with a reduced risk of hyperprolactinemia – weighing the potential risk for relapse associated with this action. Other treatment options may include lowering the dose or adding a medication to treat the condition. Use of a dopamine agonist such as bromocriptine (1.25–2.5 mg bid) or cabergoline (0.25–2 mg/week) may be considered but has the potential to exacerbate the underlying illness. Use of a D_2 partial agonist such as aripiprazole (5 mg/day, possibly increase to 10 mg/day if only partial response with 5 mg) has also been used to treat antipsychotic-associated hyperprolactinemia

- Metabolic syndrome:
  - See p. 157 for details
  - Little is known about the relative risks of FGAs with respect to causing or contributing to metabolic syndrome, as heightened awareness of the relationship between antipsychotics and this condition arose primarily during the reign of SGAs. Since weight gain, dyslipidemias, and glycemic abnormalities have been noted to occur with FGAs (though typically at a much lower rate than with many of the SGAs), it is likely that metabolic syndrome may occur especially with low-potency FGAs, albeit less commonly vs. the majority of SGAs
- Weight gain:
  - Reported in up to 40% of patients receiving treatment with FGAs. More likely to occur early in treatment (e.g., within first 6 months) and the risk appears greater with low-potency FGAs[4]
  - See relative tolerability profiles table p. 196 for a comparison of the likelihood of weight gain among antipsychotics
  - The mechanism by which antipsychotics may influence weight gain is unknown (may be a result of multiple systems including 5-HT_{1B}-, 5-HT_{2C}-, α_1-, and H_1-blockade, hyperprolactinemia, gonadal and adrenal steroid imbalance, and increase in circulating leptin; may also be due to sedation and inactivity, carbohydrate craving, and excessive intake of high-calorie beverages to alleviate drug-induced thirst and dry mouth)
  - Weight gain may contribute to or have deleterious effects on a number of conditions, including dyslipidemia, glucose dysregulation and type 2 diabetes, hypertension, coronary artery disease, stroke, osteoarthritis, sleep apnea, and self-image
  - See p. 124 for suggested monitoring guidelines and p. 157 for treatment options

| **GI Effects** | - Anorexia, dyspepsia |

- Anorexia, dyspepsia
- Constipation – see Anticholinergic Effects p. 153
- Dysphagia – (difficulty swallowing) and aspiration have been reported with antipsychotic use. Use all agents cautiously in individuals at risk for developing aspiration pneumonia (e.g., advanced Alzheimer's disease)
- Dry mouth – see Anticholinergic Effects p. 153
- Pancreatitis – rare reports of pancreatitis with haloperidol
- Peculiar taste, glossitis
- Sialorrhea, difficulty swallowing, gagging [see p. 158 for additional information on management
- Vomiting common after prolonged treatment, especially in smokers

Urogenital & Sexual Effects

- Sexual effects may result from altered dopaminergic (including hyperprolactinemia – main cause of sexual dysfunction in women), serotonergic, ACh, α_1, or H_1 activity
- An estimated 25–60% of patients on FGAs report sexual dysfunction
- Treatment options may include: 1) dosage reduction, 2) waiting 1–3 months to see if tolerance develops, 3) switching antipsychotics, or 4) adding a medication to treat the problem (see below for treatment suggestions regarding specific types of dysfunction; evidence for their use is based primarily on open-label studies and case reports)
- *Anorgasmia* [Management: Bethanechol (10 mg tid or 10–25 mg prn before intercourse), neostigmine (7.5–15 mg prn), cyproheptadine (4–16 mg/day), amantadine (100–300 mg/day)]

- *Ejaculation dysfunction* (incl. inhibition of ejaculation, abnormal ejaculation, retrograde ejaculation – especially thioridazine) – reported to be the most common sexual disturbance associated with FGAs [Management suggestions: For retrograde ejaculation – imipramine (25–50 mg at bedtime), yohimbine (5.4 mg 1–3 × daily, 1–4 h prior to intercourse), or cyproheptadine (4–16 mg/day)]
- *Erectile dysfunction, impotence* – ED is reported to occur in 23–54% of males on FGAs [Management suggestions: Bethanechol (10 mg tid or 10–50 mg prn before intercourse), yohimbine (5.4 mg 1–3 × daily, 1–4 h prior to intercourse), sildenafil (25–100 mg prn), amantadine (100–300 mg/day)]
- *Libido* – decreased libido [Management: Neostigmine (7.5–15 mg prn) or cyproheptadine (4–16 mg prn 30 min before intercourse)]
- *Priapism* – rare case reports of priapism occurring in patients on FGAs (i.e., chlorpromazine, fluphenazine, perphenazine, prochlorperazine, thioridazine, thiothixene, and trifluoperazine). Antagonism of α-adrenergic receptors is believed to play a role in this effect
- *Urinary retention* – see Anticholinergic Effects p. 154

Ocular Effects

- Blurred vision/dry eyes – see Anticholinergic Effects p. 153
- Cataracts/lens changes: Association reported between phenothiazine use and cataract formation. Though eye examination (e.g., slit lamp exam) has been recommended at baseline and 6-month intervals thereafter, this recommendation is controversial
- Lenticular pigmentation
  - Related to long-term use of antipsychotics (primarily chlorpromazine)
  - Presents as glare, halos around lights or hazy vision
  - Granular deposits in eye
  - Vision is usually not impaired; may be reversible if drug stopped
  - Often present in patients with antipsychotic-induced skin pigmentation or photosensitivity reactions
- Pigmentary retinopathy (retinitis pigmentosa)
  - Primarily associated with chronic use/higher doses of the low-potency FGAs thioridazine or chlorpromazine [annual ophthalmological examination recommended]
  - Recommended to NOT exceed a maximum dose of 800 mg per day of thioridazine
  - Reduced visual acuity (may occasionally reverse if drug stopped)
  - Blindness can occur
- With chronic use, chlorpromazine can cause pigmentation of the endothelium and Descemet's membrane of the cornea; it may cause a slate-bluish discoloration of the conjunctiva, sclera, and eyelids – may not be reversible when drug stopped

Hematological Effects

- Blood dyscrasias, including those affecting erythropoiesis, granulopoiesis, and thrombopoiesis, reported with most antipsychotics
- The development of any blood abnormalities in individuals on antipsychotics, especially other than clozapine, should undergo rigorous medical assessment to determine the underlying cause
- *Aplastic anemia* – reported primarily with chlorpromazine and trifluoperazine. Also noted to have occurred in patients treated with fluphenazine, flupenthixol, haloperidol, perphenazine, and thioridazine
- *Eosinophilia* – not typically of clinical significance unless severe. Reported with chlorpromazine and trifluoperazine
- *Leukopenia* [defined as WBC $< 4 \times 10^9$/l] and *neutropenia/agranulocytosis* [neutropenia (defined as ANC $< 1.5 \times 10^9$/L) may be subclassified as mild (ANC $= 1$–1.5×10^9/L), moderate (ANC $= 0.5$–1×10^9/L) or severe (also termed agranulocytosis – defined as ANC $< 0.5 \times 10^9$/L or sometimes as ANC $< 0.2 \times 10^9$/L)].
  - Mild neutropenia may be transient (returning to normal without a change in medication/dose), or progressive (continuing to drop, leading to agranulocytosis)
  - Reported incidence of severe neutropenia in 1 study was 0.02% with phenothiazines and 0.003% with butyrophenones
- *Thrombocytopenia* – reported with a number of FGAs, including chlorpromazine, prochlorperazine, and thioridazine. In most cases withdrawal of the medication was reported to result in normalization of platelet counts

Hepatic Effects

- Cholestatic jaundice
  - Occurs in less than 0.1% of patients within first 4 weeks of treatment, with most antipsychotics
  - Noted to occur in 0.1–0.5% of patients taking chlorpromazine
- Transient asymptomatic transaminase elevations (ALT 2–3 times the upper limit of normal) reported with haloperidol (up to 16% of patients)

Hypersensitivity Reactions

- Usually appear within the first few months of therapy (but may occur after the drug is discontinued)

First-Generation Antipsychotics/FGAs (cont.)

- Photosensitivity and photoallergy reactions including sunburn-like erythematous eruptions that may be accompanied by blistering. Occurs most commonly with low-potency phenothiazines. Patients should be advised to avoid excess exposure to sunlight and wear appropriate clothing/sunscreen
- Loxapine inhalation powder has been associated with bronchospasm which has the potential to lead to respiratory distress and respiratory arrest. This product is only available through a restricted program in the USA – Adasuve Risk Evaluation and Mitigation Strategy (REMS) – in which the health care facility must have immediate access to advanced airway management personnel and equipment. This product is contraindicated in patients with asthma, COPD or other respiratory disease associated with bronchospasm or in patients with a known hypersensitivity to loxapine or amoxapine
- Hypersensitive reactions at injection site (especially haloperidol decanoate 100 mg/mL); indurations reported with higher doses (see p. 211)
- Cases of systemic lupus erythematosus reported with chlorpromazine

Temperature Regulation
- Altered ability of body to regulate response to changes in temperature and humidity; may become hyperthermic or hypothermic in temperature extremes due to inhibition of the hypothalamic control area. Patients should be advised to avoid temperature extremes, dress appropriately, and maintain adequate hydration

Other Adverse Effects
- Low-potency antipsychotics associated with increased risk of fatal pulmonary embolism (highest risk with thioridazine)

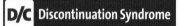 **Discontinuation Syndrome**
- Abrupt discontinuation of an antipsychotic occurs primarily in situations involving a sudden/severe adverse reaction to the drug (e.g., hepatic failure with chlorpromazine) or when patients become nonadherent by stopping their antipsychotic medication abruptly
- Abrupt discontinuation (or in some cases large dose reductions) of an antipsychotic may be associated with a number of withdrawal or discontinuation effects (see below). Prolonged antagonism of (dopaminergic, muscarinic, histaminic, adrenergic) receptors by the antipsychotic, resulting in a compensatory up-regulation, which then produces a rebound-type reaction when the antagonist is removed and the supersensitized receptors are exposed, has been proposed as a pharmacological explanation for these effects:
  1. Discontinuation syndromes – typically characterized by development of a number of symptoms including nausea, vomiting, diarrhea, diaphoresis, cold sweats, muscles aches and pains, insomnia, anxiety, and confusion. Many are believed to be the result of cholinergic and histaminergic rebound. Usually appear within days of discontinuation [Management: Mild cases may only require comfort and reassurance; for more severe symptoms consider restarting the antipsychotic followed by slow taper if possible; or, if rebound cholinergic effects present, consider adding an anticholinergic agent short term]
  2. Psychosis – exacerbation or precipitation of psychosis including a severe, rapid onset or supersensitivity psychosis, most notable with clozapine and possibly quetiapine vs. FGAs. Most likely to occur within the first 2–3 weeks post discontinuation or sooner [Management: Restart antipsychotic]
  3. Movement disorders – withdrawal dyskinesias noted to appear, usually around 2–4 weeks post abrupt withdrawal [Management: Restart antipsychotic and taper slowly]. Rebound dystonia, parkinsonism, and akathisia also reported to occur, usually within days to the first week post discontinuation [Management: Restart antipsychotic and taper or treat with appropriate anti-EPS medication]
- Abrupt cessation of a long-acting or depot antipsychotic is of less concern as plasma concentrations decline slowly (i.e., drug tapers itself)
- Clinicians should be cognizant of the potential for withdrawal effects to occur from a discontinued agent when switching to a new antipsychotic, in order to avoid misinterpreting them as adverse effects of the new agent and subsequently discontinuing it unnecessarily
- ☞ **AFTER PROLONGED USE, THESE MEDICATIONS SHOULD BE WITHDRAWN GRADUALLY WHERE POSSIBLE.** If switching to another antipsychotic, see pp. 216–217 for specific recommendations

 Precautions
- Hypotension occurs most frequently with parenteral use, especially with high doses; the patient should be in supine position during short-acting IM administration and remain supine or seated for at least 30 min; measure BP before and following each IM dose
- IM injections should be administered slowly
- Use with caution in the elderly, in the presence of cardiovascular disease, chronic respiratory disorder, hypoglycemia or convulsive disorders (see Use in Dementia p. 126)
- Should be used very cautiously/avoided in patients with narrow-angle glaucoma, BPH, decreased gastrointestinal motility, urinary retention, prolactin-dependent tumors or Parkinson's disease

- Prior to prescribing thioridazine or pimozide, a baseline ECG and serum potassium and magnesium should be done and monitored periodically during the course of therapy. DO NOT USE these drugs in patients with QTc interval over 450 msec or with significant risk factors for QTc prolongation/development of torsades de pointes (see p. 154)
- Monitor if QT interval exceeds 420 msec and discontinue drug if 500 msec exceeded; do not exceed 800 mg thioridazine or 20 mg pimozide daily
- Allergic cross-reactivity (rash) between chlorpromazine and clozapine reported

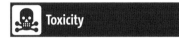 **Toxicity**

- In the majority of cases, overdose is associated with a low mortality and morbidity rate as FGAs have a high therapeutic index
- Symptoms may include nausea and vomiting, confusion, hallucinations, agitation, drowsiness progressing to coma, hypotension, respiratory depression, electrolyte imbalances, ECG changes and arrhythmias, and/or EPS

Management

- See p. 161 for further details on antipsychotic toxicity and management

 Use in Pregnancy◊

- General:
  - For each individual, consider the risks of not treating/undertreating (e.g., illness relapse, self-harm, poor adherence with prenatal care, poor nutrition, exposure to additional medication or herbal remedies, increased alcohol, tobacco or recreational drug use, deficits in mother-infant bonding) vs. the risks of continuing or starting an antipsychotic
  - Pregnancy-related changes (i.e., increased body weight, blood volume, and body fat, altered drug metabolism, and increased drug excretion) may require the use of higher drug doses to maintain efficacy. Postpartum dose tapering may be needed as liver metabolism and fluid volumes return to baseline levels. Monitor for FGA adverse effects and reduce dose as needed
  - Available data suggests most FGAs do not increase the risk of teratogenic effects in humans. However, human data for some FGAs is limited
  - Early data suggests *in utero* exposure to FGAs may decrease infant birth weight, increase the risk of small size for gestational age, and slightly increase the risk of preterm birth. However, data is conflicting and complicated by differences in study design, study population (e.g., use of concurrent medications, psychiatric diagnosis), and the inherent difficulties in studying medication use during pregnancy
  - Consider the potential effects on delivery (e.g., maternal hypotension with chlorpromazine) and for withdrawal effects in the newborn if used during the third trimester. There are case reports of fetal and neonatal toxicity including NMS, dyskinesia, EPS (manifested by heightened muscle tone and increased rooting and tendon reflexes persisting for several months), neonatal jaundice, and postnatal intestinal obstruction. In 2011, the US FDA and Health Canada asked manufacturers to update their prescribing information to warn clinicians and patients that third-trimester use of antipsychotics is associated with risk of EPS and withdrawal symptoms in newborns. Symptoms in the neonate may include: Feeding disorder, hypertonia, hypotonia, tremor, respiratory distress, and agitation. Signs related to atropinic properties of phenothiazines such as meconium ileus, delayed meconium passage, abdominal bloating, tachycardia, and feeding disorders in neonates can occur
  - Use of the long-acting injection formulation near delivery likely to prolong any withdrawal effects in the neonate
  - Avoid, if possible, FGAs that have no or very limited human pregnancy data (e.g., flupenthixol, loxapine, periciazine, pimozide, pipotiazine, thiothixene, and zuclopenthixol). FGAs with a larger reproductive safety profile include chlorpromazine, fluphenazine, haloperidol, perphenazine, and thioridazine
  - High-potency FGAs (e.g., haloperidol) may yield the best therapeutic benefit with the least anticholinergic and sedative effects; however, comparative safety with other FGAs in pregnancy is unavailable
- **Chlorpromazine** was initially used for nausea and vomiting during pregnancy. This data suggests chlorpromazine is safe if used in low doses during pregnancy. However, when given near term, particularly in doses of 500 mg or greater, chlorpromazine may cause an increased incidence of respiratory distress in the neonate and has been implicated in producing lethargy and EPS in the neonate
- **Flupenthixol**: Limited human data. No relevant animal data
- **Fluphenazine**: Limited human data. Human data suggest risk in 3rd trimester. Case reports of withdrawal effects (e.g., EPS, irritability) that developed up to 6 weeks post delivery with in utero exposure to the long-acting injection form
- **Haloperidol**: Limited human data. Animal data suggest moderate risk. Although the rates of major malformations in humans do not appear to be greater than baseline there have been cases of limb defects after first-trimester (time of greatest risk for malformations) exposure in humans to haloperidol. If haloperidol is required during pregnancy, ultrasound with particular attention to limb formation should be considered in first-trimester exposures. Two case reports of neonate tardive dyskinesia. Case report of NMS with third-trimester exposure to haloperidol and risperidone

◊ See p. 473 for further information on drug use in pregnancy and effects on breast milk

First-Generation Antipsychotics/FGAs (cont.)

- **Loxapine**: Manufacturer reports outcomes from only 3 pregnancies with loxapine exposure – one child born with achondroplasia, one child born with multiple unspecified malformations, and one child with tremors at 15 weeks of age
- **Methotrimeprazine**: Limited human data; probably compatible. No relevant animal data. Initially used in obstetric analgesia
- **Perphenazine**: Limited human data. Sporadic cases of both fetal malformations and gestational metabolic complications also emerged from a recent retrospective study investigating the use of perphenazine during pregnancy
- **Periciazine**: No published human data. No relevant animal data
- **Pimozide**: Limited human data (fewer than 5 case reports). Animal data suggest low risk
- **Thioridazine**: Limited human data. No relevant animal data
- **Thiothixene**: Limited human data. No teratogenic effects seen in animals
- **Trifluoperazine**: Limited human data. Animal data suggest low risk. Studies indicate no causal relationship between trifluoperazine exposure and congenital malformations
- **Zuclopenthixol**: Published human data (fewer than 10 case reports). Not teratogenic in animals

Breast Milk

- For each individual, consider the benefits of breastfeeding vs. the risks of infant drug exposure via breastmilk and possible effects on milk production
- Antipsychotics, like most medications, pass into breast milk however, antipsychotic amounts found are generally low. Antipsychotics have been detected in breast milk in concentrations of 0.1–11%. Long-term effects on the infant are largely unknown
- If used while breastfeeding, use lowest effective dose and monitor infant's progress
- Very limited data. Single or small numbers of case reports have found no short-term adverse effects of breastfed infants exposed to flupenthixol, perphenazine or zuclopenthixol. One report of drowsiness and lethargy with chlorpromazine. Cases of a decline in mental and psychomotor development at age 12–18 months with higher dose haloperidol (20–40 mg/day) and chlorpromazine (200–600 mg/day). Long-term effects on neurodevelopment are largely unknown. A 5-year follow-up study of 7 breastfed infants exposed to chlorpromazine found no developmental deficits
- Phenothiazines given directly to infants and children for sedation or cough and cold symptoms have been associated with apnea and sudden infant death syndrome (SIDS); however, phenothiazine exposure via breast milk is significantly lower
- Hale's lactation risk category = L3 (give only if the potential benefit outweighs the potential risk to the infant): chlorpromazine, fluphenazine, haloperidol, perphenazine, trifluoperazine, zuclopenthixol; risk category = L4 (no information available): loxapine, pimozide, thioridazine, thiothixene
- A review categorized chlorpromazine, haloperidol, and zuclopenthixol as possible for breastfeeding under medical supervision and categorized fluphenazine, flupenthixol, perphenazine, pimozide, trifluoperazine, and thiothixene as currently cannot be recommended for breastfeeding[8]
- Refer to the Drugs and Lactation Database (LactMed) website (https://www.ncbi.nlm.nih.gov/books/NBK501922/) for more information

Nursing Implications

- See pp. 126–128

Oral

- AVOID grapefruit juice with pimozide (See Drug Interactions p. 144)
- Oral solutions should be diluted just prior to administration to improve palatability. Not compatible with all beverages. Dilute fluphenazine and perphenazine solution with water, 7-Up, milk, V-8, or pineapple, apricot, prune, orange or tomato juice. Dilute haloperidol oral liquid with water or an acidic beverage such as juice; DO NOT mix with tea or coffee. Dilute loxapine with orange or grapefruit juice
- Some liquids such as chlorpromazine and methotrimeprazine have local anesthetic effects and should be well diluted to prevent choking
- If patient is suspected of not swallowing tablet medication, liquid medication can be given
- AVOID skin contact with liquid forms of fluphenazine as it may result in contact dermatitis
- Loxapine oral inhalation is given via a single-use inhaler. Once activated, the inhaler should be used within 15 min. An indicator light on the inhaler device will turn off once the full dose is delivered. It may take several breaths to deliver the full dose. Patient should hold their breath for as long as possible (up to 10 sec) after inhaling the dose. Can only be given in enrolled healthcare facilities with immediate, on-site resources to manage bronchospasm and/or respiratory distress

Short-acting IM	
	• Watch for orthostatic hypotension, especially with parenteral administration of chlorpromazine or methotrimeprazine; keep patient supine or seated for 30 min afterwards; monitor BP before and after each injection
	• Give IM into upper outer quadrant of buttocks or in the deltoid (deltoid offers faster absorption as it has better blood perfusion); alternate sites, charting (L) or (R); massage slowly after, to prevent sterile abscess formation; tell patient injection may sting
	• Prevent contact dermatitis by keeping drug solution off patient's skin and clothing and injector's hands, AVOID contact with fluphenazine, in particular
	• Do not let drug stand in syringe for longer than 15 min as plastic may adsorb drug
	• If irritation at the chlorpromazine IM injection site occurs, dilute drug with 0.9% sodium chloride injection or 2% procaine HCl
	• Haloperidol lactate can be administered IM in the same syringe as lorazepam
	• Storage: Room temperature and protected from light (chlorpromazine HCl, fluphenazine HCl, haloperidol lactate, loxapine HCl, methotrimeprazine HCl)

Long-acting IM	
	• Recommended to establish tolerability with an oral form prior to initializing a long-acting IM dosage form
	• Short-acting preparations may be required for supplementation while dosage titration is taking place
	• Use a needle of at least 21 gauge; give deep IM into large muscle (e.g., buttock, using Z-track method); rotate sites and specify in charting
	• As with all oily injections, it is important to ensure, by aspiration before injection, that inadvertent intravascular injection does not occur
	• Do not let drug stand in syringe for longer than 15 min as plastic may adsorb drug
	• DO NOT massage injection site
	• SC administration can be used for fluphenazine decanoate
	• AVOID skin contact with liquid forms of fluphenazine as it may result in contact dermatitis
	• Storage: Room temperature and protected from light – haloperidol decanoate, flupenthixol decanoate, fluphenazine decanoate

Intravenous	
	• Some short-acting injection formulations can be administered intravenously. Long-acting formulations CANNOT be administered via this route.
	• IV administration generally occurs in the intensive care or surgical setting
	• Haloperidol lactate and chlorpromazine can be given via direct IV injection or IV infusion
	• Haloperidol administered IV is associated with higher rates of sudden death, torsades de pointes, and QT prolongation
	• Methotrimeprazine injection diluted with 5% dextrose can be given as a slow infusion (20–40 drops per min) to potentiate anesthetics during surgery

▶◀ Drug Interactions

- Clinically significant interactions are listed below
- For more interaction information on any given combination, also see the corresponding chapter for the second agent

Class of Drug	Example	Interaction Effects
Acetylcholinesterase inhibitor (central)	General	Increase in mortality in elderly patients with dementia taking antipsychotics irrespective of acetylcholinesterase inhibitor use. Deaths were related to cardiac disease and cancer
	Donepezil, galantamine, rivastigmine	May enhance neurotoxicity of antipsychotics, presumably due to a relative acetylcholine/dopamine imbalance (i.e., increased acetylcholine in the presence of dopamine receptor blockade) in the CNS. Case reports of severe EPS (e.g., generalized rigidity, shuffling gate, facial grimacing) in elderly patients within a few days of starting an antipsychotic (risperidone or haloperidol) and an acetylcholinesterase inhibitor (donepezil). Symptoms resolved after discontinuing the antipsychotic agent, the acetylcholinesterase inhibitor, or both
Adsorbent	Activated charcoal, attapulgite (kaolin-pectin), cholestyramine	Oral absorption decreased significantly when used simultaneously; give at least 1 h before or 2 h after the antipsychotic
α_1-adrenergic blocker	Doxazosin, prazosin, terazosin	Additive hypotension, particularly with low-potency FGAs like chlorpromazine. Antipsychotics generally cause hypotension via α_1 blockade
Anesthetic	Enflurane	Additive hypotension, particularly with low-potency FGAs such as chlorpromazine
Amylinomimetic	Pramlintide	Pramlintide slows the rate of gastric emptying. Antipsychotics with significant anticholinergic effects can further reduce GI motility. Use drugs with minimal anticholinergic effects at the lowest effective dose. See frequency of adverse effects table p. 198

First-Generation Antipsychotics/FGAs (cont.)

Class of Drug	Example	Interaction Effects
Antiarrhythmic	General	DO NOT COMBINE with chlorpromazine, fluphenazine, pimozide, or thioridazine. NOT recommended with phenothiazines or zuclopenthixol. CAUTION with all other FGAs. Possible additive prolongation of QTc interval and associated life-threatening cardiac arrhythmias. Factors that further increase the risk include uncompensated heart failure, recent acute MI, eating disorders (e.g., anorexia), bradycardia, electrolyte imbalances (e.g., hypokalemia, hypomagnesemia), and a family history of sudden death. Also see FGA Cardiovascular Effects p. 132
	Amiodarone, quinidine	With quinidine, increased peak plasma level and AUC of haloperidol by ~2-fold due to inhibited metabolism via CYP2D6 and/or displacement from tissue binding With amiodarone and quinidine, likely to increase chlorpromazine, fluphenazine, pimozide, and thioridazine levels via inhibition of CYP2D6; further increasing risk of QT prolongation
Antibiotic Macrolide	Clarithromycin, erythromycin, telithromycin	DO NOT COMBINE with pimozide or thioridazine. NOT recommended with phenothiazines or zuclopenthixol. CAUTION with all other FGAs. Possible additive prolongation of QTc interval and associated life-threatening cardiac arrhythmias. Factors that further increase the risk include anorexia, bradycardia, hypokalemia, and hypomagnesemia. Also see Cardiovascular Effects p. 132 With clarithromycin, decreased clearance of pimozide by 46% due to inhibition of metabolism via CYP3A4. Two reports of deaths occurring within days of adding clarithromycin to pimozide. Azithromycin (which does not inhibit CYP3A4) may have a lower risk when used with pimozide, although all macrolides including azithromycin are specifically listed as contraindicated in the US pimozide product monograph Clarithromycin may decrease clearance of chlorpromazine and haloperidol. Similar interaction with erythromycin and telithromycin likely. Increased antipsychotic adverse effects including prolonged QT interval possible
Quinolone	Ciprofloxacin, levofloxacin, moxifloxacin	DO NOT COMBINE with pimozide or thioridazine. NOT recommended with phenothiazines or zuclopenthixol. CAUTION with all other FGAs. Possible additive prolongation of QTc interval and associated life-threatening cardiac arrhythmias. Factors that further increase the risk include anorexia, bradycardia, hypokalemia, and hypomagnesemia. Also see Cardiovascular Effects p. 132. Ciprofloxacin is thought to have less potential for QTc prolongation but there are isolated cases of increased QTc CAUTION. Potential to exacerbate psychiatric conditions as quinolone-induced psychosis has been reported With ciprofloxacin, may increase plasma levels of trifluoperazine due to inhibition of metabolism via CYP1A2. Clinical significance unknown
Anticholinergic	Antidepressants, antihistamines, antiparkinsonian drugs	Increases the risk of anticholinergic adverse effects (e.g., dry mouth, urinary retention, inhibition of sweating, blurred vision, constipation, paralytic ileus, confusion, toxic psychosis)
Anticoagulant	Warfarin	Decreased INR possible with chlorpromazine or haloperidol
Anticonvulsant	General	All FGAs may lower seizure threshold. At usual dosage ranges, seizure rates are less than 1%. Risk greater with low-potency FGAs and is dose related
	Carbamazepine	Decreased antipsychotic plasma levels via potent induction of CYP3A4, CYP1A2, CYP2D6, and/or possibly UGT1A4. Note it may take 2–4 weeks to reach maximum induction and an equivalent period to return to baseline after discontinuation of an inducer With haloperidol, decreased plasma levels of carbamazepine (40%). Conflicting reports on haloperidol levels likely a result of a dose-dependent interaction (i.e., the interaction is more significant with increasing carbamazepine doses). Carbamazepine 100 mg daily reduced haloperidol levels by 15% while carbamazepine 600 mg daily reduced haloperidol levels by 75%. Adjust dose as needed Likely to decrease levels of chlorpromazine, fluphenazine, flupenthixol, thiothixene, and zuclopenthixol With loxapine, increased plasma levels of carbamazepine epoxide metabolite
	Lamotrigine	Chlorpromazine may inhibit metabolism of lamotrigine, resulting in increased lamotrigine levels. Clinical significance unknown

Class of Drug	Example	Interaction Effects
	Phenobarbital, phenytoin	Decreased plasma levels of antipsychotics due to potent induction of metabolism; for phenytoin via CYP2C9 and CYP3A4; for phenobarbital primarily via CYP1A2, CYP2C9, and CYP3A4
		With phenytoin, reduced levels of chlorpromazine, haloperidol, and thioridazine reported. With phenobarbital, reduced levels of chlorpromazine (by 25%) and haloperidol reported. Limited data available; interactions with other FGAs probable. Adjust antipsychotic dose as needed
		Loxapine decreased phenytoin levels in one case report
	Valproate (divalproex, valproic acid)	Chlorpromazine inhibits the metabolism of valproate, resulting in increased valproate levels. Clinical significance unknown
Antidepressant	General	DO NOT COMBINE with pimozide or thioridazine and CAUTION with all other FGAs applies to the majority of antidepressants, due to possible additive prolongation of QT interval and associated life-threatening cardiac arrhythmias. Factors that further increase the risk include anorexia, bradycardia, hypokalemia, and hypomagnesemia. Also see Cardiovascular Effects p. 132 and Antipsychotic Augmentation Strategies p. 218
SSRI	Citalopram, escitalopram, fluoxetine, fluvoxamine, paroxetine, sertraline	Case report of QT prolongation and patient collapsing with concurrent chlorpromazine and fluoxetine
		Case report of galactorrhea and amenorrhea with loxapine and fluvoxamine possibly via additive increase in prolactin levels
		Increased EPS and akathisia
		Increased plasma levels of antipsychotics due to inhibition of metabolism of CYP1A2 (potent – fluvoxamine), 2D6 (potent – fluoxetine and paroxetine), and/or 3A4 (fluvoxamine). Adjust antipsychotic dose as needed
		DO NOT COMBINE with pimozide or thioridazine; CAUTION with all other FGAs due to additive prolongation of QTc interval. A single dose of pimozide added to citalopram did not alter the kinetics of pimozide, but did cause a prolongation of QTc by ~10 ms
		Pimozide levels: With paroxetine, 151% higher AUC and 62% higher peak level. With sertraline, 40% higher AUC and peak level. Case reports of bradycardia with concurrent use of pimozide and fluoxetine
		Haloperidol levels: With fluoxetine, 20–35% higher levels. With fluvoxamine, 23–60% higher. With sertraline, 28% higher
		Phenothiazine levels: With fluvoxamine, thioridazine levels 3-fold higher. With paroxetine, perphenazine peak levels 2- to 13-fold higher
SNRI	Desvenlafaxine, duloxetine, venlafaxine	DO NOT COMBINE with pimozide or thioridazine; CAUTION with all other FGAs; due to additive prolongation of QTc interval. Increased plasma levels of thioridazine and other phenothiazines possible due to inhibition of CYP2D6 by duloxetine
		Venlafaxine increased AUC (70%) and peak plasma level (88%) of haloperidol; case report of urinary retention developing when venlafaxine was added to haloperidol
SARI	Nefazodone	DO NOT COMBINE with pimozide or thioridazine; CAUTION with all other FGAs; due to additive prolongation of QTc interval. Increased plasma levels of pimozide possible due to inhibition of CYP3A4 by nefazodone
		Increased AUC (36%) and peak plasma level (13%) of haloperidol. Clinical significance likely minor
	Trazodone	Case reports of hypotension in combination with chlorpromazine or trifluoperazine, and fatal hepatic necrosis via additive hepatotoxicity of trazodone and phenothiazines
SMS	Vortioxetine	Serotonin modulators may enhance the dopamine blockade of antipsychotics and increase the risk of side effects
Cyclic	Amitriptyline, clomipramine, maprotiline, trimipramine	DO NOT COMBINE with pimozide or thioridazine. NOT recommended with phenothiazines or zuclopenthixol. CAUTION with all other FGAs. Possible additive prolongation of QT interval and associated life-threatening cardiac arrhythmias
		Additive sedation, hypotension, and anticholinergic effects
		Haloperidol and phenothiazines may increase plasma levels of cyclic antidepressants (TCAs). TCAs may increase plasma level of chlorpromazine. Clinical significance unknown
Irrev. MAOI, RIMA	Tranylcypromine, moclobemide	Additive hypotension, particularly with low-potency FGAs such as chlorpromazine

First-Generation Antipsychotics/FGAs (cont.)

Class of Drug	Example	Interaction Effects
Antifungal	Fluconazole, itraconazole, ketoconazole, voriconazole	DO NOT COMBINE with pimozide or thioridazine. NOT recommended with phenothiazines or zuclopenthixol. CAUTION with all other FGAs. Possible additive prolongation of QT interval and associated life-threatening cardiac arrhythmias
		Increased plasma levels of antipsychotics due to inhibition of metabolism via CYP3A4 and possibly P-glycoprotein. Increased plasma level of haloperidol (by 30% with itraconazole)
Antihypertensive	Losartan, metoprolol, ramipril	Additive hypotensive effect particularly with low-potency FGAs such as chlorpromazine. Antipsychotics generally cause hypotension via α_1 blockade (see receptor table p. 194 and frequency of adverse effects table p. 198). Start with a lower dose of antipsychotic, titrate slowly, and monitor for orthostatic hypotension
	β-blocker	See Class of Drug "β-blocker" p. 143
	Calcium channel blocker	See Class of Drug "Calcium channel blocker" p. 143
	Clonidine	Clonidine lowers blood pressure by having agonistic effects on presynaptic α_2-adrenergic receptors. FGAs that are potent α_2-adrenergic receptor antagonists can block clonidine's antihypertensive effects (see receptor table p. 194); additive hypotensive effects also possible
	Diuretic	See Class of Drug "Diuretic" p. 144
Antiparkinsonian	Levodopa, pramipexole, ropinirole	Potential for reduced therapeutic effect of antiparkinson agents. Antipsychotics reduce dopamine while antiparkinson agents increase dopamine in the CNS
Antipsychotic combination	General	Increased risk of adverse effects (e.g., EPS, elevated prolactin levels, sedation, hypotension, anticholinergic effects), increased cost, and potential for decreased adherence with use of multiple antipsychotic agents
		CAUTION – possible additive prolongation of QTc interval and associated life-threatening cardiac arrhythmias. DO NOT COMBINE with pimozide or thioridazine. Factors that further increase the risk include anorexia, bradycardia, hypokalemia, and hypomagnesemia. Also see Cardiovascular Effects p. 132
	Haloperidol + aripiprazole	See TGA Drug Interactions, p. 189
	Haloperidol + SGAs	See SGA Drug Interactions, p. 172
	Phenothiazines (e.g., chlorpromazine, thioridazine) + SGAs	Possible additive QT prolongation (see above). DO NOT COMBINE with asenapine, iloperidone, paliperidone, or ziprasidone. See SGA Drug Interactions, p. 172 for further information
	Pimozide + SGAs	Possible additive QT prolongation (see above). DO NOT COMBINE with asenapine, iloperidone, paliperidone, or ziprasidone
	Thioridazine + SGAs	Possible additive QT prolongation (see above). DO NOT COMBINE with asenapine, iloperidone, paliperidone, or ziprasidone. See SGA Drug Interactions, p. 172 for further information
	Pimozide, thioridazine + FGAs	DO NOT COMBINE. Possible additive QT prolongation (see above)
Antiretroviral		See [9]
Non-nucleoside reverse transcriptase inhibitor (NNRTI)	Delavirdine, efavirenz, etravirine, nevirapine	CAUTION. Possible interactions as NNRTIs inhibit and induce CYP enzymes (e.g., delavirdine is a strong inhibitor of 2D6, nevirapine weakly inhibits 2D6, efavirenz and etravirine induce 3A4 moderately, nevirapine weakly induces it)
		Delavirdine may increase levels of perphenazine, chlorpromazine, and zuclopenthixol due to CYP2D6 inhibition
		Efavirenz and etravirine may decrease levels of haloperidol and pimozide due to CYP3A4 induction

Class of Drug	Example	Interaction Effects
Protease inhibitor	Atazanavir, boceprevir, darunavir, fosamprenavir, indinavir, lopinavir, nelfinavir, ritonavir, saquinavir, simeprevir telaprevir, tipranavir	CAUTION. Complex interactions likely as various protease inhibitors potently inhibit as well as induce a variety of CYP enzymes (e.g., on CYP3A4, ritonavir is a potent inhibitor; atazanavir, boceprevir, darunavir, saquinavir, and telaprevir are strong inhibitors; indinavir and fosamprenavir are mild to moderate inhibitors; tipranavir is an inducer). Low boosting doses of ritonavir have little effect on CYP2D6 but higher doses cause inhibition AVOID with pimozide and thioridazine. Increased plasma levels of pimozide/thioridazine possible due to inhibition of metabolism via CYP3A4 or CYP2D6, respectively, which increases the risk of cardiotoxicity (QT prolongation, cardiac arrest) Increased levels of FGAs metabolized by CYP3A4 (i.e., haloperidol, loxapine, phenothiazines, flupenthixol, and zuclopenthixol) possible. Higher doses of ritonavir may cause a significant increase even for FGAs that are weak substrates of CYP3A4 and/or are metabolized by CYP2D6 (e.g., potentially increased chlorpromazine levels with higher doses of ritonavir, but unlikely with lower boosting doses of ritonavir). With unboosted tipranavir, levels of the FGAs may be decreased. Clinical significance unknown. Adjust antipsychotic dose as needed
Antitubercular drug	Isoniazid	Limited data suggest some may experience increased plasma levels of haloperidol. Adjust antipsychotic dose as needed
	Rifabutin, rifampin, rifapentine	Decreased plasma levels of haloperidol (by 30–70%) due to induction via CYP3A4 and/or P-glycoprotein with rifampin and accompanying increase in psychiatric symptoms. Adjust antipsychotic dose as needed
Anxiolytic Azapirone, benzodiazepines	Buspirone, clonazepam, diazepam, lorazepam	Synergistic effect with antipsychotics; used to calm agitated patients Potential for additive CNS adverse effects (e.g., dizziness, sedation, confusion, respiratory depression) and hypotension May increase extrapyramidal reactions Conflicting information with respect to effects on haloperidol levels from no change to increased levels (by 19%). Likely not clinically significant Haloperidol lactate can be administered IM in the same syringe as lorazepam
Belladonna alkaloid	Atropine, hyoscyamine, scopolamine	Additive anticholinergic effects (e.g., dry mouth, urinary retention, inhibition of sweating, blurred vision, constipation, paralytic ileus, confusion, toxic psychosis)
β-blocker		Also see Class of Drug "Antihypertensive" p. 142
	Pindolol	DO NOT COMBINE with thioridazine. Increased plasma level of thioridazine due to inhibition of metabolism via CYP2D6, thus increasing the risk of cardiotoxicity (QT prolongation, cardiac arrest) and pindolol levels may be increased. Pindolol may increase plasma levels of other phenothiazines
	Propranolol	DO NOT COMBINE with thioridazine. Increased plasma level of thioridazine (3- to 5-fold) due to inhibition of metabolism via CYP2D6, thus increasing the risk of cardiotoxicity (QT prolongation, cardiac arrest) Increased plasma level of both chlorpromazine (5-fold) and propranolol (decreased clearance by 25–32%). Case report of delirium and seizures. With haloperidol, case report of a severe hypotensive reaction
Betel (areca) nut		Two case reports of severe EPS following a period of heavy betel nut consumption in those who were maintained on a depot FGA (fluphenazine decanoate and flupenthixol, respectively). Symptoms occurred within 2 weeks and resolved 4–7 days after stopping betel nut. Betel nut's potent cholinergic effects potentially counteracted procyclidine, the anticholinergic agent both patients were taking to control EPS
Calcium channel blocker		Also see Class of Drug "Antihypertensive," p. 142
	Diltiazem, verapamil	DO NOT COMBINE with pimozide or thioridazine. Increased risk of cardiotoxicity (QT prolongation, cardiac arrest) due to possible additive calcium-channel blocking effects and increased plasma levels of pimozide due to inhibition of metabolism via CYP3A4
Caffeine	Coffee, tea, cola, energy drinks, guarana or mate-containing products	Increased akathisia/agitation/insomnia Haloperidol oral liquid is incompatible with tea or coffee (see Nursing Implications, p. 138)

First-Generation Antipsychotics/FGAs (cont.)

Class of Drug	Example	Interaction Effects
Cannabis/marijuana		Drugs with anticholinergic and α_1-adrenergic properties (e.g., chlorpromazine) can cause marked hypotension and increased disorientation
CNS depressant	Alcohol, antihistamines, hypnotics, opioids	CAUTION. Increased CNS effects (e.g., sedation, fatigue, impaired cognition). Additive orthostatic hypotension Alcohol may worsen EPS
Diuretic		Also see Class of Drug "Antihypertensive" p. 142 above
	Furosemide, hydrochlorothiazide	CAUTION with all FGAs. Diuretics can cause electrolyte disturbances resulting in additive QTc interval prolongation and risk of associated life-threatening cardiac arrhythmias. Monitor for dehydration, hypokalemia, and hypomagnesemia. Also see Cardiovascular Effects, p. 132
Disulfiram		CAUTION. Case reports of disulfiram-induced psychosis, possibly due to blockade of dopamine β-hydroxylase; however, no increased psychotic features seen in small studies of participants with psychotic disorders Case report of decreased plasma level of perphenazine, increased level of its metabolite, and clinical decline; potentially due to inhibition of CYP2E1
Grapefruit juice		AVOID with pimozide. Increased plasma level of pimozide possible due to inhibition of metabolism via CYP3A4, which increases the risk cardiotoxicity (QT prolongation, cardiac arrest) Haloperidol levels not affected by consumption of grapefruit juice 600 mL/day for 7 days
H_2 antagonist	Cimetidine	Both elevated and decreased chlorpromazine plasma levels have been reported. Chlorpromazine absorption may be decreased at higher doses of cimetidine, possibly due to increased gastric pH. Chlorpromazine metabolism may be decreased by inhibition of CYP2D6. Case reports of excessive sedation with the addition of cimetidine to chlorpromazine. May interact with other phenothiazines
Hormone	Oral contraceptive	Estrogen potentiates hyperprolactinemic effect of antipsychotics Case report of increased plasma level of chlorpromazine (6-fold) and development of severe tremor and dyskinesias after the addition of an oral contraceptive (ethinyl estradiol [50 micrograms]/norgestrel [0.5 mg]). Mechanism unknown; ethinyl estradiol is known to be an inhibitor of CYP1A2 and CYP2C19 and substrate of CYP3A4
Kava kava		Case report of atrial flutter and hypoxia after administration of IM haloperidol and lorazepam for severe aggression; suggested due to kava inhibition of CYP2D6
Lithium		CAUTION with all FGAs. Avoid toxic lithium plasma levels when used concurrently with pimozide or thioridazine, since both pimozide/thioridazine and toxic lithium levels are associated with QT prolongation Although numerous studies indicate lithium and FGAs can be safely used together, there are rare cases of severe neurotoxicity (e.g., delirium, dyskinesias, seizures, encephalopathic syndrome, NMS) and EPS with concurrent lithium and haloperidol and other FGAs (i.e., loxapine, thiothixene or phenothiazines). Factors that may increase the risk of developing neurotoxicity are the presence of acute mania, pre-existing brain damage, infection, fever, dehydration, a history of EPS, and high doses of one or both agents Decreased plasma levels of chlorpromazine (by 40%) and both increased and decreased lithium levels reported
Opioid		CAUTION. Additive CNS effects. See Class of Drug "CNS depressant" p. 144
	Codeine	Inhibition of conversion of codeine to its active metabolite, morphine, with haloperidol and phenothiazines. Monitor for efficacy of pain control. Switch to an analgesic which does not require CYP2D6 conversion if needed
	Methadone	DO NOT COMBINE with pimozide or thioridazine. NOT recommended with phenothiazines or zuclopenthixol. CAUTION with all other FGAs. Possible additive prolongation of QT interval and associated life-threatening cardiac arrhythmias. Factors that further increase the risk include anorexia, bradycardia, hypokalemia, and hypomagnesemia. Also see Cardiovascular Effects p. 132
	Tramadol	CAUTION. Tramadol lowers the seizure threshold; potential additive lowering of seizure threshold with FGAs

Class of Drug	Example	Interaction Effects
Prokinetic agent/Antiemetic	Metoclopramide	CAUTION. Metoclopramide is a potent central dopamine receptor antagonist that can cause EPS, hyperprolactinemia, and rarely NMS. Concurrent use of an FGA may increase the risk of these adverse effects
QT-prolonging agent	Antiarrhythmics (e.g., amiodarone, sotalol), antimalarials (e.g., chloroquine, mefloquine), antiprotozoals (e.g., pentamidine), arsenic trioxide, contrast agents (e.g., gadobutrol), dolasetron, droperidol, methadone, pazopanib, ranolazine, tacrolimus	DO NOT COMBINE with pimozide or thioridazine. NOT recommended with phenothiazines or zuclopenthixol. CAUTION with all other FGAs. Possible additive prolongation of QT interval and associated life-threatening cardiac arrhythmias. A study suggests ziprasidone causes less QT prolongation than thioridazine but about twice that of quetiapine, risperidone, haloperidol, and olanzapine. Factors that further increase the risk include anorexia, bradycardia, hypokalemia, and hypomagnesemia. Also see Cardiovascular Effects, p. 132
Smoking (tobacco)		Smoking induces CYP1A2; polycyclic aromatic hydrocarbons in tobacco smoke are believed to be responsible for this induction, not nicotine. Decreased plasma levels of chlorpromazine (by 24%), fluphenazine (by 51%), and thioridazine (by 46%) and increased clearance of haloperidol (by 44–61%), perphenazine (by 33%), and thiothixene (by 36%) due to the induction of CYP1A2. Similar interaction with other phenothiazines possible. Case report of marked worsening of adverse effects and increased chlorpromazine plasma levels after abrupt smoking cessation. Discuss with patient the effects of and assess on a regular basis any changes in smoking behavior
Stimulant	Amphetamine, methylphenidate	Antipsychotic agents may impair the stimulatory effect of amphetamines
		Case reports of worsening of tardive movement disorders and prolongation or exacerbation of withdrawal dyskinesia following antipsychotic discontinuation
		Concurrent use not recommended
Sympathomimetic	Cocaine	Increased risk of EPS (especially dystonia) with concurrent use, possibly via dopamine depletion from chronic use of cocaine
	Epinephrine/adrenaline, dopamine	AVOID using for the treatment of FGA-induced hypotension. May result in paradoxical fall in blood pressure as antipsychotics block peripheral α_1-adrenergic receptors, thus inhibiting α_1-vasoconstricting effects of epinephrine and leaving β-vasodilator effects relatively unopposed
		Norepinephrine and phenylephrine are safe substitutes for severe hypotension unresponsive to fluids
Zileuton		AVOID with pimozide. Zileuton is an inhibitor of CYP3A4 and may increase pimozide levels, increasing the risk of QTc interval prolongation and associated life-threatening cardiac arrhythmias. Factors which further increase the risk include anorexia, bradycardia, hypokalemia, and hypomagnesemia. Also see Cardiovascular Effects p. 132

Second-Generation Antipsychotics/SGAs

℞ Product Availability*

Generic Name	Chemical Class	Neuroscience-based Nomenclature* (Pharmacological Target/ Mode of Action)	Trade Name[A]	Dosage Forms and Strengths
Asenapine	Dibenzo-oxepino pyrrole	Dopamine, serotonin, norepinephrine/Antagonist	Saphris	Sublingual tablets: 2.5 mg[B], 5 mg, 10 mg
Clozapine	Dibenzodiazepine	Dopamine, serotonin, norepinephrine/Antagonist	Clozaril FazaClo ODT[B] Versacloz[B]	Tablets: 12.5 mg[B], 25 mg, 50 mg, 100 mg, 200 mg Oral disintegrating tablets: 12.5 mg, 25 mg, 100 mg, 150 mg, 200 mg Oral suspension: 50 mg/mL
Iloperidone[B]	Benzisoxazole	Dopamine, serotonin/Antagonist	Fanapt	Tablets: 1 mg, 2 mg, 4 mg, 6 mg, 8 mg, 10 mg, 12 mg
Lumateperone[B]	Butyrophenone	Not listed	Caplyta	Capsules: 42 mg
Lurasidone	Benzisothiazol	Dopamine, serotonin/Antagonist	Latuda	Tablets: 20 mg, 40 mg, 60 mg, 80 mg, 120 mg
Olanzapine	Thienobenzodiazepine	Dopamine, serotonin/Antagonist	Zyprexa Zyprexa Relprevv[B] Zyprexa Zydis Symbyax[B]	Tablets: 2.5 mg, 5 mg, 7.5 mg, 10 mg, 15 mg, 20 mg Short-acting IM injection (olanzapine tartrate): 10 mg/vial Long-acting IM injection (olanzapine pamoate): 210 mg/vial, 300 mg/vial, 405 mg/vial Oral disintegrating tablets: 5 mg, 10 mg, 15 mg, 20 mg Capsules (fluoxetine/olanzapine): 25 mg/3 mg, 25 mg/6 mg, 25 mg/12 mg, 50 mg/6 mg, 50 mg/12 mg
Paliperidone	Benzisoxazole	Dopamine, serotonin, norepinephrine/Antagonist	Invega Invega Sustenna Invega Trinza Invega Hafyera[B]	Extended-release tablets: 1.5 mg[B], 3 mg, 6 mg, 9 mg Long-acting 1-monthly IM (paliperidone palmitate) (PP1M): US labeling indicates the amount of paliperidone palmitate – 39 mg/0.25 mL, 78 mg/0.5 mL, 117 mg/0.75 mL, 156 mg/mL, 234 mg/1.5 mL; Canadian labeling indicates only the amount of paliperidone (not the palmitate base) – 50 mg/0.5 mL, 75 mg/0.75 mL, 100 mg/mL,150 mg/1.5 mL Long-acting 3-monthly IM (paliperidone palmitate) (PP3M): US labeling indicates the amount of paliperidone palmitate – 273 mg/0.875 mL, 410 mg/1.315 mL, 546 mg/1.75 mL, 819 mg/2.625mL; Canadian labeling indicates only the amount of paliperidone (not the palmitate base) – 175 mg/0.875 mL, 263 mg/1.315 mL, 350 mg/1.75 mL, 525 mg/2.625 mL Long-acting 6-monthly IM (paliperidone palmitate) (PP6M): US labeling indicates the amount of paliperidone palmitate – 1,092 mg/3.5 mL, 1,560 mg/5 mL
Quetiapine	Dibenzothiazepine	Dopamine, serotonin, norepinephrine/Antagonist	Seroquel Seroquel XR	Tablets: 25 mg, 50 mg[B], 100 mg, 150 mg, 200 mg, 300 mg, 400 mg[B] Extended-release tablets: 50 mg, 150 mg, 200 mg, 300 mg, 400 mg

Generic Name	Chemical Class	Neuroscience-based Nomenclature* (Pharmacological Target/ Mode of Action)	Trade Name[A]	Dosage Forms and Strengths
Risperidone	Benzisoxazole	Dopamine, serotonin, norepinephrine/Antagonist	Risperdal Risperdal M-Tab Risperdal Consta Perseris	Tablets: 0.25 mg, 0.5 mg, 1 mg, 2 mg, 3 mg, 4 mg Oral solution: 1 mg/mL Oral disintegrating tablets: 0.5 mg, 1 mg, 2 mg, 3 mg, 4 mg Long-acting IM injection: 12.5 mg/vial, 25 mg/vial, 37.5 mg/vial, 50 mg/vial Extended-release SC injection (RBP-7000): 90 mg/0.6 mL, 120 mg/0.8 mL
Ziprasidone	Benzothiazolylpiperazine	Dopamine, serotonin/Antagonist	Geodon[B], Zeldox[C]	Capsules (ziprasidone HCl): 20 mg, 40 mg, 60 mg, 80 mg Short-acting injection (ziprasidone mesylate)[B]: 20 mg/mL

* Refer to Health Canada's Drug Product Database or the FDA's Drugs@FDA for the most current availability information. • Developed by a taskforce consisting of representatives from the American College of Neuropsychopharmacology (ACNP), the Asian College of Neuropsychopharmacology (AsCNP), the European College of Neuropsychopharmacology (ECNP), the International College of Neuropsychopharmacology (CINP), and the International Union of Basic and Clinical Pharmacology (IUPHAR) (see https://nbn2r.com), [A] Generic preparations may be available,   [B] Not marketed in Canada,   [C] Not marketed in the USA

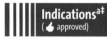

Indications[a‡]
(👍 approved)

Schizophrenia & Psychotic Disorders

Schizophrenia
- 👍 Treatment (asenapine, lumateperone, lurasidone, olanzapine, paliperidone, paliperidone long-acting 1-monthly (PP1M) injection, quetiapine, quetiapine XR, risperidone, risperidone long-acting injection, ziprasidone – Canada and USA; paliperidone long-acting 3-monthly (PP3M) injection after stabilized on PP1M injection – Canada and USA; iloperidone, olanzapine long-acting injection, paliperidone long-acting 6-monthly (PP6M) injection after stabilized on PP1M or PP3M injection, risperidone RBP-7000 long-acting injection – USA)
- 👍 Acute agitation (olanzapine short-acting IM – Canada and USA; ziprasidone short-acting IM – USA)
- 👍 Treatment resistant (clozapine – Canada and USA)
- 👍 Reduction of recurrent suicidal behavior in those at chronic risk (clozapine – USA)

Schizophrenia-related psychotic disorders
- 👍 Treatment (paliperidone, olanzapine, risperidone long-acting injection, ziprasidone – Canada)
- 👍 Acute agitation (olanzapine short-acting IM – Canada)

Schizoaffective disorder
- 👍 Monotherapy treatment (paliperidone – USA; PP1M injection – Canada and USA)
- 👍 Adjunctive therapy to mood stabilizers and/or antidepressants (paliperidone, PP1M injection – USA)
- 👍 Risk reduction of recurrent suicidal behavior in those at chronic risk (clozapine – USA)

Other psychotic disorders
- Psychosis/hallucinations associated with Parkinson's disease treatment (most evidence for clozapine)
- Drug-induced (e.g., amphetamines) psychosis treatment
- Monotherapy and co-therapy with an antidepressant for psychotic symptoms associated with PTSD (most evidence for risperidone)
- Delusional infestation/ parasitosis treatment (anecdotal reports – olanzapine, risperidone)
- Postpartum psychosis

Bipolar Disorder

Manic episodes
- 👍 Acute monotherapy treatment (asenapine, olanzapine, quetiapine, quetiapine XR, risperidone, ziprasidone – Canada and USA)
- 👍 Acute adjunctive therapy (e.g., with lithium or divalproex/valproate) (asenapine, olanzapine – Canada and USA; quetiapine, quetiapine XR, risperidone – USA)
- 👍 Acute agitation (olanzapine short-acting IM – Canada and USA)

[a] Adult population unless otherwise stated [‡] Indications listed here do not necessarily apply to all SGAs or all countries. Please refer to a country's regulatory database (e.g., US Food and Drug Administration, Health Canada Drug Product Database) for the most current availability information and indications

Second-Generation Antipsychotics/SGAs (cont.)

Mixed episodes
- ♠ Acute monotherapy treatment (asenapine, olanzapine, ziprasidone – Canada and USA; quetiapine, risperidone – USA
- ♠ Acute adjunctive therapy (e.g., with lithium or divalproex/valproate) (asenapine, olanzapine – Canada and USA; quetiapine XR, risperidone – USA)

Depressive episodes
- ♠ Acute monotherapy treatment (lurasidone, quetiapine, quetiapine XR – Canada and USA; fluoxetine/olanzapine combination – USA)
- ♠ Acute adjunctive therapy (e.g., with lithium or divalproex/valproate) (lurasidone – Canada and USA)

Maintenance treatment
- ♠ Monotherapy treatment (olanzapine, risperidone long-acting injection – Canada and USA)
- ♠ Adjunctive therapy to lithium or divalproex/valproate (quetiapine, quetiapine XR, risperidone long-acting injection, ziprasidone – USA)

Other bipolar
- • Refractory and rapid-cycling bipolar disorder

| **Delirium** |
- • Treatment of delirium

| **Dementia** |
- ♠ In severe dementia of the Alzheimer type, for short-term symptomatic management of inappropriate behavior due to aggression and/or psychosis. Risks and benefits in this population should be considered (risperidone – Canada; other agents not approved but some evidence for use)
- • Management of Lewy-body dementia: Psychosis (olanzapine: Small RCT; quetiapine: Case series); inappropriate sexual behavior; reducing visual hallucinations refractory to donepezil without worsening motor effects (quetiapine: Case reports)

| **Depression** |
- ♠ Treatment-resistant major depressive disorder (quetiapine XR – Canada; fluoxetine/olanzapine combination – USA)
- ♠ Adjunctive therapy to antidepressants (quetiapine XR – USA)
- • Adjunct therapy for major depressive disorder (olanzapine, risperidone, ziprasidone)
- • Adjunct therapy for major depressive disorder with psychotic features (olanzapine, quetiapine)
- • Monotherapy for major depressive disorder (olanzapine)
- • Monotherapy for combined depression and anxiety (case series: Low-dose quetiapine, low-dose risperidone)

| **Movement Disorders** |
- • Levodopa-induced dyskinesias (clozapine)
- • Tardive dyskinesia; improved symptoms (clozapine, olanzapine, quetiapine, risperidone)
- • Movement disorders; decreased motor symptoms in disorders such as tremor, dyskinesia and bradykinesia of Parkinson's disease, essential tremor, akinetic disorders, Huntington's chorea, blepharospasm, and Meige syndrome

| **Other** |
- • Addictive behaviors (e.g., smoking, alcoholism, drug abuse) in dual diagnosis individuals (clozapine, olanzapine, quetiapine, risperidone)
- • Anorexia nervosa (olanzapine, quetiapine, risperidone; all data comes from poor-quality clinical trials)
- • Generalized anxiety disorder (quetiapine – limited evidence)
- • Borderline personality disorder (olanzapine, quetiapine, risperidone; early data)
- • Insomnia refractory to other hypnotics/sedatives (quetiapine, olanzapine; limited data)
- • Delirium in hospitalized patients (limited data with olanzapine, quetiapine, and risperidone)
- • Nausea related to advanced cancer and associated pain (olanzapine, risperidone)
- • Obsessive-compulsive disorder (OCD): Augmentation in treatment-resistant OCD (olanzapine, quetiapine, paliperidone: Case report, risperidone, ziprasidone); occasional reports of worsening of OCD symptoms, usually in individuals with primary psychotic disorders
- • Pervasive developmental disorders (clozapine, olanzapine, quetiapine, risperidone, ziprasidone)
- • Posttraumatic stress disorder: Treatment-resistant PTSD; some improvement in flashbacks, hyperarousal, and intrusive symptoms (olanzapine, risperidone)
- • Tic disorders, Tourette's syndrome, and trichotillomania (olanzapine, quetiapine, risperidone, ziprasidone)

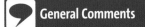 **General Comments**
- • Clozapine has consistently demonstrated superiority over other antipsychotic agents for treatment-resistant schizophrenia
- • Versus the high-potency FGA haloperidol, SGAs are generally associated with a lower incidence of EPS and tardive dyskinesia. Of the SGAs, risperidone appears to have the highest frequency of EPS
- • Unwanted metabolic effects of SGAs may include weight gain, dyslipidemias, glucose intolerance, and diabetes. The risk appears greatest with olanzapine and clozapine and lowest with ziprasidone, lurasidone, and asenapine. Individuals may also meet the criteria for metabolic syndrome

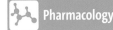

Pharmacology	<ul><li>See p. 124 and the charts listing effects on neurotransmitters/receptors (p. 194 and p. 195)</li><li>SGAs and TGAs are frequently referred to as "atypical" agents because of a lower incidence of EPS vs. FGAs. Although several mechanisms have been postulated to account for these differences, none are without confounding factors:<ul><li>Unlike FGAs, most SGAs have greater affinity for 5-HT$_{2A}$ vs. D$_2$ receptors. (Note: Amisulpride, not currently available in Canada or the USA, does not share this feature). Antagonism of 5-HT$_{2A}$ receptors in dopaminergic pathways outside the limbic system is believed to enhance dopaminergic transmission, thereby reducing EPS and hyperprolactinemia and potentially improving (or not exacerbating) negative, cognitive, and mood symptoms</li><li>Regionally selective binding to the D$_2$ receptor in mesolimbic/cortical areas has also been proposed to account for the atypical features of some SGAs</li><li>Receptor dissociation – the relative lower affinity of some SGAs for the D$_2$ receptor determines, at least in part, their faster rate of dissociation (i.e., unbinding) from the D$_2$ receptor. Rapid dissociation from the D$_2$ receptor (aka "Fast-off D$_2$ theory") allows the receptor to periodically accommodate endogenous dopamine, thus providing another explanation for why "atypical" agents may be less likely to cause EPS. Clozapine and quetiapine have the fastest dissociation rates, whereas other SGAs (e.g., asenapine, olanzapine, risperidone, ziprasidone) appear to dissociate more slowly from the D$_2$ receptor</li></ul></li></ul>
Dosing	<ul><li>For dosing of individual oral and short-acting agents for schizophrenia and psychosis, see table pp. 203–207. For long-acting agents, see table pp. 212–216</li><li>For administration details, please see the implications for nursing section pp. 165–165</li><li>In general, lower doses are recommended in the elderly, children, and patients with compromised liver or renal function</li><li>Lower doses shown to be effective as augmentation therapy of acute mania</li><li>Initial doses should be lower, and titration slower in patients prone to hypotension or with mental retardation</li><li>Dose titration recommended to minimize orthostatic hypotension: Clozapine (also minimizes sedation, and seizures); iloperidone, quetiapine, risperidone</li><li>Prescribing **restrictions apply for clozapine** – dependent on results of absolute neutrophil count (see p. 162 for details): Weekly for 26 weeks, then every 2nd week for 26 weeks, monthly thereafter</li><li>*Bipolar:*<ul><li>*Acute manic episodes (monotherapy):* Asenapine – 5–10 mg twice daily; olanzapine oral – 10–15 mg once daily; quetiapine – day 1 = 50 mg twice daily, day 2 = 100 mg twice daily, day 3 = 150 mg twice daily, day 4 = 200 mg twice daily, further dosage adjustments up to 800 mg/day by day 6 should be in increments of no greater than 200 mg/day; quetiapine XR – day 1 = 300 mg/day, day 2 = 600 mg/day, day 3 = 400–800 mg/day as needed; risperidone oral – start with 2–3 mg once daily, increase or decrease by 1 mg/day as needed to a maximum of 6 mg/day; ziprasidone – day 1 = 40 mg twice daily with a meal, day 2 = 60–80 mg twice daily</li><li>*Acute manic episodes (adjunctive therapy):* Asenapine – start with 5 mg twice daily, increase to 5–10 mg twice daily as needed; olanzapine oral – 10 mg once daily; quetiapine (USA) – day 1 = 50 mg twice daily, day 2 = 100 mg twice daily, day 3 = 150 mg twice daily, day 4 = 200 mg twice daily, further dosage adjustments up to 800 mg/day by day 6 should be in increments of no greater than 200 mg/day; quetiapine XR – day 1 = 300 mg/day, day 2 = 600 mg/day, day 3 = 400–800 mg/day as needed; risperidone oral (USA) – start with 2–3 mg once daily, increase or decrease by 1 mg/day as needed, to a maximum of 6 mg/day</li><li>*Depressive episodes (acute monotherapy):* Lurasidone (Canada) – start with 20 mg once daily (dosage range 20-60 mg/day); olanzapine oral in combination with fluoxetine (USA) – start with 5 mg/day of olanzapine (with 20 mg/day of fluoxetine), titrate up to 12.5 mg/day of olanzapine (with 50 mg/day of fluoxetine) if needed; quetiapine – day 1 = 50 mg at bedtime, day 2 = 100 mg at bedtime, day 3 = 200 mg at bedtime, day 4 = 300 mg at bedtime; quetiapine XR – day 1 = 50 mg/day, day 2 = 100 mg/day, day 3 = 200 mg/day, day 4 = 300 mg/day</li></ul></li></ul>

Second-Generation Antipsychotics/SGAs (cont.)

- Maintenance (monotherapy):
  Asenapine – 5–10 mg twice daily;
  olanzapine – 5–20 mg/day;
  risperidone Consta – 25 mg IM every 2 weeks, if needed increase no sooner than in 4 weeks to maximum of 50 mg IM every 2 weeks
- Maintenance (adjunctive therapy) (USA):
  Olanzapine oral – 5–20 mg/day;
  quetiapine – 200–400 mg twice daily;
  quetiapine XR – 400–800 mg/day;
  risperidone Consta – 25 mg IM every 2 weeks, if needed increase no sooner than in 4 weeks to maximum of 50 mg IM every 2 weeks;
  ziprasidone – 40–80 mg twice daily with food
- Depression:
  Olanzapine oral in combination with fluoxetine (USA) – start with 5 mg/day, titrate up to 20 mg/day if needed;
  quetiapine XR – day 1 and 2 = 50 mg/day, day 3 and 4 = 150 mg/day, recommended range 150–300 mg/day
- Dementia (behavioral disturbances in severe dementia) (Canada):
  Risperidone oral – start with 0.25 mg daily, increase by 0.25 mg, if needed, no sooner than every 7 days to an optimal dose of 0.5 mg twice daily or a maximum dose of 1 mg twice daily

Renal Impairment	<ul><li>Clozapine: For patients with mild–moderate impairment (i.e., CrCl 50–79 mL/min), recommended initial dose is 12.5 mg/day</li><li>Lurasidone: Dose adjustment recommended in moderate (CrCl 30–< 50 mL/min) and severe (CrCl < 30 mL/min) impairment. Recommended starting dose is 20 mg/day and should not exceed 80 mg/day</li><li>Paliperidone: In mild impairment (CrCl ≥ 50 mL/min to < 80 mL/min), recommended initial dose is 3 mg once daily; may be increased to maximum of 6 mg once daily if needed. For patients with moderate–severe impairment (CrCl ≥ 10 mL/min to < 50 mL/min), recommended initial dose is 1.5 mg once daily; may be increased to maximum of 3 mg once daily</li><li>Paliperidone palmitate 1-monthly IM: For patients with mild impairment (CrCl ≥ 50 mL/min to < 80 mL/min):<ul><li>Canadian product: day 1 = 100 mg IM, day 8 = 75 mg IM, followed by 50 mg IM q monthly, then transition to an equivalent 3-monthly dose as required</li><li>US product: day 1 = 156 mg IM, day 8 = 117 mg IM, followed by 78 mg IM q monthly; stabilize patient using paliperidone 1-monthly injectable, then transition to an equivalent 3-monthly or 6-monthly dose as required</li></ul></li><li>Risperidone: For patients with severe impairment, recommended initial dose is 0.5 mg twice daily. Increases should be in increments of no more than 0.5 mg twice daily</li><li>Risperidone long-acting injection: Treat patients with impairment with titrated doses of oral risperidone prior to initiating risperidone long-acting. Recommended oral starting dose is 0.5 mg twice daily during first week, can be increased to 1 mg twice daily or 2 mg once daily during second week. If total oral daily dose of at least 2 mg is well tolerated, an injection of 25 mg risperidone long-acting can be administered q 2 weeks</li></ul>
Hepatic Impairment	<ul><li>Asenapine: Contraindicated in patients with severe impairment (Child-Pugh C); asenapine exposure ~7 times higher in severe impairment</li><li>Clozapine: Contraindicated in active liver disease associated with nausea, anorexia or jaundice, progressive liver disease or hepatic failure. Caution advised in patients with concurrent hepatic disease</li><li>Iloperidone: Not recommended</li><li>Lumateperone: Avoid in patients with moderate (Child-Pugh B) or severe (Child-Pugh C) impairment</li><li>Lurasidone: Dose adjustment recommended in patients with moderate (Child-Pugh B) or severe (Child-Pugh C) impairment. Recommended starting dose is 20 mg/day. Dose should not exceed 80 mg/day in moderate impairment and 40 mg/day in severe impairment</li><li>Quetiapine: Start with 25 mg/day, increase daily by 25–50 mg/day as needed</li><li>Quetiapine XR: Start with 50 mg/day, increase daily by 50 mg/day as needed</li><li>Risperidone: For patients with severe impairment, recommended initial dose is 0.5 mg twice daily. Dose increases should be in increments of no more than 0.5 mg twice daily</li></ul>

- Risperidone long-acting injection: Treat patients with impairment with titrated doses of oral risperidone prior to initiating risperidone long-acting. Recommended oral starting dose is 0.5 mg twice daily during first week, can be increased to 1 mg twice daily or 2 mg once daily during second week. If total oral daily dose of at least 2 mg is well tolerated, an injection of 25 mg risperidone long-acting can be administered q 2 weeks
- Risperidone RBP-7000: Stabilize patient on risperidone oral 3 mg/day. If this is tolerated, a 90 mg dose of RBP-7000 may be considered

Pharmacokinetics

- See tables pp. 203–207 and p. 214 for kinetics of individual agents
- **Hepatic** primary route of metabolism (i.e., $\geq 50\%$): Asenapine, clozapine, iloperidone, lumateperone, lurasidone, olanzapine, quetiapine, risperidone, ziprasidone
- Hepatic impairment: Asenapine's exposure ~7 times higher in severe impairment; quetiapine's AUC and C_{max} increased by 40%, clearance reduced by 25%, and half-life increased to prolonged by 45% in mild impairment; lurasidone's AUC increased 1.5, 1.7, and 3-fold in mild, moderate, and severe impairment, respectively, with C_{max} 1.3-fold higher in all levels of impairment; risperidone's free fraction in the plasma increased by ~35%; ziprasidone's AUC increased by 19% and 34%, respectively, in mild to moderate impairment – half-life prolonged by ~2.3 h
- **Renal** primary route of excretion (i.e., $\geq 50\%$)[11]: Asenapine, clozapine, iloperidone, olanzapine, paliperidone, quetiapine, risperidone
- Renal impairment: Lurasidone's C_{max} increased by 40%, 92%, and 54%, and AUC increased by 53%, 91%, and 2-fold in mild, moderate, and severe impairment, respectively; paliperidone's clearance 32%, 64%, and 71% lower and half-life increased to 24 h, 40 h, and 51 h in mild, moderate, and severe impairment, respectively; risperidone's and metabolite's C_{max} and AUC increased by ~40% and 160%, respectively – half-life prolonged and clearance reduced by 60%

Oral

- Once-daily dosing is appropriate for most drugs because of long elimination half-life; recommended that doses of clozapine above 200–300 mg be divided due to seizure risk; manufacturer recommends quetiapine (immediate release) and ziprasidone be given twice daily (due to short half-life)
- Lumateperone: Ingestion of a high-fat meal with lumateperone lowers mean C_{max} by 33% and increases mean AUC by 9%. Median T_{max} was delayed about 1 h
- Lurasidone C_{max} and AUC increased 3- and 2-fold, respectively, when given with food. These increases were independent of meal size (i.e., 350–1000 calories) and meal fat content
- Quetiapine XR dosed once daily at steady state has comparable bioavailability, C_{max}, and AUC to an equivalent total daily dose of quetiapine regular release tablets administered bid
- Quetiapine XR can be taken with or without food. When given with a high-fat meal (~800–1000 calories), it had increases in C_{max} (44–52%) and AUC (20–22%). In comparison, a light meal (~300 calories) had no effect. Suggest taking consistently with respect to food
- The following agents can be taken with or without meals: Clozapine, iloperidone, olanzapine, paliperidone, risperidone (tablets, M-Tabs, and solution)
- Ziprasidone's bioavailability increased 2-fold with food. The calorie count, not the fat content, of food influences ziprasidone's bioavailability. Optimal bioavailability when given with a meal of at least 500 calories
- Ziprasidone suspension yields a lower C_{max} (~10–17%) and AUC (4–13%) than ziprasidone capsules. Not clinically significant

Disintegrating and Sublingual Tablets

- Asenapine sublingual tablets' absolute bioavailability is 35%; however, this is greatly reduced when swallowed (less than 2% with an oral tablet formulation) due to extensive first-pass metabolism
- Asenapine, when administered with water or food, results in reduced drug exposure. Reduced exposure following water administration at 2 min (19% decrease) and 5 min (10% decrease); food consumption immediately prior to or following asenapine decreases exposure by 20% and 4 h after asenapine decreases exposure by ~10%
- Supralingual preparations (orally disintegrating tablets) of olanzapine (Zydis) and risperidone (M-Tab) dissolve in saliva within 15 sec (can be swallowed with or without liquid) – bioequivalent to oral tablet

Short-acting IM

- Olanzapine short-acting IM C_{max} occurs in 15–45 min (compared to 5–8 h with oral form) and is 4–5 times higher than for the same oral dose. Half-life for IM and oral forms is similar
- Ziprasidone short-acting IM peak plasma level reached within 60 min and is dose related

Long-acting IM

- See table p. 214
- Long-acting antipsychotics provide improved bioavailability and more consistent blood levels without the peaks and troughs observed with short-acting oral therapy

Second-Generation Antipsychotics/SGAs (cont.)

- Treatment with olanzapine pamoate IM for ~3 months may be required to re-establish steady-state levels when switching from oral olanzapine. Olanzapine plasma concentrations during the first injection interval may be lower than those maintained by a corresponding oral dose. Steady-state olanzapine plasma concentrations for doses of 150–405 mg q 2–4 weeks are within the range of steady-state concentrations achieved with oral doses of 5–20 mg olanzapine once daily
- Following a single IM dose of paliperidone palmitate 1-monthly IM, plasma concentrations gradually rise to reach maximum at a median T_{max} of 13 days. Release of the drug starts as early as day 1 and lasts for as long as 126 days. The median apparent half-life after a single dose increased over the dose range of 39–234 mg of paliperidone palmitate 1-monthly IM (i.e., 25–150 mg of paliperidone) to 25–49 days
- Paliperidone palmitate 1-monthly IM's C_{max} is 28% higher where administered into the deltoid vs. gluteal muscle (deltoid offers faster absorption as it has better blood perfusion). Two initial deltoid injections on day 1 and day 8 help attain therapeutic concentrations rapidly without the need for oral supplementation
- Following a single IM dose of paliperidone palmitate 3-monthly IM, plasma concentrations gradually rise to reach a maximum at a median T_{max} of 30–33 days. Release of the drug starts as early as day 1 and lasts for as long as 18 months. The median apparent half-life after a single dose increased over the dose range of 273–819 mg (175–525 mg of paliperidone), ranging from 84–95 days following deltoid injections and 118–139 days following gluteal injections
- Paliperidone palmitate 3-monthly IM's C_{max} is 11–12% higher where administered into the deltoid vs. gluteal muscle (deltoid offers faster absorption as it has better blood perfusion)
- Following a single IM dose of paliperidone palmitate 6-monthly IM, plasma concentrations gradually rise to reach a maximum at a median T_{max} of 29–32 days. Release of the drug starts as early as day 1 and lasts longer than 18 months. The median apparent half-life after a single dose increased over the dose range: 1,092 mg leads to 148 days and 1,560 mg to 159 days
- Immediately after injection of the risperidone long-acting formulation, a negligible amount of risperidone is released (less than 1%, mostly from the surface of the microspheres). Over several weeks, the microspheres are gradually hydrolyzed and release a steady amount of risperidone, producing therapeutic levels within 3–4 weeks for most patients. Oral antipsychotic supplementation should be given during the first 3 weeks to maintain therapeutic levels until risperidone long-acting injection reaches therapeutic plasma concentration. When administered q 2 weeks, steady-state plasma concentrations are reached after the 4th injection and maintained for 4–6 weeks after the last injection. Complete elimination occurs approximately 7–8 weeks after the last injection
- Following a single SC dose of risperidone RBP-7000, first peak (T_{max}) of risperidone occurs at 4-6 h due to initial drug release during the depot formation processs. Second peak seen at 10-14 days post dose, is associated with the slow release of risperidone from the SC depot. Both peaks are similar in magnitude

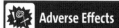 Adverse Effects

- See chart on p. 199 for incidence of adverse effects
- While a relative lower incidence of EPS may make them more tolerable to patients, metabolic effects may be a contributing factor to the significant degree of premature cardiovascular mortality noted among individuals with schizophrenia
- Some adverse effects may be preventable by employing simple strategies (e.g., slow upwards titration, dosing schedule manipulation – e.g., dosing a sedating drug at bedtime or dividing up the daily dose to minimize adverse effects related to higher peak levels)
- Certain adverse effects may be more common and/or problematic in females (e.g., weight gain, metabolic syndrome, hyperprolactinemia)

CNS Effects

- Activation, insomnia, disturbed sleep, nightmares, vivid dreams – activation reported with lower doses of ziprasidone, may subside with dosage increase. Although complaints of sedation are more common with most SGAs, insomnia has been reported with many agents including asenapine, clozapine (may be more common following withdrawal), olanzapine, paliperidone, risperidone, and ziprasidone. Disturbed sleep, nightmares, or vivid dreams occasionally reported for some of these agents (clozapine, olanzapine, quetiapine, risperidone)
- Confusion, disturbed concentration, disorientation (more common with high doses or in the elderly); toxic delirium reported with clozapine. Concomitant anticholinergic agents may exacerbate. Post-injection delirium sedation syndrome (PDSS) with olanzapine pamoate injection – see post-injection delirium sedation syndrome below
- EPS – acute onset: A result of antagonism at dopamine D_2 receptors in the nigrostriatal tract (extrapyramidal reactions correlate with D_2 binding above 80%)

- Generally speaking, extrapyramidal reactions are less common with SGAs vs. FGAs but may still occur (see p. 198 to compare incidence of EPS associated with these agents). See the relative tolerability profiles table p. 196 for a comparison of the likelihood of EPS among antipsychotics
  - Dose-related akathisia, dystonia, and parkinsonism commonly reported with lurasidone
  - Asenapine also associated with dose-related akathisia and parkinsonism
- EPS – late onset or tardive movement disorders (TD)
  - Includes tardive akathisia, tardive dyskinesia, and tardive dystonia (see p. 226 for onset, symptoms, and therapeutic management options)
  - Late onset movement disorders usually develop after months or years of treatment
  - May be irreversible, so prevention is key – use lowest possible doses and assess for signs of movement disorders regularly. Dyskinetic symptoms are not alleviated and may be exacerbated by antiparkinsonian medications
  - Annual risk of TD with FGAs estimated to be 4–5%, with a cumulative risk of up to 50%. Risk of TD lower with SGA and TGAs antipsychotics
  - Clozapine has lowest TD risk and its use has been associated with a significant reduction in existing TD (especially tardive dystonia), often within 1–4 weeks (sometimes up to 12 weeks)
- Sedation, somnolence, and fatigue – common, especially following treatment initiation and dosage increase. Usually transient, but some individuals may complain of persistent effects. See the relative tolerability profiles table p. 196 for a comparison of the likelihood of sedating effects among antipsychotics [Management: Evening/bedtime administration; lower dose, if feasible; minimize use of concomitant CNS depressants, if possible]
- Headache – reported with clozapine, olanzapine, paliperidone, quetiapine, risperidone, and asenapine at an incidence of 5–15%
- Neuroleptic malignant syndrome (NMS) – rare disorder characterized by autonomic dysfunction (e.g., tachycardia and hypertension), hyperthermia, altered consciousness, and muscle rigidity with an increase in creatine kinase (CK) and myoglobinuria. Fatalities from NMS are rare if syndrome identified early
  - Can occur with any class of antipsychotic agent, at any dose, and at any time (although usually occurs early in the course of treatment). Risk factors may include dehydration, young age, male sex, organic brain syndromes, exhaustion, agitation, and rapid or parenteral antipsychotic administration
  - Potentially fatal unless recognized early and medication stopped. Supportive therapy (e.g., maintain hydration, correct electrolyte imbalances, control fever) must be instituted as soon as possible. Additional treatment with dopamine agonists such as amantadine and bromocriptine may be helpful (controversial – may reduce muscle rigidity without an effect on overall outcome); ECT has also been used successfully to improve symptoms. Treatment with an antipsychotic agent may recommence several weeks post recovery
- Paresthesias – or "burning sensations" reported with risperidone. Oral paresthesia/hypesthesia reported to occur in about 5% of patients treated with asenapine. The effect occurs immediately following sublingual administration, is 15–25 mm in diameter, and lasts approximately 10-30 min
- Post-injection delirium sedation syndrome (PDSS) – associated with olanzapine pamoate long-acting injection. CNS symptoms may include sedation (ranging from mild sedation to coma), delirium, dizziness, weakness, dysarthria, and seizures. Injection must be administered in a facility with access to emergency services. Patients should be assessed every 30 min for 3 h post each injection for signs of post-injection syndrome
- Seizures – all antipsychotics may lower seizure threshold, resulting in seizures ranging from myoclonus to grand mal type. May occur if dose increased rapidly or may also be secondary to hyponatremia associated with SIADH. See the relative tolerability profiles table p. 196 for a comparison of the likelihood of seizures among antipsychotics
- Stroke – higher incidence of transient ischemic attacks and stroke reported in placebo-controlled trials of elderly patients with dementia treated with risperidone, olanzapine or aripiprazole. The relationship, if any, between antipsychotic medication and these events is uncertain

Anticholinergic Effects

- See the relative tolerability profiles table p. 196 for a comparison of the likelihood of anticholinergic effects among antipsychotics
- Many of these adverse effects are often dose related and may resolve over time without treatment
- Blurred vision [Management: Use adequate lighting when reading; pilocarpine 0.5% eye drops]
- Constipation – [Management/prevention: Increase dietary fiber and fluid intake, increase exercise or use an osmotic laxative (e.g., polyethylene glycol (PEG)) or bulk laxative (e.g., psyllium, polycarbophil)] occasionally associated with olanzapine and quetiapine. Clozapine has been associated with varying degrees of impairment of peristalsis ranging from constipation to intestinal obstruction, fecal impaction, and paralytic ileus (potentially fatal if undetected)
- Delirium – characterized by agitation, confusion, disorientation, visual hallucinations, tachycardia, etc. May result with use of high doses or combination anticholinergic medication. Drugs with high anticholinergic activity have also been associated with impaired cognition and selective impairments of learning and memory[4]
- Dry eyes [Management: Artificial tears, wetting solutions]

Second-Generation Antipsychotics/SGAs (cont.)

- Dry mouth/mucous membranes – if severe or persistent, may predispose patient to candida infection [Management: Sugar-free gum and candy oral lubricants (e.g., MoiStir, OraCare D), pilocarpine mouth wash – see p. 57]
- Urinary retention – may be more problematic for older patients, especially males with benign prostatic hypertrophy [Management: bethanechol]

Cardiovascular Effects

- CVD is the leading cause of death in individuals with schizophrenia, with an estimated 2/3 dying from coronary heart disease. There may be a number of contributing factors to CVD in this population, including smoking, sedentary lifestyles, poverty, poor nutrition, reduced access to health care, and a number of interrelated metabolic abnormalities including obesity, dyslipidemias, glucose intolerance, insulin resistance and diabetes, and hypertension. Please see p. 155 for more details on these endocrine and metabolic effects and their role in CVD
- Arrhythmias and ECG changes:
  - Bradycardia reported with IM olanzapine, often accompanied by decreased resting BP or an orthostatic drop. Caution in patients who have received other medications associated with hypotensive or bradycardic effects
  - ECG changes (e.g., T-wave inversion, ST segment depression, QTc lengthening – may increase risk of arrhythmias) reported with many antipsychotic medications, the clinical significance of which is unclear for many. A QTc of more than 500 msec or an increase from baseline of more than 60 msec is associated with an increased risk for torsades de pointes (TdP), ventricular fibrillation, and sudden cardiac death. Prominent risk factors for QTc prolongation include congenital long QT syndrome, elderly age, female sex, heart failure, myocardial infarction (MI), and concomitant use of medications that prolong the QT interval or inhibit the metabolism of a drug known to prolong QT (see Drug Interactions pp. 167–176). Other risk factors may include altered nutritional status (e.g., eating disorders, alcoholism), bradycardia, cerebrovascular disease, diabetes, electrolyte imbalances (e.g., hypokalemia, hypomagnesemia, hypocalcemia), hypertension, hypothyroidism, and obesity. The presence of risk factors for QT prolongation should be controlled (e.g., electrolyte imbalances corrected, interacting drugs or use of concomitant drugs that prolong QT avoided), where possible, before initiation of treatment with a SGA. A list of drugs associated with QT prolongation and ranking with respect to risk for causing TdP can be found at https://www.crediblemeds.org
  - In 2006, Health Canada adopted new guidelines regarding QT/QTc, including the requirement to submit a thorough QT/QTc study. This may have translated into more stringent warnings and precautions appearing in the product monographs for antipsychotics approved since this time:
    - Ziprasidone is contraindicated in patients with recent MI, uncompensated heart failure, and a known history of QT prolongation. The product monograph also includes warnings against using it in combination with drugs known to prolong QT, as well as recommendations regarding its use in patients with stable heart disease, at risk of significant electrolyte disturbances or who develop cardiac symptoms while taking the drug
    - There are warnings advising cautious use of antipsychotics in patients with known CVD and reports of arrhythmias and sudden cardiac death
  - See the relative tolerability profiles table p. 196 for a comparison of the likelihood of QTc prolongation among antipsychotics
  - Caution is advised when directly comparing approximate QTc prolongation times among the various agents as differences exist with respect to various methods used to calculate the QTc as well as the characteristics of the study population (e.g., concomitant medications, comorbidities, antipsychotic dosage, etc.)
  - Credible Meds Worldwide[7] categorizes risk of developing TdP as follows:
    - Risk of TdP (QT prolongation and clear association of risk of TdP even when used as directed): chlorpromazine, haloperidol, pimozide, thioridazine
    - Possible Risk of TdP (can cause QT prolongation but insufficient evidence of associated risk of TdP when used as directed): aripiprazole, asenapine, clozapine, flupenthixol, iloperidone, paliperidone, perphenazine, risperidone, zuclopenthixol
    - Conditional risk of TdP (associated with a risk of TdP but only under certain conditions – e.g., excessive dose, hypokalemia, congenital long QT syndrome, drug-drug interaction): amisulpride, olanzapine, quetiapine, ziprasidone
  - Tachycardia reported with clozapine, iloperidone, olanzapine, paliperidone, quetiapine, risperidone, and ziprasidone. Tachycardia may occur as a compensatory mechanism to orthostatic hypotension caused by α_1-adrenergic antagonism. On the other hand, persistent sinus tachycardia results from antagonism of presynaptic α_2 receptors as well as antagonism of M_2 receptors located on the sinoatrial node. Persistent tachycardia at rest accompanied by other signs of heart failure requires cardiology consultation. Treating tachycardia (with β-blockers, non-dihydropyridine calcium channel blockers or I(f) current inhibitors) without further investigation might mask underlying pathology (such as cardiomyopathy, pericarditis, heart failure, myocardial infarction, myocarditis, etc.)
  - Collapse/respiratory/cardiac arrest reported with clozapine alone and in combination with benzodiazepines and other psychotropics

- Cardiomyopathy, pericarditis, myocardial effusion, heart failure, myocardial infarction, mitral valve insufficiency, and myocarditis reported with clozapine. Deaths have been reported. Drug should be promptly discontinued and not rechallenged. Rare reports of arrhythmias and myocardial infarction with olanzapine
  - A 2020 meta-analysis of clozapine-induced myocarditis found a seven-fold difference between Australia and other countries with an event rate of 2% in 9 Australian samples and 0.3% in 15 non-Australian samples. High rates of clozapine-induced myocarditis reported in some countries may be due to rapid titration. The risk of myocarditis appears greatest in the first 3–4 weeks of therapy. Concurrent valproate use seems to increase the risk of myocarditis. DO NOT USE in patients with severe cardiac disease. The clinical presentation of myocarditis may be nonspecific. Investigate patients who develop persistent tachycardia at rest and/or fatigue, flu-like symptoms, hypotension, and unexplained fever. Patients with myocarditis may also have new onset symptoms of respiratory, gastrointestinal or urinary tract infections. Some will also exhibit symptoms of heart failure (e.g., chest pain, shortness of breath, edema or arrhythmia). Myocarditis may also be asymptomatic. A suggested monitoring protocol would be as follows:
    - At least every second day for the first 4 weeks: BP, pulse, body temperature, respiration rate
    - Days 7, 14, 21, and 28: CRP, Troponin I or T
    - Also: Ask patients (and advise carers if outpatients) to report feelings of unwellness and any symptoms of illness, including fever, cough, chest pain, shortness of breath, diarrhoea, vomiting, nausea, sore throat, myalgia, headache, sweatiness, and urinary discomfort or frequency
  - Clozapine-induced cardiomyopathy can present much later during clozapine therapy, with most cases occurring between 6–9 months of therapy but some reported as late as 4 years. Patients with a significant history of heart disease or abnormal cardiac findings on physical exam should be assessed by a physician or cardiologist before starting clozapine therapy. Clinical presentation of cardiomyopathy includes shortness of breath, orthopnea palpitations, cough, fatigue, edema, and chest pain. Patients should be assessed for the presence of these signs and symptoms regularly (e.g., four times per year). Patients with new symptoms consistent with heart failure should receive an ECG, chest x-ray and, where possible, an echocardiogram. There may be a role for routine monitoring of serum B-type brain natriuretic (BNP) or echocardiograms serially for patients on long-term clozapine therapy although this has not been evaluated with controlled studies
- Increased risk of mortality in dementia patients (see p. 126)
- Dyslipidemia (see p. 155)
- Orthostatic hypotension/compensatory tachycardia/dizziness/syncope – may occur as a result of α_1-adrenergic antagonism. See the relative tolerability profiles table p. 196 for a comparison of the likelihood of orthostatic effects among antipsychotics. Individuals receiving treatment with agents associated with a higher incidence of postural hypotension should be advised to rise slowly for the first few weeks of treatment and following dosage increases to minimize risk of falls. DO NOT USE EPINEPHRINE, as it may further lower the blood pressure (see Drug Interactions, p. 176). Risperidone, quetiapine, clozapine, and iloperidone dosing increases should be gradual to minimize hypotension as well as sinus and reflex tachycardia – may result in falls in the elderly. [Management: Rise slowly, divide the daily dose, increase fluid and salt intake, use support hose; treatment with fluid-retaining corticosteroid – fludrocortisone]
- Thromboembolism – case reports of pulmonary and/or venous thromboembolism with asenapine, clozapine, lurasidone, olanzapine, and quetiapine

Endocrine & Metabolic Effects

- Antidiuretic hormone dysfunction:
  - Disturbances in antidiuretic hormone function: PIP (polydipsia, intermittent hyponatremia, and psychosis syndrome); prevalence in schizophrenia estimated at 6–20% – can range from mild cognitive deficits to seizures, coma, and death; increased risk in the elderly, smokers, and alcoholics. Monitor sodium levels in chronically treated patients (especially with clozapine) to help identify patients at risk for seizure [Management: Fluid restriction, demeclocycline up to 1200 mg/day (note: Not currently available in Canada), captopril 12.5 mg/day, propranolol 30–120 mg/day; correct any electrolyte imbalances]
- Metabolic abnormalities associated with SGAs include dyslipidemia, glucose intolerance/diabetes, metabolic syndrome, and weight gain. A 2010 head-to-head meta-analysis suggested clozapine and olanzapine are associated with the highest overall metabolic liability (most elevation in weight, cholesterol, and glucose). Quetiapine and risperidone had more of an intermediate risk (except for cholesterol, for which quetiapine had a greater risk than risperidone). Ziprasidone and the TGA, aripiprazole, had the lowest risk. The SGAs lurasidone and ziprasidone appear to have the lowest overall metabolic risk potential but it is difficult to rank these agents according to their propensity to cause metabolic effects for a number of reasons (e.g., lack of comparative RCTs assessing metabolic abnormalities as primary outcome, differences in how metabolic effects are defined and measured, differences in trial duration, etc.)
- A network meta-analysis (100 RCTs, 25,952 patients) examining metabolic dysregulation of antipsychotics found olanzapine and clozapine to exhibit the worst profiles and aripiprazole, brexpiprazole, cariprazine, lurasidone, and ziprasidone the most benign profiles. Increased baseline weight, male sex, and non-white ethnicity were predictors of susceptibility to antipsychotic-induced metabolic changes[13]

Second-Generation Antipsychotics/SGAs (cont.)

- Dyslipidemia:
  - Lipid abnormalities (increases in fasting total cholesterol, LDL cholesterol, and triglycerides) have been associated with SGAs. Overall the risk appears greatest with clozapine and olanzapine; moderate with quetiapine; lower with risperidone, paliperidone, and ziprasidone. A 2012 systematic review and meta-analysis of asenapine, iloperidone, lurasidone, and paliperidone reported that these agents did not appear to have a clinically significant effect on cholesterol. No longer-term trials were available for iloperidone and lurasidone. A recent network meta-analysis also shows no significant increase with iloperidone, lurasidone, paliperidone, risperidone, and ziprasidone[13]
  - This risk appears to be associated with, but not dependent on, weight gain. Weight gain and obesity, dietary changes, glucose intolerance, and insulin resistance have all been proposed as possible causes/contributors to lipid dysregulation
  - See p. 124 for suggested monitoring guidelines. The 2016 Canadian Cardiovascular Society guidelines for the diagnosis and treatment of dyslipidemia and prevention of cardiovascular disease may be accessed online at https://www.onlinecjc.ca/article/S0828-282X(16)30732-2/fulltext[14]
  - Treatment options may include lifestyle and dietary modifications; switching to another antipsychotic associated with a lower potential for lipid dysregulation; adding cholesterol-lowering medication (e.g., statins, fibrates, salmon oil, etc.)
- Glucose intolerance/insulin resistance/hyperglycemia/type 2 diabetes mellitus (DM):
  - Treatment with SGAs has been associated with an increased risk for insulin resistance, hyperglycemia, and type 2 diabetes (new onset, exacerbation of existing DM, ketoacidosis)
  - Overall the risk of developing disturbances in glucose metabolism appear greatest with clozapine and olanzapine; moderate with quetiapine; lowest with risperidone and ziprasidone. A 2012 meta-analysis reported no clinically significant increases in glucose levels seen in short- (under 12 weeks) or long-term (more than 12 weeks) trials of asenapine and paliperidone; no clinically significant increases in glucose reported in short-term trials of iloperidone or lurasidone (long-term trials not available)
  - Treatment options may include lifestyle and dietary modifications; switching to another antipsychotic associated with a lower potential for glucose dysregulation; adding a hypoglycemic agent such as metformin
  - Diabetic ketoacidosis and diabetic hyperosmolar coma are very rare adverse effects of antipsychotics, but have been reported with clozapine
  - The Diabetes Canada 2018 clinical practice guidelines may be accessed online at https://guidelines.diabetes.ca/docs/cpg/Ch18-Diabetes-and-Mental-Health.pdf
- Hyperprolactinemia:
  - Prolactin level may be elevated – increases occur several hours after dosing and normalize by 12–24 h with clozapine, olanzapine, quetiapine, and ziprasidone; elevation persists during chronic administration with risperidone (incidence greater than 30% – less with long-acting IM risperidone) and paliperidone; increased plasma prolactin level related to dose of olanzapine (higher if more than 20 mg/day). Prolactin elevation has been reported to occur in individuals receiving iloperidone in short-term clinical trials. Chronic elevation of prolactin levels reported with asenapine. Dose-dependent increases in serum prolactin concentrations reported with lurasidone but no reports of associated adverse effects
  - See the relative tolerability profiles table p. 196 for a comparison of the hyperprolactinemia effects among antipsychotics
  - *Clinical consequences* of elevated prolactin levels may include short-term risks such as galactorrhea, gynecomastia, menstrual irregularities, and sexual dysfunction, and potential long-term risks such as osteoporosis (as a result of decreased bone density secondary to chronic hypogonadism), pituitary tumors, and breast cancer (data conflicting)
  - *Effects in women:* Breast engorgement and lactation (may be more common in women who have previously been pregnant), amenorrhea (with risk of infertility), menstrual irregularities, changes in libido, hirsutism (due to increased testosterone), and possibly osteoporosis (due to decreased estrogen). Recommended that women with hyperprolactinemia or amenorrhea for more than 12 months have a bone mineral density evaluation
  - *Effects in men:* Gynecomastia, rarely galactorrhea, decreased libido, and erectile or ejaculatory dysfunction
  - *Risk of breast cancer:* A nationwide nested case-control study in Finland reported that exposure to prolactin-increasing antipsychotics for 5 or more years was significantly associated with increased odds of breast cancer in comparison with minimal exposure (less than 1 year). On the other hand, exposure to prolactin-sparing antipsychotics (including clozapine, quetiapine, or aripiprazole) for 5 or more years was not associated with an increased risk of breast cancer in comparison with minimal exposure (less than 1 year)
  - *Monitoring/investigation:* The fasting morning serum prolactin level is recommended as it is least variable and best correlated with disease states. In cases where an antipsychotic medication is strongly suspected as the cause, discontinuing the suspected agent (or switching to

another antipsychotic agent with less potential for prolactin elevation) for a short period of time (e.g., 3–4 days) if clinically feasible and follow-up monitoring to determine if prolactin levels have fallen may be a simple means to confirm suspicions and avoid MRI or CT of the hypothalamic/pituitary region

- *Treatment options:* Assuming discontinuation of antipsychotic therapy is not an option, the preferred treatment is to switch to another antipsychotic agent with a reduced risk of hyperprolactinemia – weighing the potential risk for relapse associated with this action. Other treatment options may include lowering the dose or adding a medication to treat the condition. Use of a dopamine agonist such as bromocriptine (1.25–2.5 mg bid) or cabergoline (0.25–2 mg/week) may be considered but has the potential to exacerbate the underlying illness. Meta-analyses support use of low-dose adjunctive aripiprazole (5 mg/day has been shown to reduce prolactin levels)

- Metabolic syndrome:
  - Metabolic syndrome is an interrelated cluster of CVD risk factors that include abdominal obesity, dyslipidemia, hypertension, and impaired glucose tolerance. Using the International Diabetes Federation (IDF) criteria, individuals must have central obesity, which is defined according to ethnicity (e.g., for Europoids a waist circumference of 94 cm or more in males and 80 cm or more in females is required), in addition to at least 2 of the following characteristics:
    1. Triglycerides: > 1.7 mmol/L (150 mg/dl)
    2. HDL cholesterol: Men < 1.03 mmol/L (40 mg/dl)/Women < 1.3 mmol/L (50 mg/dl)
    3. Blood pressure: $\geq 130/> 85$ mmHg (or treatment for hypertension)
    4. Fasting glucose: > 5.6 mmol/L (100 mg/dl)
  - Shown to be an important risk factor in the development of type 2 diabetes and CVD. Individuals with metabolic syndrome are 5 times more likely to develop type 2 diabetes and 2–3 times more likely to experience heart attack or stroke
  - The risk of developing metabolic syndrome appears to be greater with clozapine and olanzapine, followed by risperidone, asenapine, iloperidone, and quetiapine. Ziprasidone and lurasidone appear to have a lower risk

- Thyroid hormone effects – dose-dependent decrease in total T_4 and free T_4 concentrations reported with quetiapine; clinical significance unknown

- Weight gain:
  - Approximately 50% of patients gain an average of 20% of their weight (primarily adipose tissue)
  - Four meta-analyses in 2013, 2017, 2020, and 2022 that included indirect and direct comparisons of antipsychotics suggested that clozapine, olanzapine, and iloperidone have the highest amounts of weight gain; quetiapine, risperidone, paliperdone, and asenapine intermediate amounts; and lurasidone and ziprasidone the lowest amounts (comparable to placebo rates)[13]
  - A dose-response meta-analysis of RCTs of patients with acute exacerbation (97 studies involving 36,326 patients, median duration = 6 weeks) reported that amisulpride, aripiprazole, brexpiprazole, cariprazine, haloperidol, lumateperone, and lurasidone produced mild weight gain in comparison to placebo (mean difference (MD) ≤ 1 kg for any dose). Dose-response curves did not plateau for clozapine, olanzapine, and paliperidone, with these having MDs in weight gain of 3.75 kg, 3.62 kg, and 1.95 kg, respectively. Quetiapine and ziprasidone showed a bell-shaped relationship with maximal weight gain centered around 600 mg/day (MD in weight gain = 1.48 kg) and 80 mg/day (MD in weight gain = 1.24 kg)
  - There may be temporal differences in the weight gain that occurs with antipsychotic therapy: A rapid initial gain in the first three months of treatment (phase 1); a continued steady gain over the following year (phase 2); and finally a stable weight plateau with ongoing therapy (phase 3)
  - Risk factors for antipsychotic-induced weight gain appear to be baseline lower BMI of the patient, younger age, being treatment naïve with antipsychotics, higher parental BMI, and non-smoking status
  - The mechanism by which antipsychotics may influence weight gain is unknown (may be a result of multiple systems including 5-HT$_{1B}$, 5-HT$_{2C}$, α_1, and H$_1$ blockade, prolactinemia, gonadal and adrenal steroid imbalance, and increase in circulating leptin; may also be due to sedation and inactivity, carbohydrate craving, and excessive intake of high-calorie beverages to alleviate drug-induced thirst and dry mouth)
  - See the relative tolerability profiles table p. 196 for a comparison of the likelihood of weight gain among antipsychotics
  - Treatment options: Since it is often challenging to lose weight, preventative strategies that focus on healthy lifestyles (e.g., diet and exercise) are recommended. May not be dose dependent, so the efficacy of dosage reduction strategies is uncertain. Treatment options may include healthy lifestyle strategies; switching from an antipsychotic with higher weight gain liability to one of lower liability (may result in significant reductions in body weight); or use of medications to promote weight loss. Treatment with the following agents has been tried with varying degrees of success based on case reports and randomized controlled trials: Amantadine (100–300 mg/day), bromocriptine (2.5 mg/day), famotidine (40 mg/day), topiramate (up to 200 mg/day), nizatidine (300 mg bid), orlistat (120 mg tid), and metformin (850–1000 mg bid). The bulk of evidence is for metformin and topiramate with studies typically reporting a gradual loss of weight up to 5–10 kg over 12–16 weeks

Second-Generation Antipsychotics/SGAs (cont.)

GI Effects	<ul><li>Constipation – see Anticholinergic Effects p. 153. Clozapine and olanzapine have high affinity for M_1 receptors; quetiapine has moderate affinity; the remaining SGAs are categorized as low to negligible affinity for these receptors</li><li>Dysphagia (difficulty swallowing) and aspiration have been reported with antipsychotic use. Use all agents cautiously in individuals at risk for developing aspiration pneumonia (e.g., advanced Alzheimer's disease)</li><li>Dry mouth – see Anticholinergic Effects, p. 153</li><li>GI obstructions – do not administer paliperidone to patients with pre-existing severe GI narrowing (e.g., esophageal motility disorders, small bowel inflammatory disease, short gut syndrome, etc.) due to its OROS formulation. Clozapine associated with varying degrees of impaired intestinal peristalsis, including bowel obstruction, ischemia, perforation, and aspiration; 102 cases of suspected life-threatening hypomotility disorder reviewed, resulting in mortality rate of 27.5% and considerable morbidity, largely due to bowel resection – see Anticholinergic Effects p. 153</li><li>Oral hypoesthesia – decreased oral sensitivity reported with asenapine</li><li>Parotitis reported with clozapine</li><li>Reflux esophagitis (approximately 11% incidence reported with clozapine)</li><li>Sialorrhea (most commonly associated with clozapine), with difficulty swallowing/gagging that is most profound during sleep; dose related – may lead to aspiration pneumonia. May be due to stimulation of M_4 muscarinic or α_2 receptors in salivary glands. [Management: Chew sugarless gum, cover pillow with towels, reduce dose. Preliminary evidence suggests benefit with: Amitriptyline (25–100 mg), benztropine (1–4 mg) or trihexyphenidyl (5–15 mg per day) – caution: Additive anticholinergic effects; pirenzepine (25–100 mg), clonidine (0.05–0.4 mg once daily orally or transdermal patch 0.1–0.2 mg applied weekly) – caution: Additive hypotension; terazosin (2 mg daily), scopolamine patch (1.5 mg/2.5 cm^2 patch applied every 72 h), atropine "eye" drops (1 drop sublingually 1–2 times a day), tropicamide "eye" drops (1–2 drops bilaterally sublingually once daily; case reports), ipratropium nasal (given as 2 sprays under the tongue tid)]</li></ul>
Urogenital & Sexual Effects	<ul><li>Sexual effects may result from altered dopamine (D_2), serotonergic, ACh, α_1 or H_1 activity; hyperprolactinemia is the main cause of sexual dysfunction in women</li><li>Treatment options may include: 1) dosage reduction, 2) waiting 1–3 months to see if tolerance develops, 3) switching antipsychotics or 4) adding a medication to treat the problem. (See below for treatment suggestions regarding specific types of dysfunction; evidence for their use based primarily on open-label studies and case reports)</li><li>Treatment options with lower rates of sexual dysfunction reported include quetiapine, ziprasidone, and aripiprazole</li><li>*Anorgasmia* [Management: Bethanechol (10 mg tid or 10–25 mg prn before intercourse), neostigmine (7.5–15 mg prn), cyproheptadine (4–16 mg/day), amantadine (100–300 mg/day)]</li><li>*Ejaculation dysfunction* (including inhibition of ejaculation, abnormal ejaculation, retrograde ejaculation – especially risperidone) [Management suggestions for retrograde ejaculation: Imipramine (25–50 mg at bedtime), yohimbine (5.4 mg 1–3 × daily, 1–4 h prior to intercourse) or cyproheptadine (4–16 mg/day)]</li><li>*Erectile dysfunction (ED)*, impotence. The incidence with SGAs is unclear but appears to be lower than with the FGAs (especially with agents other than risperidone) [Management suggestions: Bethanechol (10 mg tid or 10–50 mg prn before intercourse), yohimbine (5.4 mg 1–3 × daily, 1–4 h prior to intercourse), sildenafil (25–100 mg prn), amantadine (100–300 mg/day)]</li><li>*Libido* – decreased [Management: Neostigmine (7.5–15 mg prn) or cyproheptadine (4–16 mg prn) 30 min before intercourse]; monitor prolactin</li><li>Priapism – has been reported in patients on most SGAs, including newer SGAs such as iloperidone. Antagonism of α_1-adrenergic receptors is believed to play a role. See p. 194 for information on which agents have more α_1-antagonistic effects</li><li>Renal dysfunction – rare reports of interstitial nephritis and acute renal failure with clozapine</li><li>Urinary incontinence (overflow incontinence)/enuresis (nocturnal enuresis) reported with clozapine (up to 42%); case reports with olanzapine and risperidone. Appears to be more frequent with clozapine but the relative risks of the various SGAs for causing this effect are unknown. [Management strategies: Dosage reduction; limiting fluid intake in the evening, especially caffeine-containing beverages or alcohol; voiding directly before bed; and setting an alarm to wake up and void during the night. Case reports of successful treatment with a wide array of pharmacological treatments including amitriptyline 25 mg/day, aripiprazole 10–15 mg/day, or ephedrine 25–150 mg/day, oxybutynin 5–15 mg/day, pseudoephedrine 60 mg, trihexyphenidyl 5–6 mg/day or tolterodine 1–4 mg/day; verapamil 80 mg/day]</li><li>Urinary retention – see Anticholinergic Effects p. 153</li></ul>

Ocular Effects	

- Blurred vision/dry eyes: see Anticholinergic Effects p. 153
- Esotropia: Case report of esotropia (form of strabismus) with olanzapine
- Intraoperative floppy iris syndrome (IFIS) – a complication during eye surgery (cataract removal) characterized by a flaccid iris and progressive intraoperative pupil constriction that may result in damage to the eye has been associated with the use of risperidone

Hematological Effects	

- Blood dyscrasias, including those affecting erythropoiesis, granulopoiesis, and thrombopoiesis, have been reported with most antipsychotics
- Clinically significant hematological abnormalities with antipsychotics are, with the exception of clozapine, rare. Accordingly, the development of any blood abnormalities in individuals on antipsychotic medication, especially other than clozapine, should undergo rigorous medical assessment to determine the underlying cause
- **Anemia** – reported with asenapine, clozapine, iloperidone, lurasidone, and ziprasidone
- **Aplastic anemia** – reported with risperidone and clozapine
- **Eosinophilia** – not typically of clinical significance unless severe. Transient elevations in eosinophil counts without clinical sequelae reported with olanzapine, quetiapine, and ziprasidone. Eosinophilia reported with clozapine frequently between weeks 3 and 5 of treatment; higher incidence in females. Neutropenia can occur concurrently. In most case reports, withdrawal of the drug resulted in normalization of the hematological profile
- **Leukocytosis** – 41% risk of transient leukocytosis reported with clozapine. Leukocytosis also reported with ziprasidone
- **Leukopenia** [defined as WBC $< 4 \times 10^9$/L] and **neutropenia/agranulocytosis** [neutropenia (defined as ANC $< 1.5 \times 10^9$/L) may be subclassified as mild (ANC $= 1–1.5 \times 10^9$/L), moderate (ANC $= 0.5–1 \times 10^9$/L) or severe (also termed agranulocytosis – defined as ANC $< 0.5 \times 10^9$/L or sometimes as ANC $< 0.2 \times 10^9$/L)]
  - Transient neutropenia occurring only in the morning (with an afternoon ANC count returning to normal) has been reported with clozapine
  - Recurrence of previous clozapine-induced neutropenia reported after olanzapine started
  - Agranulocytosis can occur with all antipsychotics but is generally rare (incidence less than 0.1%) except with clozapine (occurs in approximately 1% of patients; 0.38% risk with monitoring). The rate of occurrence is highest in the first 26 weeks of clozapine therapy. Fatalities typically resulting from infections due to compromised immune status have been reported. Patients treated with clozapine must consent to routine hematological monitoring (see p. 162 for guidelines). Risk factors include older age, female gender, and certain ethnic groups (i.e., Ashkenazi Jews). Do not use clozapine in patients with myeloproliferative disorders, granulocytopenia or ANC $< 2 \times 10^9$/L. Monitor for, and advise patients to immediately report, any signs of infection or flu-like symptoms (e.g., fever, sore throat, chills, malaise, etc.). Individuals on clozapine may develop transient, benign fever, especially during the first few weeks of treatment. Fever due to underlying blood dyscrasia/infection, neuroleptic malignant syndrome or myocarditis must be ruled out. Avoid concomitant use of other medications associated with blood dyscrasias (see Drug Interactions pp. 167–176)
  - A recent meta-analysis of 108 studies determined that the incidence of clozapine-associated neutropenia was 2.8% and severe neutropenia 0.9%. Incidence of death related to neutropenia was 0.013%. The case fatality rate of severe neutropenia was 2.1%
- **Pancytopenia** – case report with quetiapine, hematological profile normalized within 7 days of discontinuing drug
- **Thrombocytopenia** – platelet abnormalities reported infrequently. Case reports of thrombocytopenia with asenapine, clozapine, olanzapine, quetiapine, risperidone, and ziprasidone
- **Thrombocytosis** – case reports with clozapine. In most cases, withdrawal of the medication resulted in normalization of platelet counts

Hepatic Effects	

- Acute liver failure – 2013 Health Canada Advisory regarding 3 reports of liver failure in females (aged 58–77 years) associated with quetiapine use. The duration of quetiapine exposure in these cases was relatively short (9 days – 6 weeks) and although not all the cases included information about dosing, those that did involved low doses (25–100 mg/day) of quetiapine. Two of the three cases had fatal outcomes
- Cholestatic jaundice (reversible if drug stopped). Occurs in less than 0.1% of patients on antipsychotics within first 4 weeks of treatment. Reported with clozapine, olanzapine, and ziprasidone
- Hepatomegaly/steatohepatitis – case reports of nonalcoholic steatohepatitis (i.e., fatty liver with inflammation, necrosis, and hepatomegaly, with mild to moderate increase in ALT/SGPT and/or AST/SGOT) reported with olanzapine and risperidone; risk factors include weight gain, hyperlipidemia, type 2 diabetes mellitus, and polypharmacy – usually benign but can progress to cirrhosis. Hepatomegaly and fatty liver deposits also reported with ziprasidone
- Pancreatitis – reports of pancreatitis with risperidone, olanzapine, quetiapine, and clozapine; generally occurred within first 6 months of therapy (possibly associated with hyperglycemia or hypertriglyceridemia); hyperamylasemia reported with risperidone
- Transaminase elevations – elevations in ALT, AST and/or gamma-GT have been reported typically within the first 2–6 weeks of treatment. Up to 40% of clozapine patients experience alanine transaminase levels above 2 times the upper limit of normal. May be asymptomatic and transient in nature

Second-Generation Antipsychotics/SGAs (cont.)

with rare/very rare reports of hepatitis/hepatic failure. Increases in levels beyond 3 times the normal upper limit usually warrant discontinuation; icteric hepatitis observed in only 0.06% of clozapine patients
- See p. 150 for dosing in hepatic impairment

Hypersensitivity Reactions
- Usually appear within the first few months of therapy (but may occur after the drug is discontinued)
- Photosensitivity and photoallergy reactions including sunburn-like erythematous eruptions which may be accompanied by blistering
- Skin reactions, rashes, and, rarely, abnormal skin pigmentation (risperidone); rash (5%) and urticaria reported with ziprasidone, potentially dose related, improved with antihistamine/steroid administration and/or discontinuation of ziprasidone in most cases
- Rarely, asthma, laryngeal, angioneurotic or peripheral edema, and anaphylactic reactions occur. Serious allergic reactions (Type 1 hypersensitivity) have been reported in patients treated with asenapine. Patients should be informed and advised to seek emergency medical treatment if they develop signs and symptoms of a serious reaction (swelling of face, tongue, or throat, difficulty breathing, feeling lightheaded or faint, itching)

Temperature Regulation
- Altered ability of body to regulate response to changes in temperature and humidity; may become hyperthermic or hypothermic; more likely in temperature extremes due to inhibition of the hypothalamic control area. Patients should be counseled to avoid becoming overheated or dehydrated, and to avoid prolonged exposure to freezing temperatures
- Transient temperature elevation can occur with clozapine in up to 55% of patients, usually within the first 3 weeks of treatment and lasting several days; not correlated with dose; older individuals at higher risk; may be accompanied by respiratory and gastrointestinal symptoms, mild creatine kinase elevation, and an elevation in WBC

D/C Discontinuation Syndrome
- Abrupt discontinuation of an antipsychotic occurs primarily in situations involving a sudden/severe adverse reaction to the drug (e.g., agranulocytosis with clozapine) or when patients become nonadherent by stopping their antipsychotic medication abruptly
- Abrupt discontinuation (or in some cases large dosage reduction) of an antipsychotic may be associated with several withdrawal or discontinuation effects (see below). Prolonged antagonism of (dopaminergic, muscarinic, histaminic, adrenergic) receptors by the antipsychotic, resulting in a compensatory up-regulation which then produces a rebound-type reaction when the antagonist is removed and the supersensitized receptors are exposed, has been proposed as a pharmacological explanation for these effects
  1. Discontinuation syndromes – typically characterized by development of several symptoms including nausea, vomiting, diarrhea, diaphoresis, cold sweats, muscles aches and pains, insomnia, anxiety, and confusion. Many are believed to be the result of cholinergic rebound. Usually appear within days of discontinuation [Management: Mild cases may only require comfort and reassurance; for more severe symptoms, consider restarting the antipsychotic, followed by slow taper if possible; or, if rebound cholinergic effects present, consider adding an anticholinergic agent short term]
  2. Psychosis – exacerbation or precipitation of psychosis including a severe, rapid onset or supersensitivity psychosis, most notable with clozapine and quetiapine. Most likely to occur within the first 2–3 weeks of discontinuation or sooner [Management: Restart antipsychotic]
  3. Movement disorders – withdrawal dyskinesias noted to appear usually around 2–4 weeks post abrupt withdrawal [Management: Restart antipsychotic and taper slowly] Rebound dystonia, parkinsonism, and akathisia also reported to occur, usually within days to the first week post discontinuation [Management: Restart antipsychotic and taper or treat with appropriate anti-EPS medication]
- Abrupt cessation of a long-acting or depot antipsychotic is of less concern, as plasma concentrations decline slowly
- Clinicians should be cognizant of the potential for withdrawal effects to occur from a discontinued agent when switching to a new antipsychotic in order to avoid misinterpreting them as adverse effects of the new agent and subsequently discontinuing it unnecessarily
- If planning to discontinue clozapine, a gradual dose reduction over 1–2 weeks is recommended. However, if a patient's medical condition requires abrupt discontinuation (e.g., severe leukopenia, cardiovascular toxicity), observe for recurrence of psychotic symptoms and symptoms related to cholinergic rebound such as headache, diaphoresis, nausea, vomiting, and diarrhea
- ☞ **AFTER PROLONGED USE, THESE MEDICATIONS SHOULD BE WITHDRAWN GRADUALLY where possible.** If switching to another antipsychotic, see pp. 216–217 for specific recommendations. Readers may find the website http://switchrx.com helpful

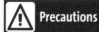 **Precautions**
- Use of SGAs in elderly patients with dementia is associated with increased risk of death, stroke, and TIA (see Geriatric Considerations p. 125)
- Dysphagia and aspiration have been associated with use of antipsychotic medications. These agents should be used cautiously in patients at risk for aspiration pneumonia (e.g., advanced Alzheimer's disease)

- Assess patients routinely for presence of significant risk factors for cardiovascular disease, including a family history of premature CVD, smoking, hypertension, dyslipidemias, diabetes, and metabolic syndrome. See pp. 124 and 161 for suggested monitoring guidelines. Control risk factors and consider SGAs with lower metabolic liabilities where possible
- SGAs may lower the seizure threshold (especially clozapine at doses exceeding 600 mg per day); use with caution in individuals with a history of seizures or with comorbidities or concomitant medications that may also increase vulnerability to seizure development
- Agents with higher affinities for the antagonizing M_1 receptor (e.g., clozapine, olanzapine, quetiapine) should be used very cautiously in patients with narrow-angle glaucoma or prostatic hypertrophy or in other conditions that may be exacerbated by anticholinergic actions
- Patients at high risk of suicide should be followed closely. Consider clozapine
- Evaluate clinical status and vital signs prior to IM olanzapine administration and monitor for oversedation and cardiorespiratory depression. DO NOT ADMINISTER within one hour of an IM benzodiazepine (see Drug Interactions, p. 173)
- Rapid elimination of clozapine and quetiapine from plasma and brain following abrupt discontinuation may result in early and severe relapse
- Allergic cross-reactivity (rash) between chlorpromazine and clozapine reported
- Quetiapine immediate release can be used as a street drug for its sedative and anxiolytic effects – called "quell," "Susie-Q," "baby heroin," or "Q-ball"

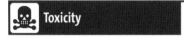 Toxicity

- May occur as a consequence of an acute ingestion, intentional or accidental, or with chronic use. In general, signs and symptoms of toxicity present as exaggerations of known adverse effects within a few hours post ingestion
- Serious toxicity primarily involves the cardiovascular and central nervous systems
- Antipsychotics with a high affinity for muscarinic receptor blockade may produce potent anticholinergic effects such as tachycardia, urinary retention, dry mouth (may see hypersalivation with clozapine), decreased/absent sweating (may cause mild temperature elevations), agitation, and delirium
- Impaired consciousness (ranging from somnolence to coma), tachycardia, and hypotension are common
- ECG manifestations include prolongation of the QRS complex and QT interval
- Dystonic reactions and other extrapyramidal adverse effects as well as neuroleptic malignant syndrome (NMS) may also occur
- Convulsions occur late, except with clozapine; symptoms may persist as drug elimination may be prolonged following intoxication

Management

- Any patient experiencing signs or symptoms other than mild drowsiness should be transported to an emergency department. Local poison control centers should be contacted
- Gastric lavage and/or activated charcoal may be considered if less than 1 h has elapsed since ingestion and airways are not compromised. Syrup of ipecac should not be administered due to concerns of additive sedation and potential for aspiration pneumonia. Hemoperfusion/hemodialysis not recommended due to large volumes of distribution and high plasma protein binding profiles of antipsychotics
- No specific antidotes; provide supportive treatment for symptomatic patients – establish/maintain airway, ensure adequate oxygenation/ventilation. Monitor vital signs and ECG for at least 6 h and admit the patient for at least 24 h if significant intoxication apparent. Agents with extended-release technologies such as paliperidone may require longer supervision/monitoring
- Hypotension and circulatory collapse treated with IV fluids (0.9% NaCl solution). Intravenous vasopressors may be considered if there is no response to fluids (caution – use of epinephrine or dopamine or other sympathomimetics with β-agonist activity may worsen hypotension in the presence of antipsychotic-induced α_1 blockade; see Drug Interactions pp. 167–176; norepinephrine or phenylephrine are preferred)
- Sodium bicarbonate (1-2 mEq/kg) should be considered for ventricular dysrhythmias or QRS prolongation above 0.12 sec
- QT prolongation should be monitored and hypokalemia or hypomagnesemia corrected. TdP is treated with IV magnesium sulfate. Avoid co-administration of drugs that produce additive QT prolongation (see Drug Interactions pp. 167–176)
- Seizures may not require treatment if short-lived. Multiple or refractory seizures may be treated with lorazepam or diazepam
- Acute dystonias may be treated with benztropine (2 mg IV or IM)
- NMS treatment may include oxygenation/ventilation, correction of hyperthermia with cooling blankets, ice-water bath, etc., and correction of hypotension (see above)

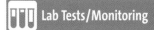 Lab Tests/Monitoring

- See p. 124 for suggested monitoring guidelines
- Iloperidone and risperidone: On initiation and with dose increases, monitor for orthostatic hypotension
- Olanzapine: Threshold plasma level may be important for response to olanzapine in acutely ill patients with schizophrenia (9 ng/mL or 27 nmol/L)

Second-Generation Antipsychotics/SGAs (cont.)

- Olanzapine injection: Recommend clinical status and vital signs be evaluated prior to and as clinically indicated post olanzapine IM (short-acting or long-acting) administration; monitor for orthostatic hypotension, oversedation, delirium, and cardiorespiratory depression. Olanzapine IM long-acting: Observe for at least 3 h and instruct patient not to drive or operate heavy machinery for remainder of the day
- Quetiapine: May result in false-positive methadone urine drug screen. Consult your lab
- Ziprasidone: Patients at risk of significant electrolyte disturbances should have baseline serum potassium and magnesium measurements. Low serum potassium and magnesium should be replaced before proceeding with treatment. Patients who are started on diuretics during ziprasidone therapy need periodic monitoring of serum potassium and magnesium

Clozapine monitoring

- Threshold plasma level suggested for response to clozapine (in the range of 350–550 nanograms/mL or 1050–1650 nanomol/L)
- On initiation and with dose increases, monitor for hypotension, sedation, and seizures

USA: Summary of ANC monitoring requirements for patient without benign ethnic neutropenia

ANC Level	Treatment Recommendations	ANC Monitoring

Normal range ($\geq$ 1500/microliter)	• Initiate treatment
	• If treatment interrupted
	  – less than 30 days: continue monitoring as before
	  – $\geq$ 30 days: monitor as if new patient
		• Weekly from initiation to 6 months
		• Every 2 weeks from 6 to 12 months
		• Monthly after 12 months

• Mild neutropenia (1000–1499/microliter)*	• Continue treatment	• Three times per week until ANC $\geq$ 1500/microliter • Once ANC $\geq$ 1500/microliter, return to patient's last "normal range" ANC monitoring (if clinically appropriate)
• Moderate neutropenia (500–999/microliter)*	• Recommend hematology consultation • Interrupt treatment for suspected clozapine-induced neutropenia • Resume treatment once ANC $\geq$ 1000/microliter	• Daily until ANC $\geq$ 1000/microliter • Then three times per week until ANC $\geq$ 1500/microliter • Once ANC $\geq$ 1500/microliter, check ANC weekly for 4 weeks, then return to patient's last "normal range" ANC monitoring (if clinically appropriate)
Severe neutropenia (less than 500/microliter)*	• Recommend hematology consultation • Interrupt treatment for suspected clozapine-induced neutropenia • Do not rechallenge unless prescriber determines benefits outweigh risk	• Daily until ANC $\geq$ 1000/microliter • Then three times per week until ANC $\geq$ 1500/microliter • If patient rechallenged, resume treatment as new patient under "normal range" monitoring once ANC $\geq$ 1500/microliter

* Confirm all initial reports of ANC less than 1500/microliter with a repeat ANC measurement with 24 h

USA: Summary of ANC monitoring requirements for patient with benign ethnic neutropenia (BEN)

ANC Level	Treatment Recommendations	ANC Monitoring

Normal BEN range (established ANC baseline $\geq$ 1000/microliter)	• Obtain at least two baseline ANC levels before initiating treatment
	• If treatment interrupted
	  – less than 30 days: continue monitoring as before
	  – $\geq$ 30 days: monitor as if new patient
		• Weekly from initiation to 6 months
		• Every 2 weeks from 6 to 12 months
		• Monthly after 12 months

BEN neutropenia (500–999/microliter)*	• Recommend hematology consultation • Continue treatment	• Three times per week until ANC $\geq$ 1000/microliter or $\geq$ patient's known baseline • Once ANC $\geq$ 1000/microliter or at patient's known baseline, check ANC weekly for 4 weeks, then return to patient's last "normal BEN range" ANC monitoring (if clinically appropriate)

ANC Level	Treatment Recommendations	ANC Monitoring
BEN severe neutropenia (less than 500/microliter)*	• Recommend hematology consultation • Interrupt treatment for suspected clozapine-induced neutropenia • Do not rechallenge unless prescriber determines benefits outweigh risk	• Daily until ANC ≥ 150/microliter • Then three times per week until ANC ≥ patient's baseline • If patient rechallenged, resume treatment as new patient under "normal BEN range" monitoring once ANC ≥ 1000/microliter or at patient's baseline

* Confirm all initial reports of ANC less than 1500/microliter with a repeat ANC measurement with 24 h

Canada: Summary of ANC monitoring requirements

Hematological Parameters (non-BEN patients)	Hematological Parameters (BEN patients)	Monitoring and Treatment Implications
≥ 2.0 × 10⁹/L	≥ 1.0 × 10⁹/L	Continue clozapine treatment
≥ 1.5 × 10⁹/L and < 2.0 × 10⁹/L	≥ 0.5 × 10⁹/L and < 1.0 × 10⁹/L	Continue clozapine treatment, sample blood at least twice weekly until counts stabilize or increase
< 1.5 × 10⁹/L	< 0.5 × 10⁹/L	Immediately withhold clozapine and monitor patient closely. Confirmation of hematological values is recommended. STOP clozapine therapy immediately if results are confirmed and assign the patient **"non-rechallengeable status"** for clozapine-associated neutropenia If patient should develop a further decrease in ANC to below 0.5 × 10⁹/L, it is recommended that patient be placed in protective isolation with close observation and be watched for signs of infection by their physician. Should evidence of infection develop, appropriate cultures should be performed and an appropriate antibiotic regimen instituted

Note: Blood monitoring for neutropenia should occur at least twice weekly following discontinuation of clozapine therapy until ANC ≥ 2.0 × 10⁹/L (≥ 1.0 × 10⁹/L for BEN patients

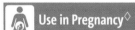 **Use in Pregnancy◊**

• General:
  – For each individual, consider the risks of not treating/undertreating (e.g., illness relapse, self-harm, poor adherence with prenatal care, poor nutrition, exposure to additional medication or herbal remedies, increased alcohol, tobacco or recreational drug use, deficits in mother-infant bonding) vs. the risks of continuing or starting an antipsychotic
  – Pregnancy-related changes (i.e., increased body weight, blood volume, and body fat, altered drug metabolism and increased drug excretion) may require the use of higher drug doses to maintain efficacy. Postpartum dose tapering may be needed, as liver metabolism and fluid volumes return to baseline levels. Monitor for SGA adverse effects and reduce dose as needed
  – Data suggest most SGAs do not significantly increase the risk of teratogenic effects in humans; however, some data suggest otherwise (e.g., major malformations 5.1% in SGA cohort vs. 2.5% in comparison cohort found in one study). Animal data suggest there may be at least a moderate risk with some agents but animal reproduction studies are not always predictive of human response. The greatest risk of fetal malformations is associated with use during the first trimester
  – There may be increased weight gain and risk of gestational diabetes (irrespective of the amount of weight gain) in pregnant women taking SGAs (particularly clozapine and olanzapine and possibly quetiapine) during gestation
  – In 2011, the US FDA and Health Canada asked manufacturers to update their prescribing information to warn clinicians and patients that third trimester use of antipsychotics is associated with risk of EPS and withdrawal symptoms in newborns. Symptoms in the neonate may include: Feeding disorder, hypertonia, hypotonia, tremor, respiratory distress, and agitation
• **Asenapine**: No published human data. Animal data suggest potential for fetal risk (i.e., death and decreased weight)
• **Clozapine**: Limited human data. Animal data suggest low risk. Possible increased incidence of maternal excessive weight gain and gestational diabetes. A case report suggests the concentration of clozapine in fetus plasma can exceed (by 2-fold) that in the mother and potential adverse effects have had reported (i.e., floppy infant syndrome, neonatal seizures, and rare cases of congenital malformations). Monitor WBC of newborn

◊ See p. 473 for further information on drug use in pregnancy and effects on breast milk

Second-Generation Antipsychotics/SGAs (cont.)

infants if mother on clozapine. One case report of delayed peristalsis in a newborn. One case report of delayed speech acquisition after in utero and breast milk exposure to clozapine
- **Iloperidone**: No published human data. Animal data suggest moderate risk (i.e., death and decreased weight)
- **Lumateperone**: Insufficient data to establish any drug-associated risks for birth defects, miscarriage, or adverse maternal or fetal outcomes. Animal data did not find malformations during organogenesis. Third trimester exposure may cause EPS and/or withdrawal symptoms in neonates
- **Lurasidone**: No human data. Potential risk in third trimester due to antipsychotics potential to cause EPS and withdrawal symptoms in newborn. No adverse developmental or teratogenic effects seen in animals
- **Olanzapine**: Human data suggest there is low risk from in utero exposure; however, there is a potential for excessive weight gain and gestational diabetes. A preliminary study found olanzapine use associated with infants who were large for gestational age however, there is conflicting data. Another preliminary study found ~72% (CI 47–98%) of human maternal olanzapine levels in umbilical cord blood; however, there was considerable variability in the range (7–167%). In clinical trials, 7 pregnancies occurred, which resulted in 2 normal births, 1 neonatal death due to cardiovascular defect, 3 therapeutic abortions, and 1 spontaneous abortion
- **Paliperidone**: No published human data. Animal data suggest low risk. As paliperidone is the active metabolite of risperidone, also consult risperidone information
- **Quetiapine**: Limited human data. Animal data suggest risk (i.e., delays in skeletal development seen in rats and rabbits using doses slightly below and above the corresponding maximum human dose). However, no pattern of issues in humans seen to date with at least 65 cases of no major malformations with quetiapine exposure. Potential for excessive weight gain and gestational diabetes. A preliminary study found ~24% (CI 19–30%; range 9–47%) of human maternal quetiapine levels in umbilical cord blood
- **Risperidone**: Limited human data. Reversible EPS (e.g., tremor, jitteriness, irritability) seen in neonates with third trimester risperidone exposure. Four retrospective reports of poorly defined developmental syndromes exist; however, relationship to risperidone use unclear. Case report of maternal NMS with third-trimester exposure to haloperidol and risperidone. Case report of maternal tardive dyskinesia with first trimester exposure to low-dose, short-term risperidone. A preliminary study found ~49% (CI 14–85%) of human maternal risperidone levels in umbilical cord blood however, there was considerable variability in the range (17–105%)
- **Ziprasidone**: Limited human data. Animal data suggest risk, including possible teratogenic effects at doses similar to human therapeutic doses. One case report of ziprasidone use throughout pregnancy (in combination with citalopram) reports no adverse effects to mother or infant at 6-month follow-up, while another report describes malformations of the face and extremities in an infant

| Breast Milk | |

- For each individual, consider the benefits of breastfeeding (e.g., clinical and psychosocial advantages for mother and infant, cost savings) vs. the risks of infant drug exposure via breast milk and possible effects on milk production
- Antipsychotics, like most medications, pass into breast milk however, antipsychotic amounts found are generally low. Long-term effects on neurodevelopment are largely unknown
- If used while breastfeeding, use lowest effective dose and monitor infant's progress
- **Asenapine**: Hale's lactation risk category = L3 (give only if the potential benefit outweighs the potential risk to the infant). No human data available
- **Clozapine**: Hale's lactation risk category = L3 (give only if the potential benefit outweighs the potential risk to the infant). Experience in breastfeeding is limited to a few case reports. In one case report, clozapine concentrations in breast milk exceeded that in the mother's plasma. Case reports of exposed infants developing agranulocytosis, and lethargy. One case report describes delay in speech developmental milestones in a child who was exposed to clozapine via breastfeeding for one year. If the mother does breastfeed, recommend monitoring for excessive sedation and regular monitoring of infant's WBC
- **Iloperidone**: Hale's lactation risk category = L3 (give only if the potential benefit outweighs the potential risk to the infant). No human data available
- **Lumateperone**: Hale's lactation risk category = Not listed. Breastfeeding not recommended
- **Lurasidone**: Hale's lactation risk category = L3 (give only if the potential benefit outweighs the potential risk to the infant). No human data available
- Reports suggest low levels of olanzapine (0–4% of mother's plasma level), quetiapine (0.09–6%), risperidone/paliperidone (0.84-4.7%), and ziprasidone (1.2% – from a single case report) pass into breast milk
- **Olanzapine**: Hale's lactation risk category = L2 (risk likely remote). Categorized as acceptable for breastfeeding. Experience limited to case reports (more than 100) and a prospective observational study involving 22 mothers who took olanzapine while breastfeeding. Case reports of breastfed

infants developing diarrhea, sedation, lethargy, sleep disorder, shaking, jaundice, and temporary motor development delay; however, many also had in utero exposure and/or exposure to other psychotropic medications. Rate of adverse effects suggested to be 16%, with somnolence (4%), irritability (2%), tremor (2%), and insomnia (2%) being the most common
- **Paliperidone**: Hale's lactation risk category = L3 (give only if the potential benefit outweighs the potential risk to the infant). No case reports specifically with paliperidone; however, risperidone data indicate that concentrations of paliperidone (9-hydroxyrisperidone) in breast milk are low
- **Quetiapine**: Hale's lactation risk category = L2 (risk likely remote). Categorized as acceptable for breastfeeding. Experience limited to fewer than 20 case reports. Case reports of breastfed infants developing excessive drowsiness and mild neurodevelopmental delay (infants also exposed to paroxetine and neither quetiapine nor paroxetine was detectable in the breast milk)
- **Risperidone**: Hale's lactation risk category = L3 (give only if the potential benefit outweighs the potential risk to the infant). Categorized as possible for breastfeeding under medical supervision. Experience limited to fewer than 10 case reports. No adverse effects reported
- **Ziprasidone**: Hale's lactation risk category = L2 (risk likely remote). However, experience in breastfed infants limited to a single case report in which no negative outcomes were seen
- Refer to the Drugs and Lactation Database (LactMed) website (https://www.ncbi.nlm.nih.gov/books/NBK501922/) for more information

Nursing Implications

- See pp. 126–128

Oral

- **With or without food?**
  - Clozapine, iloperidone, olanzapine, paliperidone, and risperidone (tablets, M-Tabs, and solution) may be taken with or without meals
  - Asenapine should be taken without food or drink for at least 10 min post dose
  - Lumateperone should be taken with food
  - Lurasidone should be taken with food (at least 350 calories), food increases lurasidone bioavailability 2-fold
  - Quetiapine can be taken with or without food, however, high-fat meals (~800–1000 calories) increase quetiapine exposure, which may be clinically relevant for some patients. Suggest taking consistently with respect to food, particularly for once daily dosing
  - Ziprasidone must be taken with food, ideally with a meal of at least 500 calories[12]. Food increases ziprasidone's bioavailability 2-fold
- **Compatibility with beverages**
  - CAUTION: Grapefruit juice may increase the levels of clozapine, iloperidone, quetiapine, and ziprasidone (see Drug Interactions p. 174)
  - Risperidone solution is compatible with water, coffee, orange juice, and low-fat milk. It is NOT compatible with cola or tea
  - Olanzapine Zydis is compatible with water, milk, coffee, orange juice, and apple juice. The mixture should be consumed promptly after mixing
- **Oral formulation considerations – sublingual, oral disintegrating tablets, extended release, suspensions**
  - Asenapine sublingual tablets dissolve in saliva within seconds when placed under the tongue. DO NOT swallow tablets as absorption is significantly reduced. DO NOT push tablet through foil backing as this could damage tablet. Use dry hands to remove tablet and immediately place tablet under the tongue
  - Oral disintegrating tablets (ODT) (clozapine ODT, risperidone M-Tabs, and olanzapine Zydis) disintegrate rapidly in saliva and can be taken with or without liquid. These products are not absorbed sublingually but swallowed, then absorbed enterally. Because they start to disintegrate upon contact with moisture, ODT tablets should be handled carefully with dry hands (direct contact with hands should be avoided as much as possible)
  - If half tablets of olanzapine Zydis are required, break tablet carefully and wash hands after the procedure. Avoid exposure to powder as dermatitis, eye irritation, and hypersensitivity reactions reported. Store broken tablet in tight, light-resistant container (tablet discolors) and use within 7 days
  - Asenapine, paliperidone, quetiapine XR, and risperidone M-Tabs must not be chewed, divided or crushed
  - Paliperidone is supplied in a non-absorbable shell that may appear in the stool and is not a cause for concern
  - Use liquid (risperidone, ziprasidone), oral disintegrating tablets (clozapine ODT, olanzapine, risperidone) or asenapine sublingual tablets if patient has difficulty swallowing or is suspected of nonadherence. However, more challenging individuals can cheek disintegrating tablets. Time to dissolution may vary by product and also by patient (e.g., dry mouth may impede dissolution times)
  - Ziprasidone suspension – shake well prior to use
  - Storage: Room temperature, protected from light and moisture – clozapine ODT, olanzapine Zydis, risperidone solution and M-Tabs, ziprasidone suspension

Second-Generation Antipsychotics/SGAs (cont.)

Short-acting IM	• Olanzapine

- Olanzapine
  - Olanzapine IM is reconstituted using the provided 2.1 mL of sterile water for injection to yield a clear, yellow 5 mg/mL solution. Use within 1 h of mixing. Inject slowly, deep into the muscle mass
  - Concomitant administration of olanzapine IM and parenteral benzodiazepine is NOT RECOMMENDED (see Drug Interactions p. 173)
  - Prior to olanzapine IM administration, evaluation of vital signs is recommended. Post-injection monitor for hypotension, oversedation, and cardiorespiratory depression
  - Storage: Room temperature (pre-mixing and reconstituted stable for a maximum of 1 h)
- Ziprasidone
  - Ziprasidone short-acting IM is reconstituted into a suspension using the provided 1.2 mL of sterile water for injection. Shake vial vigorously until all of the drug is dissolved. Following reconstitution, any unused portion should be discarded after 24 h, since no preservative or bacteriostatic agent is present in this product
  - Storage: Room temperature (protect from light; pre-mixing and reconstituted stable for a maximum of 24 h)

Long-acting IM

- It is recommended to establish tolerability with an oral form prior to initializing a long-acting IM dosage form
- Rotate administration sites. Document in charting the muscle and location (e.g., left or right) of each injection
- Storage: Room temperature – olanzapine pamoate (pre-mixing and reconstituted stable for a maximum of 24 h), paliperidone palmitate, risperidone (pre-mixing stable for a maximum of 7 days and reconstituted stable for a maximum of 6 h); refrigerate – risperidone (pre-mixing)
- Olanzapine pamoate IM
  - Can cause a post-injection sedation (including coma)/delirium syndrome. Administer where emergency services are readily accessible. Observe for at least 3 h. Instruct patient not to drive or operate heavy machinery for remainder of the day. Risk less than 0.1% at each injection
  - Wear gloves when reconstituting to prevent skin irritation. Reconstitute with supplied diluent. Inject slowly, deep into the gluteal muscle. Use 1.5-inch 19-gauge needle provided for non-obese patients. In the obese, may use 2-inch 19-gauge or larger needle. To prevent clogging, a 19-gauge or larger needle must be used. If not administered immediately, use within 24 h and shake vigorously to resuspend prior to administration. After insertion of the needle into the muscle, aspirate for several seconds to ensure that no blood appears. If any blood is drawn into the syringe, discard the syringe and the dose and begin with a new kit
    - The injection should be performed with steady, continuous pressure
    - DO NOT massage injection site
- Paliperidone palmitate 1-, 3- and 6-monthly IM
  - Paliperidone palmitate 1-monthly IM
    - Suspension in a prefilled syringe. Shake the syringe vigorously for a minimum of 10 sec to ensure a homogeneous suspension
    - Initial dose (day 1) and second dose (day 8) should be administered intramuscularly into the deltoid muscle. These two initial injections help attain therapeutic concentrations rapidly without need for oral supplementation. Further doses can be administered into the deltoid or upper outer quadrant of the gluteal muscle. (See Pharmacokinetics, p. 151). Inject slowly, deep into the muscle. Alternate injections between arms or buttocks and specify in charting. For deltoid injection, use 1.5-inch 22-gauge needle for patients ≥ 90 kg (≥ 200 lb) or 1-inch 23-gauge for patients less than 90 kg (less than 200 lb). For gluteal injection, use 1.5-inch 22-gauge needle regardless of patient weight. Needles are provided in the kit
  - Paliperidone palmitate 3-monthly IM
    - Suspension in a prefilled syringe. With the syringe tip pointed upwards, shake the syringe vigorously for a minimum of 15 sec to ensure a homogenous suspension. Ensure the dose is administered within 5 min or the syringe must be shaken again for 15 sec (note it takes longer to redisperse this suspension compared to the paliperidone 1-monthly injection syringe). The suspension should appear uniform and milky white in color
    - May be administered into the deltoid or gluteal muscle. Needle selection is based on patient weight. For deltoid injection, use 1.5-inch 22-gauge needle for patients ≥ 90 kg (≥ 200 lb) or 1-inch 22-gauge for patients less than 90 kg (200 lb). For gluteal injection, use 1.5-inch 22-gauge needle regardless of patient weight. Needles are provided in the kit

- Paliperidone palmitate 6-monthly IM
  - Suspension in a prefilled syringe. With the syringe tip pointed upwards, shake the syringe vigorously for a minimum of 15 sec, then rest briefly, then complete the mixing with ANOTHER 15 sec shake for a total of 30 sec to ensure a homogenous suspension. Ensure the dose is administered within 5 min or the syringe must be shaken again for 30 sec (note it takes longer to redisperse this suspension compared to the paliperidone 1- and 3-monthly injection syringe). The suspension should appear uniform and milky white in color
  - Should be administered into the gluteal muscle only. Use 1.5-inch 20-gauge needle regardless of patient weight. Needles are provided in the kit
- Risperidone Consta
  - Risperidone Consta is a powder for reconstitution; dose pack should be allowed to come to room temperature before reconstitution and injection. Reconstitute with diluent provided. Should be used as soon as possible – shelf life is 6 h; some clinicians recommend a test oral dose of 1–2 mg/day for 2 days if the patient has never taken risperidone
    - Only use needles supplied with the kit as use of a higher gauge may impede the passage of microspheres. Needle detachments have been reported; to prevent, follow the accompanying instructions and recheck the syringe-needle attachment prior to injection
    - Shake the preparation vigorously for at least 10 sec within 2 min before administering; give deep IM into deltoid (1-inch needle) or gluteal (2-inch needle) muscle; alternate injections between arms or buttocks and specify in charting
    - DO NOT massage injection site
- Risperidone extended-release injectable suspension for subcutaneous injection (RBP-7000)
  - Risperidone RBP-7000 is a powder for reconstitution in a syringe; allow dose pack to come to room temperature before reconstitution and injection. Reconstitute with diluent provided. Use as soon as possible. Establish tolerance with a test oral dose of 1–2 mg/day for 2 days if patient has never taken risperidone
    - The first step of premixing (5 cycles) should be done more gently to avoid spillage of the powder. An additional 55 cycles of mixing is warranted to have a ready-to-inject uniform suspension. When fully mixed, the product should be a cloudy suspension that is uniform in color. If you see clear areas in the mixture, continue to mix until color distribution is uniform. Prior to injection, the syringe should be held upright for air bubbles to rise and then to be pushed out
    - The subcutaneous injection should be done between the transpyloric and transtubercular plane. Use the 18-gauge, 5/8-inch needle included in kit
    - Advise patient that they may have a lump for several weeks that will decrease in size over time. It is important that the patient not rub or massage the injection site and to be aware of the placement of any belts or clothing waistbands

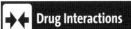 **Drug Interactions**

- Clinically significant interactions are listed below
- For more interaction information on any given combination, also see the corresponding chapter for the second agent

Class of Drug	Example	Interaction Effects
Acetylcholinesterase inhibitor (central)	General	Increase in mortality in elderly patients with dementia taking antipsychotics irrespective of acetylcholinesterase inhibitor use. Deaths largely either cardiovascular or infectious in nature
	Donepezil, galantamine, rivastigmine	May enhance neurotoxicity of antipsychotics, presumably due to a relative acetylcholine/dopamine imbalance (i.e., increased acetylcholine in the presence of dopamine receptor blockade) in the CNS. Case reports of severe EPS (e.g., generalized rigidity, shuffling gait, facial grimacing) in elderly patients within a few days of starting an antipsychotic (risperidone or haloperidol) and an acetylcholinesterase inhibitor (donepezil). Symptoms resolved after discontinuing the antipsychotic, the acetylcholinesterase inhibitor or both. Case reports of NMS with concurrent use of olanzapine and an acetylcholinesterase inhibitor (donepezil and rivastigmine).
Adsorbent	Activated charcoal, attapulgite (kaolin-pectin), cholestyramine	Gastrointestinal absorption decreased significantly when used simultaneously; give at least 1 h before or 2 h after the antipsychotic. Charcoal (1 g) reduced the C_{max} and AUC of olanzapine by 50–60%
α_1-adrenergic receptor blocker	Doxazosin, prazosin, terazosin	Additive hypotensive effect possible. Antipsychotics generally cause hypotension via α_1 blockade (see Effects of Antipsychotics on Receptors table p. 194)
Amylinomimetic	Pramlintide	Pramlintide slows the rate of gastric emptying. Antipsychotics with significant anticholinergic effects can further reduce GI motility

Second-Generation Antipsychotics/SGAs (cont.)

Class of Drug	Example	Interaction Effects
Antiarrhythmic	General	Possible additive prolongation of QT interval and associated life-threatening cardiac arrhythmias. DO NOT COMBINE with asenapine, iloperidone, paliperidone, or ziprasidone. CAUTION with all other SGAs. Also see Cardiovascular Effects of SGAs section p. 154
	Amiodarone, quinidine	CYP2D6 is inhibited by amiodarone and potently by quinidine. With amiodarone and quinidine, increased plasma levels of asenapine, clozapine (case report with amiodarone), iloperidone, and risperidone likely
Antibiotic		
Quinolone	Ciprofloxacin, levofloxacin, moxifloxacin, norfloxacin	DO NOT COMBINE with asenapine, iloperidone, paliperidone, or ziprasidone. CAUTION with all other SGAs. Possible additive prolongation of QT interval and associated life-threatening cardiac arrhythmias. Also see Cardiovascular Effects of SGAs section p. 154
		CAUTION. Potential to exacerbate psychiatric conditions, as quinolone-induced psychosis has been reported
		Ciprofloxacin and norfloxacin inhibit CYP1A2. With ciprofloxacin, increased clozapine and norclozapine levels (by 29–100%; case report of a 5-fold increase); increased olanzapine level (by more than 2-fold in a case report). Increased levels of asenapine likely. Case report of sudden-onset dystonia in a patient taking asenapine and ciprofloxacin. Norfloxacin likely to cause similar SGA level increases. Adjust antipsychotic dose as needed
Macrolide	Clarithromycin, erythromycin, telithromycin	DO NOT COMBINE with asenapine, iloperidone, paliperidone, or ziprasidone. CAUTION with all other SGAs. Possible additive prolongation of QT interval and associated life-threatening cardiac arrhythmias. See quinolone above p. 168 for further discussion
		CYP3A4 is inhibited potently by clarithromycin and telithromycin, and moderately by erythromycin. With erythromycin, decreased clearance of quetiapine (by 52%) and with clarithromycin, a case report of ∼7-fold increase in quetiapine levels. Consider reducing quetiapine dose by 50% with concurrent use of strong CYP3A4 inhibitors and by 25% with moderate CYP3A4 inhibitors. Although a pharmacokinetic study suggests no significant interaction between erythromycin and clozapine, there are case reports of increased clozapine levels (by ∼2- to 3-fold) and associated symptoms (e.g., disorientation, seizures, neutropenia, somnolence, slurred speech). Reduce iloperidone dose by 50% with concurrent use of strong CYP3A4 inhibitors. Lurasidone should NOT be used concurrently with strong CYP3A4 inhibitors and reduce its dose by 50% in the presence of moderate CYP3A4 inhibitors. Ziprasidone levels increased by ∼40% in the presence of strong CYP3A4 inhibitors Adjust antipsychotic dose as needed
Tetracycline	Tetracycline	Case report of increased motor and vocal tics when tetracycline added to risperidone and sertraline; mechanism unknown
Anticholinergic	Antidepressants, antihistamines, antiparkinsonian drugs	Increased risk of anticholinergic adverse effects (e.g., dry mouth, urinary retention, inhibition of sweating, blurred vision, constipation, paralytic ileus, confusion, toxic psychosis)
Anticoagulant	Warfarin	Two case reports of increased INR with the addition of quetiapine to warfarin
Anticonvulsant	General	All SGAs may lower seizure threshold. May occur if dose is increased rapidly or may also be secondary to hyponatremia. Potential additive risk for hyponatremia as both SGAs and carbamazepine/oxcarbazepine can cause low sodium levels. Risk of seizures is greatest with clozapine and is dose related: 1% (doses below 300 mg), 2.7% (300–599 mg), and 4.4% (above 600 mg)
	Carbamazepine	Decreased antipsychotic plasma levels via potent induction of CYP3A4, CYP1A2, CYP2D6, and/or possibly UGT1A4. Note it may take 2–4 weeks to reach maximum induction and an equivalent period to return to baseline after discontinuation of an inducer. Adjust antipsychotic dose as needed
		Clozapine levels reduced by 50%. AVOID due to potential additive risk for agranulocytosis. Case report of fatal pancytopenia
		Olanzapine levels reduced by 36–71%.
		Paliperidone's C_{max} level reduced by 37% with 400 mg/day of carbamazepine
		Quetiapine levels reduced by up to 80% with other reports of undetectable levels. Two case reports of 3- to 4-fold increase in the ratio of carbamazepine epoxide/carbamazepine resulting in ataxia and agitation in one case. AVOID combination if possible

Class of Drug	Example	Interaction Effects
		Risperidone and 9-hydroxyrisperidone levels reduced by 50%. Risperidone causes a modest, clinically insignificant increase in carbamazepine level
		Ziprasidone AUC reduced by 36% with 400 mg/day of carbamazepine. Higher carbamazepine doses may have a greater effect
	Lamotrigine	Lamotrigine is a weak UGT inducer. A significant reduction (58%) of quetiapine levels suggested by one study; however, a larger study found a clinically insignificant (17%) reduction. Studies suggest low dose lamotrigine ($\leq$ 200 mg/day) does not significantly affect the levels of clozapine, olanzapine or risperidone. However, there are case reports of clinically significant increases in levels of clozapine and risperidone, and a study found an increase in olanzapine levels (35%) in smokers taking lamotrigine. Mechanism unknown. With concurrent clozapine, monitor CBC as both drugs can depress bone marrow function. Case report of fatal agranulocytosis within 6 weeks of starting concurrent quetiapine, lamotrigine, mirtazapine, and venlafaxine. Monitor for reduced antipsychotic efficacy as well as antipsychotic toxicity (e.g., sedation, dizziness), particularly with higher doses of lamotrigine
	Oxcarbazepine	Oxcarbazepine is a weak CYP3A4 inducer and does not appear to significantly affect the levels of clozapine, olanzapine, quetiapine or risperidone; however, consider the potential for additive bone marrow suppression with clozapine and possibility of more significant SGA level reductions with high doses of oxcarbazepine ($\geq$ 1500 mg/day)
	Phenobarbital, phenytoin	Decreased levels of SGAs due to potent induction of metabolism; for phenytoin via CYP2C9 and CYP3A4; for phenobarbital primarily via CYP1A2, CYP2C9, and CYP3A4. Note it may take 2–4 weeks to reach maximum induction and an equivalent period to return to baseline after discontinuation of an inducer. Adjust antipsychotic dose as needed
		Iloperidone level likely to decrease by 2-fold based on interaction with potent inducers. Iloperidone dose may need to be increased by 50% Lurasidone levels decreased by 5-fold in the presence of other potent CYP3A4 inducers (i.e., rifampin). Recommended to avoid lurasidone with concurrent potent CYP3A4 inducers
		Paliperidone, risperidone, and ziprasidone levels reduced by other potent CYP3A4 inducers (i.e., carbamazepine); similar interaction anticipated
		With phenytoin, clozapine level decreased by 65–85%, which resulted in re-emergence of psychotic symptoms, and a case report of phenytoin intoxication after IV phenytoin loading possibly due to clozapine inhibition of CYP2C9. Quetiapine level decreased by 80%
		With phenobarbital, clozapine level decreased by 35% Olanzapine level significantly reduced by other potent CYP1A2 inducers (i.e., carbamazepine); similar interactions anticipated
	Topiramate	Topiramate is a weak CYP3A4 inducer and CYP2C19 inhibitor. Modest reduction of risperidone's C_{max} (by 23–29%) with no effect on 9-hydroxyrisperidone. Likely not clinically significant. One study found no significant changes to the levels of clozapine, norclozapine, olanzapine, risperidone, 9-hydroxyrisperidone, or quetiapine. The effects of higher doses of topiramate (more than 400 mg/day) are unknown
	Valproate (divalproex, valproic acid)	Valproate inhibits CYP2C9 and UGT and weakly inhibits CYP1A2, CYP2D6, and CYP2E1. Adjust antipsychotic dose as needed Asenapine: Product monograph states no dose adjustment required based on a single dose of asenapine and 9 days of valproate
		Clozapine: Conflicting information. Both increased and decreased clozapine levels reported. Possibly a clinically significant reduction in clozapine levels in smokers. Case reports of hepatic encephalopathy, onset of seizures in nonepileptic patients, and delirium. Reports suggest a greater risk of agranulocytosis with concurrent valproate and clozapine than with either alone. Concurrent valproate with rapid clozapine dose titration may increase risk of myocarditis
		Olanzapine: Most studies found no clinically significant change in the levels of either medication. However, reduced olanzapine levels found in one study (by ~20%) and seen in case reports (by ~50%). Incidence of hepatic enzyme elevations may increase the risk of hepatic adverse effects
		Paliperidone: C_{max} of a single dose of paliperidone increased by 50% with no effect on valproate level. Consider reduction of paliperidone dose

Second-Generation Antipsychotics/SGAs (cont.)

Class of Drug	Example	Interaction Effects
		Quetiapine: Case reports of adverse effects possibly due to increased quetiapine levels. Case report of severe cervical dystonia with the addition of valproic acid. Case report of drug-induced parkinsonism and cognitive decline with concurrent use of quetiapine (800 mg/day) and valproic acid (1500 mg/day). Two case reports of delirium in patients with mild renal impairment after the addition of valproate to quetiapine. A case report of severe hypertriglyceridemia in the absence of weight gain with the addition of valproate to quetiapine that resolved on valproate discontinuation. Cases of hyperammonemia induced by interaction with valproate and quetiapine reported. Four case reports of neutropenia with concurrent quetiapine and valproate, with one also having thrombocytopenia. Monitor CBC at baseline, in 1–2 weeks, and after any dose increases
		Risperidone: No effect on risperidone levels with a modest (20%) increase in valproate levels. A case report of elevated and another of reduced valproate levels. Two case reports of generalized edema. Case report of neutropenia resolving after valproic acid stopped. Two cases in children of hyperammonemia, and one case of catatonia with the addition of valproic acid to risperidone and sertraline. Monitoring of serum ammonia levels may be warranted if new or increased manic behavior occurs
Antidepressant SSRI	General Citalopram, escitalopram, fluoxetine, fluvoxamine, paroxetine, sertraline	Case reports of serotonin syndrome with concurrent use of antidepressants that increase serotonin and SGAs
		CAUTION with paliperidone and ziprasidone; possible additive prolongation of QT interval and associated life-threatening cardiac arrhythmias
		Increased plasma levels of antipsychotics possible due to inhibition of CYP1A2 (potent – fluvoxamine), 2D6 (potent – fluoxetine and paroxetine), and/or 3A4 (fluvoxamine). Adjust antipsychotic dose as needed
		Asenapine's C_{max} (+ 13%) and AUC (+ 29%) increased by fluvoxamine based on an asenapine single-dose study. Asenapine (a weak inhibitor of CYP2D6) increased exposure to a single dose of paroxetine by ~2-fold
		Clozapine levels: With citalopram, no change to increased. With fluoxetine, 41–76% higher levels plus 38–45% higher norclozapine levels; one fatality reported; case report of acute myocarditis after addition of clozapine to fluoxetine and lithium. With fluvoxamine, 3–11-fold higher levels. With paroxetine, no change to 41% increase plus 45% norclozapine increase. With sertraline, 41-76% increase plus 45% norclozapine increase; one fatal arrhythmia reported but causality unclear
		Iloperidone's AUC increased by ~1.6- to 3-fold in the presence of fluoxetine or paroxetine. Reduce iloperidone dose by 50% if fluoxetine or paroxetine added
		Olanzapine levels: With fluoxetine, 16% increase in C_{max}; not clinically significant. With fluvoxamine, 2.3- to 4-fold increase in olanzapine levels. Case reports of fatal hyponatremia, marked hyperglycemia, and acute pancreatitis with long-term use of paroxetine + fluphenazine + haloperidol + olanzapine
		Quetiapine levels: With fluvoxamine, may be increased by up to 159%. Case reports of NMS/serotonin syndrome with quetiapine and SSRIs (i.e., citalopram, fluvoxamine). Monitor for symptoms (e.g., fever, myoclonus, and tremor)
		Risperidone levels: With fluoxetine, 2.5- to 8-fold increased levels and case report of tardive dyskinesia. With paroxetine, 3- to 9-fold higher levels and cases of serotonin syndrome. Case reports of serotonin syndrome and/or NMS with fluvoxamine and trazodone + sertraline Case of gynecomastia and galactorrhea without elevated prolactin level in a male taking risperidone and fluvoxamine
		Ziprasidone: Case report of serotonin syndrome with ziprasidone and citalopram
NDRI	Bupropion	Risperidone: Potential for additive seizure risk due to increased plasma levels of risperidone due to competitive inhibition of CYP2D6
SNRI	Venlafaxine	Clozapine: Increased levels of both clozapine and venlafaxine possible due to competitive inhibition of CYP2D6 and/or CYP3A4. A study with venlafaxine doses of 150 mg/day or less suggests no clinically significant interaction. Case report of NMS/serotonin syndrome
		Quetiapine: Case report of fatal agranulocytosis within 6 weeks of starting concurrent quetiapine, lamotrigine, mirtazapine, and venlafaxine

Class of Drug	Example	Interaction Effects
SARI	Nefazodone, trazodone	Potential for additive adverse effects (e.g., sedation, orthostatic hypotension). Nefazodone is a potent CYP3A4 inhibitor Increased plasma levels of clozapine (case report) and quetiapine (in vitro data) possibly due to inhibited metabolism via CYP3A4 and associated adverse effects (e.g., dizziness, hypotension) Lurasidone is contraindicated with concomitant use of potent CYP3A4 inhibitors Case report of NMS with nefazodone and olanzapine. Case report of serotonin syndrome with trazodone, sertraline, and risperidone
SMS	Vortioxetine	Serotonin modulators may enhance the dopamine blockade of antipsychotics and increase the risk of side effects. Antipsychotics may enhance the serotonergic effects of serotonin modulators and increase the risk of serotonin syndrome
NaSSA	Mirtazapine	Potential for additive metabolic adverse effects (e.g., increased cholesterol, weight), and increased appetite and sedation. Case report of status epilepticus with mirtazapine and olanzapine. Case report of serotonin syndrome with mirtazapine, tramadol, and olanzapine and another within 7 weeks of adding quetiapine and mirtazapine to venlafaxine and donepezil. Case report of fatal agranulocytosis within 6 weeks of starting concurrent quetiapine, lamotrigine, mirtazapine, and venlafaxine
Cyclic	Amitriptyline, clomipramine, maprotiline, trimipramine	Additive sedation, hypotension, and anticholinergic effects. Potential for additive seizure risk DO NOT COMBINE with asenapine, iloperidone, paliperidone, or ziprasidone. CAUTION with all other SGAs. Possible additive prolongation of QT interval and associated life-threatening cardiac arrhythmias Potential for increased SGA levels as CYP2D6 is moderately inhibited by amitriptyline, clomipramine, desipramine, and imipramine Asenapine: Imipramine caused modest (17%) increase in C_{max} of a single dose of asenapine. No adjustment of asenapine dose required Clozapine: Case report of serotonin syndrome after withdrawal of clozapine in a patient taking clomipramine. Case report of 2-fold increase in nortriptyline levels after the addition of clozapine. Patient developed delirium, which was preceded by extreme fatigue and slurred speech. Case report of increased clomipramine levels and myoclonic jerks followed by seizures, possibly due to competitive inhibition for CYP1A2 and/or CYP2D6 Olanzapine: Case report of NMS/serotonin syndrome with clomipramine. Suggest using lowest doses possible if olanzapine and clomipramine used concurrently Quetiapine: Case report of 17-fold increase in quetiapine levels with concurrent doxepin and pantoprazole; mechanism unknown Risperidone: Case reports of increased maprotiline levels (40–60%) and anticholinergic effects with risperidone, possibly due to competitive inhibition of CYP2D6
Irreversible MAOI, RIMA	Moclobemide, phenelzine, tranylcypromine	Additive hypotension Case report of serotonin syndrome with quetiapine and phenelzine and another with ziprasidone and tranylcypromine
Antidiarrheal	Loperamide	Case report of fatal gastroenteritis with clozapine. Potentially anticholinergic effects of clozapine added to antimotility effects of loperamide lead to toxic megacolon
Antifungal	Fluconazole, itraconazole, ketoconazole, voriconazole	Ketoconazole and itraconazole are potent, while fluconazole and voriconazole are moderate CYP34A inhibitors. Increased iloperidone (level by 57% with ketoconazole), lurasidone (C_{max} 6- to 9-fold and AUC 9-fold), 9-hydroxyrisperidone (level by 70% in a study of risperidone with itraconazole), quetiapine (C_{max} by 335% with ketoconazole), risperidone (level by ~80% with itraconazole), and ziprasidone (AUC and C_{max} by 35–40% with ketoconazole). Adjust antipsychotic dose as needed. Recommended to AVOID concurrent use of lurasidone and ketoconazole or itraconazole CAUTION – possible additive prolongation of QT interval and associated life-threatening cardiac arrhythmias with antipsychotics
	Terbinafine	Increased plasma levels of iloperidone and risperidone possible due to inhibited metabolism via CYP2D6. Any interaction will be prolonged (up to 3 months) due to terbinafine's long half-life (200–400 h)
Antihistamine	Diphenhydramine, hydroxyzine	See Class of Drug "Anticholinergic" above (p. 168) and "CNS depressant" below (p. 174)
Antihypertensive		Additive hypotensive effect possible. Antipsychotics generally cause hypotension via α_1 blockade (see receptor table p. 194 and frequency of adverse effects table pp. 198–199). Start with a lower dose of antipsychotic, titrate slowly, and monitor for orthostatic hypotension

Second-Generation Antipsychotics/SGAs (cont.)

Class of Drug	Example	Interaction Effects
	Calcium channel blockers	Also see Class of Drug "calcium channel blocker" p. 173
	Clonidine	SGAs that are potent α_2-adrenergic receptor antagonists may block clonidine's antihypertensive effects via α_2-adrenergic receptor agonism (see receptor table p. 194). Additive hypotensive effects also possible
	Diuretic	Also see Class of Drug "diuretic" p. 174
	Lisinopril	Case report of significantly increased plasma levels of clozapine and norclozapine. Case report of pancreatitis 3 months after lisinopril added to olanzapine
Antiparkinsonian agent	Levodopa, pramipexole, ropinirole	Potential for reduced therapeutic effect of antiparkinson drugs. Antipsychotics reduce dopaminergic activity while antiparkinson agents increase dopamine in the CNS. If a SGA is necessary, consider using clozapine or quetiapine, which have been reported to be less likely to cause worsening control of movement disorders than other antipsychotics
Antipsychotic combination	General	Increased risk of adverse effects (e.g., EPS elevated prolactin levels, sedation hypotension, and anticholinergic effects), increased cost, and potential for decreased adherence with use of multiple antipsychotic agents
	Aripiprazole + SGAs	See p. 189 in TGA interaction section
	Clozapine + olanzapine	Case reports of NMS. Potential for additive metabolic effects and weight gain Case report of delayed recovery of clozapine-induced agranulocytosis when given olanzapine
	Clozapine + quetiapine	Clozapine increased serum concentration of quetiapine by 82% (unknown mechanism but suggested to be clinically significant); consider starting at a lower than usual dose of quetiapine
	Clozapine + risperidone	Isolated case reports suggest increased clozapine and risperidone levels with concurrent use. However, kinetic studies found no effects on levels. Discrepancy potentially due to genetic variability in metabolism. Chronic concurrent administration may increase risperidone levels. Most common adverse effects with concurrent use are EPS (e.g., akathisia), higher fasting glucose, sedation, hyperprolactinemia, and hypersalivation. Case reports of NMS
	Haloperidol + SGAs	With clozapine, a case of significantly elevated haloperidol decanoate levels and cases of NMS; including one after a single IM dose of haloperidol following abrupt clozapine discontinuation, another after abrupt discontinuation of both medications With olanzapine, a case of extreme parkinsonism potentially due to competitive inhibition of CYP2D6 and/or additive adverse effects Case report of fatal hyponatremia, marked hyperglycemia, and acute pancreatitis with long-term use of paroxetine + fluphenazine + haloperidol + olanzapine
	Phenothiazines (e.g., chlorpromazine) + SGAs	Possible additive QT prolongation (see Cardiovascular Effects p. 154). DO NOT COMBINE with asenapine, iloperidone, paliperidone, or ziprasidone Case reports of NMS including with olanzapine + fluphenazine; olanzapine + chlorpromazine; after several years of olanzapine + clozapine + fluphenazine. Case report of fatal hyponatremia, marked hyperglycemia, and acute pancreatitis with long-term use of paroxetine + fluphenazine + haloperidol + olanzapine
	Pimozide + SGAs	Possible additive QT prolongation (see above). DO NOT COMBINE with asenapine, iloperidone, paliperidone, or ziprasidone
	Thioridazine + SGAs	Possible additive QT prolongation (see above). DO NOT COMBINE with asenapine, iloperidone, paliperidone, or ziprasidone Increased clearance (i.e., decreased plasma levels) of quetiapine (by 65%). Increased plasma levels of risperidone (by ~5-fold) with reduced 9-hydroxyrisperidone levels due to inhibition of metabolism via CYP2D6. Increased levels of other SGAs (e.g., iloperidone, clozapine) possible. Increased SGA levels have the potential to further increase the risk of QT prolongation
	Quetiapine + ziprasidone	Case report of increased QTc prolongation with cardiac arrhythmia, possibly due to increased plasma level of either drug as a result of competitive inhibition via CYP3A4

Class of Drug	Example	Interaction Effects
Antiretroviral		See [16] for additional information
Non-nucleoside reverse transcriptase inhibitor (NNRTI)	Delavirdine, efavirenz, etravirine, nevirapine	CAUTION. Possible interactions as NNRTIs inhibit and induce CYP enzymes (e.g., delavirdine is a strong inhibitor of 2D6, nevirapine weakly inhibits 2D6, efavirenz and etravirine induce 3A4 moderately, nevirapine weakly induces it) Delavirdine may increase levels of risperidone and iloperidone due to CYP2D6 inhibition Efavirenz and etravirine may decrease levels of quetiapine and lurasidone due to CYP3A4 induction
Protease inhibitor	Atazanavir, boceprevir, darunavir, fosamprenavir, indinavir, lopinavir, nelfinavir, ritonavir, saquinavir, simeprevir, telaprevir, tipranavir	CAUTION. Complex interactions likely as various protease inhibitors (PI) potently inhibit as well as induce a variety of CYP enzymes (e.g., on CYP3A4, ritonavir is a potent inhibitor; atazanavir, boceprevir, darunavir, saquinavir, and telaprevir are strong inhibitors; fosamprenavir and indinavir are mild to moderate inhibitors; tipranavir is an inducer. Low boosting doses of ritonavir have little effect on CYP2D6 but higher doses cause inhibition) Increased plasma level of clozapine possible due to inhibition of CYP3A4; however, ritonavir may also decrease levels via induction of CYP1A2. Net effect of ritonavir difficult to predict.[9] AVOID if possible due to potential for clozapine toxicity and additive effects on cardiac conduction. Consider monitoring clozapine levels if used concurrently
Antitubercular drug	Rifabutin, rifampin, rifapentine	Decreased clozapine (plasma levels by 6-fold), lurasidone (C_{max} by 86% and AUC by 80%), risperidone (C_{max} by up to 50%), and 9-hydroxyrisperidone (i.e., paliperidone; C_{max} by 46%) due to induction via CYP3A4, CYP2C9/19, and/or P-glycoprotein with rifampin. Coadministration of lurasidone and rifampin NOT recommended. Reduced levels of iloperidone and quetiapine likely
Anxiolytic		
Benzodiazepines	Clonazepam, diazepam, flurazepam, lorazepam, midazolam	Synergistic effect with antipsychotics; used to calm agitated patients Potential for additive CNS adverse effects (e.g., dizziness, sedation, confusion, respiratory depression) and hypotension Increased incidence of dizziness, hypotension, sedation, excessive salivation, and ataxia when combined with clozapine; cases of ECG changes, delirium, cardiovascular or respiratory arrest, and deaths reported – more likely to occur early in treatment when clozapine added to benzodiazepine regimen Lurasidone (120 mg/day) slightly increased levels of midazolam (C_{max} by 21% and AUC by 44%). May not be clinically significant Concomitant administration of short-acting IM olanzapine and parenteral benzodiazepine and/or other drugs with CNS depressant activity has been associated with serious adverse events (e.g., hypotension, bradycardia, respiratory or CNS depression), including fatalities; thus, it is NOT RECOMMENDED
	Buspirone	Case report of GI bleeding and hyperglycemia with clozapine
Aprepitant		Case report of 11-fold increase in quetiapine levels with accompanying somnolence. Quetiapine dose reduced by 50% with subsequent aprepitant courses and somnolence did not occur
Belladonna alkaloid	Atropine, hyoscyamine, scopolamine	Additive anticholinergic effects (e.g., dry mouth, urinary retention, inhibition of sweating, blurred vision, constipation, paralytic ileus, confusion, toxic psychosis). The elderly are particularly vulnerable to these effects. See frequency of adverse reactions table p. 199 Caution is advised
Calcium channel blocker	Diltiazem, verapamil	Increased lurasidone (C_{max} 2.1-fold and AUC 2.2-fold) with diltiazem. If coadministered, maximum dose of lurasidone should be 40 mg/day Increased risperidone (C_{max} 1.8-fold), and 9-hydroxyrisperidone (i.e., paliperidone; slight increase) with verapamil. Interactions likely due to diltiazem's/verapamil's ability to inhibit metabolism via CYP3A4 and/or to increase intestinal absorption via inhibition of P-glycoprotein. Increased quetiapine possible
Caffeine	Coffee, tea, cola, energy drinks, guarana or mate containing products	Increased akathisia/agitation/insomnia Increased plasma levels of clozapine due to competition for metabolism via CYP1A2. Clozapine and norclozapine levels decreased by a mean of 47% and 31%, resepctively, following a 5-day caffeine-free period More likely to be clinically relevant in those who are nonsmokers or consuming more than 400 mg of caffeine/day (e.g., more than 4 cups of caffeinated coffee/day). Variations in caffeine intake should be considered when clozapine concentrations fluctuate Risperidone solution is incompatible with cola or tea, but it is compatible with coffee

Second-Generation Antipsychotics/SGAs (cont.)

Class of Drug	Example	Interaction Effects
CNS depressant	Alcohol, antihistamines, hypnotics, opioids	CAUTION. Increased CNS effects (e.g., sedation, fatigue, impaired cognition) and orthostatic hypotension. Alcohol may worsen EPS. Monitor for adverse effects when starting a SGA or increasing the dose; recommended to avoid alcohol during these times
Disulfiram		CAUTION. Case reports of disulfiram-induced psychosis, possibly due to blockade of dopamine β-hydroxylase; however, no increased psychotic features seen in small studies of participants with psychotic disorders. Decreased metabolism and increased plasma level of clozapine possible due to inhibition of CYP2E1
Diuretic	General	CAUTION. Diuretics can cause electrolyte disturbances resulting in additive QT interval prolongation and risk of associated life-threatening cardiac arrhythmias. Monitor for dehydration, hypokalemia, and hypomagnesemia. Also see Cardiovascular Effects p. 154
	Furosemide	In risperidone placebo-controlled trials in elderly patients with dementia, a higher incidence of mortality was observed in patients treated with furosemide plus risperidone (7.3%) when compared to patients treated with risperidone alone (3.1%), furosemide alone (4.1%), or placebo without furosemide (2.9%). The increase in mortality with furosemide plus risperidone was observed in two of four clinical trials. No pathophysiological mechanism has been identified to explain this finding and no consistent pattern for cause of death observed
Ginkgo biloba		Case report of priapism with recent addition of ginkgo to long-standing risperidone. Mechanism unclear; potentially due to additive vessel-dilating properties. In theory, reduction of clozapine levels may occur via induction of CYP2E1
Glucocorticoid	Betamethasone, hydrocortisone, prednisone	CAUTION. Potential to exacerbate psychiatric conditions as glucocorticoid-induced psychiatric disorders, such as psychosis, can occur. Glucocorticoids can induce metabolism via CYP3A4. Higher doses of antipsychotics metabolized via CYP3A4 (e.g., clozapine, iloperidone, lurasidone, quetiapine or ziprasidone) may be needed
Grapefruit		CAUTION. Increased plasma levels of clozapine, iloperidone, lurasidone, quetiapine, and ziprasidone possibly due to inhibition of metabolism via intestinal CYP3A4 and inhibition of intestinal transporters, such as P-glycoprotein. Grapefruit's inhibitory effects may be prolonged (i.e., 24–48 h). Data with clozapine suggests 500 mL or less of grapefruit juice daily may not result in clinical changes Pertinent to avoid or minimize grapefruit and grapefruit juice until more information is available
H₂ antagonist	Cimetidine	Increased plasma levels of clozapine (case reports), possibly due to inhibited metabolism via CYP1A2, 2D6, and/or 3A4. Effect on quetiapine and ziprasidone not clinically significant. Increased bioavailability of risperidone (by 64%); however, no effect on AUC, and thus unlikely to be clinically significant
	Nizatidine	Case report of higher doses (600 mg/day) of nizatidine in combination with quetiapine and paroxetine resulting in akathisia, bradykinesia, mild rigidity, and bilateral tremor in upper extremities
	Ranitidine	Increased bioavailability of risperidone (26%) and AUC of risperidone plus 9-hydroxyrisperidone (20%). Not clinically significant
Hormone	Oral contraceptive, ethinyl estradiol	Estrogen potentiates hyperprolactinemic effect of antipsychotics Ethinyl estradiol is an inhibitor of CYP1A2 and CYP2C19 and substrate of CYP3A4, which are the main enzymes that metabolize clozapine. Case report of ~2-fold increase in clozapine levels and marked drowsiness, anergy, and dizziness with the addition of an ethinyl estradiol-containing oral contraceptive (OC). Another report of increased plasma level of clozapine with an OC (ethinyl estradiol [35 micrograms]/norethindrone [0.5 mg]). Case report of seizures with addition of lithium 900 mg/day to clozapine 300–600 mg/day and an OC (ethinyl estradiol [35 micrograms]/norethindrone [0.5/0.75/1 mg])
Lithium		CAUTION. Monitor plasma levels of lithium closely when it is used concurrently with SGAs, since both SGAs (in particular ziprasidone) and high lithium levels are associated with QT prolongation. Also see Cardiovascular Effects p. 154

Class of Drug	Example	Interaction Effects
		Although studies indicate lithium and SGAs can be safely used together, there are cases of severe adverse effects. Factors that may increase the risk of developing neurotoxicity are the presence of acute mania, pre-existing brain damage, infection, fever, dehydration, a history of EPS, and high doses of one or both agents With clozapine: Asterixis (+ zuclopenthixol), diabetic ketoacidosis (no history of hyperglycemia and no signs of lithium toxicity), acute myocarditis (+ fluoxetine), rhabdomyolysis, and seizures (one case also taking an oral contraceptive and exhibiting mild jerking of the arms 2 days prior to the seizure) With olanzapine: Encephalopathy, NMS, nonketotic hyperosmolar syndrome (+ valproic acid), priapism, and somnambulism (+ valproic acid) With quetiapine: Delirium and tonic-clonic seizure With risperidone: Diabetic ketoacidosis + NMS + MI, encephalopathy, EPS (acute rabbit syndrome), NMS, and priapism Potential for additive adverse effects (e.g., weight gain) Monitor patients closely, especially during the first 3 weeks and after dose increases. In particular, monitor for EPS, NMS, and hyperglycemia. Monitor lithium levels; however, note that in the case reports of severe adverse effects listed above, lithium levels were within therapeutic range Case reports of adding lithium in those who developed neutropenia with clozapine or olanzapine. Lithium resulted in normalization of WBC (via its ability to induce leukocytosis) and permitted continued use of clozapine or olanzapine
Opioid	General	CAUTION. Additive CNS effects
	Methadone	DO NOT COMBINE with asenapine, iloperidone, paliperidone, or ziprasidone. CAUTION with all other SGAs. Possible additive prolongation of QT interval and associated life-threatening cardiac arrhythmias. Also see Cardiovascular Effects p. 154 Quetiapine modestly increased methadone levels (7–30%), possibly via inhibition of CYP2D6 and/or P-glycoprotein; this may be clinically significant for some patients. Quetiapine may result in a false-positive methadone urine drug screen.
	Tramadol	CAUTION. Tramadol lowers the seizure threshold; potential additive lowering of seizure threshold with SGAs (in particular clozapine); case report of a fatal seizure in a complicated patient who was taking tramadol and clozapine. Tramadol blocks reuptake of serotonin; potential additive increase in serotonin with SGAs, which could result in serotonin syndrome; case report with mirtazapine, tramadol, and olanzapine
Prokinetic agent/antiemetic	Metoclopramide	CAUTION. Metoclopramide is a potent central dopamine receptor antagonist that can cause EPS, hyperprolactinemia, and rarely NMS. Concurrent use of an SGA may increase the risk of these adverse effects. Case report of Pisa syndrome after addition of metoclopramide to clozapine
Proton pump inhibitor	Esomeprazole, omeprazole	Case reports of decreased plasma level of clozapine (by ~40%) likely due to induction of metabolism via CYP1A2 and/or CYP3A4 with omeprazole. Similar interaction likely with the S-isomer of omeprazole (i.e., esomeprazole). Increase clozapine dose as needed or use an alternative proton pump inhibitor. The interaction may be more clinically relevant in nonsmokers. Decreased levels of asenapine and olanzapine possible
QT-prolonging agent	Antiarrhythmics (e.g., amiodarone, sotalol), antimalarials (e.g., chloroquine, mefloquine), antiprotozoals (e.g., pentamidine), arsenic trioxide, contrast agents (e.g., gadobutrol), dolasetron, droperidol, methadone, pazopanib, ranolazine, tacrolimus	DO NOT COMBINE with asenapine, iloperidone, paliperidone, or ziprasidone. CAUTION with all other SGAs. Possible additive prolongation of QT interval and associated life-threatening cardiac arrhythmias

Second-Generation Antipsychotics/SGAs (cont.)

Class of Drug	Example	Interaction Effects
Smoking (tobacco)		Smoking induces CYP1A2; polycyclic aromatic hydrocarbons in tobacco smoke are believed to be responsible for this induction, not nicotine. Decreased plasma levels of clozapine/norclozapine and olanzapine due to induction of metabolism via CYP1A2. Dosage modifications not routinely recommended; however, some patients, in particular males who are heavy smokers, may require higher doses of clozapine for efficacy. Caution when patients stop smoking as levels of antipsychotics will increase; case reports suggest after smoking cessation symptoms from increased antipsychotic levels emerge after 4–10 days with olanzapine and 2–4 weeks with clozapine. Case reports of serious clozapine toxicity and EPS with olanzapine following smoking cessation; serum clozapine increases of 72–261% reported. Smoking induces olanzapine clearance by ~55%.
Statin	Lovastatin	Case report of prolonged QTc interval with quetiapine, possibly due to competitive inhibition of CYP3A4
	Simvastatin	Case report of rhabdomyolysis with quetiapine; however, an interaction between simvastatin and clarithromycin may have been the cause
		Three case reports of rhabdomyolysis with simvastatin plus risperidone; possibly due to competitive inhibition of CYP3A4; in one case, cyclosporine may also have contributed to the event
Stimulant	Amphetamine, methylphenidate	Antipsychotic agents may impair the stimulatory effect of amphetamines. Concurrent use not recommended
		Case reports of acute EPS, agitation, irritability, worsening of tardive movement disorder, and prolongation or exacerbation of withdrawal dyskinesia following the abrupt discontinuation of risperidone with the concurrent start of methylphenidate
		Case reports of rebound dystonia when a stimulant medication was withdrawn from patients taking risperidone. These reactions may be due to supersensitivity of dopamine receptors
		Two case reports of priapism with concurrent use of stimulants and SGAs (quetiapine, olanzapine)
	Armodafinil	Decreased C_{max} and AUC of quetiapine by 45% and 42%, respectively
	Modafinil	CAUTION. Potential to exacerbate psychosis. Case report of re-emergence of psychotic symptoms after the addition of modafinil to clozapine
		Case report of an almost 2-fold increase in clozapine levels and related toxicity (dizziness, gait disturbance, tachycardia, and hypoxia). Modafinil may inhibit clozapine metabolism via inhibition of CYP2C19
St. John's wort		Potential for additive increase in serotonin resulting in serotonin syndrome
		St. John's wort induces P-glycoprotein, CYP1A2, CYP3A4 (to a lesser extend), and possibly CYP2C19. Decreased plasma levels of SGAs (in particular asenapine, clozapine, quetiapine, risperidone, and olanzapine) reported (mechanism unclear)
Sympathomimetic	Epinephrine/adrenaline, dopamine	AVOID using for the treatment of SGA-induced hypotension. May result in paradoxical fall in blood pressure, as antipsychotics block peripheral α_1-adrenergic receptors, thus inhibiting α-vasoconstricting effects of epinephrine and leaving β-vasodilator effects relatively unopposed
		Case reports of severe hypotension in those with quetiapine overdose who were given IV epinephrine. Substitution with norepinephrine resolved the problem. Case report of severe hypotension with olanzapine and venlafaxine overdose unresponsive to IV dopamine but responsive to norepinephrine
		Norepinephrine and phenylephrine are safe substitutes for severe hypotension unresponsive to fluids
		Benefits may outweigh risk in anaphylaxis
	Cocaine	Case reports of EPS, particularly dystonia, with concurrent use of ziprasidone and risperidone, possibly via dopamine depletion from chronic use of cocaine; case report of clozapine causing a dose-dependent increase in plasma concentration of intranasal cocaine dose, though the positive effects of cocaine were reduced

Product Availability*

Generic Name	Chemical Class	Neuroscience-based Nomenclature* (Pharmacological Target/ Mode of Action)	Trade Name	Dosage Forms and Strengths
Aripiprazole	Phenylpiperazine	Dopamine, serotonin/Partial agonist and antagonist	Abilify	Tablets: 2 mg, 5 mg, 10 mg, 15 mg, 20 mg, 30 mg Oral solution[(B)]: 1 mg/mL Short-acting injection[(B)]: 9.75 mg/1.3 mL (7.5 mg/mL)
			Abilify Discmelt[(B)]	Oral disintegrating tablets: 10 mg, 15 mg, 20 mg, 30 mg
			Abilify Maintena	Long-acting injection: 300 mg/vial, 400 mg/vial
			Aristada[(B)]	Prolonged-release injectable suspension in pre-filled syringe: 441 mg/1.6 mL, 662 mg/2.4 mL, 882 mg/3.2 mL
			Aristada Initio[(B)]	Extended-release injectable suspension in single-dose pre-filled syringe: 675 mg/2.4 mL
Brexpiprazole	N-arylpiperazine	Dopamine, serotonin/Partial agonist and antagonist	Rexulti	Tablets: 0.25 mg, 0.5 mg, 1 mg, 2 mg, 3 mg, 4 mg,
Cariprazine	Phenylpiperazine	Dopamine, serotonin/Partial agonist and antagonist	Vraylar	Capsules: 1.5 mg, 3 mg, 4.5 mg, 6 mg

* Refer to Health Canada's Drug Product Database or the FDA's Drugs@FDA for the most current availability information * Developed by a taskforce consisting of representatives from the American College of Neuropsychopharmacology (ACNP), the Asian College of Neuropsychopharmacology (AsCNP), the European College of Neuropsychopharmacology (ECNP), the International College of Neuropsychopharmacology (CINP), and the International Union of Basic and Clinical Pharmacology (IUPHAR) (see https://nbn2r.com), [(B)] Not marketed in Canada

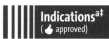 **Indications[a‡]**
(👍 approved)

Schizophrenia & Psychotic Disorders

👍 Schizophrenia:
  – Treatment in adults (aripiprazole, aripiprazole long-acting injection, aripiprazole prolonged-release injectable, brexpiprazole, cariprazine)
  – Agitation associated with schizophrenia (aripiprazole short-acting injection – USA)
• Schizoaffective disorder (subpopulation in RCTs)

Bipolar Disorder

👍 Bipolar I disorder:
  – Acute manic/mixed episodes (aripiprazole as monotherapy or as adjunctive therapy with lithium or valproate in adults, cariprazine as monotherapy)
  – Maintenance treatment (aripiprazole, aripiprazole long-acting injection as monotherapy)
  – Treatment of depressive episodes (cariprazine as monotherapy)
  – Agitation associated with manic/mixed episodes (aripiprazole short-acting injection – USA)

Depression

👍 Adjunctive treatment to antidepressants (aripiprazole, brexpiprazole)

[a] Adult population unless otherwise stated [‡] Indications listed here do not necessarily apply to all countries. Please refer to a country's regulatory database (e.g., US Food and Drug Administration, Health Canada Drug Product Database) for the most current availability information and indications

Third-Generation Antipsychotics/TGAs (cont.)

Other	

- Addiction: Alcohol, amphetamines, cocaine (aripiprazole – limited studies, some suggest a lack of efficacy and potential for increased drug abuse)
- Anxiety disorders (aripiprazole – small, open studies in a variety of anxiety disorders suggesting benefit)
- Borderline personality disorder (aripiprazole – small, short-term RCT)
- Delirium (aripiprazole – small open or cohort studies)
- Dementia-related psychosis or agitation (aripiprazole – meta-analysis: small but statistically significant effect). Product monographs highlight safety concerns in the elderly with dementia
- Parkinson's disease: Dyskinesia due to levodopa (aripiprazole – small open-label study using very low doses); psychosis (aripiprazole – open study with mixed results)
- Tourette's syndrome and tic disorders (aripiprazole – small studies suggesting benefit)

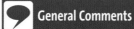 **General Comments**

- TGAs may be classified as atypical antipsychotics and are sometimes referred to as second-generation antipsychotics although they have distinct pharmacological profiles (see below)
- TGAs have comparable efficacy to other antipsychotic agents in the treatment of positive symptoms
- TGAs are associated with a lower overall risk of:
  - Metabolic adverse effects (such as weight gain, dyslipidemias, and glucose intolerance/diabetes mellitus) vs. many SGAs – monitoring for such effects is still advised
  - EPS (most notably, akathisia has been reported)
  - Hyperprolactinemia
  - Sedation
  - Anticholinergic effects
- Most notable adverse effects of TGAs:
  - May cause dizziness and/or orthostatic hypotension during initiation or dosage increase
  - Insomnia
  - Activation/akathisia
- TGAs have long half-lives which may result in delayed-onset adverse events (see Pharmacokinetics pp. 182 and 207). They require dosage adjustment with potent inhibitors of CYP2D6 and/or 3A4 (see Dosing with concomitant medications p. 181 and Drug Interactions pp. 187–190
- Aripiprazole long-acting injection: In a 12-month study aimed at assessing aripiprazole long-acting injectable in the treatment of first-episode psychosis (50 patients, aged 18–26), aripiprazole long-acting was associated with progressive improvement, compared to baseline, of both positive and negative symptoms and in general psychopathology and decreased global severity. Progressive improvement in quality of life and social and personal functioning was also reported. Treatment adherence was 78% at study endpoint
- A meta-analysis (14 studies with 2,494 patients) that compared aripiprazole to D_2 receptor antagonists in patients with early stages of schizophrenia found no difference between the treatment groups for overall symptom reduction or all-cause discontinuation. However, aripiprazole was more favorable than D_2 antagonist for depressive symptoms, prolactin levels, and triglyceride levels, but less favorable than second-generation D_2 antagonists for akathisia
- Results from a nested case-control study (219 patients) suggested that first-episode psychosis patients with a gambling history, problematic or not, may be at increased risk of developing problem gambling when receiving aripiprazole
- Aripiprazole and brexpiprazole: A dose response meta-analysis of antipsychotics for acute schizophrenia (69 studies) was conducted for all placebo-controlled dose-finding studies. The 95% effective doses were 11.5 mg/day for aripiprazole and 3.36 mg/day for brexpiprazole. The authors state that doses higher than the identified 95% effective doses may on average not provide more efficacy
- Brexpiprazole: A meta-analysis of 14 RCTs reported significant improvements in schizophrenia and MDD and good tolerability. Associated side effects included akathisia, weight increase, and somnolence. Compared to 4 mg brexpiprazole, 2 mg was associated with less risk of akathisia and somnolence
- Cariprazine: Data from 3 randomized, double-blind, placebo-controlled trials (1383 participants) in patients with bipolar depression were pooled and showed significant improvement in depressive symptoms for 1.5–3 mg/day vs. placebo. Coupled with efficacy in manic symptoms, cariprazine appears to be effective across the range of bipolar disorder symptoms

- In a randomized, double-blind, controlled trial (461 patients), cariprazine (target dose 4.5 mg) compared to risperidone (target dose 4 mg) was more efficacious in the treatment of predominant negative symptoms of schizophrenia. Improvement in negative symptoms associated with cariprazine was correlated with improvement in functioning that included self-care, personal and social relationships, and socially useful activities
- Aripiprazole and cariprazine: A network meta-analysis (50 trials, 11,488 participants) comparing efficacy and tolerability for treatment of acute bipolar depression reported that cariprazine, divalproex, lamotrigine, olanzapine, olanzapine/fluoxetine, and quetiapine appear to be effective as compared to placebo. Aripiprazole showed higher discontinuation rates vs. placebo due to adverse events

Pharmacology

- TGAs act as partial agonists with high affinity at pre- and post-synaptic D_2 receptors and serotonin ($5\text{-}HT_{1A}$) receptors, and as antagonists at $5\text{-}HT_{2A}$ receptors
- Aripiprazole exhibits high affinity for dopamine D_2 and D_3, serotonin $5\text{-}HT_{1A}$, and $5\text{-}HT_{2A}$ receptors and moderate affinity for dopamine D_4, serotonin $5\text{-}HT_{2C}$ and $5\text{-}HT_7$, α_1, and histamine H_1 receptors as well as for the serotonin reuptake site. It has no appreciable affinity for cholinergic muscarinic receptors
- Brexpiprazole acts as a partial agonist at the $5HT_{1A}$, D_2 (high affinity), and D_3 (high affinity) receptors and as an antagonist at $5\text{-}HT_{2A}$, $5\text{-}HT_{2B}$, $5\text{-}HT_7$, α_{1A}, α_{1B}, α_{1D}, and α_{2C} receptors. It also exhibits affinity for histamine H_1 and muscarinic M_1 receptors
- Cariprazine acts as a partial agonist at dopamine D_2 and D_3 receptors with high binding affinity and at serotonin $5\text{-}HT_{1A}$ receptors. It acts as an antagonist at $5\text{-}HT_{2A}$ (moderate affinity) and $5\text{-}HT_{2B}$ (high affinity) receptors as well as binding to histamine H_1 receptors. It shows lower binding affinity to the serotonin $5HT_{2C}$ and α_{1A}-adrenergic receptors and has no appreciable affinity for cholinergic muscarinic receptors
- As a partial dopamine agonist, the intensity of interaction with the dopamine receptor is less than that of endogenous dopamine (intrinsic activity = 100%). Accordingly, the net effect of dopamine partial agonism depends on whether a hypo- or hyperdopaminergic state exits. In areas of hypodopaminergic activity, partial D_2 agonism results in an increase in overall dopaminergic function (postulated as an explanation for benefit in negative symptoms and affective symptoms, and less EPS). Conversely, in areas of hyperdopaminergic activity, partial D_2 agonism results in a net decrease in dopaminergic function (postulated as explanation for improvement of positive symptoms)

⚖ Dosing

- See table p. 207 for more information on dosing for schizophrenia and psychosis
- Activation, agitation, akathisia and /or insomnia may occur on initiation of TGAs. Some practitioners recommend dosing in the morning and starting with a lower dose than is recommended by the monograph
- *Schizophrenia:*
  - Aripiprazole: Begin at 10 or 15 mg orally once daily. If needed, increase at intervals of 2 weeks or greater, up to 30 mg/day. Doses greater than 10–15 mg/day not shown to be more effective than 10–15 mg/day
  - Aripiprazole long-acting injection (Abilify Maintena):
    - One-injection start based on clinical study data: For patients naïve to aripiprazole, establish tolerability with oral aripiprazole prior to initiating treatment. On day of treatment initiation, administer one injection of 400 mg and continue treatment with 10–20 mg oral aripiprazole for 14 consecutive days to maintain therapeutic antipsychotic concentrations during initiation of therapy. For patients switching from oral antipsychotics other than aripiprazole, continue treatment with current oral antipsychotic for 14 days. Maintenance dose is 400 mg every 4 weeks. If adverse events occur, dose may be reduced to 300 mg every 4 weeks. Dosing interval should be no shorter than 26 days
      · Known CYP2D6 poor metabolizers: 300 mg at initiation and 300 mg every 4 weeks for maintenance
      · Known CYP2D6 poor metabolizer taking strong concomitant CYP3A4 inhibitors: 200 mg at initiation and 200 mg every 4 weeks for maintenance
    - Two-injection start based on modeling and simulation study data: Approved by the European Medicines Agency (November 2020) and Health Canada (March 2021): For patients naïve to aripiprazole, establish tolerability with oral aripiprazole prior to initiating treatment. On day of treatment initiation, administer two separate injections of 400 mg at separate injection sites, along with one 20 mg dose of oral aripiprazole. Patients must discontinue their current oral antipsychotic upon initiation of the two-injection start of aripiprazole long acting. Maintenance dose is 400 mg every 4 weeks. If adverse events occur, dose may be reduced to 300 mg every 4 weeks. Dosing interval should be no shorter than 26 days
      · Known CYP2D6 poor metabolizers: 2 separate injections of 300 mg at initiation and 300 mg every 4 weeks for maintenance
      · Known CYP2D6 poor metabolizer taking strong concomitant CYP3A4 inhibitors: Two-injection start not recommended
  - Aripiprazole lauroxil (Aristada): For patients naïve to aripiprazole, establish tolerability with oral aripiprazole prior to initiating treatment. Starting dose can be 441 mg, 662 mg or 882 mg administered monthly, 882 mg dose every 6 weeks, or 1064 mg dose every 2 months. There are two ways to initiate treatment with aripiprazole lauroxil (Aristada):

Third-Generation Antipsychotics/TGAs (cont.)

- Option 1: Administer one injection of 675 mg of Aristada Initio (in either the deltoid or gluteal muscle) and one 30 mg dose of oral aripiprazole in conjunction with the first aripiprazole lauroxil (Aristada) injection. The first aripiprazole lauroxil (Aristada) injection may be administered on the same day as Aristada Initio or up to 10 days thereafter. Avoid injecting both Aristarda Initio and aripiprazole lauroxil (Aristada) concomitantly into the same deltoid or gluteal muscle
- Option 2: Administer 21 consecutive days of oral aripiprazole in conjunction with the first aripiprazole lauroxil (Aristada) injection
  - IM dose of 441 mg every month: Concomitant oral aripiprazole 10 mg/day for 21 days
  - IM dose of 662 mg every month or 882 mg every 6 weeks or 1064 mg every 2 months: Concomitant oral aripiprazole 15 mg/day for 21 days
  - IM dose of 882 mg every month: Concomitant oral aripiprazole 20 mg/day for 21 days
- Dose adjustments are required for 1) known CYP2D6 poor metabolizers and 2) patients taking CYP2D6 inhibitors, CYP3A4 inhibitors or CYP3A4 inducers for more than 2 weeks
  - Brexpiprazole: Begin at 1 mg orally once daily (days 1–4). Increase to 2 mg once daily (days 5–7), then 4 mg on day 8 based on patient's clinical response and tolerability. Recommended target dose is 2–4 mg once daily
  - Cariprazine:
    - USA: Begin at 1.5 mg orally daily. Can be increased to 3 mg on day 2. Depending on clinical response and tolerability, further dose adjustments can be made in 1.5 mg or 3 mg increments. Recommended dose range is 1.5–6 mg once daily
    - Canada: Begin at 1.5 mg orally daily. Recommended dose range is 1.5–6 mg once daily. Depending upon clinical response and tolerability, dosage can be increased gradually in 1.5 mg increments
- *Bipolar I:*
  - Aripiprazole:
    - Acute manic and mixed episodes: Starting dose is 15 mg (monotherapy) or 10–15 mg (adjunctive with lithium or valproate) orally once daily; target dose is 15 mg orally once daily; range is 10–30 mg/day
  - Aripiprazole long-acting injection (Abilify Maintena):
    - Maintenance monotherapy: See dosing for schizophrenia
  - Cariprazine:
    - USA:
      - Manic or mixed episodes: Starting dose is 1.5 mg orally once daily. Can be increased to 3 mg on day 2. Depending on clinical response and tolerability, further dose adjustments can be made in 1.5 mg or 3 mg increments. Recommended dose range is 3–6 mg once daily
      - Bipolar depression: Starting dose is 1.5 mg orally once daily. Can be increased to 3 mg once daily on day 15. Maximum recommended dose is 3 mg orally once daily
    - Canada:
      - Manic or mixed episodes: Starting dose is 1.5 mg, can be increased thereafter by 1.5 mg increments, based on clinical response and tolerability. The recommended dosage range is 1.5–6 mg once daily
      - Bipolar depression: Starting dose is 1.5 mg orally once daily. Can be increased to 3 mg once daily on day 15. Maximum recommended dose is 3 mg orally once daily
- *Major depression (adjunctive treatment):*
  - Aripiprazole: Begin at 2 or 5 mg orally once daily. If needed, increase by up to 5 mg at intervals of one week or greater. Usual treatment range is 2–15 mg/day
  - Brexpiprazole: Begin at 0.5 or 1 mg orally once daily. Further dose increases should be done at weekly intervals based on clinical response and tolerability, up to the target dose of 2 mg orally once daily. Maximum recommended dose is 3 mg once daily
- *Agitation (schizophrenia or bipolar mania/mixed episode):*
  - Aripiprazole short-acting IM injection: Usual dose is 9.75 mg IM as a single dose; range is 5.25–15 mg IM; maximum total daily dose is 30 mg. Wait at least 2 h between doses as shorter intervals have not been studied
  - Aripiprazole oral solution can be substituted for tablets on a mg-per-mg basis up to the 25 mg dose level. Patients receiving 30 mg tablets should receive 25 mg of the solution as plasma levels achieved with solution are slightly higher than with the tablet formulation

- Dose adjustment NOT required in smokers or the elderly
- *Concomitant medications:*
  - Strong inhibitors of CYP2D6 (e.g., paroxetine)
    - Reduce dose of short-acting aripiprazole formulations to one half (50%)
    - If taking a strong inhibitor for more than 14 days, reduce maintenance dose of aripiprazole long-acting injection from 400 mg to 300 mg every 4 weeks, or from 300 mg to 200 mg every 4 weeks
    - Reduce dose of brexpiprazole to half the usual dose (50%)
  - Strong inhibitors of CYP3A4 (e.g., clarithromycin)
    - Reduce dose of short-acting aripiprazole formulations to one half (50%)
    - If taking a strong inhibitor for more than 14 days, reduce maintenance dose of aripiprazole long-acting injection from 400 mg to 300 mg every 4 weeks, or from 300 mg to 200 mg every 4 weeks
    - Reduce dose of brexpiprazole to half the usual dose (50%)
    - · USA: Reduce current dose of cariprazine by 50%. For patients taking 4.5 mg daily, reduce dose to 1.5 mg or 3 mg daily. For patients taking 1.5 mg daily, adjust dose to every other day. Cariprazine dose may need to be increased if CYP3A4 inhibitor is withdrawn

      Canada: Concomitant use of strong (and moderate) CYP3A4 inhibitors is contraindicated during treatment with cariprazine and for at least 2 weeks after cariprazine discontinuation
  - Strong inhibitors of CYP2D6 **and** CYP3A4
    - Reduce dose of short-acting aripiprazole formulations to one quarter (25%)
    - If taking strong inhibitors for more than 14 days, reduce maintenance dose of aripiprazole long-acting injection from 400 mg to 200 mg every 4 weeks, or from 300 mg to 160 mg every 4 weeks
    - Reduce dose of brexpiprazole to one quarter of the usual dose (25%)
  - Strong inducers of CYP3A4 (e.g., carbamazepine)
    - Double the dose of short-acting aripiprazole formulations
    - If taking a strong inducer for more than 14 days, avoid use of aripiprazole long-acting injection
    - Double the usual dose of brexpiprazole over 1–2 weeks
    - · USA: Concomitant use of cariprazine not recommended

      Canada: Concomitant use of a strong (or moderate) CYP3A4 inducer is contraindicated during treatment with cariprazine
  - Increase the dose appropriately if a strong inhibitor is stopped
  - Decrease the dose appropriately if a strong inducer is stopped
- *Pharmacogenetics:*
  - CYP poor metabolizers may be at increased risk of adverse drug events at usual doses and lower starting doses or avoidance of specific agents may be recommended. CYP intermediate metabolizers have some degree of metabolic activity and have often not been described as "clinically important" with regard to drug dosing adjustments. CYP ultra-rapid metabolizers may be at increased risk of therapeutic failure when certain agents are used; avoiding agents that are substrates for certain CYP isoenzymes or using therapeutic drug monitoring is usually warranted. See https://www.pharmgkb.org for updated clinical guidelines and dosing recommendations when utilizing pharmacogenetic testing
  - For administration details, please see Nursing Implications p. 186

Renal Impairment	<ul><li>Aripiprazole: No dosage adjustment required (however, based on a small, single-dose study)</li><li>Brexpiprazole: If CrCl less than 60 mL/min, administer maximum dose of 2 mg once daily for major depressive disorder; maximum dose of 3 mg once daily for schizophrenia</li><li>Cariprazine: If CrCl less than 30 mL/min, use is not recommended (has not been studied), no dosage adjustment necessary if CrCl $\geq$ 30 mL/min</li></ul>
Hepatic Impairment	<ul><li>Aripiprazole: No dosage adjustment required (however, based on a small, single-dose study)</li><li>Brexpiprazole: In moderate to severe impairment (Child-Pugh class B or C), administer maximum dose of 2 mg once daily for major depressive disorder; maximum dose of 3 mg once daily for schizophrenia; no dose adjustment necessary for mild impairment</li><li>Cariprazine: In moderate to severe impairment (Child-Pugh class of B or C) use is not recommended; no dose adjustment necessary for mild impairment</li></ul>

Third-Generation Antipsychotics/TGAs (cont.)

 Pharmacokinetics

- Also see table pp. 207–**??**

Absorption

- All TGAs can be taken with or without food
- Oral:
  - Bioavailability of aripiprazole tablet is 87%. At equivalent doses, peak plasma concentrations from the oral solution are higher (by ~22%) than from the tablet formulation
  - Time to peak plasma concentration (T_{max}) is 3–5 h when taken on an empty stomach, and up to 6 h if taken with a high-fat meal
  - Bioavailability of brexpiprazole is 95%. After single dose administration of brexpiprazole tablets, peak plasma concentrations occurred within 4 h
  - Bioavailability of cariprazine is high and after single dose administration of cariprazine, peak plasma concentrations occurred in approximately 3–6 h
- Aripiprazole disintegrating tablet:
  - Bioequivalent to oral tablet. Dissolves in saliva within 15 sec. Recommended to be taken without liquid, but can be given with liquid if needed
- Aripiprazole short-acting IM injection:
  - Bioavailability is 100%
  - Time to peak plasma concentration T_{max} is 1–3 h
- Aripiprazole long-acting IM injection:
  - Time to peak plasma concentration T_{max} is 5–6 days

Distribution

- Protein binding of aripiprazole and dehydro-aripiprazole (major, active metabolite) is more than 99% (primarily to albumin). Volume of distribution at steady state is high (404 L or 4.9 L/kg), indicating extensive extravascular distribution
- Brexpiprazole is highly protein bound in plasma (over 99%) to serum albumin and α_1-acid glycoprotein, and its protein binding is not affected by renal or hepatic impairment. Volume of distribution following intravenous administration is high (1.56 ± 0.42 L/kg), indicating extravascular distribution
- Cariprazine and its major active metabolites are highly bound (91–97%) to plasma proteins

Metabolism & Elimination

- Aripiprazole:
  - Metabolism of aripiprazole is hepatic, primarily via the P450 isozymes CYP2D6 (dehydrogenation, hydroxylation) and CYP3A4 (dehydrogenation, hydroxylation, N-dealkylation)
  - Dehydro-aripiprazole is the major metabolite of aripiprazole. It is active, represents 40% of parent drug exposure in plasma, and has similar affinity for D_2 receptors
  - Mean half-lives are about 75 h and 94 h for aripiprazole and dehydro-aripiprazole, respectively. Steady-state concentrations for oral doses are attained within 14 days for both active moieties while they take 3–4 months to reach with aripiprazole long-acting injections
  - Half-life and aripiprazole exposure are influenced by capacity to metabolize CYP2D6 substrates. Aripiprazole exposure increases by about 80% and dehydro-aripiprazole exposure decreases by about 30% in poor CYP2D6 metabolizers. In extensive CYP2D6 metabolizers, aripiprazole's half-life = 75 h vs. poor metabolizers = 146 h. Steady-state concentrations may take 28 days to be attained in poor metabolizers. The majority of the population are extensive CYP2D6 metabolizers. Approximately 8% of Caucasians, 3–8% of Black/African Americans, 3–6% of Hispanics, 0–4% of Native Americans, and 0.3–1% East Asians are poor CYP2D6 metabolizers
  - Excretion of an oral dose is via feces (55%, with about 18% as unchanged aripiprazole) and urine (25%, with less than 1% as unchanged aripiprazole)
- Brexpiprazole:
  - Metabolism of brexpiprazole is hepatic, primarily via CYP2D6 and CYP3A4
  - Its major metabolite is not considered to contribute to the therapeutic effects of brexpiprazole
  - CYP2D6 poor metabolizers have higher brexpiprazole concentrations than normal metabolizers of CYP2D6. Approximately 8% of Caucasians and 3–8% of Black/African Americans cannot metabolize CYP2D6 substrates and are classified as poor metabolizers

- Cariprazine:
  - Extensively metabolized by CYP3A4 and, to a lesser extent, by CYP2D6 to two major active metabolites: desmethyl cariprazine (DCAR) and didesmethyl cariprazine (DDCAR). DCAR is further metabolized into DDCAR by CYP3A4 and CYP2D6. DDCAR is then metabolized by CYP3A4 to a hydroxylated metabolite
  - DCAR and DDCAR are pharmacologically equipotent to cariprazine
  - Half-lives based on time to reach steady state, estimated from the mean concentration-time curves, are 2–4 days for cariprazine and approximately 1–3 weeks for DDCAR
  - CYP2D6 poor metabolizer status does not have clinically relevant effect on pharmacokinetics of cariprazine, DCAR, or DDCAR

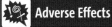 Adverse Effects

- See General Comments (p. 178) and p. 199 for a quick summary
- Adverse events may first appear several weeks after the initiation of TGA treatment, probably because plasma levels of TGAs and their major metabolites accumulate over time. As a result, the incidence of adverse reactions in short-term trials may not reflect the rates after longer-term exposure
- A 2013 study of the long-term safety and tolerability of aripiprazole long-acting injection reported a tolerability profile comparable to oral aripiprazole. Treatment-emergent adverse effects occurring at rate of 5% or more were anxiety, akathisia, headache, nausea, and weight gain
- Most common adverse reactions (over 5% and at least twice the rate of placebo) for brexpiprazole in two pooled 6-weeks, placebo-controlled, MDD trials (dose range 1–4 mg once daily) were akathisia and weight gain; however, incidence of these adverse events was lower (less than 5%) in two short-term (up to 6 weeks) schizophrenia trials
- Based on four placebo-controlled, 6-week schizophrenia trials with cariprazine doses ranging from 1.5 mg to 12 mg once daily, the most common adverse effects (over 5% and at least twice the rate of placebo) were EPS and akathisia. The pooled data from three short-term cariprazine trials with dose range of 3–12 mg once daily in bipolar mania (duration of 3 weeks) suggested the most common adverse effects (over 5% and at least twice the rate of placebo) are EPS, akathisia, dyspepsia, vomiting, somnolence, and restlessness

CNS Effects

- Aripiprazole commonly reported adverse effects include: Headache (more than 20%), agitation (more than 15%), anxiety (more than 25%), insomnia (more than 15%), nervousness, lightheadedness, and dizziness (more than 10%), somnolence (more than 10%), and asthenia. Many of these develop during the first week of treatment and resolve over time. A lower starting dose of 2–5 mg once daily may minimize many of these adverse effects
- Based on pooled data from short-term trials, brexpiprazole and cariprazine seem to cause less agitation, insomnia, and sedation (less than 10%)
- EPS – acute onset
  - Aripiprazole has a favorable EPS profile, though dystonia, akathisia reported; tremor (mostly described as mild intensity, limited duration) reported (more than 2%); case report of exacerbation of Parkinson's disease and 2 case reports of rabbit syndrome
  - Based on pooled data from short-term trials, brexpiprazole appears to cause less akathisia (less than 10%) compared to aripiprazole and cariprazine (more than 10%)
- EPS – late onset or tardive movement disorders (TD): Risk of TD appears highest among the elderly, especially elderly women, but it is not possible to predict which patients are likely to develop the syndrome. Whether TGA drug products differ in their potential to cause TD is unknown. Case reports of tardive movement disorders associated with aripiprazole in literature
- Neuroleptic malignant syndrome has been reported in patients treated with aripiprazole. Also rhabdomyolysis in the absence of a diagnosis of NMS
- Seizure incidence in patients receiving TGAs is reported to be less than 2% – use cautiously in individuals with a history of seizures, poorly controlled seizures, or medications and/or conditions known to lower the seizure threshold

Cardiovascular Effects

- Arrhythmias and ECG changes
  - ECG changes (e.g., T-wave inversion, ST segment depression, QTc lengthening – may increase risk of arrhythmias) reported with many antipsychotic medications, the clinical significance of which is unclear for many. See p. 154
  - One published case report associated aripiprazole with the development of torsades de pointes (TdP). CredibleMeds risk category rated as "possible risk of TdP" – (see p. 154 for more information)
- Cardiomyopathy – 1 case report noting eosinophilic myocarditis and elevated levels of aripiprazole found on autopsy of a 36-year-old male with schizophrenia
- Dyslipidemias – see Endocrine & Metabolic Effects
- Orthostatic hypotension/compensatory tachycardia/dizziness/syncope – antagonism of α_1-adrenergic receptors may result in orthostatic hypotension, dizziness, and reflex tachycardia. Incidence appears low with TGAs

Third-Generation Antipsychotics/TGAs (cont.)

Endocrine & Metabolic Effects	• Antidiuretic hormone dysfunction – a few cases of hyponatremia/SIADH documenting resolution within 7–10 days of aripiprazole discontinuation have been reported • Dyslipidemias – risk appears low with TGAs; monitoring still suggested – see p. 124 for suggested monitoring guidelines – In long-term, open-label schizophrenia studies, shifts in normal baseline fasting triglyceride were observed in 13% of patients on brexpiprazole (to triglyceride level of less than 500 mg/dL); less than 1% patients had increase in triglyceride resulting in level of more than 500 mg/dL • Glucose dysregulation, ketoacidosis, type 2 diabetes mellitus; risk appears low with TGAs; case reports of hyperglycemia and of diabetic ketoacidosis in patients treated with aripiprazole, so monitoring still suggested – see p. 124 for suggested monitoring guidelines • Hyperprolactinemia – partial D_2 agonists appear to have minimal effect on prolactin and, in some cases, a drop in prolactin levels has been reported. However, a few cases of galactorrhea have been reported; assess for signs and symptoms routinely. For more information on hyperprolactinemia symptoms, monitoring, and treatment options see p. 156 • A dose-response meta-analysis of RCTs of patients with acute exacerbation (97 studies involving 36,326 patients, median duration = 6 weeks) reported that amisulpride, aripiprazole, brexpiprazole, cariprazine, haloperidol, lumateperone, and lurasidone produced mild weight gain in comparison to placebo (mean difference (MD) ≤ 1 kg for any dose). Dose-response curves did not plateau for clozapine, olanzapine, and paliperidone, with these having MDs in weight gain of 3.75 kg, 3.62 kg, and 1.95 kg, respectively. Quetiapine and ziprasidone showed a bell-shaped relationship with maximal weight gain centered around 600 mg/day (MD in weight gain = 1.48 kg) and 80 mg/day (MD in weight gain = 1.24 kg) • See relative tolerability profiles table p. 196 for a comparison of the likelihood of weight gain among antipsychotics
GI Effects	• Constipation incidence reported to be more than 10% in aripiprazole-treated patients. Based on pooled short-term data, incidence seems to be lower in brexpiprazole-treated patients (2–3%). 6% incidence reported in cariprazine-treated patients in short-term trials • Dysphagia and aspiration reported with antipsychotic use; use cautiously in individuals at risk for developing aspiration pneumonia (e.g., advanced Alzheimer's disease) • Nausea and vomiting reported in more than 10% of patients receiving aripiprazole, generally seen at start of therapy; appears to dissipate over the first week. Based on pooled data from short-term trials, incidence of nausea and vomiting seems to be lower with brexpiprazole (less than 10%). Incidence of nausea with cariprazine appears to be higher (more than 10%)
Urogenital & Sexual Effects	• Priapism – case report of recurrent priapism starting 6 h after the first dose of aripiprazole • Based on their pharmacological profile (D_2 partial agonist in tuberoinfundibular tract translating into less hyperprolactinemia and low affinity for cholinergic receptors), it seems unlikely that these agents would cause sexual dysfunction • The 2009 PORT treatment recommendations for schizophrenia rank the relative risk for prolactin elevation and sexual side effects with antipsychotics as follows: Risperidone = paliperidone > FGA medications > olanzapine > ziprasidone > quetiapine = clozapine > aripiprazole
Hematological Effects	• Leukopenia and neutropenia reported during treatment with antipsychotics, including TGAs. A few case reports suggest a possible association of aripiprazole and the development of leukopenia and/or neutropenia, and thrombocytopenia • Stop TGA treatment if neutrophil count drops below 1.0×10^9/L (1000/mm^3)
Hepatic Effects	• Elevations in liver function tests (ALT, AST, BUN) reported infrequently
Hypersensitivity Reactions	• Rare occurrences of allergic reaction (anaphylactic reaction, angioedema, laryngospasm, pruritus/urticaria, or oropharyngeal spasm) reported
Other Adverse Effects	• Acneiform eruption – case report of acneiform eruptions which resolved upon discontinuation of aripiprazole • Raynaud's phenomenon, epistaxis, gingival bleeding (rare) with aripiprazole • Hiccups • Blurred vision (2.5%) • Rhinitis and pharyngitis

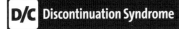 **D/C Discontinuation Syndrome**

- Withdrawal symptoms reported similar to those seen with other classes of antipsychotics. However, due to the long elimination half-lives of TGAs, these medications may self-taper with few withdrawal symptoms if promptly discontinued. See Discontinuation Syndrome p. 160 for a general discussion.
- Since aripiprazole and cariprazine have minimal affinity for cholinergic muscarinic receptors, an abrupt switch from an agent with high affinity for these receptors to aripiprazole or cariprazine could result in symptoms of cholinergic rebound upon withdrawal of the initial antipsychotic
- Utilizing the delayed withdrawal method when switching from an SGA/FGA to a TGA may be advisable. Theoretically, an abrupt switch from a D_2 antagonist to a D_2 partial agonist (aripiprazole, brexpiprazole, and cariprazine) could result in a temporary surge of dopaminergic activity as a result of unmasking upregulated D_2 receptors. In the mesolimbic tract, this could translate into a temporary exacerbation of positive symptoms. The same actions in the nigrostriatal tract could result in the onset of withdrawal dyskinesias. It may be advisable to use the delayed withdrawal method when switching to aripiprazole to minimize the occurrence of these effects
- Readers may find the website http://switchrx.com helpful for managing antipsychotic switching

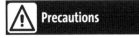 **Precautions**

- Caution in patients with known cardiovascular disease, cerebrovascular disease, seizure disorders or conditions that predispose patients to hypotension or aspiration pneumonia
- Increased risk of suicidal thinking in children, adolescents, and young adults. Monitor for worsening and emergence of suicidal thoughts and behaviors
- Aripiprazole: Post-marketing case reports suggest that patients can experience intense urges, particularly for gambling. Other compulsive urges, reported less frequently, include: sexual urges, shopping, eating or binge eating, and other impulsive or compulsive behaviors. It should be noted that impulse-control symptoms can be associated with the underlying disorder. In some cases, urges were reported to have stopped when dose was reduced or medication discontinued

 Toxicity

- Aripiprazole:
  - A retrospective study of 286 cases of isolated aripiprazole exposures found 55% of patients reported symptoms – somnolence (56%), sinus tachycardia (20%), nausea/vomiting (18%), dystonia (13%), tremor (6%), agitation, dizziness (2%), paresthesias, headache (1%)
  - A 2009 review of atypical antipsychotic overdoses suggested cardiovascular toxicity with aripiprazole ingestion was minimal
  - Acute ingestions of up to 1080 mg aripiprazole reported with no fatalities
- There is limited clinical trial experience with brexpiprazole and cariprazine overdose

Management

- No specific antidote is available. Close medical supervision, monitoring of vital signs and functions including cardiac function, and supportive therapy to maintain airways and oxygenation and manage symptoms is required. Early administration of charcoal may help in partially preventing absorption of aripiprazole or brexpiprazole. Hemodialysis is not deemed likely to be of benefit due to aripiprazole's or brexpiprazole's high plasma protein binding
- No specific antidotes for cariprazine are known. In managing overdose, provide supportive care, including close medical supervision and monitoring, and consider the possibility of multiple drug involvement. Consult a Certified Poison Control Center for up-to-date guidance and advice

 Lab Tests/Monitoring

- Therapeutic range not established for TGAs
- One study suggests best efficacy for schizophrenia with serum aripiprazole levels between 150 and 300 ng/mL and minimal adverse effects when levels are between 110 and 249 ng/mL. A target plasma level range between 150 and 210 ng/mL has also been proposed. Therapeutic drug monitoring suggested to be of limited value other than assessing adherence, optimizing efficacy

 Use in Pregnancy◇

- Aripiprazole:
  - Pregnancy alters the pharmacokinetic profile of aripiprazole, a 52% decrease of serum aripiprazole concentrations was observed in the third trimester. Pregnancy induces CYP2D6 and 3A4 enzymes, therefore TGAs, which are substrates for these metabolic pathways, may have reduced concentrations in late pregnancy. Consider therapeutic drug monitoring if indicated
  - Aripiprazole is considered a drug with "Limited human data – Animal data suggest risk"
  - Chemical properties (e.g., small molecular weight) and measurement of umbilical cord blood levels of aripiprazole and dehydro-aripiprazole at delivery in case reports indicate aripiprazole and dehydro-aripiprazole both cross the human placenta
  - No teratogenicity or developmental toxicity were seen in eight cases. Five of them involved exposure at some point during the first trimester, the

◇ See p. 473 for further information on drug use in pregnancy and effects on breast milk

trimester most sensitive to structural malformations. There was increased risk of malformations, in particular cardiovascular defects, in a cohort study of SGAs where 60 of 561 patients were taking aripiprazole at some time during pregnancy
- The following adverse events have been reported with third-trimester exposure to aripiprazole: Fetal distress (i.e., tachycardia) during labor with subsequent failure to establish lactation, mild respiratory distress 10 min post-delivery, and no spontaneous breath with poor muscle tone just after birth requiring short-term (1 min) resuscitation
- Brexpiprazole:
  - Adequate and well-controlled studies with brexpiprazole have not been conducted in pregnant women to inform drug-associated risks. In animal reproduction studies, no teratogenicity was observed with oral administration of brexpiprazole to pregnant rats and rabbits during organogenesis at doses up to 73 and 146 times, respectively, of the maximum recommended human dose (MRHD) of 4 mg/day on a mg/m^2 basis. However, when brexpiprazole was administered to pregnant rats during the period of organogenesis through lactation, the number of perinatal deaths of pups was increased at 73 times the MRHD. The background risk of major birth defects and miscarriage for the indicated population(s) is unknown
- Cariprazine:
  - There is a pregnancy exposure registry that monitors pregnancy outcomes in women exposed to cariprazine during pregnancy. For more information, contact the National Pregnancy Registry for Atypical Antipsychotics at 1-866-961-2388 or visit http://womensmentalhealth.org/clinical-and-researchprograms/pregnancyregistry/
  - No available data on cariprazine use in pregnant women to inform any drug-associated risks for birth defects or miscarriage
  - Based on animal data, cariprazine may cause fetal harm. Administration of cariprazine to rats during the period of organogenesis caused malformations, lower pup survival, and developmental delays at drug exposures less than the human exposure at the maximum recommended human dose (MRHD) of 6 mg/day

Breast Milk	

- Aripiprazole:
  - Case reports indicate aripiprazole likely transfers to breast milk with the relative infant dose estimated to be less than 0.7% to 8.3%
  - Possibility of somnolence in breastfed infants
  - Hale's lactation risk category = L3 (give only if the potential benefit outweighs the potential risk to the infant)
- Brexpiprazole: Lactation studies have not been conducted to assess the presence of brexpiprazole in human milk, the effects of the drug on the breastfed infant, or the effects on milk production
- Cariprazine: Lactation studies have not been conducted to assess the presence of cariprazine in human milk, the effects of the drug on the breastfed infant, or the effects on milk production
- The development and health benefits of breastfeeding should be considered along with the mother's clinical need for TGAs and any potential adverse effects on the breastfed infant from the medication or from the underlying maternal condition. Refer to the Drugs and Lactation Database (LactMed) website (https://www.ncbi.nlm.nih.gov/books/NBK501922/) for more information

 Nursing Implications

- See p. 126

Oral	

- TGAs can be taken with or without food
- AVOID grapefruit juice (see Drug Interactions p. 190)
- Aripiprazole disintegrating tablets dissolve rapidly in saliva; recommended to be taken WITHOUT liquid, but if needed can be taken with liquid
- Aripiprazole disintegrating tablets break easily. Do NOT push the tablet through the foil backing as this could damage the tablet. Use dry hands to remove the tablet and immediately place tablet on the tongue
- Aripiprazole oral solution can be used for up to 6 months after opening, but not beyond the expiration date on the bottle. Store at room temperature
- Each mL of oral solution contains 400 mg of sucrose and 200 mg of fructose

Aripiprazole Short-Acting IM Injection	

- Available as a ready-to-use solution of 9.75 mg/1.3 mL in a single-dose vial for IM administration only. Discard any unused portion of the vial
- Inject slowly, deep into the muscle mass
- Wait at least 2 h between doses

| Aripiprazole Long-Acting IM Injection | <ul><li>Abilify Maintena:<ul><li>Reconstitute powder with provided diluent. Shake vial vigorously for 30 sec until the suspension appears uniform</li><li>Can store the reconstituted mixture in the vial at room temperature for up to 4 h. Reshake vial vigorously for at least 60 sec before use</li><li>Inject slowly, deep into the deltoid or gluteal muscle</li><li>For deltoid administration: Use 23 gauge, 1-inch needle for non-obese patients and 22 gauge, 1.5 inch needle for obese patients</li><li>For gluteal administration: Use 22 gauge, 1.5-inch needle for non-obese patients and 21 gauge, 2-inch needle for obese patients</li><li>Do NOT massage the injection site</li><li>Rotate sites</li></ul></li><li>Aristada:<ul><li>Supplied as injectable suspension in pre-filled syringe</li><li>Can be stored at room temperature (20–25 degrees Celsius)</li><li>Tap syringe at least 10 times to dislodge any material which may have settled</li><li>Shake syringe vigorously for a minimum of 30 sec to ensure a uniform suspension. If syringe is not used with 15 min, shake again for 30 sec</li><li>The 441 mg (1.6 mL) strength kit contains a 1-inch 21 gauge, a 1.5-inch 20 gauge, and a 2-inch 20 gauge needle. Can be given in deltoid or gluteal muscle</li><li>The 662 mg (2.4 mL), 882 mg (3.2 mL), and 1064 mg (3.9 mL) strength kits contain a 1.5-inch 20 gauge and a 2-inch 20 gauge needle. For gluteal administration only</li><li>Do NOT massage the injection site</li><li>Rotate sites</li></ul></li><li>Aristada Initio:<ul><li>Supplied as injectable suspension in pre-filled syringe</li><li>Can be stored at room temperature (20–25 degrees Celsius)</li><li>Tap syringe at least 10 times to dislodge any material which may have settled</li><li>Shake syringe vigorously for a minimum of 30 sec to ensure a uniform suspension. If syringe is not used with 15 min, shake again for 30 sec</li><li>The 675 mg (2.4 mL) kit contains a 1-inch 21 gauge, a 1.5-inch 20 gauge, and a 2-inch 20 gauge needle. Can be given in deltoid (using a 1-inch 21 gauge or a 1.5-inch 20 gauge needle) or gluteal (using a 1.5-inch 20 gauge or a 2-inch 20 gauge needle</li><li>Do NOT massage the injection site</li></ul></li></ul> |

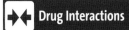

Drug Interactions

- Clinically significant interactions are listed below
- For more interaction information on any given combination, also see the corresponding chapter for the second agent

Class of Drug	Example	Interaction Effects
Acetylcholinesterase inhibitor (central)	General	Increase in mortality in elderly patients with dementia taking antipsychotics irrespective of acetylcholinesterase inhibitor use. Deaths largely either cardiovascular or infectious in nature. Also see p. 126
	Donepezil, galantamine, rivastigmine	May enhance neurotoxicity of antipsychotics, presumably due to a relative acetylcholine/dopamine imbalance (i.e., increased acetylcholine in the presence of dopamine receptor blockade) in the CNS
Antiarrhythmic	General	Possible additive prolongation of QT interval and associated life-threatening cardiac arrhythmias. However, aripiprazole, brexpiprazole, and cariprazine appear to have low potential to prolong the QT interval compared to other antipsychotics. Also see TGA Cardiovascular Effects p. 183
	Amiodarone	Amiodarone is a CYP2D6 inhibitor. Increased plasma levels of aripiprazole and brexpiprazole possible
	Quinidine	Quinidine is a potent CYP2D6 inhibitor resulting in an increased AUC of aripiprazole by 107–112% (i.e., doubled). AUC of active metabolite decreased by 32–35%. Due to aripiprazole's long half-life, interaction effects may be delayed for up to 10–14 days. Brexpiprazole's AUC was approximately 2-fold higher with concurrent use of quinidine (brexpiprazole's major metabolite is inactive). Cariprazine does not get metabolized extensively by CYP2D6, consequently the interaction with quinidine might not be clinically significant

Third-Generation Antipsychotics/TGAs (cont.)

Class of Drug	Example	Interaction Effects
Antibiotic	Clarithromycin, erythromycin, telithromycin	CYP3A4 is inhibited potently by clarithromycin and telithromycin, and moderately by erythromycin. Increased plasma levels of aripiprazole, brexpiprazole, and cariprazine likely to occur. Effects may be delayed due to their long half-lives
Anticonvulsant	General	As with other antipsychotics, aripiprazole, brexpiprazole, and cariprazine may lower seizure threshold. Monitor for increased seizure frequency and increase anticonvulsant medication as needed. See also Antipsychotic Augmentation Strategies p. 218
	Carbamazepine, oxcarbazepine	CYP3A4 is induced potently by carbamazepine and weakly by oxcarbazepine Carbamazepine reduces C_{max} and AUC of aripiprazole and its active metabolite by about 70% with concurrent use and one week after discontinuing carbamazepine. Brexpiprazole prescribing information recommends increase in dose when used concomitantly with strong CYP3A4 inducer. Cariprazine prescribing information recommends concomitant use to be avoided Note it may take 2–4 weeks to reach maximum induction and an equivalent period to return to baseline after discontinuation of an inducer. Oxcarbazepine at higher dose (i.e., $\geq$ 1500 mg/day) may result in a clinically relevant induction of aripiprazole
	Clobazam	Clobazam may cause potent CYP2D6 inhibition and weak CYP3A4 induction
	Lamotrigine	No clinically significant pharmacokinetic changes. Case reports of adverse effects with concurrent use: Three cases of Stevens-Johnson syndrome within 2–4 weeks after adding lamotrigine to aripiprazole; one case of disabling intention tremor 2 months after the addition of aripiprazole to lamotrigine which resolved upon lamotrigine discontinuation; one case of false-positive diagnosis of pheochromocytoma
	Phenobarbital, phenytoin	Phenobarbital and phenytoin are potent CYP3A4 inducers. Degree of induction likely similar to the interaction between TGAs and carbamazepine Case report of leucopenia and thrombocytopenia with addition of aripiprazole (10 mg/day) to phenytoin (300 mg/day)
	Valproate (divalproex, valproic acid)	Mild reductions of aripiprazole's C_{max} and AUC (by up to 25%). Not clinically significant. No dose adjustment required. Approved for concurrent use in the management of bipolar disorder. Adverse effects reported with concurrent use include: More frequent – akathisia, increased triglyceride levels, tiredness, tremor, weight gain; serious – one case of severe abdominal pain
Antidepressant	General	Increased rates of akathisia and fatigue with concurrent antidepressant use Serotonin syndrome theoretically possible with antidepressants that increase serotonin (e.g., SNRIs, SSRIs)
SSRI	Citalopram, escitalopram, sertraline	No clinically significant pharmacokinetic changes to escitalopram, sertraline or aripiprazole. Adverse effect case reports with citalopram and aripiprazole include one of urinary obstruction and one of EPS. Adverse effect case reports with sertraline (at 200 mg/day) and aripiprazole include one each of severe akathisia, acute dystonia, and myxedema coma
	Fluoxetine, paroxetine	Fluoxetine and paroxetine are significant CYP2D6 inhibitors. Increased aripiprazole levels (30–70%) reported. Effects may be delayed due to the antipsychotic's long half-life. Small changes in fluoxetine (18% increase), norfluoxetine (36% increase), and paroxetine (27% decrease) levels reported. Case reports with fluoxetine and aripiprazole of: NMS 2 weeks after starting the combination; leucopenia that resolved upon aripiprazole discontinuation and reoccurred upon rechallenge Secondary to strong inhibition of CYP2D6, dosage decrease has been recommended for brexpiprazole
	Fluvoxamine	Fluvoxamine is a weak CYP2D6 and CYP3A4 inhibitor. Clearance of aripiprazole may be reduced by 40%. Clinical significance unknown
NDRI	Bupropion	CAUTION. Potential for additive risk of seizures. No published reports of seizures with concurrent use; however, data limited to six patients. Bupropion is an inhibitor of CYP2D6, which could increase aripiprazole and brexpiprazole levels. No published reports of aripiprazole levels with concurrent bupropion. In the six cases of concurrent use, akathisia and/or insomnia occurred in at least three

Class of Drug	Example	Interaction Effects
SNRI	Duloxetine	Duloxetine is a moderate CYP2D6 inhibitor; however, a study found no significant change in aripiprazole levels. Case report of high aripiprazole levels, confusion, and loss of coordination in a patient taking high-dose aripiprazole (50 mg/day) with darunavir and ritonavir (modest CYP2D6 and potent CYP3A4 inhibitors) and duloxetine. Case report of hypertensive crisis within 2 weeks of adding aripiprazole to duloxetine; blood pressure decreased upon aripiprazole dose reduction
	Venlafaxine	No clinically significant pharmacokinetic changes. Case report of hypertensive crisis with confusion and agitation 2 days after adding aripiprazole to venlafaxine which resolved upon aripiprazole discontinuation. Two case report of parkinsonism with concurrent use of venlafaxine and aripiprazole
Antifungal	Fluconazole, itraconazole, ketoconazole, voriconazole	Ketoconazole and itraconazole are potent, while fluconazole and voriconazole are moderate CYP3A4 inhibitors. AUC of aripiprazole and its metabolite increased by 63% and 77% with ketoconazole and 48% and 39% with itraconazole, respectively AUC of brexpiprazole approximately 2-fold higher with concurrent administration of ketoconazole. Refer to dosing recommendations for concurrent administration of strong CYP3A4 inhibitors AUC of cariprazine on average 4-fold higher with concurrent administration of ketoconazole. Refer to dosing recommendations for concurrent administration of strong CYP3A4 inhibitors
	Terbinafine	Increased plasma levels of aripiprazole and brexpiprazole possible due to inhibited metabolism via CYP2D6. Any interaction will be prolonged (up to 3 months) due to terbinafine's long half-life (200–400 h)
Antihistamine	Trimeprazine (aka alimemazine)	Increased serum level of aripiprazole (by 56%) but not of dehydro-aripiprazole found in a pharmacokinetic study. Mechanism and clinical significance unknown
Antiparkinsonian agent	Levodopa, pramipexole, ropinirole	Worsening of motor symptoms reported in some patients with Parkinson's disease. Antipsychotics reduce dopaminergic activity while antiparkinson agents increase dopamine in the CNS. If an antipsychotic is necessary, consider using clozapine or quetiapine, which have been reported to be less likely to cause worsening control of movement disorders than other antipsychotics. Note: A pilot study of very low-dose aripiprazole (0.625 mg/day) found improvement in levodopa-induced dyskinesias. Case report of hypoglycemia 10 days after adding aripiprazole to levodopa
Antipsychotic combination	General	When combining antipsychotics, consider the risks (e.g., additive adverse effects, cost, increased pill burden) vs. potential and evidence for efficacy
	Clozapine	Preliminary data on adding aripiprazole to clozapine to improve efficacy and/or mitigate adverse effects of clozapine (e.g., weight gain, enuresis)
	Haloperidol	Resolution of haloperidol-induced hyperprolactinemia with addition of aripiprazole (15–30 mg/day) in a small RCT. No significant change in serum haloperidol levels. Case report of asymptomatic QTc prolongation (by 75 ms) when haloperidol (5 mg/day) was added to aripiprazole (30 mg/day)
	Olanzapine	Case report of NMS with the addition of aripiprazole (10 mg/day) to olanzapine (10 mg/day). Case reports of worsening hallucinations, paranoia, and delusions with addition of aripiprazole (10–30 mg/day)
	Paliperidone, risperidone	Preliminary data on adding aripiprazole to resolve risperidone- or paliperidone-induced hyperprolactinemia. Case report of improvement in tardive dyskinesia with addition of aripiprazole (15 mg/day)
	Quetiapine	Case report of worsening irritation, grandiosity, and hallucinations with the addition of aripiprazole (15–30 mg/day) to quetiapine (800 mg/day)
	Ziprasidone	Case report of worsening psychosis with addition of aripiprazole (30 mg/day)

Third-Generation Antipsychotics/TGAs (cont.)

Class of Drug	Example	Interaction Effects
Antiretroviral Protease inhibitor	 Atazanavir, boceprevir, darunavir, fosamprenavir, indinavir, lopinavir, nelfinavir, ritonavir, saquinavir, simeprevir telaprevir, tipranavir	See [16] for additional information CAUTION. Complex interactions likely as various protease inhibitors potently inhibit as well as induce a variety of CYP enzymes (e.g., on CYP3A4 ritonavir is a potent inhibitor; atazanavir, boceprevir, darunavir, saquinavir, and telaprevir are strong inhibitiors; indinavir and fosamprenavir are mild to moderate inhibitors; tipranavir is an inducer. Low boosting doses of ritonavir have little effect on CYP2D6 but higher doses cause inhibition) Increased levels of TGAs possible with enzyme-inhibiting protease inhibitors (e.g., ritonavir, indinavir). Decreased levels possible with unboosted tipranavir Case report of high aripiprazole levels, confusion, and loss of coordination in a patient taking high-dose aripiprazole (50 mg/day) with darunavir and ritonavir (modest CYP2D6 and potent CYP3A4 inhibitors) and duloxetine
Antitubercular	Rifampin	Decreased brexpiprazole AUC (70%) and C_{max} (20%) via CYP3A4 induction
Benzodiazepine	Lorazepam	Increased incidence of sedation and orthostatic hypotension
β-blocker	Metoprolol, propranolol	Increased serum levels of aripiprazole and dehydro-aripiprazole found in one study, possibly due to inhibition of metabolism via CYP2D6 Metoprolol may increase serum levels of brexpiprazole
Cardiac	Ranolazine	CAUTION. In theory, increased plasma levels of aripiprazole and brexpiprazole possible due to inhibited metabolism via CYP2D6
CNS depressant	General (e.g., alcohol, hypnotics, opioids) Alcohol	CAUTION. Potentiation of CNS effects (e.g., sedation, hypotension, respiratory depression) May worsen EPS
Glucocorticoid	Betamethasone, methylprednisolone, hydrocortisone, prednisone	CAUTION. Potential to exacerbate psychiatric conditions, as glucocorticoid-induced psychiatric disorders such as psychosis can occur Glucocorticoids can induce metabolism via CYP3A4. In theory, higher TGA doses may be needed
Grapefruit		Grapefruit juice is a moderate CYP3A4 inhibitor. In theory, increased plasma level of TGAs possible
H₂ antagonist	Famotidine Cimetidine	Decreased rate of absorption (C_{max}) by 37% and 21% and extent of absorption (AUC) by 13% and 15% of aripiprazole and its active metabolite, respectively. Of low clinical significance; no dose adjustment required Cimetidine is a moderate CYP2D6 and CYP3A4 inhibitor. In theory, increased plasma levels of TGAs possible
Lithium		Increased rates of akathisia and tremor generally occur within 6 weeks and resolve with continued use. Case reports of adverse effects with concurrent use, including NMS, Pisa syndrome, and tardive dyskinesia
Metoclopramide		CAUTION. Metoclopramide is a potent central dopamine receptor antagonist that can cause EPS, hyperprolactinemia, and rarely NMS. Concurrent use of an antipsychotic may increase the risk of these adverse effects
Opioid	Methadone	Methadone is a moderate CYP2D6 inhibitor and weak CYP3A4 inhibitor. Potential for increased aripiprazole and brexpiprazole levels
Stimulant	Amphetamine, methylphenidate	CAUTION. Potential to exacerbate psychiatric conditions as stimulant-induced psychosis can occur Antipsychotics can counteract many signs of stimulant toxicity (e.g., anxiety, aggression, visual or auditory hallucinations, psychosis), may impair the stimulatory effect of amphetamines, and have additive adverse effects (e.g., insomnia, restlessness, tremor) Case report of acute dystonia on abrupt discontinuation of methylphenidate. Case report of acute dystonia with recreational amphetamine use

5-HT$_{2A}$ Inverse Agonist Antipsychotic

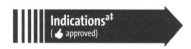 **Product Availability***

Generic Name	Chemical Class	Neuroscience-based Nomenclature*(Pharmacological Target/Mode of Action)	Trade Name	Dosage Forms and Strengths
Pimavanserin	Not part of a class	Serotonin/Antagonist	Nuplazid[(B)]	Tablets: 17 mg

* Refer to Health Canada's Drug Product Database or the FDA's Drugs@FDA for the most current availability information   * Developed by a taskforce consisting of representatives from the American College of Neuropsychopharmacology (ACNP), the Asian College of Neuropsychopharmacology (AsCNP), the European College of Neuropsychopharmacology (ECNP), the International College of Neuropsychopharmacology (CINP), and the International Union of Basic and Clinical Pharmacology (IUPHAR) (see https://nbn2r.com),
[(B)] Not marketed in Canada

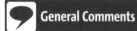 **Indications**[a‡]
(👍 approved)

👍 Parkinson's disease: For the treatment of hallucinations and delusions associated with Parkinson's disease psychosis

General Comments

- Pimavanserin is the first and only medication approved by the FDA for the treatment of hallucinations and delusions associated with Parkinson's disease psychosis
- A Phase 3, double-blind, RCT was stopped early for efficacy but showed that patients with dementia-related psychosis (i.e., Alzheimer's disease, Parkinson's disease, dementia, dementia with Lewy bodies, frontotemporal dementia, or vascular dementia) who had a response to pimavanserin had a lower risk of relapse with continuation of the drug than with discontinuation
- A Phase 2, 26-week, RCT (403 patients) involving stable outpatients with schizophrenia with predominant negative symptoms found a significant change in total 16-item Negative Symptom Assessment scores from baseline for pimavanserin vs. placebo. However, given the small effect size, further investigation is warranted
- In a meta-analysis (4 studies, 680 patients), pimavanserin was found to show a significant improvement in psychotic symptoms in patients with Parkinson's disease compared with placebo[18]
- In a Phase 2 study of Alzheimer's disease psychosis, pimavanserin significantly improved psychosis at week 6 vs. placebo on the Neuropsychiatric Inventory Nursing Home Psychosis Score. In a subgroup of patients with a baseline NPI-NH PS > 12, a substantially larger treatment effect was observed vs. participants with a baseline NPI-NH-PS < 12. Further studies required to determine efficacy and safety of pimavanserin as a potential treatment for hallucinations and delusions of dementia-related psychosis

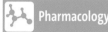 **Pharmacology**

- The mechanism of action of pimavanserin in the treatment of hallucinations and delusions associated with Parkinson's disease psychosis is unknown. However, the drug's effect could be mediated through a combination of inverse agonist and antagonist activity at serotonin 5-HT$_{2A}$ receptors and to a lesser extent at serotonin 5-HT$_{2C}$ receptors
- In vitro, pimavanserin acts as an inverse agonist and antagonist at serotonin 5-HT$_{2A}$ receptors with high binding affinity (Ki value 0.087 nM) and at serotonin 5-HT$_{2C}$ receptors with lower binding affinity (Ki value 0.44 nM). Pimavanserin shows low binding to sigma 1 receptors (Ki value 120 nM) and has no appreciable affinity (Ki value < 300 nM), to serotonin 5-HT$_{2B}$, dopaminergic (including D$_2$), muscarinic, histaminergic, or adrenergic receptors, or to calcium channels

 Dosing

- Recommended dose is 34 mg, taken orally as two 17 mg tablets once daily, without titration
- *Concomitant medications:*
  - Strong inhibitors of CYP3A4 (e.g., ketoconazole): Reduce pimavanserin dose by one-half
  - Strong inducers of CYP3A4 (e.g., carbamazepine): An increase in pimavanserin dose may be needed
- An expert consensus when switching from off-label antipsychotics to pimavanserin: Aim to maintain adequate 5-HT$_{2A}$ antagonism during the switch, thus providing a stable transition with efficacy maintained. Consensus recommendation is to add pimavanserin at the full recommended daily dose of 34 mg for 2–6 weeks in most patients before beginning to taper and discontinue quetiapine or clozapine over several days to weeks

[a] Adult population unless otherwise stated   [‡] Indications listed here do not necessarily apply to all countries. Please refer to a country's regulatory database (e.g., US Food and Drug Administration, Health Canada Drug Product Database) for the most current availability information and indications

5-HT₂ₐ Inverse Agonist Antipsychotic (cont.)

Renal Impairment	• No dosage adjustment needed in patients with mild–moderate renal impairment. Use not recommended in patients with severe renal impairment
Hepatic Impairment	• Not recommended in patients with hepatic impairment

 Pharmacokinetics
- Also see table p. 209
- Ingestion of a high-fat meal had no significant effect on rate (C_{max}) and extent (AUC) of exposure
- T_{max}: 6 h (range 4–24 h)
- Approximately 95% protein bound
- Half-life: 57 h (active metabolite: 200 h)
- Volume of distribution: 2173 (307) L
- Predominantly metabolized by CYP3A4 and CYP3A5, to a lesser extent by CYP2J2, CYP2D6, and various other CYP and FMO enzymes
- Approximately 0.55% eliminated as unchanged drug in urine and 1.53% eliminated in feces after 10 days

 Adverse Effects
- Most common adverse reactions ($\geq$ 2% for pimavanserin and greater than placebo): Peripheral edema (7% vs. 2%), nausea (7% vs. 4%), confusion state (6% vs. 3%), hallucination (5% vs. 3%), constipation (4% vs. 3%), and gait disturbance (2% vs. 1%)

Cardiovascular Effects	

- Pimavanserin prolongs the QT interval. Avoid in patients with known QT prolongation or in combination with other drugs known to prolong QT interval including Class 1A antiarrhythmics (e.g., procainamide, quinidine) or Class 3 antiarrhythmics (e.g., amiodarone, sotalol), certain antipsychotic medications (e.g., chlorpromazine, ziprasidone), and certain antibiotics (e.g., gatifloxacin, moxifloxacin)
- Avoid in patients with a history of cardiac arrhythmias, as well as other circumstances that may increase the risk of the occurrence of torsades de pointes and/or sudden death, including symptomatic bradycardia, hypokalemia, or hypomagnesemia, and the presence of congenital prolongation of the QT interval

 D/C Discontinuation Syndrome
- No information available

 Precautions
- Antipsychotic drugs increase the all-cause risk of death in elderly patients with dementia-related psychosis

 Toxicity
- No information available

 Lab Tests/Monitoring
- Therapeutic range not established for pimavanserin

Use in Pregnancy◇
- No data on pimavanserin use in pregnant women that would allow assessment of the drug-associated risk of major congenital malformations or miscarriage

Breast Milk	

- No information regarding the presence of pimavanserin in human milk, effects on the breastfed infant, or effects on milk production
- The developmental and health benefits of breastfeeding should be considered along with the mother's clinical need for pimavanserin

◇ See p. 473 for further information on drug use in pregnancy and effects on breast milk

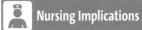
- See p. 126
- Taken once daily with or without food
- CAUTION: Grapefruit juice may increase the level of pimavanserin
- Advise patient to inform their healthcare providers if there are any changes to their current prescription or over-the-counter medications, since there is a potential for drug interactions

Drug Interactions

- Clinically significant interactions are listed below
- For more interaction information on any given combination, also see the corresponding chapter for the second agent

Class of Drug	Example	Interaction Effects
CYP3A4 inducer	Carbamazepine, phenytoin, rifampin, St. John's wort	May reduce pimavanserin exposure, resulting in a potential decrease in efficacy
CYP3A4 inhibitor	Clarithromycin, indinavir, itraconazole, ketoconazole	Increased pimavanserin exposure
QT interval prolonging agents	Class 1 A antiarrhythmics (disopyramide, procainamide, quinidine), class 3 antiarrhythmics (amiodarone, sotalol), antipsychotics (chlorpromazine, ziprasidone), antibiotics (gatifloxacin, moxifloxacin)	Concomitant use of drug that prolongs QT interval may add to QT effects of pimavanserin and increase risk of cardiac arrhythmia

Effects of Antipsychotics on Neurotransmitters/Receptors*

	FGAs												
	Chlorprom-azine	Flu-penthixol	Fluphen-azine	Haloperi-dol	Loxapine	Methotri-meprazine	Periciazine	Perphen-azine	Pimozide	Thiori-dazine	Thiothix-ene	Trifluo-perazine	Zuclo-penthixol
D_2 blockade	++++	+++++	+++++	+++++	++++	+++	++++	+++++	++++	++++	+++++	++++	+++++
H_1 blockade	+++	+++	+++	+	+++	+++++	?	++++	+	+++	+++	++	+++
M_1 blockade	+++	+++	+	+	++	?	?	+	+	++++	+	+	++
M_3 blockade	+++	?	+	+	++	?	?	+	?	+++	?	?	?
α_1 blockade	++++	+++	+++	+++	+++	?	?	+++	+++	++++	++	+++	++++
α_2 blockade	++	++	+	+	+	?	+	++	++	+	++	+	++
$5\text{-}HT_{1A}$ blockade	+	?	++	+	+	?	?	++	++	++	++	++	?
$5\text{-}HT_{2A}$ blockade	++++	++++	++++	++++	++++	++++	?	++++	+++	++++	+++	++++	++++
$5\text{-}HT_{2C}$ blockade	+++	?	++	+	+++	?	?	++	+	+++	+	++	?
$5\text{-}HT_7$ blockade	+++	?	++++	++	+++	?	?	+++	+++++	+++	+++	++	?

	SGAs										TGAs		
	Asenapine	Clozapine	Iloperidone	Lumatepe-rone	Lurasidone	Olanzapine	Paliperi-done	Quetiapine	Risperi-done	Ziprasi-done	Aripipra-zole	Brexpi-prazole	Cariprazine
D_2 blockade	++++	++	+++	+++	++++	+++	++++	++	++++	++++	+++++[a]	+++++[a]	++++++[a]
H_1 blockade	++++	++++	++	−	+	++++	+++	+++	+++	+++	+++	+++	+++
M_1 blockade	+	+++[a]	+	−	+	++++	−	++	−	−	−	+	−
M_3 blockade	?	+++	+	−	?	+++	−	+	+	+	+	?	−
α_1 blockade	++++	++++	++++	+++	+++	+++	++++	+++	++++	+++	+++	+++	++
α_2 blockade	++++	++	++	+++	+++	++	+++	+++	++	++	+++	+++	?
$5\text{-}HT_{1A}$ blockade	++++	++[a]	++[a]	−	++++[a]	+	++	++[a]	++	+++[a]	++++[a]	+++++[a]	++++[a]
$5\text{-}HT_{2A}$ blockade	+++++	+++	+++++	+++++	+++++	++++	+++++	+++	+++++	++++	++++	+++++	+++
$5\text{-}HT_{2C}$ blockade	+++++	+++	+++	++	++	++++	+++	+	+++	+++	+++	?	++
$5\text{-}HT_7$ blockade	+++++	+++	++	−	+++++	++	+++	++	++++	++++	++++	++++	++

[a] Partial agonist

Key: K_i (nM) > 10,000 = −; 1000–10,000 = +; 100–1000 = ++; 10–100 = +++; 1–10 = ++++; 0.1–1 = +++++; 0.001–0.1 = ++++++; ? = unknown

See p. 195 for Pharmacological Effects on Neurotransmitters.

Adapted from: [19, 20, 21]. See also the National Institute of Mental Health's Psychoactive Drug Screening Program. Available at http://pdsp.med.unc.edu

* The ratio of K_i values (inhibition constant) between various neurotransmitters/receptors determines the pharmacological profile for any one drug

Pharmacological Effects of Antipsychotics on Neurotransmitters/Receptor Subtypes

D_2
- Antagonism of postsynaptic D_2 receptors:
  - In mesolimbic tract – reduction in positive symptoms (note: TGAs are partial agonists at D_2 receptors, partial agonism of this receptor may also reduce positive symptoms; partial agonist behaves like an antagonist in cases where a hyperdopaminergic state exists)
  - In nigrostriatal tract – EPS (e.g., dystonias, pseudoparkinsonism, akathisia, tardive movement disorders, etc.)
  - In tuberoinfundibular tract – prolactin elevation (e.g., galactorrhea, sexual dysfunction, etc.)
  - In mesocortical tract – may exacerbate negative symptoms

H_1
- Antagonism of H_1 receptors:
  - Anti-emetic effect, anxiolytic effects
  - Sedation, drowsiness, appetite increase, weight gain

M_1
- Antagonism of M_1 receptors:
  - Mitigation of extrapyramidal adverse effects
  - Dry mouth, dry eyes, blurred vision, constipation, urinary retention, sinus tachycardia, QRS changes, confusion, worsening cognition, delirium
  - Potentiation of effects of drugs with anticholinergic properties

M_3
- Antagonism of M_3 receptors:
  - Beta cell failure, reduced insulin release, glucose intolerance, type 2 diabetes mellitus

α_1
- Antagonism of α_1 adrenergic receptors:
  - Postural hypotension, dizziness, reflex tachycardia, sedation

α_2
- Antagonism of α_2-adrenergic receptors:
  - May improve cognitive deficits and have antidepressant activity
  - Antagonism of presynaptic α_2-adrenergic receptors enhances serotonin and norepinephrine neurotransmission

$5\text{-}HT_{1A}$
- Agonism/partial agonism of $5\text{-}HT_{1A}$ serotonergic receptors:
  - Postulated to be associated with procognitive, anxiolytic, and antidepressant effects
  - Enhances dopamine release in prefrontal cortex

$5\text{-}HT_{2A}$
- Antagonism of $5\text{-}HT_{2A}$ serotonergic receptors:
  - Sedation, prodopaminergic actions may ameliorate EPS, and postulated to improve (not worsen) negative, cognitive, and mood symptoms
  - Enhances dopamine release in prefrontal cortex

$5\text{-}HT_{2C}$
- Antagonism of $5\text{-}HT_{2C}$ serotonergic receptors:
  - Increased appetite, weight gain
  - Postulated to be associated with procognitive and antidepressant effects
  - Inhibits dopamine and norepinephrine release in prefrontal cortex

$5\text{-}HT_7$
- Antagonism of $5\text{-}HT_7$ serotonergic receptors:
  - Postulated to be associated with procognitive, anxiolytic, and antidepressant effects

Relative Tolerability Profiles of Antipsychotics

Adverse Effect	Higher Likelihood	Moderate Likelihood	Lower Likelihood
Sedation	LP-FGAs Clozapine Olanzapine Quetiapine	MP-FGAs Asenapine Lurasidone Risperidone Ziprasidone	HP-FGAs TGAs Iloperidone Lumateperone Paliperidone
EPS	HP-FGAs	MP-FGAs Cariprazine Lurasidone Paliperidone Risperidone Ziprasidone	LP-FGAs Aripiprazole[a] Asenapine Brexpiprazole Clozapine Iloperidone Lumateperone Olanzapine Quetiapine
Tardive dyskinesia	FGAs	Asenapine Iloperidone Lumateperone Lurasidone Olanzapine Paliperidone Risperidone Ziprasidone	TGAs Clozapine Quetiapine
Seizures	HP-FGAs LP-FGAs Clozapine	–	TGAs Asenapine Iloperidone Lumateperone Lurasidone Olanzapine Paliperidone Quetiapine Risperidone Ziprasidone
Hyperprolactinemia	HP-FGAs Paliperidone Risperidone	MP-FGAs Asenapine Iloperidone Olanzapine Ziprasidone	LP-FGAs TGAs Clozapine Lumateperone Quetiapine

Adverse Effect	Higher Likelihood	Moderate Likelihood	Lower Likelihood
Anticholinergic effects	LP-FGAs Clozapine Olanzapine Quetiapine	MP-FGAs	HP-FGAs TGAs Asenapine Iloperidone Lumateperone Lurasidone Paliperidone Risperidone Ziprasidone
Orthostatic hypotension/ reflex tachycardia	LP-FGAs Clozapine	MP-FGAs Asenapine Iloperidone Paliperidone Quetiapine Risperidone Ziprasidone	HP-FGAs TGAs Lumateperone Lurasidone Olanzapine
Weight gain (and possibly other metabolic effects)	Clozapine Iloperidone Olanzapine	LP-FGAs MP-FGAs Asenapine Paliperidone Quetiapine Risperidone	HP-FGAs TGAs Lumateperone Lurasidone Ziprasidone
QT prolongation (CredibleMeds Worldwide rating)	Known risk of TdP: Chlorpromazine Haloperidol Pimozide Thioridazine	Possible risk of TdP: Aripiprazole Asenapine Clozapine Flupenthixol Iloperidone Lumateperone Paliperidone Perphenazine Zuclopenthixol	Conditional risk of TdP: Amisulpride Olanzapine Quetiapine Risperidone Ziprasidone

[a] Moderate likelihood of akathisia

• HP-FGAs = high-potency FGAs, LP-FGAs = low-potency FGAs, MP-FGAs = medium-potency FGAs, TdP = torsades de pointes (see p. 154 for definitions of CredibleMeds Worldwide risk categories for TdP)

Frequency (%) of Adverse Reactions to Antipsychotics at Therapeutic Doses

Reaction	FIRST-GENERATION AGENTS												
	Chlor-promazine	Flu-penthixol	Fluphen-azine	Haloperi-dol	Loxapine	Methotri-meprazine	Periciazine	Perphena-zine	Pimozide	Thiorida-zine	Thiothix-ene	Trifluoper-azine	Zuclo-penthixol
CNS Effects													
Drowsiness, sedation	> 30	> 2	> 2	> 2(a)	> 30	> 30	> 30	> 10	> 10	> 30	> 10	> 2	> 30
Insomnia, agitation	< 2	< 2	> 2	> 10	< 2	< 2	< 2	> 10	> 2	< 2	> 10	> 2	> 10
Extrapyramidal Effects													
Parkinsonism	> 10	> 30	> 30	> 30(b)	> 30	> 10	> 2	> 10	> 30	> 2	> 30	> 30	> 30
Akathisia	> 2	> 30	> 30	> 30	> 30	> 2	> 2	> 10	> 10	> 2	> 30	> 30	> 10
Dystonic reactions	> 2	> 10	> 10	> 30(b)	> 10	< 2	< 2	> 10	> 2	< 2	> 2	> 10	> 10(b)
Anticholinergic Effects	> 30	> 10	> 2	> 2	> 10	> 30	> 30	> 10	> 2	> 30	> 2	> 2	> 10(c)
Cardiovascular Effects													
Orthostatic hypotension	> 30(a)	> 2	> 2	> 2	> 10	> 30(a)(d)	> 10	> 10	> 2	> 30	> 2	> 10	> 2
Tachycardia	> 10	> 2	> 10	< 2	> 10	> 10	> 10	> 10	> 2	< 2	> 2	< 2	> 2
ECG abnormalities*	> 30(e)	> 2	< 2	< 2	< 2	> 10	< 2	> 2	> 2(f)	> 30(e)	< 2	< 2	< 2
QTc prolongation (> 450 ms)	> 2(e)	< 2	> 2(e)	> 2(e)	–	> 2	> 2	< 2	> 2(f)	> 10(e)	< 2	> 2	< 2
Endocrine Effects													
Sexual dysfunction**	> 30(g)	> 30(g)	> 30(g)	> 30(g)	> 2	> 2(g)	> 10(g)	> 10(g)	> 30	> 30(g)	> 2(g)	> 30(g)	> 30(g)
Galactorrhea	> 30	–	> 10	< 2	> 2	> 30	> 10	> 10	< 2	> 30	< 2	> 10	–
Weight gain	> 30	> 10	> 30	> 10	< 2(h)	> 10	> 10	> 10	> 2(h)	> 30	> 10	> 10	> 10
Hyperglycemia	> 30	> 10	> 10	> 10	> 2(i)	> 2(i)	> 2(i)	> 10	> 2	> 2(i)	> 2(i)	> 2	> 2(i)
Hyperlipidemia	> 30	?	?	> 2	> 10	?	?	> 2(i)	?	> 30	?	?	?
Ocular Effects*													
Lenticular pigmentation	> 2	< 2	< 2	< 2	< 2	> 2	> 2	< 2	< 2	> 2	< 2	< 2	< 2
Pigmentary retinopathy	> 2	< 2	–	–	< 2	> 2	–	< 2	–	> 10	< 2	< 2	–
Blood dyscrasias	< 2	< 2	< 2	< 2	< 2	< 2	< 2	< 2	< 2	< 2	< 2	< 2	< 2
Hepatic disorder	< 2	< 2	< 2	< 2	< 2	< 2	< 2	< 2	< 2	< 2	< 2	< 2	< 2
Seizures#	< 2(a)	< 2	< 2	< 2	< 2	< 2	< 2	< 2	< 2	< 2	< 2	< 2	< 2
Skin Reactions													
Photosensitivity	> 10	< 2	< 2	< 2	< 2	> 10	> 2	< 2	–	> 10(e)	< 2	< 2	< 2
Rashes	> 10	> 2	< 2	< 2	> 2	> 2	> 2	< 2	> 2	> 10	< 2	< 2	< 2
Pigmentation***	> 30(e)	–	–	< 2	–	< 2	–	–	–	> 2	> 2	–	< 2

Reaction	SECOND-GENERATION AGENTS										THIRD-GENERATION AGENTS		
	Asena-pine	Clozapine	Iloperi-done	Lumate-perone	Lurasi-done	Olanza-pine	Paliperi-done	Quetia-pine	Risperi-done	Ziprasi-done	Aripipra-zole	Brexpipra-zole	Caripra-zine
CNS Effects													
Drowsiness, sedation	>10	>30	>10	>2	>10	>30	>2	>30	>10[d]	>10	>10	>2	>2
Insomnia, agitation	>10	>2	>10	–	>2	>10	>10	>10	>10	>30	>10	>2	>2
Extrapyramidal Effects													
Parkinsonism	?	>2	<2	<2	>2	>2	>2	>2	>10[k]	>2	>2	>2	>2
Akathisia	?	>10	>2	<2	>10	>10	>2	>2	>10[k]	>2	>10	>2	>2
Dystonic reactions	?	<2	<2	<2	>2	<2	<2	<2	<2[k]	>2	<2	<2	<2
Anticholinergic Effects	>2	>30[c]	>2	>2	<2	>10	>2	>30	>2	>10	<2	>2	<2
Cardiovascular Effects													
Orthostatic hypotension	>10	>10–30[d]	>10	–	>2	>2	>2	>10	>10[d]	>10	>2	>2	>2
Tachycardia	<2	>10[d]	>10	–	–	>10[l]	>2	>10	<2	<2	>2	<2	<2
ECG abnormalities*	?	>30[e]	<2	–	<2	<2	<2	<2	>2	>2[e]	<2	<2	<2
QTc prolongation (>450 ms)	9	<2[e]	<2	–	–	<2	>2	<2	<2	<2[e]	–	–	–
Endocrine Effects													
Sexual dysfunction**	?	<2[g]	>2	?	<2	>30[g]	<2	>30[g]	>30[g]	<2[g]	<2[g]	<2[g]	<2[g]
Galactorrhea	?	<2	<2	?	<2	>2	<2	–	>10	>2	<2	<2	<2
Weight gain	>10	>30	>10	–	<2	>30	>10	>10	>10	>2	>2[h]	>2[h]	<2[h]
Hyperglycemia	>10	>30	?	>2	<2	>30	?	>30	>10	>2	<2	<2	<2
Hyperlipidemia	>10	>30	?	>2	<2	>30	?	>10	>10	<2	<2	<2	<2
Ocular Effects*													
Lenticular pigmentation	?	–	?	?	–	–	?	<2	–	–	–	–	–
Pigmentary retinopathy	?	–	?	?	–	–	–	–	–	–	–	–	–
Blood dyscrasias	<2	<2[m]	?	?	<2	<2	?	–	<2	<2	<2	<2	<2
Hepatic disorder	>2	>2	<2	<2	–	>2	?	>2	<2	–	<2	<2	<2
Seizures#	<2	>2[n]	<2	?	<2	<2	<2	<2	<2	–	<2	<2	<2
Skin Reactions													
Photosensitivity	?	>2	?	?	–	–	?	–	>2		<2	<2	<2
Rashes	?	>2	?	?	<2	<2	?	<2	<2	>2	>2	<2	<2
Pigmentation***	?	–	?	?	–	–	?	–	<2	–	–	–	–

Data are pooled from separate studies and are not necessarily comparable; the figures in the table cannot be used to predict the incidence of side effects in the course of usual medical practice, where patient characteristics and other factors differ from those in the clinical trials.

– = None reported in literature perused

* ECG abnormalities usually without cardiac injury including ST segment depression, flattened T waves, and increased U wave amplitude,   ** Includes impotence, inhibition of ejaculation, anorgasmia,   *** Usually seen after prolonged use,   # In nonepileptic patients

[a] More frequent with rapid dose increase,   [b] Lower incidence with depot preparation,   [c] Sialorrhea reported,   [d] May be higher at start of therapy or with rapid dose increase,   [e] Higher doses pose greater risk,   [f] Pimozide above 20 mg daily poses greater risk,   [g] Priapism reported,   [h] Weight loss reported,   [i] Reported to occur, but no definitive data published as to incidence,   [k] Increased risk with oral doses above 10 mg daily,   [l] Bradycardia frequent with IM olanzapine; often accompanied by hypotension,   [m] Risk < 2% with strict monitoring (legal requirement in North America),   [n] Risk increased with doses above 300 mg

Antipsychotic Doses and Pharmacokinetics (Oral and Short-Acting Injections)

FIRST-GENERATION AGENTS (FGAs)										
Drug	Oral CPZ Equiva-lents (mg)[1]	Monograph Doses for Psychosis	Bio-availability	Protein Binding	Peak Plasma Level (h) (T_{max})	Elimination Half-Life (h)	Metabolizing Enzymes[2] / Transporters (CYP450; other)	Enzyme Inhibition[3] / Transporters (CYP450; other)	% D_2 Receptor Occupancy[4] (dose & plasma level)	% 5-HT$_{2A}$ Occu-pancy (dose)
Chlorpromazine (Largactil[C], Thorazine[B])	100	Oral: Start: 25–75 mg daily in 2–4 divided doses; increase by 20–50 mg twice weekly. Recommended maximum: 1 g/day. Give od or bid for maintenance with larger dose at at bedtime Short-acting IM: Start: 25 mg followed by 25–50 mg in 1 h if needed, then q 3–12 h prn. Can increase over several days. Recommended maximum (acute psychosis or mania): 400 mg q 4–6 h	Oral: 25–65%	95–99% (to albumin)	Oral: 0.51	Oral: 16–30	1A2[w], **2D6**[p], 3A4[w]; UGT1A4	1A2, **2D6**[p], 3A4[w], 2C9[w], 2C19, 2E1; P-gp	78–80% (100–200 mg; 10 nmol/L)	?
Flupenthixol[C] (Fluanxol)	2	Oral: Start: 1 mg tid; increase by 1 mg q 2–3 days if needed. Usual = 3–6 mg/day in divided doses; up to 12 mg/day used in some patients	30–70%	99%	3–8	26–36	?	2D6[w]	70–74% (5–10 mg; 2–5 nmol/L)	?
Fluphenazine HCL (Moditen[C], Prolixin[B])	2	Oral: Start: 2.5–10 mg daily in divided doses q 6–8 h. Maintenance: 1–5 mg/day. Doses greater than 20 mg = use with caution Short-acting IM or SC: Start: 1.25 mg; range 2.5–10 mg daily divided q 6–8 h. Doses greater than 10 mg = use with caution	1–50%	90–99%	Oral: 0.5 Short-acting IM: 1.5–2	Oral: 13–58 Short-acting IM: 13–58	1A2, 2D6; P-gp	1A2, **2D6**[p], 3A4[w], 2E1 2C8/9; P-gp	?	?
Haloperidol (Haldol)	2	Oral: Start: 1.5–3 mg divided bid or tid (elderly 0.25–1 mg od or divided bid) Maintenance: 4–12 mg divided od–tid Usual maximum = 20 mg/day 85–100 mg daily used rarely	40–80%	92% (to α$_1$-AGP)	0.5–3	12–36	1A2[w], 2D6[w], **3A4**[p]	**2D6**, 3A4; P-gp[w]	75–89% (4–6 mg; 6–13 nmol/L)	?
Haloperidol lactate		Short-acting IM: 2–5 mg (0.5–1 mg in the elderly) q 4–8 h prn; may repeat q 1 h if required Maximum: 20 mg/day (elderly ~5 mg/day)			Short-acting IM (lactate): 10–20 min					

Drug	Oral CPZ Equiva-lents (mg)[1]	Monograph Doses for Psychosis	Bio-availability	Protein Binding	Peak Plasma Level (h) (T_{max})	Elimination Half-Life (h)	Metabolizing Enzymes[2] / Transporters (CYP450; other)	Enzyme Inhibition[3] / Transporters (CYP450; other)	% D$_2$ Receptor Occupancy[4] (dose & plasma level)	% 5-HT$_{2A}$ Occu-pancy (dose)
Loxapine (Adasuve[B], Loxapac[C], Loxitane[B])	20	Oral: Start: 10 mg bid (up to 50 mg/day if needed) Usual = 60–100 mg/day divided bid–qid Usual maintenance: 20-60 mg/day Maximum = 250 mg/day Oral inhalation: 10 mg via single-use inhaler Maximum = 10 mg/day	33%	97%	Oral = 1–2 Oral inhalation = 2 min	Oral = 3 (range 1–14); 5–19 (metabolites)	1A2, 2D6, 3A4; UGT1A4	P-gp	60–80% (15–30 mg)	58–75% (10–30 mg) 75–90% metabo-lite (> 30 mg)
Loxapine hydrochloride		Short-acting IM: 12.5–50 mg q 4–6 h prn or longer			Short-acting IM = 2–5	Short-acting IM = 12 h (range 8–23); 8–30 (metabolites)				
Methotrimeprazine/ Levomepromazine[C] (Nozinan)	50	Oral (for severe psychosis): Start: 50–200 mg daily divided into 2 or 3 doses. Caution if starting with 100 mg or greater/day. Increase up to 1 g or more a day if needed Short-acting IM: 75–100 mg daily given as 3 or 4 deep IM injections	Oral: 21–50%	?	Oral: 1–3 Short-acting IM: 30–90 min	Oral: 16–78	1A2, 2D6, 3A2; P-gp	**2D6**[p]; P-gp	?	?
Periciazine[C] (Neuleptil)	8	Oral: 5–20 mg AM + 10–40 mg PM Maintenance: 2.5–15 mg AM + 5–30 mg PM	?	?	2	~12	2D6, 3A4	P-gp	?	?
Perphenazine (Trilafon)	8	Oral: Start: 8–16 mg bid to qid. Recommended maximum: 64 mg/day	25%	91–92%	1–4	9–21	1A2, **2D6**[p], 3A4, 2C9, 2C19	1A2[w], **2D6**[p], 3A4, 2C9, 2C19; P-gp	79% (4–8 mg)	?
Pimozide (Orap)	2	Oral: Start: 2–4 mg once daily; increase by 2–4 mg q week; average dose: 6 mg/day (usual range 2–12 mg/day) Doses above 20 mg/day not recommended[x]	15–50%	97%	6–8 (range 4–12)	29–55[y]	1A2[w], **3A4**[p]	**2D6**[p], 3A4; P-gp[p]	77–79% (4–8 mg)	?

Antipsychotic Doses and Pharmacokinetics (Oral and Short-Acting Injections) (cont.)

FIRST-GENERATION AGENTS (FGAs)											
Drug	Oral CPZ Equiva-lents (mg)[1]	Monograph Doses for Psychosis	Bio-availability	Protein Binding	Peak Plasma Level (h) (T_{max})	Elimination Half-Life (h)	Metabolizing Enzymes[2] / Transporters (CYP450; other)	Enzyme Inhibition[3] / Transporters (CYP450; other)	% D_2 Receptor Occupancy[4] (dose & plasma level)	% 5-HT$_{2A}$ Occu-pancy (dose)
Thioridazine[B],[x] (Mellaril)	100	Oral: 150–400 mg daily in outpatients with severe symptoms given in 2–4 divided doses; 200–800 mg daily in hospitalized patients; Recommended maximum: 800 mg/day	10–60%	97–99%	1–4	9–30	1A2[w], 2D6[w], 2C19[w]	1A2, **2D6**[p], 2C8/9, 2E1; P-gp; Inducer of 3A4	74–81% (100–400 mg; 620–900 nmol/L)	?
Thiothixene[B] (Navane)	5	Oral: Start: 2 mg tid – 5 mg bid. Usual = 15–30 mg od; > 60 mg/day rarely increases response	50%	90–99%	1–3	34	**1A2**[p]	2D6[w]	?	?
Trifluoperazine (Stelazine)	5	Oral: Start: 2–5 mg bid or tid. Usual = 15–20 mg/day. A few may need 40 mg/day or more. 80 mg/day or more rarely necessary	?	95–99%	2–4	7–18	1A2; P-gp; UGT1A4	P-gp	75–80% (5–10 mg)	?
Zuclopenthixol[C] (Clopixol)	8	Oral: Start: 10–50 mg/day divided bid—tid; increase by 10–20 mg q 2–3 days; usual daily dose: 20–60 mg; doses above 100 mg/day not recommended	44%	98%	2–4	12–28	**2D6**[p]	2D6	> 70%	?
Zuclopenthixol acetate[C] (Clopixol Acuphase)		Usual dose: 50–150 mg IM and repeated q 2–3 days prn to a maximum cumulative dose of 400 mg and maximum of 4 injections (a 2nd injection may need to be given 1–2 days later in some patients)	–	98%	24–48	48–72	**2D6**[p]	2D6	> 70%	?

[1] Oral dose equivalents: Chlorpromazine (CPZ) equivalents: represent the doses that are equivalent to 100 mg/day chlorpromazine from multiple sources,   [2] CYP450 isoenzymes involved in drug metabolism,   [3] CYP450 isoenzymes inhibited by drug,
[4] D_2 receptor occupancy correlates better to plasma level than to dose, and appears to relate to clinical efficacy in controlling positive symptoms of schizophrenia as well as risk of extrapyramidal adverse effects (if > 80%)
[B] Not marketed in Canada,   [C] Not marketed in the USA
[p] Potent activity,   [w] Weak activity,   [x] Monitor cardiac function,   [y] Half-life longer (mean 66–111 h) in children and adults with Tourette's syndrome

		SECOND-GENERATION AGENTS (SGAs)								
Drug	Oral dose equivalents (mg)[1]	Monograph Doses for Psychosis (for doses for other indications and in renal impairment, see pp. 149–150)	Bioavaila-bility	Protein Binding	Peak Plasma Level (h) (T_{max})	Elimination Half-Life (h)	Metabolizing Enzymes[2]/ Transporters (CYP450; other)	Enzyme Inhibition[3]/ Transporters (CYP450; other)	% D_2 Receptor Occupancy[4] (dose & plasma level)	% 5-HT_{2A} Occu-pancy (dose)
Asenapine (Saphris)	Minimum effective dose method: OLA 1 mg = 1.33 (1) RIS 1 mg = 5 (2.5) HAL 1 mg = 2.5 (2.2) CPZ 100 mg = 4 (3.6) Mean dose method: OLA 1 mg = 0.89	Oral: 5 mg sublingually bid – starting and target dose Maximum: 10 mg bid	35% (< 2% if swallowed; reduced if food/drink taken within 10 min)	95% (including albumin and α_1-AGP)	0.5–1	24	**1A2**[(p)], 2D6[(w)], 3A4[(w)]; **UGT1A4**[(p)]	2D6[(w)]	79% (4.8 mg sublingual)	
Clozapine (Clozaril, FazaClo ODT[(B)])	Minimum effective dose method: OLA 1 mg = 40 (30) RIS 1 mg = 150 (75) HAL 1 mg = 75 (67) CPZ 100 mg = 120 (107) Mean dose method: OLA 1 mg = 30.62	Oral: 12.5 mg once or twice daily to start; increase gradually by 25–50 mg/day increments up to 300–450 mg/day in divided doses[(F)] by the end of 2 weeks; subsequent increases ≤ once or twice/week in increments ≤100 mg/day Usual range: 300–600 mg/day Maximum: 900 mg/day[(G)] Prescribing restrictions: see p. 149	90–95% (40–60% after 1st pass metabolism)	95–97% (to α_1-AGP)	1–6 (mean 2.5)	6–33 (mean 12; parent) 11–105 (active metabolite) Caution in the elderly Reduced in smokers (20–40% shorter)	**1A2**[(p)], 2D6[(w)], 3A4[(m)], 2C9[(w)], 2C19[(m)], 2E1[(w)]; FMO; UGT1A4; P-gp[(w)]	1A2[(w)], 2D6[(w)], 3A4, 2C9[(w)], 2C19, 2E1[(w)]	38–68% (300–900 mg; 600–2500 nmol/L)[(G)]	85–94% (> 125 mg)
Iloperidone (Fanapt)[(B)]	Minimum effective dose method: OLA 1 mg = 1.07 (1.2) RIS 1 mg = 4 (3) HAL 1 mg = 2 (2.7) CPZ 100 mg = 3.2 (4.3) Mean dose method: N/A	Oral: 1 mg bid to start and increase daily by 2–4 mg over 7 days to a target dose of 6–12 mg bid Maximum: 24 mg/day	96%	~95%	2–4	18[(K)]–33[(D)] (parent) 26[(K)]–37[(D)] and 23[(K)]–31[(D)] (active metabolites)	**2D6**[(p)], **3A4**[(p)] (Reduce dose by 50% in poor metabolizers of 2D6. Dose changes required with concurrent use of drugs that affect 2D6 and/or 3A4)	–		

Antipsychotic Doses and Pharmacokinetics (Oral and Short-Acting Injections) (cont.)

SECOND-GENERATION AGENTS (SGAs)										
Drug	Oral dose equivalents (mg)[1]	Monograph Doses for Psychosis (for doses for other indications and in renal impairment, see pp. 149–150)	Bioavaila-bility	Protein Binding	Peak Plasma Level (h) (T_{max})	Elimination Half-Life (h)	Metabolizing Enzymes[2] / Transporters (CYP450; other)	Enzyme Inhibition[3] / Transporters (CYP450; other)	% D_2 Receptor Occupancy[4] (dose & plasma level)	% 5-HT$_{2A}$ Occupancy (dose)
Lumateperone (Caplyta)[B]	Minimum effective dose method: N/A Mean dose method: N/A	Oral: 42 mg once daily with food Dose titration not required	4.4%	97.4%	1–2	18	Various UGTs, 2D6, 3A4 (Avoid concomitant use with strong CYP3A4 inhibitors or inducers)		39 (60 mg)	?
Lurasidone (Latuda[B])	Minimum effective dose method: OLA 1 mg = 5.33 (4) RIS 1 mg = 20 (10) HAL 1 mg = 10 (8.9) CPZ 100 mg = 16 (14.2) Mean dose method: N/A	Oral: 40 mg once daily to start Maximum: 160 mg once daily	9–19%	>99.8% (to albumin and α_1-AGP)	1–3	18–37 (parent) 7.5–10 (active metabolite)	**3A4**[p] (Avoid concomitant use with strong CYP3A4 inhibitors or inducers)	–	63–79% (40–80 mg)	?
Olanzapine (Zyprexa, Zyprexa Zydis)	Minimum effective dose method: RIS 1 mg = 3.75 (2.5) HAL 1 mg = 1.88 (2.2) CPZ 100 mg = 3 (3.6) Mean dose method: OLA 1 mg = 1	Oral: 5–10 mg once daily to start, with a target of 10 mg/day within several days Further dose increases of ≤ 5 mg/day at intervals of ≥ 1 week Maximum: 20 mg/day (higher doses, e.g., 40 mg/day, have safety but not efficacy data)	Oral: 57–80%	93% (to albumin and α_1-AGP)	Oral: 5–8	21–54 (30 mean) No change in hepatic disease (only based on single-dose study) or renal disease. Prolonged in the elderly (1.5 times longer) and females (30% longer – clinical significance unclear) Reduced in smokers (40% shorter)	1A2[p], 2D6[w]; FMO; UGT1A4[p]	1A2[w], 2D6[w], 3A4[w], 2C9[w], 2C19[w]	55–80% (5–20 mg; 59–187 nmol/L) 83–88% (30–40 mg)	80–90% (5–20 mg)

Drug	Oral dose equivalents (mg)[1]	Monograph Doses for Psychosis (for doses for other indications and in renal impairment, see pp. 149–150)	Bioavaila-bility	Protein Binding	Peak Plasma Level (h) (T_{max})	Elimination Half-Life (h)	Metabolizing Enzymes[2] / Transporters (CYP450; other)	Enzyme Inhibition[3] / Transporters (CYP450; other)	% D$_2$ Receptor Occupancy[4] (dose & plasma level)	% 5-HT$_{2A}$ Occu-pancy (dose)
(Zyprexa IntraMuscular)		Short-acting IM: 10 mg to start (2.5–5 mg in the elderly) If needed, give 2nd dose of 5–10 mg 2 h after 1st; if 3rd dose needed, give $\geq$ 4 h after 2nd dose Maximum: 30 mg/day (high rate of orthostatic hypotension) with no more than 3 injections in 24 h			Short-acting IM: 15–45 min (C_{max} 4–5 fold > same oral dose)					
Paliperidone (active metabolite of risperidone) (Invega)	Minimum effective dose method: OLA 1 mg = 0.4 (0.6) RIS 1 mg = 1.5 (1.5) HAL 1 mg = 0.75 (1.3) CPZ 100 mg = 1.2 (2.1) Mean dose method: N/A	Oral: 6 mg once daily (preferably in AM) If needed, increase by 3 mg q 4–5 days to a maximum of 12 mg/day	28%	74% (to albumin and α_1-AGP)	24	23 In mild, moderate, and severe renal impairment: 24, 40, and 51, respectively	2D6[w], 3A4[w], P-gp (Minimally metabolized, < 7%)	P-gp[w] (at high doses *in vitro*)	66% (6 mg) 70–80% predicted for 4.5–9 mg	?
Quetiapine (Seroquel)	Minimum effective dose method: OLA 1 mg = 20 (25) RIS 1 mg = 75 (62.5) HAL 1 mg = 37.5 (55.6) CPZ 100 mg = 60 (88.9) Mean dose method: OLA 1 mg = 32.27	Oral: 25 mg bid to start; increase by 25–50 mg bid per day, as tolerated, to a target dose of 300–400 mg/day (given bid or tid) within 4–7 days. Further increases $\geq$ 2 days. Usual daily dose: 300–600 mg/day, in divided doses Maximum[H]: 800 mg/day	~73% (relative bioavailabil-ity; absolute unknown)	83%	Oral: 0.5–3	~6–7 (parent) ~12 (active metabolite) Prolonged in hepatic disease (45% longer; based on a low-, single-dose study in those with mild disease), renal disease (25% longer; based on a low-, single-dose study in those with severe disease), and the elderly (30–50% longer)	**3A4**[p], 2D6[w]; P-gp	1A2[w], 2D6[w], 3A4[w], 2C9[w], 2C19[w]	20–44% (300–700 mg) 13–41% (150–750 mg)	21–80% (150–600 mg) 38–74% (150–750 mg)

Antipsychotic Doses and Pharmacokinetics (Oral and Short-Acting Injections) (cont.)

						SECOND-GENERATION AGENTS (SGAs)				
Drug	Oral dose equivalents (mg)[1]	Monograph Doses for Psychosis (for doses for other indications and in renal impairment, see pp. 149–150)	Bioavailability	Protein Binding	Peak Plasma Level (h) (T_{max})	Elimination Half-Life (h)	Metabolizing Enzymes[2] / Transporters (CYP450; other)	Enzyme Inhibition[3] / Transporters (CYP450; other)	% D_2 Receptor Occupancy[4] (dose & plasma level)	% 5-HT$_{2A}$ Occupancy (dose)
(Seroquel XR)		Oral (XR): 300 mg once daily in the evening to start, increase by up to 300 mg/day Maintenance: 400–800 mg/day Maximum: 800 mg/day			Oral (XR): ~6					
Risperidone (Risperdal, Risperdal M-tab)	Minimum effective dose method: OLA 1 mg = 0.27 (0.4) HAL 1 mg = 0.5 (0.9) CPZ 100 mg = 0.8 (1.4) Mean dose method: OLA 1 mg = 0.38	Oral: 1–2 mg once to twice daily and increase by 0.5–2 mg q 1–7 days Usual daily dose: 4–6 mg Doses above 10 mg/day do not usually produce further improvement Maximum: 16 mg/day with a maximum of 8 mg/dose	70%	88–90% (parent; to albumin and α_1-AGP) 77% (active metabolite) Reduced in hepatic disease	1–1.5 (parent) 3[K]–17[D] (active metabolite)	3[K]–20[D] (parent) 21[K]–30[D] (active metabolite) Increased by ~60% in moderate to severe renal disease	**2D6**[p], 3A4[m], P-gp	2D6, 3A4[w]	60–75% (2–4 mg) 63–85% (2–6 mg; 36–252 nmol/L)	60–90% (1–4 mg)
Ziprasidone (Geodon[B], Zeldox[C])	Minimum effective dose method: OLA 1 mg = 5.33 (8) RIS 1 mg = 20 (20) HAL 1 mg = 10 (17.8) CPZ 100 mg = 16 (28.4) Mean dose method: OLA 1 mg = 7.92	Oral: 20–40 mg bid to start. If needed, increase ≥ q 2 days. Doses > 80 mg bid generally not recommended. Short-term efficacy data for 100 mg bid but limited safety data	Oral: 30% (60% with food)	> 99% (to albumin and α_1-AGP)	Oral: 6–8 (C_{max} increased 32–72% in mild renal impairment)	Oral: 4–10 dose-dependent (6.6 mean) No change in the elderly or renal disease Prolonged in hepatic disease (mean in hepatic disease = 7.1 vs. 4.8 in control group)	**3A4**[m], 1A2[w], 2D6, 3C18/19; Aldehyde oxidase[w]	2D6[w], 3A4[w]	45–75% (40–80 mg)	80–90% (40–80 mg)

SECOND-GENERATION AGENTS (SGAs)										
Drug	Oral dose equivalents (mg)[1]	Monograph Doses for Psychosis (for doses for other indications and in renal impairment, see pp. 149–150)	Bioavaila-bility	Protein Binding	Peak Plasma Level (h) (T_{max})	Elimination Half-Life (h)	Metabolizing Enzymes[2]/ Transporters (CYP450; other)	Enzyme Inhibition[3]/ Transporters (CYP450; other)	% D_2 Receptor Occupancy[4] (dose & plasma level)	% 5-HT$_{2A}$ Occu-pancy (dose)
Ziprasidone mesylate[B]		Short-acting IM: 10 mg q 2 h or 20 mg q 4 h to a maximum of 40 mg/24 h for up to 3 days	Short-acting IM: 100%		Short-acting IM: ~60 min	Short-acting IM: 2–5 h (Caution in renal disease due to excipient – cyclodextrin)				

[1] Dose equivalents determined using minimum effective dose method and mean dose method: The doses in mg are equivalent to 1 mg/day olanzapine (OLA), 1 mg/day risperidone (RIS), 1 mg/day haloperidol (HAL), and 100 mg/day chlorpromazine (CPZ). Numbers in parentheses are the results of the sensitivity analysis (2 positive trials). N/A = none available,   [2] CYP450 isoenzymes involved in drug metabolism,   [3] CYP450 isoenzymes inhibited by drug,   [4] D_2 receptor occupancy correlates better to plasma level than to dose, and appears to relate to clinical efficacy in controlling positive symptoms of schizophrenia as well as risk of extrapyramidal adverse effects (if > 80%)

[B] Not marketed in Canada,   [C] Not marketed in the USA,   [D] Poor metabolizers of CYP2D6,   [F] Three times daily dosing can also be used for titration to minimize adverse effects (e.g., hypotension, sedation, and seizure). Dose can be divided unevenly such that a larger dose is given at bedtime. Maintenance doses ≤ 200 mg/day can be given as a single dose at bedtime   [G] Occasionally higher doses (i.e., 950–1400 mg/day) may be required to reach therapeutic levels, in particular in males who are heavy smokers. In such cases, monitor clozapine levels and for any signs/symptoms of toxicity,   [H] Maximum dose suggested by manufacturer. Anecdotal and preliminary data with doses > 800 mg/day, including one case report using 2400 mg/day. However, further study of efficacy and safety required,   [K] Extensive metabolizers of CYP2D6

[m] Moderate activity,   [p] Potent activity,   [w] Weak activity

THIRD-GENERATION AGENTS (TGAs)										
Drug	Oral Dose Equivalents (mg)[1]	Monograph Doses for Psychosis	Bio-availability	Protein Binding	Peak Plasma Level (h) (T_{max})	Elimination Half-Life (h)	Metabolizing Enzymes[2]/ Transporters (CYP450; other)	Enzyme Inhibition[3]/ Transporters (CYP450; other)	% D_2 Receptor Occupancy[4] (dose & plasma level)	% 5-HT$_{2A}$ Occupancy (dose)
Aripiprazole (Abilify)	Minimum effective dose method: OLA 1 mg = 1.33 (1) RIS 1 mg = 5 (2.5) HAL 1 mg = 2.5 (2.2) CPZ 100 mg = 4 (3.6)	Oral: Start and target dose: 10 or 15 mg once daily. If needed, increase q 2 weeks (up to 30 mg/day). However, greater efficacy has not been demonstrated at doses > 10 mg/day Anecdotal evidence suggests dosing in the morning and using lower starting doses to minimize activation effects Short-acting IM: Usual: 9.75 mg Range: 5.25–15 mg as a single dose Maximum: 30 mg/day with at least 2 h between doses	87% (tablet; slightly higher with oral solution form) Short-acting IM: 100%	> 99% (primarily to albumin)	Oral: 3–5 Short-acting IM: 1–3	75–146[D] (active metabolite = 94) No change in renal or hepatic impairment or in elderly	2D6[p], 3A4[p] (Reduce dose by 50% in poor metabolizers of 2D6. Dose changes required with concurrent use of drugs that affect 2D6 and/or 3A4)	–	40–95% (0.5–30 mg)	54–60% (10–30 mg)

Antipsychotic Doses and Pharmacokinetics (Oral and Short-Acting Injections) (cont.)

THIRD-GENERATION AGENTS (TGAs)										
Drug	Oral Dose Equivalents (mg)[1]	Monograph Doses for Psychosis	Bio-availability	Protein Binding	Peak Plasma Level (h) (T_{max})	Elimination Half-Life (h)	Metabolizing Enzymes[2] / Transporters (CYP450; other)	Enzyme Inhibition[3] / Transporters (CYP450; other)	% D_2 Receptor Occupancy[4] (dose & plasma level)	% 5-HT$_{2A}$ Occupancy (dose)
Brexpiprazole (Rexulti)	N/A	1 mg once daily on days 1–4. Titrate to 2 mg once daily on days 5–7, then to 4 mg on day 8 depending on response and tolerability. Recommended target dose is 2–4 mg once daily	95%	> 99%	4	91 (major metabolite = 86)	2D6[p], 3A4[p] (Reduce dose by 50% in poor metabolizers of 2D6. Dose changes required with concurrent use of drugs that affect 2D6 and/or 3A4)	–	?	?
Cariprazine[B] (Vraylar)	N/A	Starting dose is 1.5 mg; can be increased to 3 mg on day 2. Depending on response and tolerability, further dose adjustments can be made in 1.5 or 3 mg increments. Recommended dose range is 1.5–6 mg once daily	High	19–97%	3–6	2–5 days (2–3 weeks for active metabolite)	3A4[p], 2D6[w] (Reduce dose by 50% in patients initiating a strong CYP3A4 inhibitor)	–	?	?

[1] Dose equivalents determined from fixed-dose studies using the minimum effective dose method: The doses in mg are equivalent to 1 mg/day olanzapine (OLA), 1 mg/day risperidone (RIS), 1 mg/day haloperidol (HAL), and 100 mg/day chlorpromazine (CPZ). Numbers in parentheses are the results of the sensitivity analysis (2 positive trials). N/A = none available, [2] CYP450 isoenzymes involved in drug metabolism, [3] CYP450 isoenzymes inhibited by drug, [4] D_2 receptor occupancy correlates better to plasma level than to dose, and appears to relate to clinical efficacy in controlling positive symptoms of schizophrenia as well as risk of extrapyramidal adverse effects (if > 80%), [B] Not marketed in Canada, [D] Poor metabolizers of CYP2D6, [p] Potent activity, [w] Weak activity

5-HT₂ₐ INVERSE AGONIST										
Drug	Dose Equivalents (mg)[1]	Monograph Doses for Psychosis	Bioavailability	Protein Binding	Peak Plasma Level (h) (T_{max})	Elimination Half-Life (h)	Metabolizing Enzymes[2] / Transporters (CYP450; other)	Enzyme Inhibition[3] / Transporters (CYP450; other)	% D₂ Receptor Occupancy (dose & plasma level)	% 5-HT₂ₐ Occupancy (dose)
Pimavanserin (Nuplazid)	–	34 mg, taken orally as two 17 mg tablets once daily, without titration	N/A. High-fat meal had no significant effect on C_{max} and AUC	~95%	6 (range 4–24)	57 (active metabolite = 200)	3A4, 3A5	–	No appreciable affinity for D₂ receptors	–

[1] N/A = none available   [2] CYP450 isoenzymes involved in drug metabolism,   [3] CYP450 isoenzymes inhibited by drug

NOTES:
- Comparable doses are only approximations. Generally doses used are higher in the acute stage of the illness than in maintenance. Each patient's medication dosage must be individualized
- Plasma levels are available for some antipsychotics but their clinical usefulness is limited
- For CYP activity data, see: [23, 24, 25]; product monographs of individual agents; [*Note: data regarding CYP450 profiles may not be consistent among references*]
- Abbreviations: α₁-AGP = α₁-acid glycoprotein; bid = twice daily; FMO = flavin monooxygenase enzyme involved in *N*-oxidation reactions; od = once daily; P-gp = P-glycoprotein [*a transporter of hydrophobic substances in or out of specific body organs (e.g., block absorption in the gut)*]; qid = four times daily; tid = three times daily; UGT = uridine diphosphate glucuronosyl transferase [*involved in Phase II reactions (conjugation)*]

Comparison of Long-Acting IM Antipsychotics

	FIRST-GENERATION AGENTS (FGAs)			
	Flupenthixol decanoate[C] (Fluanxol)	Fluphenazine decanoate (Modecate, Prolixin)	Haloperidol decanoate (Haldol LA)	Zuclopenthixol decanoate[C] (Clopixol Depot)
Chemical class	Thioxanthene	Piperazine phenothiazine	Butyrophenone	Thioxanthene
Form	Esterified with decanoic acid (a 10-carbon chain fatty acid) and dissolved in vegetable oil; must be hydrolyzed to free flupenthixol; metabolites inactive	Esterified with decanoic acid and dissolved in sesame oil; must be hydrolyzed to free fluphenazine	Esterified with decanoic acid and dissolved in sesame oil; must be hydrolyzed to free haloperidol	Esterified with decanoic acid in coconut oil; must be hydrolyzed to free zuclopenthixol
Strength supplied	20 mg/mL (2%) 100 mg/mL (10%)	25 mg/mL 100 mg/mL[C]	50 mg/mL 100 mg/mL	200 mg/mL
Administration	Gluteal muscle Deep IM injection	Gluteal muscle (IM) Deltoid muscle (SC) SC or deep IM injection	Gluteal muscle Deep IM injection	Gluteal muscle Deep IM injection
Overlap with oral formulation	1 week	1 week	None to 4 weeks	2 weeks
Starting dose	Long-acting IM naive: Test dose of 5–20 mg; assess over next 5–10 days Non-naive: 20–40 mg Increase in increments not exceeding 20 mg Continue oral for first week in a diminishing dose	IM or SC: 2.5–12.5 mg	50 mg or 10–20 times previous oral dose (10–15 times if elderly, debilitated or on stable oral doses of ≤ 10 mg/d) to a max. of 100 mg Continue oral in a diminishing dose if starting with a low IM dose	100–200 mg Supplemental oral in diminishing dosage may be needed for the first 2 weeks
Usual dose range	20–80 mg	12.5–50 mg	50–200 mg or 10–15 times previous oral dose	150–300 mg
Maximum dose [D]	Doses above 80 mg generally unnecessary	Doses above 50 mg generally unnecessary; doses up to 100 mg q 2 weeks have been used in some cases	450 mg/month	400 mg q 2 weeks
Usual duration of action	2–4 weeks	2–5 weeks	4 weeks	2–4 weeks
CPE	16–40 mg q 2 weeks	10–25 mg q 2 weeks	40–100 mg q 4 weeks	80–200 mg q 2 weeks
OLE	40 mg q 2 weeks	25 mg q 2 weeks	150 mg q 4 weeks	200 mg q 2 weeks
Pharmacokinetics				
Time to peak plasma level[G]	3–7 days	First peak in 8–10 h (due to presence of hydrolyzed "free" fluphenazine); level drops, then peaks again in 8–12 days	3–9 days	3–7 days
Elimination half-life[H]	8 days (after single injection), 17 days (multiple dosing)	6.8–9.6 days (single injection), up to 14.3 days (multiple dosing)	18–21 days	19 days
Time to steady state	2 months	2 months	2–3 months	2 months

	FIRST-GENERATION AGENTS (FGAs)			
	Flupenthixol decanoate[(C)] **(Fluanxol)**	**Fluphenazine decanoate (Modecate, Prolixin)**	**Haloperidol decanoate (Haldol LA)**	**Zuclopenthixol decanoate**[(C)] **(Clopixol Depot)**
Adverse effects: Generally similar to oral drugs in same class	Flupenthixol (see p. 198)	Fluphenazine (see p. 198)	Haloperidol (see p. 198)	Zuclopenthixol (see p. 198)
CNS	Both sedating and alerting effects reported; may have energizing effects at low doses	Both drowsiness and insomnia reported	Both drowsiness and insomnia reported	Both drowsiness and insomnia reported (less frequent than with oral zuclopenthixol)
Extrapyramidal	Frequent; more frequent with first few injections, diminish thereafter	Less frequent than with oral preparation. Tend to occur in the first few days after an injection. Increased frequency of dystonia noted with use of "older" multipunctured multidose vials due to presence of "free" fluphenazine	Frequent, however, reported less often than with oral haloperidol	Reported in 5–15% of patients
Skin and local reactions	Indurations rarely seen (at high doses) Photosensitivity and hyperpigmentation very rare; dermatological reactions seen Pain at injection site	One case of induration seen at a high dose; dermatological reactions have been reported Pain at injection site	Local dermatological reactions; Inflammation and nodules at injection site (may be more common with 100 mg/mL preparation or with higher volumes); less common if deltoid used One case of photosensitization reported; "tracking" reported Pain at injection site can continue for 2 days after administration	No indurations but local dermatological reactions reported Pain at injection site
Laboratory changes	Rarely leukopenia, eosinophilia	Dose-dependent rise in prolactin; one case of jaundice reported; rarely agranulocytosis; ECG changes seen in some patients	Dose-dependent rise in prolactin; rarely jaundice, leukopenia, agranulocytosis	Transient changes in liver function seen Rarely neutropenia, agranulocytosis

[(C)] = Not marketed in the USA, [(D)] Typical maximal doses based on product monographs. Some clinicians may use higher doses if they are effective with minimal adverse effects, [(G)] Important as indicator when maximum adverse effects will occur, [(H)] Useful for determining dosing interval; steady state will be reached in approximately 5 half-lives

Comparison of Long-Acting IM Antipsychotics (cont.)

	SECOND-GENERATION AGENTS (SGAs)[1]						THIRD-GENERATION AGENTS (TGAs)	
	Olanzapine pamoate[B] (Zyprexa Relprevv)	Paliperidone palmitate 1-monthly (Invega Sustenna)	Paliperidone palmitate 3-monthly (Invega Trinza)	Paliperidone palmitate 6-monthly (Invega Hafyera)	Risperidone (Risperdal Consta)	Risperidone RBP-7000 (Perseris[B])	Aripiprazole (Abilify Maintena)	Aripiprazole lauroxil (Aristada[B])
Chemical class	Thienobenzodiazepine	Benzisoxazole	Benzisoxazole	Benzisoxazole	Benzisoxazole	Benzisoxazole	Phenylpiperazine	Phenylpiperazine
Form	Yellow solid of olanzapine pamoate monohydrate crystals forming a yellow, opaque suspension on reconstitution with provided aqueous diluent	White to off-white sterile, aqueous, extended-release suspension in prefilled syringes	White to off-white sterile, aqueous, extended-release suspension in prefilled syringes	White to off-white sterile, aqueous, extended-release suspension in prefilled syringes	White to off-white, free-flowing powder with risperidone encapsulated in a polymer as extended-release microspheres. Must be reconstituted with provided aqueous base just prior to use	White to off-white powder, to be mixed with colorless to yellow solution. Forms viscous suspension white to yellow-green once reconstituted	White to off-white lyophilized powder forming an opaque, milky-white suspension on reconstitution with provided sterile water for injection	White to off-white sterile aqueous extended-release suspension in prefilled syringe, supplied as a kit with safety needles
Strength supplied	210 mg/vial, 300 mg/vial, 405 mg/vial	Strengths vary in different countries, e.g., US labeling indicates the amount of pali-peridone palmitate: 39 mg/0.25 mL, 78 mg/0.5 mL, 117 mg/0.75 mL, 156 mg/mL, 234 mg/1.5 mL Canadian labeling indicates only the amount of paliperidone (not the palmitate base): 50 mg/0.5 mL, 75 mg/0.75 mL, 100 mg/mL, 150 mg/1.5 mL	Strengths vary in different countries, e.g., US labeling indicates amount of paliperidone palmitate: 273 mg/0.875 mL, 410 mg/1.315 mL, 546 mg/1.75 mL, 819 mg/2.625 mL Canadian labeling indicates only the amount of paliperidone (not the palmitate base): 175 mg/0.875 mL, 263 mg/1.315 mL, 350 mg/1.75 mL, 525 mg/2.625 mL	US labeling indicates amount of paliperidone palmitate: 1,092 mg/3.5 mL and 1,560 mg/5 mL	12.5 mg/vial, 25 mg/vial, 37.5 mg/vial, 50 mg/vial	90 mg/0.6 mL syringe, 120 mg/0.8 mL syringe	300 mg/vial, 400 mg/vial	441 mg, 662 mg, 882 mg, 1064 mg prefilled syringe

	SECOND-GENERATION AGENTS (SGAs)[1]						THIRD-GENERATION AGENTS (TGAs)	
	Olanzapine pamoate[B] (Zyprexa Relprevv)	Paliperidone palmitate 1-monthly (Invega Sustenna)	Paliperidone palmitate 3-monthly (Invega Trinza)	Paliperidone palmitate 6-monthly (Invega Hafyera)	Risperidone (Risperdal Consta)	Risperidone RBP-7000 (Perseris[B])	Aripiprazole (Abilify Maintena)	Aripiprazole lauroxil (Aristada[B])
Administration	Gluteal muscle Deep IM injection	Deltoid muscle for days 1 and 8. Deltoid or gluteal muscle thereafter Deep IM injection	Deltoid or gluteal muscle Single, deep IM injection (not divided)	Gluteal muscle Single, deep IM injection (not divided)	Deltoid or gluteal muscle Deep IM injection	Abdominal subcutaneous injection	Deltoid or gluteal muscle Deep IM injection	Deltoid (441 mg dose only) or gluteal muscle (all strengths) Deep IM injection
Overlap with oral formulation	None	None	None	None	3 weeks	None	2 weeks	3 weeks
Starting dose[A]	For 1st 8 weeks: If previously on 10 mg/day oral = 210 mg IM/q 2 weeks or 405 mg/q 4 weeks; 15–20 mg/day oral = 300 mg/q 2 weeks. In patients who are debilitated or prone to hypotension, start with 150 mg IM/q 4 weeks	Day 1: 234 mg IM of paliperidone palmitate (150 mg of paliperidone) Day 8: 156 mg IM of paliperidone palmitate (100 mg of paliperidone) For dosing in renal or hepatic impairment see SGA Dosing section p. 150	Only to be used after treatment with paliperidone 1-monthly IM has been established as an adequate treatment for at least 4 months Initiate paliperidone 3-monthly IM when the next paliperidone 1-monthly IM dose is due (+/- 7days), using a 3.5-fold higher dose than that of the previous 1-monthly formulation injection	Only to be used after treatment with paliperidone 1-monthly IM has been established as an adequate treatment for at least 4 months OR after treatment with paliperidone 3-monthly IM has been established as an adequate treatment for at least 3 months Initiate paliperidone 6-monthly IM when the next paliperidone 1- or 3-monthly IM dose is due (+/- 7days) Use the following conversions: PP1M 156 mg → PP6M 1,092 mg PP1M 234 mg → PP6M 1,560 mg PP3M 546 mg → PP6M 1,092 mg PP3M 819 mg → PP6M 1,560 mg	25 mg IM q 2 weeks Continue oral risperidone for the first 3 weeks For dosing in renal or hepatic impairment see SGA Dosing section p. 150	Depending on patient's needs: 90 mg corresponds to 3 mg/day of oral risperidone; 120 mg corresponds to 4 mg/day of oral risperidone	One-injection start based on clinical study data: One injection of 400 mg IM and continue with 10–20 mg oral aripiprazole for 14 days, OR continue with current oral antipsychotic for 14 days Two-injection start based on modeling and simulation study data: 2 separate injections of 400 mg at separate injection sites, along with one 20 mg dose of oral aripiprazole. Discontinue current oral antipsychotic	Depending on patient's needs. Can be initiated at 441 mg, 662 mg or 882 mg IM q 4 weeks, 882 mg IM q 6 weeks or 1064 mg IM q 2 months. (Continue oral aripiprazole for the first 21 days OR administer one injection of 675 mg Aristada Initio and one 30 mg dose of oral aripiprazole in conjunction with the first dose of Aristada (see Dosing p. 179))

Comparison of Long-Acting IM Antipsychotics (cont.)

	SECOND-GENERATION AGENTS (SGAs)[1]						THIRD-GENERATION AGENTS (TGAs)	
	Olanzapine pamoate[B] (Zyprexa Relprevv)	Paliperidone palmitate 1-monthly (Invega Sustenna)	Paliperidone palmitate 3-monthly (Invega Trinza)	Paliperidone palmitate 6-monthly (Invega Hafyera)	Risperidone (Risperdal Consta)	Risperidone RBP-7000 (Perseris[B])	Aripiprazole (Abilify Maintena)	Aripiprazole lauroxil (Aristada[B])
Usual dose range[A]	After 1st 8 weeks: If previously on 10 mg/day oral = 150 mg IM/q 2 weeks or 300 mg/q 4 weeks; 15 mg/day oral = 210 mg/q 2 weeks or 405 mg/q 4 weeks; 20 mg/day oral = 300 mg/q 2 weeks	117 mg IM pali-peridone palmitate (75 mg paliperidone) q 4 weeks Dose can be higher or lower within the recommended range of 78–234 mg of paliperidone palmitate (50–150 mg paliperidone) based on individual patient tolerability and/or efficacy	273–819 mg paliperidone palmitate (175–525 mg paliperidone) q 3 months. Dose can be adjusted within the range every 3 months based on tolerability and/or efficacy	1,092–1,560 mg paliperidone palmitate q 6 months. Dose can be adjusted within the range every 6 months based on tolerability and/or efficacy	25–50 mg q 2 weeks	90–120 mg q 4 weeks Patients on stable oral risperidone doses < 3 mg/day or > 4 mg/day may not be candidates for injectable	400 mg IM q 4 weeks. If adverse effects, can reduce to 300 mg q 4 weeks. Interval should be no shorter than 26 days and no longer than 5 weeks for the 2nd and 3rd dose or 6 weeks for the 4th and sub-sequent doses. Dose varies if known CYP2D6 poor meta-bolizer or if taking strong 2D6 or 3A4 inhibitors – see monograph	441 mg IM q 4 week to 1064 mg q 2 months. Dose varies if known CYP2D6 poor metabolizer or if taking strong 2D6 or 3A4 inhibitors (see Dosing p. 179)
Maximum dose[A], [D]	300 mg IM q 2 weeks/ 405 mg IM q 4 weeks	234 mg IM of pali-peridone palmitate (150 mg paliperidone) q 4 weeks	819 mg paliperidone palmitate (525 mg paliperidone) q 3 months	1,560 mg paliperidone palmitate q 6 months	50 mg q 2 weeks[E]	120 mg q 4 weeks	400 mg IM q 4 weeks	1064 mg q 2 months
Usual duration of action	2–4 weeks	4 weeks	3 months	6 months	2 weeks	4 weeks	4 weeks	441 mg, 662 mg: 4 weeks 882 mg: 4–6 weeks 1064 mg: 2 months
OLA equivalents[2]	210 mg q 2 weeks = 1 mg	25 mg q 4 weeks = 0.06 mg	?	?	25 mg q 2 weeks = 0.12 mg	90 mg q 4 weeks = 0.21 mg	400 mg q 4 weeks = 0.95 mg	441 mg q 4 weeks = 0.71 mg
Pharmacokinetics Time to peak plasma level[G]	2–4 days	13 days	Median: 30–33 days	Median: 29–32 days	30 days[26]	First peak: 4-6 h Second peak: 10-14 days	Following multiple injections: 4 days (deltoid), 7 days (gluteal)	Not in monograph. Reaches systemic circulation after 5–6 days
Elimination half-life[H]	~30 days	25–49 days Increased in renal disease	Median: 84–95 days following deltoid injection, 118–139 days following gluteal injection	Median: 148–159 days	3–6 days Elimination complete by 7–8 weeks Increased in hepatic or renal disease	9–11 days	30 days (300 mg), 47 days (400 mg)	53.9–57.2 days

	SECOND-GENERATION AGENTS (SGAs)[1]						THIRD-GENERATION AGENTS (TGAs)	
	Olanzapine pamoate[B] (Zyprexa Relprevv)	Paliperidone palmitate 1-monthly (Invega Sustenna)	Paliperidone palmitate 3-monthly (Invega Trinza)	Paliperidone palmitate 6-monthly (Invega Hafyera)	Risperidone (Risperdal Consta)	Risperidone RBP-7000 (Perseris[B])	Aripiprazole (Abilify Maintena)	Aripiprazole lauroxil (Aristada[B])
Time to steady state	2–3 months	2–3 months	?	?	2 months	By end of second injection	3–4 months	4 months
Adverse effects[I]: Generally similar to oral drugs in same class	Olanzapine (see p. 199)	Paliperidone (see p. 199)	As per paliperidone 1-monthly IM, except where noted	As per paliperidone 1- and 3-monthly IM, except where noted	Risperidone (see p. 199)	Risperidone (see p. 199)	Aripiprazole (see p. 183)	Aripiprazole (see p. 183)
CNS	Post-injection delirium sedation syndrome (PDSS). Administer when ER services readily accessible. Observe for at least 3 h. Instruct not to drive/operate heavy machinery for remainder of the day. Risk < 0.1% at each injection Headache ≤ 18%, sedation ≤ 13%	Insomnia, headache ≤ 15%; anxiety ≤ 8%; drowsiness ≤ 7%			Adverse effects increase with dose over 50 mg q 2 weeks Drowsiness 3–6%, anxiety 25%, insomnia 23%, headache 13%, depression 16%	Sedation (4.7%)	Sedation (IM: 2.4%, oral: 1.1%, placebo: 0.7%)	Headache (IM: 3–4%, placebo: 3%) Insomnia (IM: 2–4%, placebo: 2%)
Extrapyramidal		Akathisia (100 mg IM: 11%, 50 mg IM: 5%, placebo: 5%); parkinsonism (100 mg IM: 18%, 50 mg IM: 9%, placebo: 7%)	Akathisia 4%; parkinsonism 6%	Akathisia 3%; parkinsonism 5%	Akathisia (50 mg IM: 9%, 25 mg IM: 2%, placebo: 4%); parkinsonism (50 mg IM: 10%, 25 mg IM: 4%, placebo: 3%)	Akathisia (90 mg SC: 2.6%, 120 mg SC: 6.8%, placebo: 4.2%)	Akathisia (IM: 8.2%, oral: 6.8%, placebo: 6%); parkinsonism (IM: 6.9%, oral: 4.1%, placebo: 3%)	Akathisia (IM: 11%, placebo: 4%); parkinsonism (IM: 5–7% placebo: 4%)
Skin and local reactions	At injection site: Pain, induration or site mass ≤ 3.6%	At injection site: Pain, redness, swelling or induration ≤ 10% (more common with 1st injection; reduced incidence with subsequent injections)	At injection site: Pain, redness, and swelling 2%	At injection site: Pain, redness, and swelling 11%, worse at first dose	At injection site: Pain, redness, swelling or induration (more than 10%) [ensure solution is at room temperature and inject into alternate buttocks]	At injection site: erythema (5.2%), pain (19%) (decreased frequency and intensity with subsequent injections)	At injection site: Pain (5%), redness, swelling, induration of mild to moderate severity (decreased frequency and intensity with subsequent injections)	At injection site: Pain (IM: 3–4%, placebo: 2%); redness, swelling, induration: 1% (decreased frequency and intensity with subsequent injections)

Comparison of Long-Acting IM Antipsychotics (cont.)

	SECOND-GENERATION AGENTS (SGAs)[1]						THIRD-GENERATION AGENTS (TGAs)	
	Olanzapine pamoate[B] (Zyprexa Relprevv)	Paliperidone palmitate 1-monthly (Invega Sustenna)	Paliperidone palmitate 3-monthly (Invega Trinza)	Paliperidone palmitate 6-monthly (Invega Hafyera)	Risperidone (Risperdal Consta)	Risperidone RBP-7000 (Perseris[B])	Aripiprazole (Abilify Maintena)	Aripiprazole lauroxil (Aristada[B])
Other	Orthostatic hypotension 0.1%; weight gain ≤ 7% (mean gain = 11.2 kg after at least 24 weeks)	Orthostatic hypotension < 2%	Weight gain 9%; headache 9%	Weight gain 9%; headache 9%	Hypotension < 2%	Weight gain (12,9%) (Mean gain placebo: 2.8 kg, 90 mg: 5.1 kg, 120 mg: 4.7 kg)		

[1] See the relevant sections in Second-Generation Antipsychotics/SGAs (pp. 146—162) for further information   [2] Dose equivalents determined from acute phase studies using minimum effective dose method: Doses in mg are equivalent to 1 mg/day olanzapine (OLA). Since risperidone RBP-7000 is administered by SC injection, differenct equivalent doses may result due to different metabolism in comparison to other long-acting injectables given IM   [A] For schizophrenia and related psychotic disorders. See Dosing section p. 150 for dosing in renal and hepatic impairment,   [B] Not marketed in Canada,   [D] Typical maximal doses based on product monographs. Some clinicians may use higher doses if they are effective with minimal adverse effects,   [E] Maximum dose suggested by manufacturer. Increase in adverse effects without any increase in efficacy reported with 75 mg q 2 weeks,   [G] Important as indicator when maximum adverse effects will occur,   [H] Useful for determining dosing interval; steady state will be reached in approximately 5 half-lives,   [I] Incidences are not from head to head trials of agents thus incidences may not be comparable

Abbreviations: CNS = central nervous system; q X weeks = every X weeks

Switching Antipsychotics

 Switching Antipsychotics

Reasons for Considering a Switch	• 1. A switch may be considered in cases of nonresponse, partial or less than optimal response, or relapse despite adherence. Motivating factors may include:
	  − Persistent positive symptoms (consider a FGA or a SGA; switching to clozapine may offer additional response in up to a further 50% of patients)
	  − Persistent negative symptoms (consider alternate SGA, lowering dose, or a TGA)
	  − Persistent cognitive or affective symptoms (consider SGA)
	  − Persistent suicidal ideation or behaviors (consider clozapine)
	  − A request for change from patient or family member
	  − A change in patient's medical or psychiatric condition warranting a change in treatment
	• 2. To relieve or decrease a bothersome adverse effect (e.g., sexual dysfunction, sedation, EPS) or one that may be associated with short- or long-term morbidity (e.g., TD, metabolic effects). These are often major contributors to nonadherence and eventual treatment failure
	• A combination of 1. and 2.

When Switching Therapies	• Reaffirm diagnosis and rationale for switching makes sense
	• Address any confounding or complicating factors. For example:
	  − Attempt to rule out partial adherence or nonadherence. If present, identify and address barriers to adherence if possible (e.g., some adverse effects may be resolved by lowering the dose, changing the administration schedule or waiting for tolerance to develop)
	  − Ensure adequate trial period was employed – adequate dose for adequate duration [at least 4–6 weeks at maximally tolerated dose (longer for clozapine)]
	  − Determine if any drug interactions may be impacting on efficacy or adverse effects

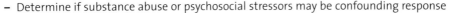

- Determine if substance abuse or psychosocial stressors may be confounding response
  - Give thoughtful consideration to the pros and cons of making a change
  - Establish a thorough plan including how to make the switch and what to expect. How long will it take to work? What unwanted effects might occur and how to monitor for them
  - Confirm the patient is agreeable to the change and discuss the switching plan with them
- Potential problems that may be anticipated during a switch are:
  - Withdrawal effects related to discontinuation of the initial antipsychotic
  - Adverse effects that result from the addition of a new agent
- These, coupled with a time lag to response, may discourage the patient and negatively impact on adherence unless the patient is educated as to what to expect

Withdrawal Effects

- Abrupt withdrawal of a medication that strongly antagonizes one or more receptors results in the exposure of sensitized receptors, leaving them potentially vulnerable to excessive stimulation. This may result in:
  - Dopaminergic rebound – if a high D_2 affinity medication (e.g., risperidone) is abruptly replaced with a low D_2 affinity medication or a rapid on/off fast-dissociating antipsychotic (e.g., quetiapine) or a partial D_2 agonist (e.g., aripiprazole), dopaminergic rebound may result. In the mesolimbic tract, this could lead to supersensitivity psychosis; in the nigrostriatal tract, treatment-emergent EPS and TD may materialize
  - Cholinergic rebound – if a high-affinity cholinergic antagonist (e.g., olanzapine) is abruptly replaced by an antipsychotic with little affinity for blocking cholinergic receptors, cholinergic rebound may ensue, causing the patient to complain of flu-like symptoms such as nausea, vomiting, diarrhea, diaphoresis, blurred vision, and insomnia
  - Histaminic rebound – abrupt replacement of a high-affinity histamine antagonist (e.g., clozapine) with a low-affinity agent (e.g., aripiprazole) may see improvement in several metabolic parameters such as weight gain, glucose intolerance, and dyslipidemias. Sedation may also improve, but some individuals may experience distressing rebound insomnia and anxiety which may be interpreted as a sign of relapse
  - Serotonergic rebound – it has been suggested that abrupt discontinuation of a high-affinity serotonin 5-HT$_{2A}$ antagonist may result in serotonin syndrome (agitation, diaphoresis, fever, tremor, confusion, etc.) or NMS-like symptoms (e.g., switching from SGA to FGA)
  - In the absence of any strong scientific evidence, empirical recommendations favor a slow cross-taper method to minimize rebound and the addition/continuation of adjunctive treatments (e.g., anticholinergics for cholinergic rebound or benzodiazepines for insomnia) when necessary

Switching Methods

- Four options (no clear evidence to support one method over another)
  1. Washout/start:
     - Withdraw the first drug gradually and begin the second drug following a suitable washout period. May minimize withdrawal-emergent reactions. Not clinically practical when patient is symptomatic. May increase the risk of relapse
  2. Stop/start:
     - Abruptly discontinue the first drug, then start the second drug at its usual initial dose; increase the dose to a therapeutic range accordingly. This technique is often used when the patient has a significant/serious adverse reaction to the initial drug (e.g., agranulocytosis, NMS, ketoacidosis). Potential drawbacks include an increased risk of relapse and withdrawal-emergent reactions
  3. Cross-taper:
     - Taper the dose of the first medication while simultaneously increasing the dose of the second drug. Commonly used when stable patients are experiencing bothersome adverse effects and require a medication change. Consider using at least 2 weeks for tapering down or titrating up antipsychotics that have higher likelihood of sedation or anticholinergic effects (see table Relative Tolerability Profiles of Antipsychotics p. 196) to allow for patient tolerability and to minimize potential for withdrawal-emergent effects. Generally the most well accepted or preferred strategy, thought to minimize the potential for withdrawal-emergent effects and relapse. Drawbacks of this strategy include an increased risk of relapse should the patient spend time with subtherapeutic doses of both antipsychotics, an increased risk of polypharmacy should the patient improve during the switch and the practitioner become reluctant to make further changes, and an increased risk of additive or synergistic effects from both drugs
  4. Delayed withdrawal:
     - Establishing the patient on a therapeutic dose of the second drug before reducing the existing medication. The strategy may be preferred in situations for which relapse is a significant concern. There is an increased risk for polypharmacy with this method if the changeover is not completed. There is also an increased risk of additive or synergistic effects from both drugs during the procedure
- Rate of switching/cross-tapering should be slow in the elderly and in young patients

Antipsychotic Augmentation Strategies

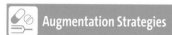 **Augmentation Strategies**

- The addition of another pharmacological agent or treatment to an antipsychotic in an attempt to augment or improve the response to the initial antipsychotic
- The goal is to combine different mechanisms of action to create a synergistic effect that will enhance efficacy while minimizing the potential for increased adverse effects and drug interactions
- Most of the literature on augmentation strategies evaluates augmentation of clozapine therapy, the assumption being that monotherapy with clozapine would often be attempted first before less well-studied alternatives such as augmentation strategies with other antipsychotics would be employed. There are still circumstances in which augmentation of other antipsychotics may be considered before a clozapine trial. In many of these cases, the target symptom is something other than residual psychotic symptoms – e.g., benzodiazepines for agitation and hostility, antidepressants for depressive symptomatology, mood stabilizers for affective lability
- An estimated one third of individuals with schizophrenia do not achieve an adequate response to antipsychotic treatment. The superiority of clozapine in treatment-resistant schizophrenia (commonly defined as inadequate response to sequential trials of two or more antipsychotics) is well established. Estimates of improvement when switched to clozapine vary from 30% to 60%
- Before concluding that a trial of clozapine monotherapy has been unsuccessful, the following is suggested
  - An adequate trial has been employed for at least 3 months (trials of up to 6 months are often suggested)
  - Rule out nonadherence (including partial adherence) to clozapine
  - Rule out substance abuse as a contributing factor
  - Rule out presence of an untreated depression
  - Rule out inadequate dosing (Note: On average, smokers require a 50% greater dose to achieve the same clozapine plasma level as nonsmokers – see also p. 176 for interactions of smoking with SGAs. Some CYP hyperfunction polymorphisms might mandate higher doses for same drug effects)
  - Consider obtaining a clozapine plasma level to confirm adherence/adequate dosing
- Should a decision to employ an augmentation strategy be made, a detailed plan should be documented that clearly states the agent to be used, the planned dosage strategy, the target symptoms to be evaluated, and the anticipated time to see effect/trial period (e.g., 3–4 months), and how and when to monitor for efficacy and safety. The plan should also include a strategy for discontinuing the augmenting agent should it prove to be ineffective. An adequate trial period of at least 10 weeks has been suggested when augmenting clozapine with a second antipsychotic
- An overview of augmentation strategies for clozapine-refractory schizophrenia is presented below
- In addition to the information provided below, refer to the corresponding drug interaction section

In General

- A consensus among members of the Treatment Response and Resistance in Psychosis (TRRIP) working group (63 members) is as follows:
  1. For clozapine-refractory positive symptoms, combination with a second antipsychotic (amisulpride or oral aripiprazole) or augmentation with ECT achieved consensus,
  2. For negative symptoms, waiting for a delayed response was recommended; as an intervention for clozapine-refractory negative symptoms, clozapine augmentation with an antidepressant, a mood stabilizer, or ECT met consensus criteria, and
  3. For clozapine-refractory aggression, augmentation with a mood stabilizer or a second antipsychotic achieved consensus
- A pair-wise meta-analysis of 46 studies of 25 interventions found that the most effective augmentation agents for total psychosis symptoms were aripiprazole, fluoxetine, and sodium valproate. Memantine was effective for negative symptoms

Anticonvulsants

- A meta-analysis of 22 RCTs (1227 participants) with 4 agents (topiramate [5 RCTs, 270 participants], lamotrigine [8 RCTs, 299 participants], sodium valproate [6 RCTs, 430 participants], and magnesium valproate [3 RCTs, 228 participants]) found significant superiority in total psychopathology for topiramate, lamotrigine, and sodium valproate, compared to clozapine monotherapy. After removing outliers, the positive effect of sodium valproate remained but that of lamotrigine disappeared. Significantly improved efficacy in positive and general symptom severity was observed for topiramate and sodium valproate. Topiramate augmentation had a too-high discontinuation rate

Lamotrigine

- Lamotrigine augments the anti-aggression effects of clozapine, particularly verbal aggression
- Caution – both lamotrigine and clozapine have the potential to depress bone marrow function

<table>
<tr>
<td>Lithium</td>
<td>

- May be of benefit for schizoaffective patients (rather than with schizophrenia), with improvements in negative and cognitive symptoms
- Has been used for clozapine rechallenge in patients with previous clozapine-induced neutropenia
- Tremors, involuntary movements, and seizures, reversible leukocytosis and rhabdomyolysis reported when combined with clozapine

</td>
</tr>
<tr>
<td>Topiramate</td>
<td>

- Augmenting with topiramate may cause memory impairment and deficits in cognitive processing
- Augmenting with topiramate will offset some of the weight gain resulting from clozapine

</td>
</tr>
<tr>
<td>Valproic acid</td>
<td>

- There is conflicting evidence regarding the use of valproic acid as augmentation agent. Case reports suggest benefit in refractory patients on clozapine. A meta-analysis of five randomized controlled trials examining valproate as an add-on to various antipsychotics did not report beneficial results
- Reduces hostility and anxiety
- Caution – there are conflicting reports that valproic acid may increase serum clozapine levels and worsen the severity of weight gain (see Drug Interactions p. 169)

</td>
</tr>
</table>

Antidepressants

- Clozapine has anti-serotonergic effects that may be associated with the development of obsessive-compulsive symptoms. SSRIs could alleviate this to some extent
- Fluvoxamine inhibits CYP1A2, thereby increasing the clozapine/norclozapine ratio. Reduction of norclozapine levels results in improved metabolic profile
- Citalopram may be the antidepressant of choice to treat depressive symptoms in clozapine-treated patients due to its limited effect on serum clozapine levels
- Mirtazapine may improve avolition and anhedonia

Antipsychotics

- Augmentation of clozapine with a number of antipsychotics (amisulpride, aripiprazole, haloperidol, quetiapine, risperidone, and ziprasidone) has been studied. There is currently insufficient evidence to conclude superior efficacy of combination therapy over monotherapy
- In a nationwide cohort study of patients with schizophrenia in Finland (62,260 participants), certain combinations of antipsychotics showed reduced risk of psychiatric rehospitalization compared to monotherapy as follows: clozapine + aripiprazole (compared to clozapine monotherapy); aripiprazole + clozapine (compared to aripiprazole monotherapy); olanzapine + any long-acting injectable or clozapine (compared to olanzapine monotherapy); risperidone + clozapine, olanzapine, or quetiapine (compared to risperidone monotherapy); quetiapine + any antipsychotic (compared to quetiapine monotherapy); any long-acting injectable + olanzapine (compared to any long-acting injectable monotherapy). The combination associated with lowest risk of rehospitalization was clozapine + aripiprazole[27]

<table>
<tr>
<td>Amisulpride</td>
<td>

- Open retrospective study showed beneficial effects in ameliorating positive and negative symptoms. Allowed for a 24% reduction in clozapine dose and thus a better side effect profile
- Comparison study: Clozapine augmented with amisulpride was superior to clozapine augmented with quetiapine at 8 weeks using BPRS
- Another study showed improvement in global psychopathology with doses up to 600 mg amisulpride
- An RCT (768 participants) of amisulpride augmentation of clozapine reported that, compared with participants randomized to placebo, those receiving amisulpride (up to 800 mg/day) had a greater chance of being a responder (20% reduction in total PANSS score) by the 12-week follow-up and a greater improvement in negative symptoms. However, these numerical differences were not statistically significant and only evident at 12 weeks. Amisulpride was associated with a greater side effect burden, including cardiac side effects
- May reduce clozapine-induced hypersalivation

</td>
</tr>
<tr>
<td>Aripiprazole</td>
<td>

- Has resulted in improvements in waist circumference, BMI, body weight, and serum lipids
- A 24-week study showed significant improvements in positive symptoms
- Clozapine + aripiprazole was the antipsychotic combination associated with the lowest risk of rehospitalization and was superior to clozapine monotherapy in a cohort study[27]
- May help improve negative symptoms

</td>
</tr>
</table>

Electroconvulsive Therapy (ECT)

- Of benefit in acute schizophrenia when a rapid reduction in symptoms is desired, especially if catatonia or affective symptoms are present
- May be more effective in schizoaffective disorder than in catatonic or hebephrenic schizophrenia
- Some reports suggest superiority with bilateral treatment; usually 12–20 treatments required for schizophrenia
- A meta-analysis of 18 RCTs (1769 participants) reported that adjunctive ECT was superior to clozapine monotherapy regarding symptomatic improvement at post-ECT assessment and endpoint assessment, separating as early as week 1–2

Antipsychotic Augmentation Strategies (cont.)

- Benefits may not be sustained upon discontinuation of ECT and the risk-to-benefit ratio of maintenance ECT in this population is unknown
- Predominant side effects include nausea, tachycardia, hypertension, memory problems, and confusion

Memantine

- A small RCT reported benefit in positive and negative symptoms when memantine 20 mg/day (a nonselective NMDA receptor antagonist) was added to clozapine in patients with refractory schizophrenia
- In an RCT crossover study in patients with clozapine-treated refractory schizophrenia, memantine addition significantly improved verbal and visual memory and negative symptoms without serious adverse effects; results were sustained in an open-label 1-year extension study
- A pair-wise meta-analysis of 46 studies of 25 interventions reported that memantine was effective for negative symptoms

Raloxifene

- Mixed results in males and females in restoring cognition or reducing symptom severity; benefits may be related to patient's age, dosage, and duration of treatment
- Shown to have beneficial effects on attention/processing speed and memory for both men and women
- Double-blind placebo-controlled studies report contradictory results with raloxifene (120 mg/day) augmentation of antipsychotics in postmenopausal women: Negative results seen in severely decompensated patients with schizophrenia, positive results reported in refractory schizophrenia
- Consideration: Small increase in the risk of venous thromboembolism and endometrial cancer

Repetitive Transcranial Magnetic Stimulation (rTMS)

- A review of the literature finds evidence that repetitive transcranial magnetic stimulation can have benefit in relieving positive and negative symptoms of schizophrenia, particularly auditory hallucinations

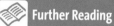 **Further Reading**

References

1 Taipale H, Tanskanen A, Mehtälä J, et al. 20-year follow-up study of physical morbidity and mortality in relationship to antipsychotic treatment in a nationwide cohort of 62,250 patients with schizophrenia (FIN20). World Psychiatry. 2020;19(1):61–68. doi:10.1002/wps.20699

2 Correll CU, Solmi M, Croatto G, et al. Mortality in people with schizophrenia: A systematic review and meta-analysis of relative risk and aggravating or attenuating factors. World Psychiatry. 2022;21(2):248–271. doi:10.1002/wps.20994

3 Elbe D, Black TR, McGrane IR, et al. Clinical handbook of psychotropic drugs for children and adolescents. (4th ed.). Boston, MA: Hogrefe Publishing, 2019.

4 American Psychiatric Association. Practice guideline for the treatment of patients with schizophrenia. (3rd ed.). Retrieved from doi:10.1176/appi.books.9780890424841

5 Miura I, Nosaka T, Yabe H, et al. Antidepressive effect of antipsychotics in the treatment of schizophrenia: Meta-regression analysis of randomized placebo-controlled trials. Int J Neuropsychopharmacol. 2021;24(3):200–215. doi:10.1093/ijnp/pyaa082

6 Sarva H, Henchcliffe C. Valbenazine as the first and only approved treatment for adults with tardive dyskinesia. Expert Rev Clin Pharmacol. 2018;11(3):209–217. doi:10.1080/17512433.2018.1429264

7 Credible Meds Worldwide. https://www.crediblemeds.org

8 Klinger G, Stahl B, Fusar-Poli P, et al. Antipsychotic drugs and breastfeeding. Pediatr Endocrinol Rev. 2013;10(3):308–317.

9 Drug interaction guide. Immunodeficiency Clinic, Toronto General Hospital. Retrieved from https://hivclinic.ca/wp-content/plugins/php/app.php

10 Azorin JM, Bowden CL, Garay RP, et al. Possible new ways in the pharmacological treatment of bipolar disorder and comorbid alcoholism. Neuropsychiatr Dis Treat. 2010;6:37–46. doi:10.2147/NDT.S6741

11 Sheehan JJ, Sliwa JK, Amatniek JC, et al. Atypical antipsychotic metabolism and excretion. Curr Drug Metab. 2010;11(6):516–525. doi:10.2174/138920010791636202#sthash.ou4XZBI4.dpuf

12 Lincoln J, Stewart ME, Preskorn SH. How sequential studies inform drug development: evaluating the effect of food intake on optimal bioavailability of ziprasidone. J Psychiatr Pract. 2010;16(2):103–114. doi:10.1097/01.pra.0000369971.64908.dc

13 Pillinger T, McCutcheon RA, Vano L, et al. Comparative effects of 18 antipsychotics on metabolic function in patients with schizophrenia, predictors of metabolic dysregulation, and association with psychopathology: A systematic review and network meta-analysis. Lancet. 2020;7(1):64–77. doi:10.1016/S2215-0366(19)30416-X

14 Anderson TJ, Grégoire J, Pearson GJ, et al. 2016 Canadian Cardiovascular Society guidelines for the management of dyslipidemia for the prevention of cardiovascular disease in the adult. Can J Cardiol. 2016;32(11):1263–1282. doi:10.1016/j.cjca.2016.07.510

15 Babu GN, Desai G, Tippeswamy H, et al. Birth weight and use of olanzapine in pregnancy: A prospective comparative study. J Clin Psychopharmacol. 2010;30(3):331–332. doi:10.1097/JCP.0b013e3181db8734

16 Toronto General Hospital HIV/HCV drug therapy guide. https://hivclinic.ca/drug-information/drug-interaction-tables/

17 Hale TW, Krutsch K. Hale's medications and mothers' milk 2023. (20th ed.) New York, NY: Springer, 2022.

18 Mansuri Z, Reddy A, Vadukapuram R, et al. Pimavanserin in the treatment of Parkinson's disease psychosis: Meta-analysis and meta-regression of randomized clinical trials. Innov Clin Neurosci. 2022;19(1–3):46–51. Retrieved from https://pubmed.ncbi.nlm.nih.gov/35382074/

19 Brunton LL, Lazo JS, Parker K. Goodman & Gillman's The pharmacological basis of therapeutics (11th ed.) New York, NY: McGraw-Hill, 2006.

20 Buckley PF. Receptor-binding profiles of antipsychotics: Clinical strategies when switching between agents. J Clin Psychiatry. 2007;68(Suppl. 6):5–9.

21 Horacek J, Bubenikova-Valesova V, Kopecek M. Mechanism of action of atypical antipsychotic drugs and the neurobiology of schizophrenia. CNS Drugs 2006;20(5):389–409. doi: 10.2165/00023210-200620050-00004

22 Leucht S, Samara M, Heres S, et al. Dose equivalents for second-generation antipsychotics: The minimum effective dose method. Schizophr Bull. 2014;40(2):314–326. doi:10.1093/schbul/sbu001

23 Flockhart DA. Drug interactions: Cytochrome P450 drug interaction table. Indiana University School of Medicine. Retrieved from http://medicine.iupui.edu/clinpharm/ddis/

24 Oesterheld JR, Osser DN. P450 Drug Interactions. Retrieved from http://www.mhc.com/Cytochromes

25 http://www.atforum.com/SiteRoot/pages/addiction_resources/P450%20Drug%20Interactions.PDF, http://mhc.daytondcs.com:8080/ddi46/resources/PgpTable.html, http://mhc.daytondcs.com:8080/ddi46/resources/UGTTable.html, http://www.psychresidentonline.com/CYP450%20drug%20interactions.htm

26 Thyssen A, Rusch S, Herben V, et al. Risperidone long-acting injection: Pharmacokinetics following administration in deltoid versus gluteal muscle in schizophrenic patients. J Clin Pharmacol. 2010;50(9):1011–1021. doi:10.1177/0091270009355156

27 Tiihonen J, Taipale H, Mehtälä J, et al. Association of antipsychotic polypharmacy vs monotherapy with psychiatric rehospitalization among adults with schizophrenia. JAMA Psychiatry. 2019;76(5):499–507. doi:10.1001/jamapsychiatry.2018.4320

Additional Suggested Reading

- Ceraso A, Lin JJ, Schneider-Thoma J, et al. Maintenance treatment with antipsychotic drugs for schizophrenia. Cochrane Database Syst Rev. 2020;8(8):CD008016. doi:10.1002/14651858.CD008016.pub3

- Gentile S. Antipsychotic therapy during early and late pregnancy. A systematic review. Schizophr Bull. 2010;36(3):518–544. doi:10.1093/schbul/sbn107

- Greenblatt HK, Greenblatt DJ. Use of antipsychotics for the treatment of behavioral symptoms of dementia. J Clin Pharmacol. 2016;56(9):1048–1057. doi:10.1002/jcph.731

- Kim DD, Barr AM, Lu C, et al. Clozapine-associated obsessive-compulsive symptoms and their management: A systematic review and analysis of 107 reported cases. Psychother Psychosom. 2020;89(3):151–160. doi:10.1159/000505876

- Lee LH, Choi C, Collier AC, et al. The pharmacokinetics of second-generation long-acting injectable antipsychotics: Limitations of monograph values. CNS Drugs. 2015;29(12):975–983. doi:10.1007/s40263-015-0295-2

- Lian L, Kim DD, Procyshyn RM, et al. Long-acting injectable antipsychotics for early psychosis: A comprehensive systematic review. PLoS One. 2022;17(4):e0267808. doi:10.1371/journal.pone.0267808

- Lindenmayer JP, Kaur A. Antipsychotic management of schizoaffective disorder: A review. Drugs. 2016;76(5):589–604. doi:10.1007/s40265-016-0551-x

- Lobo MC, Whitehurst TS, Kaar SJ, et al. New and emerging treatments for schizophrenia: A narrative review of their pharmacology, efficacy and side effect profile relative to established antipsychotics. Neurosci Biobehav Rev. 2022;132:324–361. doi:10.1016/j.neubiorev.2021.11.032

- Remington G, Foussias G, Fervaha G, et al. Treating negative symptoms in schizophrenia: An update. Curr Treat Options Psychiatry. 2016;3(2):133–150. doi:10.1007/s40501-016-0075-8

- Roy S, Charreteur R, Peries M, et al. Abuse and misuse of second-generation antipsychotics: An analysis using VigiBase, the World Health Organisation pharmacovigilance database. Br J Clin Pharmacol. 2022;88(10):4646–4653. doi:10.1111/bcp.15420

- Sabe M, Pillinger T, Kaiser S, et al. Half a century of research on antipsychotics and schizophrenia: A scientometric study of hotspots, nodes, bursts, and trends. Neurosci Biohav Rev. 2022;136, 104608. doi:10.1016/j.neubiorev.2022.104608

- Schneider-Thoma J, Chalkou K, Dörries C, et al. Comparative efficacy and tolerability of 32 oral and long-acting injectable antipsychotics for the maintenance treatment of adults with schizophrenia: A systematic review and network meta-analysis. Lancet. 2022;399(10327):824–836. doi:10.1016/S0140-6736(21)01997-8

- Ventriglio A, Gentile A, Stella E, et al. Metabolic issues in patients affected by schizophrenia: Clinical characteristics and medical management. Front Neurosci. 2015;9:297. doi:10.3389/fnins.2015.00297

- Wang M, Ma Y, Shen Z, et al. Mapping the knowledge of antipsychotics-induced sudden cardiac death: A scientometric analysis in CiteSpace and VOSviewer. Front Psychiatry. 2022;13:925583. doi:10.3389/fpsyt.2022.925583

- Yin J, Collier AC, Barr AM, et al. Paliperidone palmitate long-acting injectable given intramuscularly in the deltoid versus the gluteal muscle: Are they therapeutically equivalent? J Clin Psychopharmacol. 2015;35(4):447–449. doi:10.1097/JCP.0000000000000361

ANTIPSYCHOTIC-INDUCED EXTRAPYRAMIDAL SIDE EFFECTS AND THEIR MANAGEMENT

Extrapyramidal Adverse Effects of Antipsychotics

	Acute Extrapyramidal Effects	Tardive Syndromes
Onset	Acute or insidious (up to 30 days)	• After months or years of treatment, especially if drug dose is decreased or discontinued • Tends to persist for years or decades
Proposed mechanism	Most EPS symptoms are due to dopamine (D_2) blockade (if >80%), and positively correlate with association rates to D_2 receptor Affinity for other receptors (e.g., 5-HT_{1A}, 5-HT_{2A}, and M_1) involved in EPS	• Precise pathophysiology remains unclear • Upregulation and supersensitivity of postsynaptic dopamine receptors induced by long-term blockade • Neurotoxic effects of free radicals produced by the metabolism of excessive compensatory dopamine release, coupled with impairment of the antioxidant system • Glutamate-associated excitotoxicity • GABA dysfunction in the globus pallidus/substantia nigra • Multiple genetic associations related to schizophrenia, the dopamine system, metabolism of antipsychotics and free radicals (Nur77 deletion, ICOMT, DRD2, CYP1A2, IP5K2A gene polymorphisms) • Cholinergic deficiency
Treatment	• Respond to antiparkinsonian drugs • See p. 222 • Akathisia may be mediated by different mechanisms and is therefore more responsive to other treatments (e.g., benzodiazepines, β-blockers – see p. 233)	• **Valbenazine** and **deutetrabenazine** are FDA-approved drugs for treating tardive dyskinesia (TD). No other agents or strategies have proven efficacy in the treatment of tardive syndromes • **Valbenazine** (prodrug of the (+)α isomer of tetrabenazine): Reported to improve TD in a randomized double-blind placebo-controlled 6-week Phase III trial of 234 patients (following a Phase II trial). During the study extension, valbenazine maintained efficacy and safety for up to 46 weeks; adverse effects similar to tetrabenazine • **Deutetrabenazine** is a derivative of tetrabenazine (deuterated formulation). Deutetrabenazine improved TD in two phase III 12-week randomized, double-blind placebo-controlled studies. In the first study of 117 patients with moderate to severe TD, deutetrabenazine reduced abnormal movements (measured with AIMS). The second study of 298 patients with TD demonstrated the efficacy, safety, and tolerability of deutetrabenazine 24 mg/day and 36 mg/day • Consider the severity of TD, the degree of distress, and potential risks and benefits of any treatment strategy before taking action • Early recognition and discontinuation of the offending antipsychotic have been recommended as a means to improve the chance of remission, but discontinuation of antipsychotic treatment is not often feasible • Dosage reduction or use of lowest effective dose have also been suggested, but the success of dosage reduction or cessation has not been proven and must be weighed against the risk of relapse[1] • Slow taper recommended to avoid worsening of TD or chorea-like withdrawal-emergent syndrome. Switching to an atypical antipsychotic, such as clozapine or quetiapine, has also been recommended. However, high doses of atypical antipsychotics may cause TD and should not be used for long-term treatment of TD • Restarting or increasing the dose of the causative antipsychotic should be avoided and reserved only for the most severe cases that require immediate control of involuntary movements • The tendency for antipsychotic discontinuation to worsen TD and for antipsychotic dosage increase to suppress TD in the short term, as well as the waxing/waning nature of TD over time may bias placebo-controlled studies examining the effectiveness of antipsychotics in treating TD in favor of the antipsychotic and make interpretation of the results difficult • *Anticholinergic agents*: No benefit and may worsen tardive dyskinesias – taper and discontinuation recommended. May benefit tardive dystonia • Other experimental therapies/potential interventions (Note: large-scale clinical trials are required to confirm results) include:

	Acute Extrapyramidal Effects	Tardive Syndromes
		Benzodiazepines (indirect GABA agonist): Limited evidence – small benefit reported in 1 study. Small double-blind RCT reported benefit with clonazepam
		β-blockers: Used in tardive akathisia – insufficient evidence regarding efficacy. Low doses of propranolol suggested to have an antidyskinesia effect – very limited evidence from case reports
		Botulinum toxin: Limited studies with conflicting results – botulinum toxin has been shown to benefit patients with cervical dystonia, involuntary tongue protrusion in case reports; a small, single-blind study failed to show benefit in orofacial TD
		Branched-chain amino acids: Limited evidence demonstrating potential benefit in children and adolescents and in men. One double-blind, placebo-controlled 3-week study with 18 patients showed benefit
		Calcium channel blockers: Currently no evidence to support routine use. Diltiazem – moderate evidence against
		Clonidine: Insufficient evidence – few studies, small number of patients, poor methodology
		Deep brain stimulation (DBS): Insufficient evidence – benefits reported in tardive dystonia
		Dopamine-depleting medications: Tetrabenazine: A number of small trials with design issues suggesting potential benefit. Duration of treatment and dose-dependent serious adverse effects are concerns. TD relapse in most patients once drug is withdrawn. Reserpine: insufficient evidence, central and peripheral adverse effects. Amantadine: two small double-blind trials showed symptom improvement – weak evidence
		Essential fatty acids (omega-3): Experimental – benefit reported in animal studies. No benefit reported in recent placebo-controlled double-blind trial with 77 patients
		Fluvoxamine: Five case reports of benefit at doses of 100–200 mg/day; fluvoxamine is a potent sigma-1 receptor agonist
		Ginkgo biloba (antioxidant): Double-blind study of 157 patients showed benefit with a standardized extract of G. biloba leaves (EGb-761) vs. placebo over 12 weeks
		Levetiracetam (reduces neurotransmitter release): A number of studies reporting benefit. Most were small size, open-label design, and of short duration. One small RCT reporting benefit vs. placebo
		Melatonin (hormone with antioxidant effects, role in circadian rhythms): Two small placebo-controlled, double-blind studies showed significant improvement in a few patients with doses of 10 and 20 mg/day
		Piracetam (nootropic, structural similarity to GABA): Weak evidence – initially effective in study 30 years ago. Recent randomized DBPC study (*n* = 40) reported symptom improvement
		Pyridoxine: Low-quality evidence – may have benefit; a small DBPC crossover study (15 participants) reported benefit with vitamin B6. A more recent larger 26-week randomized DBPC (50 participants) reported efficacy with 1200 mg/day
		Resveratrol (antioxidant found in grapes, cranberries): Experimental – reported to have protective effect when co-administered with antipsychotic agent in animal models
		Vitamin E: Most studied antioxidant for improving TD; 40 trials conducted over the past 30 years – evidence is limited and contradictory. May protect against further deterioration or reduce the risk of development. Patients with TD for less than 5 years might respond better
		Zolpidem: Limited evidence from case reports
		Zonisamide (antiepileptic – enhances GABA): Small open-label study reporting significant improvement in AIMS score in some patients
		Miscellaneous (baclofen, sodium valproate, ECT, estrogen, insulin, tryptophan): No strong evidence to support use. GABA agonists (baclofen, sodium valproate) associated with adverse effects which likely outweigh any possible benefits
		See p. 226 for additional information on potential treatments

Extrapyramidal

Extrapyramidal Adverse Effects of Antipsychotics (cont.)

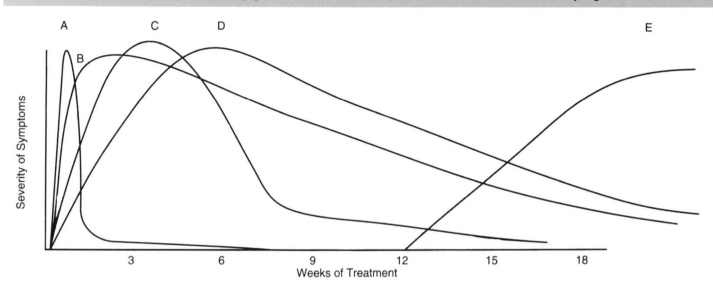

A: Dystonic reactions: uncoordinated spastic movements of muscle groups (e.g., trunk, tongue, face)
B: Akathisia: restlessness, pacing (may result in insomnia)
C: Bradykinesia: decreased muscular movements
   Rigidity: coarse muscular movement; loss of facial expression
D: Tremors: fine movement (shaking) of the extremities ("pill-rolling")
   Rabbit syndrome: involuntary movements around the lips
   Pisa syndrome: can either be acute or tardive in nature (rare; occurs more commonly in people with brain damage/abnormality)
E: Tardive syndromes: Symptoms of movement disorders that start about 3 months (or later) after therapy is initiated

Type	Physical (Motor) Symptoms	Psychological Symptoms	Onset	Proposed Risk Factors	Clinical Course	Treatment Options	Differential Diagnosis
Acute dystonias	Torsions and spasms of muscle groups; mostly affects muscles of the head and neck; muscle spasms, e.g., oculogyric crisis, trismus, laryngospasm, torti/retro/antero-collis tortipelvis, opisthotonus, blepharospasm	Anxiety, fear, panic Dysphoria Repetitive meaningless thoughts	Acute (usually within 24–48 h after the first dose); 90% occur within first week of treatment	Young males, children Antipsychotic naive High potency FGAs; low risk with SGAs and TGAs Rapid dose increase Moderate to high doses Lack of prophylactic antiparkinsonian medication Previous dystonic reaction Hypocalcemia, hyperthyroidism, hypoparathyroidism Dehydration Recent cocaine use Family history of dystonia	Acute, painful, spasmodic; oculogyria may be recurrent Acute laryngeal/ pharyngeal dystonia may be potentially life threatening	IM benztropine (1st line), IM diphenhydramine, sublingual lorazepam To prevent recurrence: prophylactic antiparkinsonian agents Reduce dose or change antipsychotic	Seizures Catatonia Hysteria Malingering Hypocalcemia Primary genetic disorders Neuro-degenerative disorders

Type	Physical (Motor) Symptoms	Psychological Symptoms	Onset	Proposed Risk Factors	Clinical Course	Treatment Options	Differential Diagnosis
Acute akathisia	Motor restlessness, fidgeting, pacing, rocking, swinging of leg, trunk rocking forward and backward, repeatedly crossing and uncrossing legs, inability to lie still, shifting from foot to foot Respiratory symptoms: Dyspnea or breathing discomfort	Restlessness, intense urge to move, irritability, agitation, violent outbursts, dysphoria, feeling "wound-up" or "antsy" or like "having a motor running inside"; sensation of skin crawling Mental unease	Acute to insidious (within hours to days); 90% occur within first 6 weeks of treatment; sometimes only with higher doses	Elderly female, young adults High caffeine intake High-potency FGAs; lower risk with SGAs TGAs: Aripiprazole and cariprazine associated with higher risk than many SGAs Brexpiprazole associated with lowest risk among TGAs Genetic predisposition Anxiety Diagnosis of mood disorder Microcytic anemia Low serum ferritin Concurrent use of SSRI	May continue through entire treatment Increases risk of tardive dyskinesia Suggested that it may contribute to suicide and/or violence	Reduce dose or change antipsychotic β-blockers (e.g., propranolol 10–20 mg bid) Mirtazapine 15 mg hs Benzodiazepines have been shown useful in small studies, anticholinergics may be considered if akathisia co-occurs with parkinsonism	Psychotic agitation/decompensation Severe agitation Anxiety Drug-intoxication Drug-seeking behavior/withdrawal Excess caffeine intake Restless leg syndrome
Acute pseudo-parkinsonism	Tremor: "pill-rolling"-type tremor (4–8 cycles per second; greater at rest and bilateral) Rigidity: cogwheel rigidity Bradykinesia: mask-like facial expression, diminished or absent arm swing, shuffling gait, stooped posture, slowness of movement	Slowed thinking Fatigue, anergia Cognitive impairment Depression	Acute to insidious (within 30 days); 90% occur within first 6 weeks of treatment	Elderly female High potency FGAs; lower risk with SGAs and TGAs Higher doses Antipsychotic polypharmacy Discontinuation of anticholinergics Concurrent neurological disorder Also seen with lithium, calcium channel blockers, SSRIs, MAOIs, and valproate	May continue through entire treatment (especially in the elderly)	Reduce dose or change antipsychotic Antiparkinsonian drug	Negative symptoms of schizophrenia Idiopathic Parkinson's disease Depression Essential tremor Vascular Parkinsonism
Pisa syndrome	Leaning to one side		Can be acute or tardive	Elderly patients Compromised brain function, dementia	Often ignored by patients	Antiparkinsonian drug (higher doses)	
Rabbit syndrome	Fine tremor of lower lip		After months of therapy	Elderly patients		Antiparkinsonian drug	

Extrapyramidal Adverse Effects of Antipsychotics (cont.)

Type	Physical (Motor) Symptoms	Psychological Symptoms	Onset	Proposed Risk Factors	Clinical Course	Treatment Options	Differential Diagnosis
Tardive akathisia	Persistent symptoms of akathisia following dose decrease or withdrawal of antipsychotic	As for akathisia, but subjective sense of restlessness may be less intense	After months of therapy; after drug withdrawal	As for akathisia Coexisting tardive dyskinesia, dystonia, and iron deficiency	Persistent; early discontinuation of antipsychotic increases chance of remission. Fluctuating course	Potential treatments (insufficient evidence for efficacy) include switch to an SGA (clozapine, also olanzapine or quetiapine despite limited evidence) or TGA (brexpiprazole associated with lowest risk of akathisia among TGAs) Suggested treatments include: anticholinergics, benzodiazepines, β-blockers (i.e., propranolol), vitamin B6	As for akathisia
Tardive dyskinesia	Involuntary abnormal movements of face (e.g., tics, frowning, grimacing), lips (pursing, puckering, smacking), jaw (chewing, clenching), tongue ("fly-catcher," rolling, dysarthria), eyelids (blinking, blepharospasm), limbs (tapping, piano-playing fingers or toes), trunk (rocking, twisting), neck (nodding), respiratory (dyspnea, gasping, sighing, grunting, forceful breathing) Often coexists with parkinsonism and akathisia. Abnormal movements disappear during sleep	Cognitive impairment, distress (talking, swallowing, eating) and embarrassment	After 3 or more months of therapy in adults and earlier in the elderly Common early sign is rapid flicking movement of the tongue ("fly-catcher tongue")	Age over 40, female, history of severe EPS early in treatment, chronic use of antipsychotics (FGAs more than SGAs/TGAs) or metoclopramide, chronic use of high doses of dopamine agonists in the treatment of Parkinson's disease, presence of a mood component, history of diabetes, cognitive impairment, alcohol and drug abuse (e.g., cannabis), organic brain damage	Persistent; early discontinuation of antipsychotic increases chance of remission Spontaneous remission in 14–24% after 5 years	Valbenazine 40 mg/day initial dose, increase to recommended dose of 80 mg/day after one week Deutetrabenazine 12 mg/day (6 mg bid) initial dose, increase at weekly intervals in increments of 6 mg/day; not to exceed 48 mg/day (24 mg bid). Dose should not exceed 36 mg/day (18 mg bid) in patients who are either poor CYP2D6 metabolizers or concomitantly taking strong CYP2D6 inhibitors Other treatment suggestions without proven efficacy include: Switch to an SGA (e.g., clozapine) or TGA Pyridoxine 300–400 mg/day Clonazepam 0.5–6 mg/day Tetrabenazine 50–150 mg/day Branched-chain amino acids (Tarvil, 222 mg/kg tid) Vitamin E 1200–1600 IU/day Vitamin B6 400–1200 IU/day Levetiracetam 1000–3000 mg Ginkgo biloba extract (EGb 761, 120–240 mg/day)	Spontaneous or withdrawal dyskinesia Stereotypic behavior Tourette's syndrome Huntington's chorea or other neurological conditions Movement disorder secondary to co-prescribed drug Systemic lupus erythematosus and other neuroimmune diseases
Tardive dystonia	Sustained muscle contractions of face, jaw, tongue, eyes, neck, limbs, back, or trunk (craniocervical area involved most frequently), e.g., blepharospasm, laryngeal dystonia, dysarthria, retroflexed hands		After months or years of therapy	Young male Genetic predisposition (?) Neurological disorder, mental retardation Coexisting tardive dyskinesia Akathisia	Persistent; early discontinuation of antipsychotic increases chance of remission	Switch to an SGA (clozapine) or TGA Suggestions for treatment include: Tetrabenazine 50–150 mg/day Higher doses of anticholinergics (e.g., trihexyphenidyl 40 mg/ day); Botulinum toxin 25–50 mg/site (multiple sites used)	Myoclonus Motor tics Idiopathic dystonia Meige syndrome

Type	Physical (Motor) Symptoms	Psychological Symptoms	Onset	Proposed Risk Factors	Clinical Course	Treatment Options	Differential Diagnosis
Tics	Motor (e.g., eye blinking, head jerking, shoulder shrugging) and/or vocal tics (e.g., throat clearing, coprolalia, barking)		After a few days to several years after antipsychotic initiation or 1 week to 3 months after antipsychotic discontinuation	FGAs: higher risk of i) tics occurring after antipsychotic discontinuation, ii) co-occurring motor and vocal tics, and iii) complex vocal tics (e.g., coprolalia)	Tics occurring during antipsychotic treatment may persist for 1–3 years and as long as 9 years Tics occurring during antipsychotic discontinuation may disappear spontaneously within 5 months to 2 years or persist for 1–2 years	Tics occurring during antipsychotic treatment: discontinue or reduce dose (may exacerbate core symptoms) or switch to an antipsychotic with a different receptor binding profile Tics occurring after antipsychotic discontinuation: reinitiate an antipsychotic Augmentation strategies: clomipramine, clonazepam, sodium valproate, clonidine, physostigmine, or biperiden	Myoclonus, obsessive-compulsive symptoms, blepharospasm, acute dystonia, stereotypes

Treatment Options for Extrapyramidal Side Effects

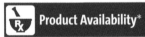 **Product Availability***

Generic Name	Chemical Class	Trade Name[A]	Dosage Forms and Strengths
Amantadine	Dopamine agonist	Symmetrel	Capsules/Tablets[B]: 100 mg Syrup: 50 mg/5 mL
Benztropine	Anticholinergic	Cogentin	Tablets: 0.5 mg[B], 1 mg, 2 mg Injection: 1 mg/mL
Biperiden[B]	Anticholinergic	Akineton[B]	Tablets[B]: 2 mg
Clonazepam	Benzodiazepine	Rivotril[C], Klonopin[B]	Tablets: 0.5 mg, 1 mg, 2 mg
Cyproheptadine	Antihistamine	Periactin	Tablets: 4 mg Syrup: 2 mg/5 mL
Deutetrabenazine	Vesicular monoamine transporter 2 (VMAT2) inhibitor	Austedo	Tablets[B]: 6 mg, 9 mg, 12 mg
Diazepam	Benzodiazepine	Diastat Diazemuls[C] Diazepam Intensol[B]	Rectal gel: 5 mg/mL Emulsion injection (IM/IV)[C]: 5 mg/mL Oral solution concentrate[B]: 5 mg/mL

Treatment Options for Extrapyramidal Side Effects (cont.)

Generic Name	Chemical Class	Trade Name(A)	Dosage Forms and Strengths
		Valium	Tablets: 2 mg, 5 mg, 10 mg Injection: 5 mg/mL Oral solution: 1 mg/mL
Diphenhydramine	Antihistamine	Benadryl	Caplets/Capsules/Liquigels/Tablets: 25 mg, 50 mg Oral liquid: 6.25 mg/5 mL(C), 12.5 mg/5 mL Injection: 50 mg/mL
Ethopropazine(C)	Anticholinergic	Parsitan(C)	Tablets(C): 50 mg
Lorazepam	Benzodiazepine	Ativan Lorazepam Intensol(B)	Tablets: 0.5 mg, 1 mg, 2 mg Sublingual tablets(C): 0.5 mg, 1 mg, 2 mg Injection: 2 mg/mL(B), 4 mg/mL Solution(B): 2 mg/mL
Orphenadrine	Skeletal muscle relaxant	Orfenace(C), Orphenadrine citrate	Extended-release tablets: 100 mg Injection(B): 30 mg/mL
Procyclidine(C)	Anticholinergic	Kemadrin(C)	Tablets(C): 2.5 mg, 5 mg
Propranolol	β-blocker	Hemangeol Hemangiol(C) Inderal(B) Inderal LA InnoPran XL(B)	Oral solution(B): 4.28 mg/mL (propranolol hydrochloride) Oral solution: 3.75 mg/mL (propranolol base) Tablets: 10 mg, 20 mg, 40 mg, 60 mg, 80 mg Sustained-release capsules: 60 mg, 80 mg, 120 mg, 160 mg Extended-release capsules: 80 mg, 120 mg
Trihexyphenidyl	Anticholinergic	Artane	Tablets: 2 mg, 5 mg Elixir(B): 2 mg/5 mL
Valbenazine	VMAT2 inhibitor	Ingrezza	Capsules(B): 40 mg, 80 mg

* Refer to Health Canada's Drug Product Database or the FDA's Drugs@FDA for the most current availability information.   (A) Generic preparations may be available,   (B) Not marketed in Canada,   (C) Not marketed in the USA

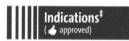

Indications‡
(👍 approved)

Indications related to EPS (see p. 233 for comparison of drugs):
- 👍 Tardive dyskinesia (valbenazine – USA; deutetrabenazine, also indicated for the treatment of chorea associated with Huntington's disease – USA)
- 👍 Pseudoparkinsonian effects (tremor, rigidity, shuffling) (benztropine, trihexyphenidyl – Canada and USA; ethopropazine – Canada; amantadine, biperiden, diphenhydramine injection – USA)
- 👍 Drug-induced extrapyramidal reactions (benztropine, trihexyphenidyl – Canada and USA; ethopropazine – Canada; amantadine, biperiden – USA)
- 👍 Musculoskeletal conditions (acute, painful) (orphenadrine – Canada and USA)
- 👍 Tremor (essential) (propranolol – USA)

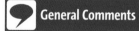

General Comments

- Individual patients may respond better, or tolerate one drug over another
- Because of the acute onset and distressing nature of acute dystonic reactions, IM benztropine is typically the preferred treatment and usually brings relief within 15 min
- Anticholinergics including benztropine may be preferred for dystonias, parkinsonism (especially rigidity); benzodiazepines most useful for akathisia; and propranolol most useful for akathisia and tremor

‡ Indications listed here do not necessarily apply to all agents for treating extrapyramidal side effects or all countries. Please refer to a country's regulatory database (e.g., US Food and Drug Administration, Health Canada Drug Product Database) for the most current availability information and indications

- Valbenazine and deutetrabenazine are the only proven treatments for tardive dyskinesia. For other tardive movement disorders, prevention (use antipsychotics at the lowest effective dose and only when necessary) and frequent assessment/early detection are important
- Controversy exists whether antiparkinsonian agents should be given prophylactically to patients at risk of developing EPS with FGAs, or whether they should only be started when EPS develop. The decision to initiate preventative agents should be made on an individual basis with consideration given to a number of factors including patient preference, history of EPS, potential of the particular antipsychotic to induce EPS, presence of comorbidities or concomitant medications, which may be exacerbated by anticholinergic effects
- There is a wide variance (e.g., 2–50%) in the reported incidence of drug-induced parkinsonian effects. Rates are higher in the elderly and in females and are dose related
- Consider dosage reduction or discontinuation of the offending antipsychotic agent (if appropriate) or switching to a newer generation antipsychotic as potential treatment options

 Pharmacology

- Centrally-active anticholinergic drugs cross the blood-brain barrier, block excitatory muscarinic pathways in the basal ganglia, and restore the dopamine/acetylcholine balance disrupted by antipsychotic drugs, thus treating EPS
- Five subtypes of muscarinic receptors have been determined; the M_1 and M_2 subtypes are the best characterized; the M_1 subtype is found centrally and peripherally, whereas the M_2 subtype is located in the heart
- Agents in order from highest to lowest affinity for the M_1 receptor as follows: Benztropine (0.2 nM), biperiden (0.48 nM), trihexyphenidyl (1.6 nM), procyclidine (4.6 nM) [values in parentheses are K_i values as determined using cloned human receptors]
- Agents in order from highest to lowest affinity for the M_2 receptor as follows: Benztropine (1.4 nM), biperiden (6.3 nM), trihexyphenidyl (7 nM), procyclidine (25 nM) [values in parentheses are K_i values as determined using cloned human receptors]
- Anticholinergic drugs also block presynaptic reuptake of dopamine (primarily benztropine), norepinephrine (primarily diphenhydramine), and serotonin (diphenhydramine, weakly)
- Valbenazine and deutetrabenazine block presynaptic monoamine uptake through reversible inhibition of the vesicular monoamine transporter 2 (VMAT2)
- Amantadine and ethopropazine have moderate NMDA (n-methyl-D-aspartate) receptor blocking properties; amantadine may exert its activity by increasing dopamine at the receptor (facilitates presynaptic release and inhibits reuptake)

 Dosing

- See chart pp. 236–238
- Dosage increases must be balanced against the risk of evoking anticholinergic adverse effects
- Dosage should be adjusted for patients with moderate–severe hepatic impairment (reduce valbenazine to 40 mg/day)
- Consider dosage reduction in CYP2D6 poor metabolizers or when given in combination with potent CYP2D6 and/or CYP3A4 inhibitors (valbenazine) or CYP2D6 inhibitors (deutetrabenazine)
- Plasma level monitoring is not currently advocated

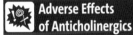 **Adverse Effects of Anticholinergics**

CNS

- CNS effects: Seen primarily in the elderly and at high doses; include cognitive impairment (including decreased memory and distractibility), somnolence, confusion, disorientation, delirium, hallucinations, restlessness, stimulation, weakness, headache
- Excess use/abuse of these drugs may lead to an anticholinergic (toxic) psychosis with symptoms of disorientation, confusion, euphoria (see Toxicity p. 230), in addition to physical signs such as dry mouth, blurred vision, dilated pupils, dry flushed skin
- Dopamine-agonist activity of amantadine can occasionally cause worsening of psychotic symptoms, nightmares, insomnia, and mood disturbances
- Tetrabenazine may cause neuroleptic malignant syndrome (NMS) due to reduced dopaminergic transmission. Patients on deutetrabenazine or valbenazine should be closely observed for any signs of NMS
- Deutetrabenazine may increase depression in patients with TD; it can also increase depression and suicidality in patients with Huntington's disease

Peripheral

- Related to anticholinergic potency (i.e., M_1 antagonism): Benztropine > biperiden > trihexyphenidyl > procyclidine > orphenadrine > diphenhydramine
- Common: Dry mouth, blurred vision, decreased bronchial secretions, constipation, dry eyes, flushed skin

Treatment Options for Extrapyramidal Side Effects (cont.)

- Occasional: Delayed micturition, urinary retention, sexual dysfunction
- Excess doses can suppress sweating, resulting in hyperthermia

Cardiovascular Effects

- Palpitations, tachycardia; high doses can cause arrhythmias
- QT prolongation (valbenazine and deutetrabenazine at higher concentrations)

GI Effects

- Nausea, vomiting, gastroesophageal reflux disease, paralytic ileus

 Precautions

- Use cautiously in patients with conditions in which excess anticholinergic activity could be harmful (e.g., benign prostatic hypertrophy, urinary retention, narrow-angle glaucoma, myasthenia gravis, GI obstruction, arrhythmias)
- Avoid valbenazine and deutetrabenazine in patients with congenital long QT syndrome or in patients with arrhythmias associated with a prolonged QT interval
- May decrease sweating; educate and monitor patients on these medications in hot weather to prevent hyperthermia
- Monitor breathing patterns in patients with respiratory difficulties since antiparkinsonian medications can dry bronchial secretions and make breathing difficult
- Caution when using amantadine in patients with peripheral edema or history of congestive heart failure (there are patients who developed congestive heart failure while receiving amantadine); the clearance of amantadine is significantly reduced in adult patients with renal insufficiency
- If withdrawn abruptly, anticholinergic drugs may cause a cholinergic rebound: Symptoms include restlessness, anxiety, dyskinesia, dysphoria, sweating, and diarrhea
- Euphorigenic and hallucinogenic properties may lead to abuse of anticholinergic agents
- Use of anticholinergic agents in patients with existing TD can exacerbate the movement disorder and may unmask latent TD
- Monitor patients on deutetrabenazine or valbenazine for signs of NMS

Toxicity

- Can occur following excessive doses, with combination therapy, in the elderly, poor metabolizers, hepatic impairment, or with drug abuse
- Symptoms of anticholinergic toxicity include:
  - Blind as a bat (mydriasis, blurred vision)
  - Dry as a bone (dry skin and mucous membranes, no sweating, urinary retention)
  - Hot as a hare (hyperthermia)
  - Mad as a hatter (confusion, delirium, hallucinations)
  - Red as a beet (flushed skin)
  - Sinus tachycardia, hypertension, decreased bowel sounds, muscle twitching, seizures, and coma may also occur

Management

- General guidelines:
  - Absorption may be delayed because of the pharmacological effects of anticholinergics on gastrointestinal motility. Effects of benztropine intoxication can persist for 2–3 days
  - Maintain an open airway and assist ventilation if required; cardiac and pulse oximetry monitoring
  - Decontamination with single-dose activated charcoal may be administered under appropriate conditions – delayed gut emptying and reduced peristalsis caused by anticholinergics may permit use of activated charcoal even when patients present hours post ingestion. Hemodialysis, hemoperfusion, and peritoneal dialysis are not effective in removing these agents
  - Following GI decontamination, many cases can be managed well with supportive care – e.g., control agitation (benzodiazepines); fever (fluids, antipyretics, active cooling measures); seizures (benzodiazepines); urinary retention (bladder catheterization), manage cardiac conduction disturbances

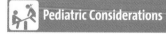 **Pediatric Considerations**

- For detailed information on the use of antiparkinsonian agents in this population, please see the *Clinical Handbook of Psychotropic Drugs for Children and Adolescents*[2]
- Doses up to 80 mg trihexyphenidyl have been employed in the treatment of hereditary dystonias in children; these were well tolerated with few side effects

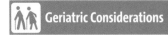

Geriatric Considerations	• The elderly are very sensitive to anticholinergic drugs. Monitor for constipation, urinary retention as well as increased confusion, memory loss, and disorientation. Avoid drugs with potent central or peripheral anticholinergic activity • Caution when using two or more drugs with anticholinergic properties • Caution with VMAT2 inhibitors, start low and go slow
Use in Pregnancy◇	• Greatest risk of malformation during first trimester use • Consider potential for withdrawal or other effects (e.g., metabolism) in newborn and effects on delivery during third trimester • Limited human data with many of these agents • See chart pp. 234–235
Breast Milk	• See chart pp. 234–235
Nursing Implications	• These drugs should be given only to relieve extrapyramidal side effects of antipsychotics; excess use or abuse can precipitate a toxic psychosis • Some adverse effects of these drugs (i.e., anticholinergic) are additive to those of antipsychotics; observe patient for signs of side effects or toxicity • Monitor patient's intake and output. Urinary retention can occur, especially in the elderly; bethanechol (Urecholine) can be used to reverse this effect • To help prevent gastric irritation, administer drug after meals • Relieve dry mouth by giving patient cool drinks, ice chips, sugarless chewing gum, or hard, sour candy. Suggest frequent rinsing of the mouth, and teeth should be brushed regularly. Patients should avoid calorie-laden beverages and sweet candy as they increase the likelihood of dental caries and promote weight gain. Formerly well-fitting dentures may cause rubbing and/or ulceration of the gums. Products that promote or replace salivation (e.g., MoiStir, Saliment) may be of benefit • Blurring of near vision is due to paresis of the ciliary muscle. This can be helped by wearing suitable glasses, reading by a bright light or, if severe, by the use of pilocarpine eye drops 0.5% • Dry eyes may be of particular difficulty to the elderly or those wearing contact lenses. Artificial tears or contact lens wetting solutions may be of benefit in dealing with this problem • Anticholinergics reduce peristalsis and decrease intestinal secretions, leading to constipation. Increasing fluids and bulk (e.g., bran, salads) as well as fruit in the diet is beneficial. If necessary, bulk laxatives (e.g., Metamucil, Prodiem) can be used; lactulose may be used for chronic constipation • Warn the patient not to drive a car or operate machinery until response to the drug has been determined • Appropriate patient education regarding medication and side effects is necessary prior to discharge
Patient Instructions	• For detailed patient instructions on antiparkinsonian agents for treating extrapyramidal side effects, see the Patient Information Sheet (details p. 474)
⏩ **Drug Interactions**	• Only clinically significant interactions are listed below • For more interaction information on any given combination, also see the corresponding chapter for the second agent • For drug interactions associated with benzodiazepines, please see p. 246

Class of Drug	Example	Interaction Effects
Adsorbent	Activated charcoal, antacids, cholestyramine, kaolin-pectin (attapulgite)	Oral absorption decreased when used simultaneously
Antiarrhythmic	Quinidine	Valbenazine: Increased exposure to valbenazine's active metabolite due to CYP2D6 inhibition; may increase risk of adverse reactions
Antibiotic	Clarithromycin	Increased exposure to valbenazine due to strong CYP3A4 inhibition; may increase risk of adverse reactions
	Co-trimoxazole (trimethoprim/sulfamethoxazole)	Amantadine: Competition for renal clearance resulting in elevated plasma level of amantadine

◇ See p. 473 for further information on drug use in pregnancy and effects on breast milk

Treatment Options for Extrapyramidal Side Effects (cont.)

Class of Drug	Example	Interaction Effects
Anticholinergic	Antidepressants, antihistamines, FGAs (low potency)	Anticholinergic agents: Increased atropine-like effects causing dry mouth, blurred vision, constipation, etc. May produce inhibition of sweating and may lead to paralytic ileus High doses can bring on a toxic psychosis
Anticonvulsant	Carbamazepine, phenytoin Topiramate	Valbenazine: Decreased exposure to valbenazine and its active metabolite due to CYP3A4 induction; may reduce efficacy Anticholinergic agents: May potentiate the risk of oligohidrosis and hyperthermia, particularly in pediatric patients
Antidepressant SSRI	 Fluoxetine, paroxetine	 Valbenazine and deutetrabenazine: Increased exposure to the active metabolites of valbenazine and tetrabenazine due to CYP2D6 inhibition; may increase risk of adverse reactions Cyproheptadine: Case reports of reversal of antidepressant and antibulimic effects of fluoxetine and paroxetine Procyclidine: Increased plasma level of procyclidine (by 40%) with paroxetine
NDRI	Bupropion	Amantadine: Case reports of neurotoxicity in elderly patients Valbenazine and deutetrabenazine: Bupropion may increase active metabolites of valbenazine and deutetrabenazine at higher doses via moderate CYP2D6 inhibition
MAOI	Isocarboxazid, phenelzine, selegiline	Deutetrabenazine: Contraindicated. Stop MAOI and wait at least 14 days before starting deutetrabenazine Valbenazine: May increase monoamine neurotransmitters in synapses, cause serotonin syndrome or reduce therapeutic effect of valbenazine
Antifungal	Itraconazole, ketoconazole	Valbenazine: Increased exposure to valbenazine due to strong CYP3A4 inhibition; may increase risk of adverse reactions
Antihypertensive	Hydrochlorothiazide, triamterene Reserpine	Reduced renal clearance of amantadine resulting in drug accumulation and possible toxicity Deutetrabenazine: Contraindicated. Stop reserpine and wait at least 20 days before starting deutetrabenazine to reduce the risk of overdosage
Antipsychotic	Aripiprazole, chlorpromazine, clozapine, flupenthixol, haloperidol, olanzapine, trifluoperazine Thioridazine	Anticholinergic agents: May aggravate tardive dyskinesia or unmask latent TD Additive anticholinergic effects may occur, resulting in paralytic ileus, hyperthermia, heat stroke, and anticholinergic intoxication syndrome Propranolol: May significantly increase thioridazine levels or cause arrhythmias Potential for additive hypotensive effects Deutetrabenazine: Increased risk of parkinsonism, NMS, and akathisia
Antitubercular	Rifampin	Valbenazine: Decreased exposure to valbenazine and its active metabolite due to CYP3A4 induction; may reduce efficacy
Caffeine		May offset beneficial effects by increasing tremor and akathisia
Cardiac glycoside	Digoxin	Anticholinergic agents: May increase bioavailability of digoxin tablets (not capsules or liquids) due to decreased gastric motility or inhibition of intestinal P-glycoprotein (valbenazine) Propranolol: May increase risk of bradycardia
Cholinesterase inhibitor	Donepezil, rivastigmine	Benztropine, diphenhydramine: Antagonism of effects
Herbal preparation	Hawthorn, kava kava, Siberian ginseng, valerian Henbane St. John's wort	Diphenhydramine: May increase effects of diphenhydramine. May enhance CNS depression Diphenhydramine: Increased anticholinergic effects with combination Valbenazine: Decreased exposure to valbenazine and its active metabolite due to CYP3A4 induction; may reduce efficacy

Class of Drug	Example	Interaction Effects
Opioid	Codeine, methadone, tramadol	Anticholinergic agents: Additive CNS effects including cognitive and psychomotor impairment Diphenhydramine: May interfere with analgesic effect of codeine due to reduced conversion of codeine to morphine via CYP2D6 inhibition
	Methadone, tramadol	Diphenhydramine: Additive respiratory depressant effects
Potassium supplement	Potassium chloride, potassium citrate	Anticholinergic agents: May potentiate the risk of upper GI injury of oral solid formulations of potassium salts, possibly due to increased GI transit time secondary to reduction of stomach and intestinal mobility
VMAT2 inhibitor	Deutetrabenazine, tetrabenazine, valbenazine	Concomitant use of two VMAT2 inhibitors is not recommended. Deutetrabenazine concomitant use with tetrabenazine or valbenazine is contraindicated. Deutetrabenazine can be initiated the following day after stopping tetrabenazine

Effects on Acute Extrapyramidal Symptoms and Tardive Dyskinesia

Agent	Tremor	Rigidity	Dystonia	Akinesia	Akathisia	Dyskinesia
Amantadine (Symmetrel)	++	++	+	+++	++	++
β-blockers (e.g., propranolol, nadolol)	++	–	–	–	+++	–
Benztropine (Cogentin)	++	+++	+++	++	++	–
Biperiden (Akineton)	++	+++	++	+++	+	–
Clonazepam (Rivotril, Klonopin)	–	+	+	–	+++	++
Cyproheptadine (Periactin)	–	–	–	–	+++	–
Deutetrabenazine (Austedo)	–	–	–	–	–	+++
Diazepam (Valium)	+	++	+++	+	+++	–
Diphenhydramine (Benadryl)	++	+	++	–	+++	–
Ethopropazine (Parsitan)	+++	++	+	+	++	–
Lorazepam (Ativan)	+	+	+++	–	+++	–
Orphenadrine (Norflex)	++	++	–	++	+	–
Procyclidine (Kemadrin)	+	++	++	++	++	–
Trihexyphenidyl (Artane)	+	++	++	+++	++	–
Valbenazine (Ingrezza)	–	–	–	–	–	+++

Based on literature and clinical observations: – effect not established, + some effect (20% response), ++ moderate effect (20–50% response), +++ good effect (over 50% response)

Comparison of Agents for Treating Acute Extrapyramidal Side Effects and Tardive Dyskinesia

Agent	Therapeutic Effects	Adverse Effects	Pregnancy	Breast Milk
Amantadine (Symmetrel)	An NMDA receptor antagonist. Pro-dopaminergic. Is not anticholinergic. Not recommended for acute dystonias – no injectable dosage form May improve akathisia (less effective than β-blockers and benzodiazepines), akinesia, rigidity, parkinsonism; may enhance the effects of other antiparkinsonian agents Tolerance to fixed dose may develop after 1–8 weeks. Long-term efficacy not established May be useful in levodopa-induced movement disorder	1–10%: Anorexia, nausea, orthostatic hypotension, peripheral edema, agitation, anxiety, ataxia, confusion, dizziness, fatigue, insomnia, hallucinations, livedo reticularis (mottled skin discoloration). Many are dose related and disappear on drug withdrawal <1%: NMS, seizures, coma, increased LFTs, respiratory failure, suicidal ideation The elderly and those with diminished renal function may be more vulnerable to CNS effects Less anticholinergic than other agents Withdrawal syndrome reported – taper dose upon discontinuation	Limited human data. Teratogenic and embryotoxic in rats but not in rabbits. In humans, possible association with cardiovascular and limb reduction defects in first trimester exposure, but the number of exposures is too small to draw a conclusion. Avoid in first trimester if possible	Excreted into breast milk in small amounts; should be used with caution because of potential adverse effects in nursing infants such as vomiting, skin rash, and urinary retention. As it can reduce prolactin levels, milk production may be reduced
Benztropine (Cogentin)	Beneficial effect on rigidity Relieves sialorrhea and drooling Powerful muscle relaxant; sedative action Cumulative and long-acting; once-daily dosing can be used (preferably in the morning) IM/IV: Dramatic effect on dystonic symptoms – drug of choice for acute dystonic reactions Does not relieve tardive dyskinesia – use not recommended	Dry mouth, dry eyes, blurred vision, urinary retention, constipation, nausea, GERD, paralytic ileus, tachycardia, decreased cognition, hallucinations, delirium, convulsions, heat stroke, hyperthermia Increased intraocular pressure Toxic psychosis when abused or overused The elderly may be more susceptible to anticholinergic (bladder, bowel, CNS) effects – avoid use were possible Also see p. 229	Limited human data. Probably compatible. Possible association with cardiovascular defects in first trimester exposure; reported small left colon syndrome in newborns exposed to the drug *in utero* at term, manifested as decreased intestinal motility, vomiting, abdominal distention, and inability to pass meconium	No human data. Unknown excretion into breast milk. As it can reduce prolactin levels, milk production may be reduced
Biperiden (Akineton)	Has effect against rigidity and akinesia	Has higher affinity for muscarinic receptors in the CNS and may be less likely to cause peripheral anticholinergic effects Also see p. 229	Limited data. Human data suggest risk in third trimester (GI toxicity in newborn)	No human data. Unknown excretion into breast milk. As it can reduce prolactin levels, milk production may be reduced
Clonazepam (Rivotril, Klonopin)	Useful for akathisia	Drowsiness, lethargy, disinhibition (see p. 244)	Crosses the placenta. Potential for increased risk of congenital anomalies with first trimester use, however, conflicting data. Potential for newborn withdrawal symptoms and floppy baby syndrome if used close to delivery	Excreted into breast milk. Potential to cause sedation, feeding difficulties, and weight loss in infant
Cyproheptadine (Periactin)	Moderate effect on akathisia Sedative and anticholinergic effects Has been used to increase appetite May help ameliorate drug-induced sexual dysfunction	Drowsiness, weight gain, anticholinergic effects (dry eyes, confusion, constipation, urinary retention, etc.) Use with caution in: the elderly, CVD, increased intraocular pressure, asthma, GI obstructions, urinary retention, thyroid dysfunction May potentiate the effects of other CNS depressants	Limited data. Possible association with hypospadias and oral clefts in first trimester exposure. Possible association with preterm delivery	Limited data. As it can reduce prolactin levels, milk production may be reduced. Potential for irritability and drowsiness in the infant

Agent	Therapeutic Effects	Adverse Effects	Pregnancy	Breast Milk
Deutetrabenazine (Austedo)	Improves symptoms of tardive dyskinesia Long-term efficacy established (up to 2 years)	>3% nasopharyngitis and insomnia 2% depression and akathisia QT prolongation at higher concentrations Binds to melanin-containing tissues and may cause long-term ophthalmic complications	Limited data	No human data
Diazepam (Valium, etc.)	Beneficial effect on akathisia and acute dystonia Muscle relaxant	Drowsiness, lethargy, disinhibition (see p. 244)	Crosses the placenta. Potential for increased risk of congenital anomalies with first trimester use, however, conflicting data. Potential for newborn withdrawal symptoms and floppy baby syndrome if used close to delivery	Excreted into breast milk. Potential to cause sedation, feeding difficulties, and weight loss in infant. Potential for prolonged effects due to diazepam's long half-life. Short-acting agents (e.g., lorazepam) are preferred
Diphenhydramine (Benadryl)	Has effect on tremor and akathisia Sedative effect may benefit tension and excitation; may enhance the effects of other antiparkinsonian agents Some effect on rigidity	Somnolence, confusion, and dizziness, especially in the elderly; delirium reported Use with caution in: the elderly, CVD, increased intraocular pressure, asthma, GI obstructions, urinary retention, thyroid dysfunction May potentiate the effects of other CNS depressants	Compatible. Use near delivery can cause neonatal withdrawal effects	Excreted into breast milk. Limited data but probably compatible. High doses or chronic use may reduce prolactin levels and milk production. Potential for irritability and drowsiness in the infant
Ethopropazine (Parsitan, Parsidol)	Has effect against rigidity; improves posture, gait, and speech Specific for tremor	Mild anticholinergic activity. See benztropine for general adverse effects profile and conditions to avoid use in Also see p. 229	No human or animal data	No human data. Unknown excretion into breast milk. As it can reduce prolactin levels, milk production may be reduced
Lorazepam (Ativan)	Beneficial effect on akathisia Excellent for acute dyskinesia (sublingual works quickest)	Drowsiness, lethargy, disinhibition (see p. 244)	Crosses the placenta. Potential for increased risk of congenital anomalies with first trimester use, however, conflicting data. Potential for newborn withdrawal symptoms and floppy baby syndrome if used close to delivery	Excreted into breast milk. Potential to cause sedation, feeding difficulties, and weight loss in infant
Orphenadrine (Norflex)	Modest effect on sialorrhea, Parkinson's disease (tremor, rigidity, bradykinesia) Beneficial effects tend to wear off in 2–6 months	See benztropine for general anticholinergic adverse effects profile and conditions to avoid use in Has some euphorigenic properties	Limited data	No human data. Unknown excretion into breast milk. May reduce prolactin levels and milk production. Potential for irritability and drowsiness in the infant
Procyclidine (Kemadrin)	Questionable effect on tremor Useful agent to use in combination when muscle rigidity is severe	See benztropine for general adverse effects profile and conditions to avoid use in Also see p. 229	No human or animal data	No human data. Unknown excretion into breast milk. As it can reduce prolactin levels, milk production may be reduced
Propranolol (Inderal)	Very useful for akathisia and tremor	Monitor pulse and blood pressure; do not stop high dose abruptly due to rebound tachycardia	Potential for growth restriction and reduced placental weight with use in second and third trimesters. Potential for β-blockade in newborn if used near delivery. Monitor for bradycardia, respiratory depression, and hypoglycemia	Excreted into breast milk. Compatible with breastfeeding. Monitor for symptoms of β-blockade

Comparison of Agents for Treating Acute Extrapyramidal Side Effects and Tardive Dyskinesia (cont.)

Agent	Therapeutic Effects	Adverse Effects	Pregnancy	Breast Milk
Trihexyphenidyl (Artane)	Mild to moderate effect against rigidity and spasm (occasionally dramatic results) Tremor alleviated to a lesser degree; as a result of relaxing muscle spasm, more tremor activity may be noted Stimulating – can be used during the day for sluggish, lethargic, and akinetic patients	See benztropine for general adverse effects profile and conditions to avoid use in Also see p. 229	Limited data	No human data. Unknown excretion into breast milk. May reduce prolactin levels and milk production
Valbenazine (Ingrezza)	Improves symptoms of tardive dyskinesia Long-term efficacy established (up to 48 weeks)	>10% somnolence, fatigue, sedation 2.7–5.4% anticholinergic adverse effects (see benztropine), balance disorders, akathisia <2.7% vomiting, nausea, arthralgia QT prolongation at higher concentrations	Limited data	No human data. Animal studies suggest excretion into milk. Women should wait at least 5 days after final dose before breastfeeding

Doses and Pharmacokinetics of Agents for Treating Acute Extrapyramidal Side Effects and Tardive Dyskinesia

Agent	Dose in Adults	Onset of Action	Time to Peak Plasma Level (T_{max})	Bioavailability	Protein Binding	Elimination Half-life ($T_{1/2}$)	Excretion	Metabolizing Enzymes (CYP450 and/or UGT*)	Enzyme Inhibition (CYP450)**
Amantadine (Symmetrel)	Oral: 100 mg bid, may increase to 300 mg/day in divided doses CrCl 30–50 mL/min: 100 mg od CrCl 15–29 mL/min: 100 mg q 48 h CrCl <15 mL/min: 200 mg q 7 days Hepatic impairment: no dosage adjustment suggested – use caution Cocaine withdrawal: 100 mg bid to tid	Within 48 h	2–4 h	86–90%	67% (normal renal function); 59% (hemodialysis)	9–31 h (normal renal function); 20–41 h (healthy, elderly); 7–10 days (end-stage renal disease)	Urine (80–90% unchanged by glomerular filtration and tubular secretion)	Minimal metabolism. 80–90% excreted unchanged by glomerular filtration and tubular secretion	–
Benztropine (Cogentin)	Oral: 1–2 mg od–tid up to 4 mg bid if needed Acute dystonia: IM/IV: 1–2 mg; may repeat in 30 min Hepatic and renal impairment: no dosage adjustment suggested – use caution	Oral: 1–2 h IM/IV: few minutes	7 h	29%	95%	1–2 h	Urine	2D6[(m)]	–
Biperiden (Akineton)	Oral: 2 mg od–tid Hepatic and renal impairment: no dosage adjustment available – use caution	Oral: 10–30 min IM/IV: few minutes	1.5 h	87%	60%	18–24 h	Primarily urine	?	?

Agent	Dose in Adults	Onset of Action	Time to Peak Plasma Level (T_{max})	Bioavailability	Protein Binding	Elimination Half-life ($T_{1/2}$)	Excretion	Metabolizing Enzymes (CYP450 and/or UGT*)	Enzyme Inhibition (CYP450)**
Clonazepam (Rivotril, Klonopin)	Oral: 0.5–6 mg/day in divided doses Hepatic and renal impairment: no dosage adjustment suggested, metabolites may accumulate – use caution	15–30 min	1–4 h	90%	86%	17–60 h	Urine (<2% as unchanged drug)	**3A4** [(p)]	–
Cyproheptadine (Periactin)	Initial: 4 mg tid up to 32 mg/day Hepatic and renal impairment: no dosage adjustment suggested – use caution	?	metabolites: 6–9 h	?	96–99%	metabolites: ~16 h	Urine (~ 40%, primarily as metabolites); feces (2–20%)	UGT1A	?
Deutetrabenazine (Austedo)	Recommended dose: 12–48 mg/day Hepatic impairment: contraindicated Geriatric use: caution, consider dose reduction CYP2D6 poor metabolizers: do not exceed 36 mg/day	?	3–4 h		82–85% Metabolites: 59–68%	9–12 h	75–86% urine (<10% of dose as active metabolites) 8–11% feces	**2D6** [(p)], 1A2, 3A4/5 [(m)]	
Diazepam (Valium, etc.)	Oral: up to 5 mg qid IV: 10 mg for acute dystonia by slow direct IV push (rate of 5 mg (1 mL)/min) Renal impairment: No dosage adjustment recommended; decrease dose if prescribed for extended periods as metabolite accumulates Hepatic impairment: Caution in moderate impairment – reducing dose by 50% recommended, contraindicated in severe impairment	Oral: rapid (15 min or less) IV: imme-diate	Oral: 15 min–2 h	93%	98%	20–50 h; 50–100 h for active major metabolite (desmethyl-diazepam); increased half-life in the elderly and those with severe hepatic disorders	Urine (very little as unchanged drug)	**2C19** [(p)], **3A4** [(p)], 1A2 [(m)], 2B6 [(m)], 2C9 [(m)]	2C19 [(w)], 3A4 [(w)] UGT
Diphenhydramine (Benadryl)	IM/IV: 50 mg for dystonia, may repeat in 20–30 min Oral: 25–50 mg tid–qid Renal impairment: No adjustment Hepatic impairment: no dosage adjustment suggested – use caution	IM/IV: 15–20 min Oral: 1–3 h	Oral: ~2 h	40–70%	78%	7–12 h (adults); 9–18 h (elderly)	Urine (as metabolites and unchanged drug)	**2D6** [(p)], 1A2 [(m)], 2C9 [(m)], 2C19 [(m)]; UGT1A3	2D6
Ethopropazine (Parsitan, Parsidol)	Starting oral dose: 100–500 mg/day as bid–tid Hepatic and renal impairment: no dosage adjustment available – use caution	?	?	Poor?	93%	1–2 h	?	?	?
Lorazepam (Ativan)	Oral: Up to 2 mg qid Sublingual: 1–2 mg up to tid IM: 1–2 mg for dystonia Renal impairment: No adjustment Hepatic impairment: mild to moderate – no adjustment; severe impairment – use caution	Oral: 15–30 min	Oral: 2 h Sublingual: 1 h IM: <3 h	90%	88–92%; free fraction may be sig-nificantly higher in the elderly	10–20 h; 32–70 h (end-stage renal disease)	Urine (88% as inactive metabolites); feces (7%)	UGT2B7, UGT2B15	–

Extrapyramidal

Doses and Pharmacokinetics of Agents for Treating Acute Extrapyramidal Side Effects and Tardive Dyskinesia (cont.)

Agent	Dose in Adults	Onset of Action	Time to Peak Plasma Level (T_{max})	Bioavailability	Protein Binding	Elimination Half-life ($T_{1/2}$)	Excretion	Metabolizing Enzymes (CYP450 and/or UGT[*]	Enzyme Inhibition (CYP450)[**]
Orphenadrine (Orfenace)	Oral: 100 mg bid Renal dosing: No adjustment Hepatic dosing not defined	20 min	2–4 h	?	20%	14–16 h	Primarily urine (8% as unchanged drug)	Metabolized extensively but not adequately characterized	?
Procyclidine (Kemadrin)	Starting oral dose: 2.5 mg bid–tid; increase by 2.5 mg/day if required Maximum 30 mg/day Hepatic and renal impairment: no dosage adjustment suggested – use caution	45–60 min	1 h	75%	100%	12 h	Minimal unchanged drug in urine	2D6 (?)	?
Propranolol (Inderal)	Oral: Akathisia: 30–120 mg/day as bid–tid Essential tremor: 40 mg bid to start (maintenance: 120–320 mg/day Hepatic and renal impairment: no dosage adjustment suggested – use caution	1–2 h	1–4 h (immediate release); 6–14 h (sustained release)	25% (high first-pass metabolism); protein-rich foods increase bioavailability by 50%	90%	3–6 h (immediate release); 8–10 h (sustained release)	Metabolites are excreted primarily in urine (96–100%) <1% excreted in urine as unchanged drug	**1A2[(p)], 2D6[(p)]**, 2C19[(m)], 3A4[(m)]	1A2[(w)], 2D6[(w)]
Trihexyphenidyl (Artane)	Oral: 1 mg/day; increase prn 5–15 mg/day as tid–qid Hepatic and renal impairment: no dosage adjustment suggested – use caution	1 h	1–1.5 h	100%	?	3.3–4.1 h	Urine and bile	?	?
Valbenazine (Ingrezza)	Oral: 40–80 mg/day Recommended dose: 80 mg Hepatic impairment: 40 mg Renal impairment: no dose adjustment Concomitant strong CYP3A4 inducers: Not recommended Concomitant strong CYP3A4 inhibitors: Reduce dose to 40 mg/day Concomitant strong CYP2D6 inhibitors or known CYP2D6 poor metabolizers: Consider reducing dose	<30 min	30 min–1 h	49%	>99% Metabolite tetra-benazine: ~64%	15–22 h	60% urine 30% feces (<2% overall as unchanged valbenazine or tetrabenazine)	**3A4/5** [(p)], 2D6[(m)]	–

[*] Cytochrome P450 isoenzymes involved in Phase I metabolism (data not consistent among references), UGT: UDP-glucuronosyltransferase is the most important Phase II (conjugative) enzyme   [**] CYP450 isoenzymes inhibited by drug,   [(m)] Minor route of metabolism   [(p)] Primary route of metabolism   [(w)] Weak inhibitor/inducer of CYP450

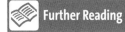
Further Reading

References

[1] Bergman H, Rathbone J, Agarwal V, et al. Antipsychotic reduction and/or cessation and antipsychotics as specific treatments for tardive dyskinesia. Cochrane Database Syst Rev. 2018;2:CD000459. doi:10.1002/14651858.CD000459.pub3

[2] Elbe D, Black TR, McGrane IR, et al. Clinical handbook of psychotropic drugs for children and adolescents. (4th ed.). Boston, MA: Hogrefe Publishing, 2019.

[3] Bergman H, Soares-Weiser K. Anticholinergic medication for antipsychotic-induced tardive dyskinesia. Cochrane Database Syst Rev. 2018;1(1):CD000204. doi:10.1002/14651858.CD000204.pub2

Additional Suggested Reading

- Caroff SN, Campbell EC. Drug-induced extrapyramidal syndromes: Implications for contemporary practice. Psychiatr Clin North Am. 2016;39(3):391–411. doi:10.1016/j.psc.2016.04.003
- Duma SR, Fung VS. Drug-induced movement disorders. Aust Prescr. 2019;42:56–61. doi:10.18773/austprescr.2019.014
- Haddad PM, Das A, Keyhani S, et al. Antipsychotic drugs and extrapyramidal side effects in first episode psychosis: A systematic review of head-head comparisons. J Psychopharmacol. 2012;26(5 Suppl):15–26. doi:10.1177/0269881111424929
- Hazari N, Kate N, Grover S. Clozapine and tardive movement disorders: A review. Asian J Psychiatr. 2013;6(6):439–451. doi:10.1016/j.ajp.2013.08.067
- Huhn M, Nikolakopoulou A, Schneider-Thoma J, et al. Comparative efficacy and tolerability of 32 oral antipsychotics for the acute treatment of adults with multi-episode schizophrenia: A systematic review and network meta-analysis. Lancet. 2019;394:939–951. doi:10.1016/S0140-6736(19)31135-3
- Kane JM, Fleischhacker WW, Hansen L, et al. Akathisia: An updated review focusing on second-generation antipsychotics. J Clin Psychiatry. 2009;70(5):627–643. doi:10.4088/JCP.08r04210
- Keks N, Hope J, Schwartz D, et al. Comparative tolerability of dopamine D2/3 receptor partial agonists for schizophrenia. CNS Drugs. 2020;34:473–507. doi:10.1007/s40263-020-00718-4
- P450 Drug Interaction Table, Indiana University School of Medicine, Division of Clinical Pharmacology. Retrieved from http://medicine.iupui.edu/clinpharm/ddis/table.asp
- Pardis P, Remington G, Panda R, et al. Clozapine and tardive dyskinesia in patients with schizophrenia: A systematic review. J Psychopharmacol. 2019;33(10):1187–1198. doi:10.1177/0269881119862535
- Pringsheim T, Gardner D, Addington D, et al. The assessment and treatment of antipsychotic-induced akathisia. Can J Psychiatry. 2018;1:706743718760288. doi:10.1177/0706743718760288

ANXIOLYTIC (ANTIANXIETY) AGENTS

Classification

- Anxiolytic agents can be classified as follows:

Chemical Class	Agent	Page
Antidepressants		
Selective serotonin reuptake inhibitors (SSRI)	Examples: Escitalopram, paroxetine, sertraline	See p. 3
Serotonin norepinephrine reuptake inhibitors (SNRI)	Example: Venlafaxine	See p. 25
Tricyclic Antidepressants (TCA)	Example: Clomipramine	See p. 54
Noradrenergic/specific serotonergic antidepressants (NaSSA)	Example: Mirtazapine	See p. 49
Monoamine oxidase inhibitors (MAOI)	Example: Phenelzine	See p. 67
Anticonvulsants		
GABA analogs	Examples: Gabapentin, pregabalin	See p. 284 and p. 438
Phenyltriazine	Example: Lamotrigine	See p. 284
Azaspirone	Example: Buspirone	See p. 253
Benzodiazepines	Examples: Alprazolam, diazepam, lorazepam	See p. 240

Benzodiazepines

Product Availability*

Generic Name	Neuroscience-based Nomenclature* (Pharmacological Target/Mode of Action)	Trade Name(A)	Dosage Forms and Strengths
Alprazolam	GABA/Benzodiazepine receptor agonist (GABA$_A$ receptor positive allosteric modulator)	Xanax	Tablets: 0.25 mg, 0.5 mg, 1 mg, 2 mg Oral concentrate: 1 mg/mL(B)
		Xanax TS(C)	Triscored tablets (TS): 2 mg
		Xanax XR(B)	Extended-release tablets: 0.5 mg, 1 mg, 2 mg, 3 mg
		Niravam(B)	Oral disintegrating tablet: 0.25 mg, 0.5 mg, 1 mg, 2 mg
Bromazepam(C)	GABA/Benzodiazepine receptor agonist (GABA$_A$ receptor positive allosteric modulator)	Lectopam	Tablets: 1.5 mg, 3 mg, 6 mg
Chlordiazepoxide	GABA/Benzodiazepine receptor agonist (GABA$_A$ receptor positive allosteric modulator)	Librium	Capsules: 5 mg, 10 mg, 25 mg

Generic Name	Neuroscience-based Nomenclature* (Pharmacological Target/Mode of Action)	Trade Name[A]	Dosage Forms and Strengths
Clonazepam	GABA/Benzodiazepine receptor agonist (GABA$_A$ receptor positive allosteric modulator)	Klonopin[B], Rivotril[C]	Tablets: 0.25 mg[C], 0.5 mg, 1 mg, 2 mg Rapidly disintegrating tablets[B]: 0.125 mg, 0.25 mg, 0.5 mg, 1 mg, 2 mg
Clorazepate	GABA/Benzodiazepine receptor agonist (GABA$_A$ receptor positive allosteric modulator)	Tranxene	Tablets[B]: 3.75 mg, 7.5 mg, 15 mg Capsules[C]: 3.75 mg, 7.5 mg, 15 mg
Diazepam	GABA/Benzodiazepine receptor agonist (GABA$_A$ receptor positive allosteric modulator)	Valium Diazepam Intensol[B] Diastat, Diastat Acudial[B]	Tablets: 2 mg, 5 mg, 10 mg Oral solution: 1 mg/ml Injection: 5 mg/mL Oral concentrate[B]: 5 mg/mL Rectal gel: 5 mg/mL
Estazolam[B]	GABA/Benzodiazepine receptor agonist (GABA$_A$ receptor positive allosteric modulator)	ProSom	Tablets: 1 mg, 2 mg
Flurazepam	GABA/Benzodiazepine receptor agonist (GABA$_A$ receptor positive allosteric modulator)	Dalmane	Capsules: 15 mg, 30 mg
Lorazepam	GABA/Benzodiazepine receptor agonist (GABA$_A$ receptor positive allosteric modulator)	Ativan Lorazepam Intensol[B]	Tablets: 0.5 mg, 1 mg, 2 mg Sublingual tablets[C]: 0.5 mg, 1 mg, 2 mg Injection: 2 mg/mL, 4 mg/mL Oral concentrate[B]: 2 mg/mL
Nitrazepam[C]	GABA/Benzodiazepine receptor agonist (GABA$_A$ receptor positive allosteric modulator)	Mogadon	Tablets: 5 mg, 10 mg
Oxazepam	GABA/Benzodiazepine receptor agonist (GABA$_A$ receptor positive allosteric modulator)	Serax	Tablets[C]: 10 mg, 15 mg, 30 mg Capsules[B]: 10 mg, 15 mg, 30 mg
Temazepam	GABA/Benzodiazepine receptor agonist (GABA$_A$ receptor positive allosteric modulator)	Restoril	Capsules: 7.5 mg[B], 15 mg, 22.5 mg[B], 30 mg
Triazolam	GABA/Benzodiazepine receptor agonist (GABA$_A$ receptor positive allosteric modulator)	Halcion	Tablets: 0.125 mg[B], 0.25 mg

* Refer to Health Canada's Drug Product Database or the FDA's Drugs@FDA for the most current availability information   • Developed by a taskforce consisting of representatives from the American College of Neuropsychopharmacology (ACNP), the Asian College of Neuropsychopharmacology (AsCNP), the European College of Neuropsychopharmacology (ECNP), the International College of Neuropsychopharmacology (CINP), and the International Union of Basic and Clinical Pharmacology (IUPHAR) (see https://nbn2r.com), [A] Generic preparations may be available,   [B] Not marketed in Canada,   [C] Not marketed in the USA

Benzodiazepines (cont.)

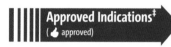

Approved Indications[‡]
(👍 approved)

		Anxiety Disorders	Panic Disorder	Insomnia	Perioperative Sedation	Seizure Disorders	Skeletal Muscle Spasticity	Alcohol Withdrawal
Short-acting	Alprazolam	👍	👍					
	Triazolam			👍				
Intermediate	Bromazepam[(C)]	👍						
	Estazolam[(B)]			👍				
	Lorazepam	👍			👍			
	Oxazepam	👍						👍
	Temazepam			👍				
Long-acting	Chlordiazepoxide	👍			👍			👍
	Clonazepam		👍			👍		
	Clorazepate	👍				👍		👍
	Diazepam	👍			👍	👍	👍	👍
	Flurazepam			👍				
	Nitrazepam[(C)]			👍		👍		

[(A)] Acute use only,   [(B)] Not marketed in Canada,   [(C)] Not marketed in the USA

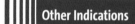

Other Indications

- Akathisia secondary to antipsychotic agents
- Abnormal movements associated with tardive dyskinesia (clonazepam)
- Sedation in severe agitation
- Mania: Often used short-term with antipsychotics or lithium to control agitation
- Social phobia (alprazolam, clonazepam, diazepam, lorazepam)
- Catatonia (parenteral and sublingual lorazepam, diazepam, clonazepam)
- Myoclonus, restless legs syndrome, Tourette's syndrome (clonazepam)
- Acute dystonia (sublingual or intramuscular lorazepam)
- Alcohol withdrawal, Delirium tremens (chlordiazepoxide, diazepam), lorazepam, oxazepam
- Delirium in older persons caused by withdrawal from alcohol/sedative–hypnotics (benzodiazepines as monotherapy)
- Neuralgic pain (clonazepam)
- Premenstrual dysphoric disorder (alprazolam)
- Status epilepticus (lorazepam)
- Rapid eye movement sleep behavior disorder (clonazepam)

[‡] Indications listed here do not necessarily apply to all countries. Please refer to a country's regulatory database (e.g., US Food and Drug Administration, Health Canada Drug Product Database) for the most current availability information and indications

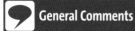

General Comments	<ul><li>The potency of a benzodiazepine is the affinity of the parent drug, or its active metabolite(s), for "benzodiazepine"-GABA$_A$ receptors in vivo. Potency does not necessarily correlate with onset of action</li><li>Benzodiazepines are suggested to relieve behavioral and somatic manifestations of anxiety, but have little effect on psychic or cognitive symptoms (e.g., worry, anger, interpersonal sensitivity, and obsessions); may be most helpful during the beginning phase of treatment; not recommended long term</li><li>A multimodal treatment approach, including medication, psychosocial therapy, and environmental interventions has shown to confer greater improvement in symptoms as compared to medication use alone</li></ul>
Pharmacology	<ul><li>Benzodiazepines are positive allosteric modulators of the GABA$_A$-chloride receptor complex. Binding of benzodiazepines to the "benzodiazepine"-GABA$_A$ receptor complex increases the frequency of opening of the chloride channels, facilitating inhibition of neuronal firing at the level of the limbic system, the brain stem reticular formation, and the cortex. Intensity of action depends on degree of receptor occupancy</li><li>Benzodiazepines bind nonselectively to various subtypes of "benzodiazepine"-GABA$_A$ receptor complexes. GABA$_A$ receptor subtypes containing an α_1 subunit are associated with sedation, ataxia, and amnesia; GABA$_A$ receptor subtypes containing α_2 and/or α_3 subunits generally have greater anxiolytic activity</li><li>As the dose of a benzodiazepine is increased (i.e., increased receptor occupancy), the anxiolytic effects are noticed first, followed by anticonvulsant effects, a reduction in muscle tone, and finally sedation and hypnosis</li><li>In addition to its activity at the "benzodiazepine"-GABA$_A$ receptor complex, clonazepam decreases the utilization of serotonin by neurons</li></ul>
Dosing	<ul><li>See pp. 249–252 for individual agents</li><li>Although the majority of indications for benzodiazepines are for short-term (less than 2 months) treatment, many patients are prescribed these agents for extended periods of time (more than 3 months). Clinicians should discuss the risks and benefits of long-term use with patients at the beginning of therapy</li><li>Following IV administration of diazepam, local pain and thrombophlebitis may occur due to precipitation of the drug, or due to an irritant effect of propylene glycol (a saline flush following the diazepam reduces the incidence)</li><li>IM use is discouraged with diazepam as absorption is slow, erratic, and possibly incomplete; local pain often occurs. Lorazepam IM is adequately absorbed (though absorption can also be erratic by this method)</li><li>When switching from immediate-release (divided dose) to XR (single dose), alprazolam 0.5 mg tid = alprazolam XR 1.5 mg daily. Alprazolam XR is administered once daily, preferably in the morning; should not be chewed, crushed, or broken. Dosage titration recommended of no more than 1 mg/day every 3–4 days. Slower absorption rate results in a relatively constant concentration that is maintained for 5–11 h after dosing. Dose reductions should be in decrements of 0.5 mg every 3 days, or slower. A high-fat meal given up to 2 h before dosing with alprazolam XR can increase the mean C_{max} by about 25%, however, the extent of exposure (AUC) and elimination half-life ($T_{1/2}$) are not affected by eating</li></ul>
Pharmacokinetics	<ul><li>See pp. 249–252 for individual agents</li><li>Marked interindividual variation (up to 10-fold) is found in all pharmacokinetic parameters. Age, liver disease, physical disorders, as well as concurrent use of other drugs may influence parameters by changing the volume of distribution, metabolism, and elimination half-life of these drugs</li><li>Well absorbed from GI tract after oral administration; food can delay the rate but not the extent of absorption; onset of action is determined by rate of absorption and lipid solubility</li><li>Lipid solubility positively correlates with enhancing benzodiazepines' (a) affinity for peripheral adipose tissue, resulting in redistribution from the vascular compartment (this increases volume of distribution), and (b) passage across the blood/brain barrier, facilitating its CNS activity. Benzodiazepines have a high volume of distribution (i.e., the tissue drug concentration is much higher than the blood drug concentration)</li><li>Elimination half-life is a contributor to, but not the sole determinant of, duration of action. The duration of action is dependent on the size of the dose, the rate of absorption, the rate and extent of drug distribution, and the rate of elimination. A benzodiazepine with a long half-life (e.g., diazepam) may have a short duration of action if the dose is small or if it undergoes rapid and extensive distribution. Conversely, a short half-life benzodiazepine (e.g., lorazepam) may have a long duration of action if the dose is large or if the drug has significant peripheral distribution</li><li>Differences in pharmacokinetics between the various benzodiazepines have been presumed to indicate clinical differences as well – this is not necessarily so. However, present rationale for selection of a benzodiazepine remains the difference in pharmacokinetic profile. Generally, short-acting agents can be used as hypnotics and for acute problems relating to anxiety, while long-acting agents can be used for chronic conditions where a continuous drug effect is needed</li></ul>

Benzodiazepines (cont.)

- The longer the half-life of a benzodiazepine, the greater the likelihood that the compound will have an adverse effect on daytime functioning (e.g., hangover effect). Conversely, shorter half-life benzodiazepines are more often associated with (a) interdose withdrawal, (b) rebound anxiety between doses, and (c) anterograde amnesia
- The major pathway of metabolism is Phase I (i.e., hepatic microsomal oxidation and demethylation). Phase II metabolism (i.e., conjugation) produces more polar (water-soluble) by-products, allowing for easier renal excretion. Phase I metabolism (e.g., oxidation) can be compromised by disease states (e.g., hepatic cirrhosis), age or drugs that inhibit various CYP450 isozymes. Drugs that only undergo Phase II metabolism (i.e., conjugation) are not affected to the same degree (e.g., lorazepam, oxazepam, temazepam)
- Renal impairment may increase the free unbound plasma concentration of benzodiazepine and reduce its clearance. Reduce dose by 25–50% in patients with CrCl less than 10 mL/min

Adverse Effects

CNS Effects

- Most common are extensions of the generalized sedative effect (e.g., fatigue, drowsiness); alprazolam XR may prolong daytime sedation
- Impaired mental speed, central cognitive processing ability, memory, and performance. Associated with increased risk of motor vehicle accidents and accidental injuries
- Tolerance to acute short-term memory impairment may not develop with time
- Anterograde amnesia (more likely with high-potency agents or higher doses); dysmnesia (e.g., IV diazepam)
- Chronic use: May impair several neurocognitive domains (e.g., speed of learning, visuospatial ability, speed of processing, verbal memory, motor control/performance and nonverbal memory)
- Paradoxical irritability, impulsivity, and agitation (increased risk in the young, the elderly, individuals with learning disabilities, and people with a neurological disorder)
- Confusion and disorientation – primarily in the elderly. Periods of blackouts or amnesia have been reported
- Treatment-emergent depression
- Excessive doses can result in respiratory depression and apnea
- Dysarthria, muscle weakness, incoordination, ataxia, nystagmus
- Headache

Other Adverse Effects

- Sexual dysfunction including decreased libido, erectile dysfunction, anorgasmia, ejaculatory disturbance, and gynecomastia
- Dizziness (up to 12% with higher doses of clonazepam)
- Falls and related injuries (e.g., fractures)
- Rare reports of purpura and thrombocytopenia with diazepam
- Few documented allergies to benzodiazepines; rarely reported skin reactions include rashes, fixed drug eruption, photosensitivity reactions, pigmentation, alopecia, bullous reactions, exfoliative dermatitis, vasculitis, and erythema nodosum

D/C Discontinuation Syndrome

- Benzodiazepines present different risks of physiological dependence at therapeutic doses, depending on the individual as well as the drug's potency and its elimination half-life. Up to 30% of patients suggested to experience withdrawal after 8 weeks of benzodiazepine treatment
- Discontinuation of a benzodiazepine can produce:
  – Withdrawal: Occurs 1–2 days (with short-acting agent) to 5–10 days (with long-acting agent) following drug discontinuation. Common symptoms include insomnia, agitation, anxiety, perceptual changes, dysphoria, headache, muscle aches, twitches, tremors, loss of appetite, diaphoresis, tachycardia, and GI distress. Catatonia and depression have also been reported. Severe reactions can occur such as grand mal or petit mal seizures, delirium, depersonalization, psychotic states, and coma
  – Rebound: Occurs hours to days after drug discontinuation; symptoms (of anxiety) are similar but more intense than those reported originally
  – Relapse: Occurs weeks to months after drug discontinuation; symptoms are similar to original symptoms of anxiety, and get progressively worse until treated

- Pseudo-withdrawal is a psychological withdrawal as a result of the patient's apprehension about discontinuing the drug – consists of anxiety symptoms unaccompanied by true withdrawal symptoms; this may be dealt with by slow withdrawal and reassurance

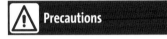

Management

- To withdraw a patient from a benzodiazepine, an equivalent dose of diazepam may be substituted (see pp. 249–252). If insomnia is a major problem, then most of the diazepam should be given at bedtime. Withdrawal schedules will be dependent on patient history and psychological issues regarding benzodiazepine use
  - A conservative schedule would be to reduce the current dose of diazepam by 10–20% every 1–2 weeks depending on patient's symptoms
- ☞ **The withdrawal schedule for alprazolam should be no faster than 0.25 mg every week; quicker withdrawal may result in delirium and seizures**
- ☞ **The above withdrawal schedule is only intended as a general guide. The rate of tapering should never be rigid but flexible, depending on the patient's individual symptoms**

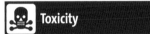

Precautions

- Concomitant use of benzodiazepines with opioids may result in profound respiratory depression, coma, and death. Avoid combination if possible, consider other alternatives
- Do not use in patients with sleep apnea
- Administer with caution to elderly or debilitated patients, those with liver disease, or those with chronic obstructive pulmonary disease
- Administer with caution to those performing hazardous tasks requiring mental alertness or physical coordination. Higher risk of injury and motor vehicle accidents has been reported with benzodiazepine use
- Benzodiazepines may diminish the therapeutic efficacy of electroconvulsive therapy (ECT) by raising the seizure threshold
- Anxiolytics lower the tolerance to alcohol, and high doses may produce mental confusion similar to alcohol intoxication
- Can cause physical and psychological dependence, tolerance, and withdrawal symptoms – correlates to dose and duration of use
- Benzodiazepines are at risk of being misused. Agents with rapid peak drug effects (e.g., diazepam, lorazepam, alprazolam) may confer higher risk, although all benzodiazepines are at risk of misuse

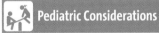

Toxicity

- Rarely, if ever, fatal when taken alone; may be lethal when taken in combination with other drugs, such as alcohol, opioids, and barbiturates
- Symptoms of overdose include hypotension, respiratory depression, and coma

Management

- Flumazenil injection (benzodiazepine antagonist) reverses the hypnotic-sedative effects of benzodiazepines. Repeated doses may be required due to flumazenil's short duration of action ($T_{1/2}$: 40–80 min)

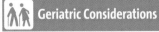

Pediatric Considerations

- For detailed information on the use of anxiolytics in this population, please see the *Clinical Handbook of Psychotropic Drugs for Children and Adolescents*[1]
- Probable indications for anxiolytics include seizure disorder, GAD, adjustment disorder, insomnia, night terrors, and somnambulism
- High-potency benzodiazepines (clonazepam) useful for panic disorder/agoraphobia, social phobia, and separation anxiety disorder
- Benzodiazepines are metabolized faster in children than in adults; may require small divided doses to maintain blood level
- Adverse effects include sedation, cognitive and motor effects; disinhibition with irritability and agitation reported in up to 30% of children – primarily in younger impulsive patients with mental retardation

Geriatric Considerations

- Caution when using drugs that are metabolized via Phase I pathways including oxidation (all but lorazepam, oxazepam, and temazepam) as they can accumulate in the elderly or in persons with liver disease
- Caution when combining with other drugs that have CNS effects; excessive sedation can cause confusion, disorientation
- The elderly are more vulnerable to adverse CNS effects, specifically with regard to balance, gait, memory, cognition, behavior – long-term use should be discouraged
- Benzodiazepine use increases incoordination, risk for falls and fractures
- Limited randomized controlled data to support the use of benzodiazepines for older adults with anxiety disorders
- A meta-analysis (980 patients, 860 adults or elderly individuals) reported that benzodiazepines can be a risk factor for developing dementia. Current evidence lacks power to infer differences between effects of Alzheimer's disease and vascular dementia, long-acting and short-acting benzodiazepines, and various exposure loads (duration and dose)
- A meta-analysis of 18 studies reported that both benzodiazepine and Z-drug use were significantly associated with an increased risk of hip fracture

Benzodiazepines (cont.)

Use in Pregnancy◊	<ul><li>Benzodiazepines and metabolites freely cross the placenta and accumulate in fetal circulation</li><li>Benzodiazepines in general are associated with increased risk of congenital anomalies if used in the first trimester and with neonatal withdrawal if used in chronic doses throughout pregnancy</li><li>Use of a benzodiazepine in the last weeks of pregnancy may cause neonatal CNS depression, poor feeding, hypothermia, flaccidity, and respiratory depression</li><li>In a prospective study involving 725 subjects, alprazolam exposure during pregnancy was associated with higher likelihood (vs. non-exposure) for spontaneous abortion, low birth weight, and Apgar score at 1 minute ≤ 7. There was no significant difference in congenital abnormalities between the exposure and non-exposure groups[2]</li></ul>
Breast Milk	<ul><li>Benzodiazepines are excreted into breast milk in levels sufficient to produce effects in the newborn, including sedation, poor feeding, weight loss, lethargy, and poor temperature regulation (e.g., infant can receive up to 13% of maternal dose of diazepam and 7% of lorazepam dose)</li><li>Metabolism of benzodiazepines in infants is slower, especially during the first 6 weeks; long-acting agents can accumulate</li><li>For breastfeeding women who require benzodiazepines, choose a short-acting agent with no active metabolite (e.g., lorazepam). Monitor newborn for poor feeding and sedation</li></ul>
Nursing Implications	<ul><li>Assess the anxiety level of patients on these drugs to determine if anxiety control has been accomplished and if oversedation has occurred</li><li>The dose should be maintained as prescribed; caution patient not to increase or decrease the dose without consulting their physician</li><li>Inform patients that activities requiring mental alertness should not be performed after taking medication; advise the patient to report any memory lapses or amnesia to their physician immediately</li><li>Caution patients not to use other CNS depressant drugs, including over-the-counter drugs (e.g., antihistamines) or alcohol, without consulting their physician</li><li>Excessive consumption of caffeinated beverages can counteract the effects of anxiolytics</li><li>Tolerance and misuse can occur; caution patient that withdrawal symptoms can occur with abrupt discontinuation after prolonged use</li><li>Inform patients that introducing grapefruit and pomegranate juice into their diet while on some benzodiazepines (i.e., alprazolam, clonazepam, diazepam, estazolam, and triazolam) can result in increased blood levels, resulting in more pronounced effects (including side effects)</li><li>Antacids delay the rate of absorption of benzodiazepines from the intestine. Separate the administration of antacids and benzodiazepines to prevent this interaction</li><li>Alprazolam XR should be administered at a consistent time once daily (preferably in the morning); a high-fat meal prior to drug administration can affect the plasma level of this drug. Alprazolam XR should not be broken, crushed, or chewed, but should be swallowed whole</li></ul>
Patient Instructions	<ul><li>For detailed patient instructions on anxiolytic drugs, see the Patient Information Sheet (details p. 474)</li></ul>
Drug Interactions	<ul><li>Many interactions; only clinically significant ones are listed below</li><li>For more interaction information on any given combination, also see the corresponding chapter for the second agent</li></ul>

Class of Drug	Example	Interaction Effects
Anesthetics	Ketamine	Prolonged recovery with diazepam due to decreased metabolism Benzodiazepines may reduce the antidepressant effects of ketamine in the treatment of depression. Possible attenuation of ketamine response from concurrent use of benzodiazepines also suggested; may be due to 1) the nonspecific central depressant effect of benzodiazepines, mediated through γ-aminobutyric acid (GABA), or 2) benzodiazepine-induced suppression of ketamine-related activation of dopamine neurons in the nucleus accumbens and striatum

◊ See p. 473 for further information on drug use in pregnancy and effects on breast milk

Class of Drug	Example	Interaction Effects
Antibiotic	Clarithromycin, erythromycin, troleandomycin	Decreased metabolism and increased plasma levels of benzodiazepines metabolized by CYP3A4, including triazolam (by 52%), alprazolam (by 60%), estazolam, and diazepam; no interaction with azithromycin
	Chloramphenicol	Decreased metabolism of benzodiazepines that are metabolized via CYP2C19 and 3A4
	Quinolones: Ciprofloxacin	Decreased metabolism of diazepam via inhibition of CYP1A2 and 3A4
	Quinupristin/dalfopristin	Decreased metabolism of diazepam via inhibition of CYP3A4
Anticonvulsant	Barbiturates, carbamazepine	Increased metabolism and decreased plasma level of benzodiazepines metabolized by CYP3A4 and 2C19, including alprazolam (more than 50%), clonazepam (19–37%), and diazepam; additive CNS effects
	Phenytoin	Both increases and decreases in phenytoin plasma levels reported. The exact mechanism of the interaction is unknown Increased phenytoin level and toxicity reported with diazepam, chlordiazepoxide, and clonazepam Increased metabolism and decreased plasma level of benzodiazepines metabolized by CYP3A4
	Valproate	Displacement by diazepam from protein binding, resulting in increased plasma level Decreased metabolism and increased pharmacological effects of clonazepam and lorazepam
Antidepressant		
Cyclic	Desipramine, imipramine	Increased plasma levels of desipramine and imipramine with alprazolam (by 20% and 31%, respectively) Desipramine and triazolam: Report of hypothermia (neither drug causes this effect alone)
SSRI	Fluoxetine, fluvoxamine, sertraline	Decreased metabolism and increased plasma level of benzodiazepines metabolized by CYP3A4, including alprazolam (increased by 100% with fluvoxamine and 46% with fluoxetine) and diazepam (13% with sertraline)
SARI	Nefazodone	Increased plasma levels of alprazolam (by 200%) and triazolam (by 500%) due to inhibited metabolism via CYP3A4
Antifungal	Fluconazole, itraconazole, ketoconazole	Decreased metabolism and increased half-life of chlordiazepoxide; decreased metabolism of triazolam (6-7 fold); reduce dose by 50–75%; AUC of alprazolam increased up to 4 fold
Antipsychotic	Clozapine	Marked sedation, increased salivation, hypotension (collapse), delirium, and respiratory depression/arrest reported; more likely to occur early in treatment when clozapine is added to benzodiazepine regimen. Benzodiazepines may increase risk of pneumonia when combined with clozapine[3]
	Olanzapine	Synergistic increase in somnolence when lorazepam given with IM olanzapine. AVOID IM olanzapine with benzodiazepines as this combination can potentiate hypotension, bradycardia, and respiratory or CNS depression
Antiretroviral		
Combination	Stribild (Elvitegravir + cobicistat + emtricitabine + tenofovir)	Decreased metabolism of benzodiazepines that are metabolized by oxidation (CYP3A4) Use with midazolam is contraindicated. Potentially increased midazolam effects (e.g., prolonged sedation, altered mental status, respiratory depression)
Protease inhibitor	Indinavir, ritonavir	Increased plasma level of benzodiazepines that are metabolized by oxidation via CYP3A4 (e.g., alprazolam, triazolam)
Antitubercular	Isoniazid	Decreased metabolism of benzodiazepines that are metabolized by oxidation (CYP3A4) (triazolam clearance decreased by 75%)
Antiviral		
Hepatitis C virus protease inhibitor	Boceprevir, grazoprevir, simeprevir	Decreased metabolism and increased plasma level of benzodiazepines metabolized by CYP3A4 (e.g., midazolam)
Anxiolytic	Buspirone	Prior treatment with benzodiazepines for generalized anxiety disorder (GAD) may reduce response to buspirone
	Rifampin	Increased metabolism of benzodiazepines that are metabolized by oxidation (e.g., diazepam by 300% and estazolam); rifampin is a pan-inducer of CYP isoenzymes
β-blocker	Propranolol	Increased half-life and decreased clearance of diazepam and bromazepam (no interaction with alprazolam, lorazepam or oxazepam)

Benzodiazepines (cont.)

Class of Drug	Example	Interaction Effects
Caffeine		May counteract sedation and anxiolytic effects and increase insomnia
Calcium channel blocker	Diltiazem	Decreased metabolism and increased plasma level of drugs metabolized by CYP3A4 (e.g., triazolam by 100%)
CNS depressant	Alcohol	Alprazolam reported to increase aggression in moderate alcohol drinkers Brain concentrations of various benzodiazepines altered by ethanol: Triazolam and estazolam concentrations decreased, diazepam concentration increased, no change with chlordiazepoxide
	Antihistamines, barbiturates	Increased CNS depression; with high doses coma and respiratory depression can occur Barbiturates are pan-inducers of CYP isoenzymes and thus may induce the metabolism of benzodiazepines
Cardiac glycoside	Digoxin	Alprazolam may increase serum levels of digoxin; mechanism unknown but may be related to reduced protein binding
Disulfiram		Decreased plasma clearance of chlordiazepoxide (by 54%) and diazepam (by 41%); no effect reported for oxazepam
Grapefruit juice		Increased absorption (bioavailability) of diazepam and triazolam due to inhibition of CYP3A4 in the gut by grapefruit juice Decreased metabolism of alprazolam, diazepam, and triazolam via inhibition of CYP3A4, resulting in increased peak concentration; clinical relevance not established based on limited case studies
H_2 antagonist	Cimetidine	Decreased metabolism of benzodiazepines that are metabolized by oxidation via CYP1A2, 2C19, 2D6, and/or 3A4; (no effect with ranitidine, famotidine or nizatidine); peak plasma concentration of alprazolam increased by 86%
Hormone	Estrogen, oral contraceptives	Decreased metabolism of benzodiazepines that are metabolized by oxidation (e.g., diazepam, chlordiazepoxide, nitrazepam); increased half-life of alprazolam by 29% Clearance of combined oral contraceptives may be reduced with diazepam due to inhibited metabolism
Kava kava		May potentiate CNS effects, causing increased side effects and toxicity
Lithium		Increased incidence of sexual dysfunction (up to 49%) when combined with benzodiazepines
L -dopa		Benzodiazepines can reduce the efficacy of L-dopa secondary to the GABA agonist effect
Opioid	Buprenorphine, methadone, morphine	Increased risk of severe side effects such as respiratory depression, coma, or death when combined with benzodiazepines
Pomegranate juice		Increased absorption (bioavailability) of diazepam and triazolam due to inhibition of CYP3A4 in the gut by pomegranate juice Decreased metabolism of alprazolam, diazepam, and triazolam via inhibition of CYP3A4, resulting in increased peak concentrations
Probenecid		Decreased clearance of lorazepam (by 50%)
Propoxyphene		Increased half-life of alprazolam (by 58%) due to inhibited hydroxylation
Proton pump inhibitor	Omeprazole	Increased ataxia and sedation due to decreased metabolism of benzodiazepines metabolized by oxidation (no effect with lansoprazole)
St. John's wort		Decreased AUC of alprazolam (by 40%) and half-life (by 24%) due to induced metabolism via CYP3A4

Drug	Approximate Equivalent Dose*	Time to Peak Plasma Level PO (T_{max})	Lipid Solubility**	Onset of Action	Protein Binding (PB) Volume of Distribution (Vd)	Elimination Half-life (Parent and Active Metabolite)	Metabolic Pathway Active Metabolite(s)	Dosage for Approved Indications
Alprazolam	0.5 mg Potency: High	Oral tablet = 1–2 h Disintegrating tablet = 1.5–2 h XR = 5–11 h (a high-fat meal increases C_{max} by 25% and decreases T_{max} by about 30%) Asians reported to reach higher C_{max}	Moderate	15–30 min	PB: 80% Rapidly and completely absorbed; absorption rate for XR preparation differs significantly depending on time of day administered Vd: 0.9–1.2 L/kg	Parent: 12–15 h Half-life increased in obese patients, in hepatic insufficiency, and in Asians; clearance in the elderly only 50–80% that of young adults Smokers: Plasma level decreased in smokers by up to 50%; half-life reduced; clearance increased by 24%	Oxidation (CYP3A4) Active metabolites: Yes	*Anxiety*: Immediate release: Effective doses are 0.5–4 mg/day in divided doses; the manufacturer recommends starting at 0.25–0.5 mg tid; titrate dose upward in increments ≤ 1 mg/day; usual maximum: 4 mg/day (however, doses as high as 10 mg/day have been used Extended release: 0.5–1 mg daily; dose may be increased every 3–4 days in increments ≤ 1 mg/day (range: 3–6 mg/day) Renal impairment: No dosage adjustment listed in product monograph but renal impairment does increase unbound alprazolam Hepatic impairment: Advanced hepatic disease: start 0.25 mg po bid-tid, 0.5 mg ER po daily; titrate gradually
Brom-azepam[(C)]	5–6 mg Potency: High	1–4 h Elderly: 2–12 h; increase in C_{max}	Low	15–30 min	PB: 70% Vd: 0.9 L/kg	Parent: 8–30 h Metabolite: 8–30 h Elderly: Half-life increased	Conjugation (glucuronidation) Active metabolites: Yes	*Anxiety*: Initial: 6–18 mg/day in divided doses Maintenance: 6–30 mg/day Renal impairment: No dosage adjustment necessary; however, since active metabolites may accumulate, dosage should be reduced during long-term administration Hepatic impairment: Contraindicated in severe hepatic impairment
Chlor-diazepoxide	25 mg Potency: Low (Parent compound less potent than metabo-lites)	0.5–4 h	Moderate	15–30 min	PB: 90–98% Vd: 3.3 L/kg	Parent: 5–30 h Metabolite: 24–96 h Half-life increased (2–3 fold) in patients with cirrhosis	Oxidation (CYP1A2) Active metabolite(s): Yes Metabolites accumulate on chronic dosing	*Anxiety*: 5–25 mg tid-qid *Alcohol withdrawal*: 50–100 mg to start, dose may be repeated in 2–4 h as necessary to a maximum of 300 mg/24 h Renal impairment: Decrease dose by 50% in patients with CrCl less than 10 mL/min Hepatic impairment: caution advised Elderly: decrease dose by 50%

Comparison of the Benzodiazepines (cont.)

Drug	Approximate Equivalent Dose*	Time to Peak Plasma Level PO (T_{max})	Lipid Solubility**	Onset of Action	Protein Binding (PB) Volume of Distribution (Vd)	Elimination Half-life (Parent and Active Metabolite)	Metabolic Pathway Active Metabolite(s)	Dosage for Approved Indications
Clonazepam	0.5 mg Potency: High	1–2 h Quickly and completely absorbed	Low	15–30 min	PB: 86% Vd: 1.5–4.4 L/kg	Parent: 18–50 h	Oxidation (CYP3A4); reduction Active metabolite(s): No	*Panic disorder:* 0.25 mg bid; increase in increments of 0.125–0.25 mg bid every 3 days; target dose: 1 mg/day (maximum: 4 mg/day) *Seizure disorders:* Initial dose not to exceed 1.5 mg given in 3 divided doses; may increase by 0.5–1 mg every third day until seizures are controlled or adverse effects seen (maximum: 20 mg/day) Renal impairment: No dosage adjustment necessary Hepatic impairment: Contraindicated in patients with significant impairment
Clorazepate	15 mg	0.5–2 h Hydrolyzed in the stomach to active metabolite (parent compound inactive); rate of hydrolysis depends on gastric acidity, therefore absorption is unreliable (one study disputes this)	High	15 min or less	PB: 80–95% Vd: 1.0–1.8 L/kg	Metabolite: 50–100 h	Oxidation Active metabolite(s): Yes Metabolite accumulates on chronic dosing	*Anxiety:* 15–60 mg/day in divided doses; maintenance: 7.5 mg tid (could be switched to 22.5 mg/day as single dose once patient is stabilized) *Seizure disorders (adjunct for partial seizures):* 7.5 mg tid; increase by no more than 7.5 mg/week (maximum: 90 mg/day) *Alcohol withdrawal:* 30–90 mg in divided doses Renal impairment: No dosage adjustment necessary Hepatic impairment: No information
Diazepam	10 mg Potency: Medium	0.5–2 h	High	15 min or less; rapid onset of action followed by redistribution into adipose tissue; IM drug erratically absorbed	PB: 98%; less in the elderly, therefore attains higher serum levels; increased free (unbound) diazepam Vd: 1 L/kg	Parent: 20–80 h Metabolite: 50–100 h Males have a shorter half-life and higher clearance rate than females; half-life increased (2–3 fold) in patients with cirrhosis; smoking associated with higher diazepam clearance, especially in the young	Oxidation (CYP1A2, 2C9, 2C19, 3A4) Active metabolite(s): Yes Accumulation with chronic dosing	*Anxiety:* 2–10 mg bid-qid (oral); 2–10 mg, may repeat in 3–4 h if needed (IV/IM) *Seizure disorders (adjunct):* 2–10 mg bid-qid *Skeletal muscle relaxant:* 2–10 mg tid-qid Muscle spasm (IM/IV): 5–10 mg initially, then 3–10 mg in 3–4 h if needed. Larger doses may be required if associated with tetanus *Alcohol withdrawal:* Oral: 10 mg tid-qid first 24 h, then 5 mg tid-qid as needed IV: 10 mg initially, then 5–10 mg in 3–4 h if needed (IM/IV) Renal impairment: No dosage adjustment necessary Hepatic impairment: Caution advised in patients with mild–moderate impairment. Contraindicated in patients with severe impairment

Drug	Approximate Equivalent Dose*	Time to Peak Plasma Level PO (T_{max})	Lipid Solubility**	Onset of Action	Protein Binding (PB) Volume of Distribution (Vd)	Elimination Half-life (Parent and Active Metabolite)	Metabolic Pathway Active Metabolite(s)	Dosage for Approved Indications
Estazolam[(B)]	1–2 mg Potency: High	2 h	Low	30–60 min	PB: 93% Vd: 0.64 L/kg	Parent: 10–24 h	Oxidation (CYP3A4) Active metabolite(s): No Metabolism impaired in the elderly and in hepatic disease	*Insomnia:* 1 mg at bedtime. Some patients may require 2 mg. Start at doses of 0.5 mg in debilitated or small elderly patients Renal impairment: No dosage adjustment necessary Hepatic impairment: Caution advised
Flurazepam	15–30 mg Potency: Low	0.5–1 h	High	15 min or less	PB: 97% Vd: 3.4 L/kg	Parent: Not significant Metabolite: 40–100 h	Oxidation (CYP2C9 and 3A4) Active metabolite(s): Yes Rapidly metabolized to active metabolite; elderly males accumulate metabolite more than young males on chronic dosing	*Insomnia:* 15–30 mg at bedtime Renal impairment: No dosage adjustment necessary Hepatic impairment: Caution advised
Lorazepam	1 mg Potency: High	Oral: 2–4 h IM: 45–75 min IV: 5–10 min SL: 1 h Well absorbed sublingually	Moderate	15–30 min	PB: 88–93% Vd: 1.3 L/kg	Parent: 10–20 h; longer elimination half-life in women; half-life and Vd doubled in patients with cirrhosis	Conjugation (glucuronidation) Active metabolite(s): No Reduced clearance (by 22%) in the elderly (one study)	*Anxiety:* 1–10 mg/day in 2–3 divided doses; usual dose: 2–6 mg/day in divided doses; largest dose at bedtime *Perioperative sedation:* IM 0.05 mg/kg at least 2 h before surgery (maximum: 4 mg) IV: 0.044 mg/kg 15–20 min before surgery (usual dose: 2 mg) *Seizure disorders (status epilepticus):* 4 mg/dose slow IV (maximum rate: 2 mg/min); may repeat in 10–15 min; usual maximum dose: 8 mg *Insomnia caused by anxiety or transient situational stress:* 2–4 mg at bedtime Renal impairment: No dosage adjustment necessary if given orally. If given IV, there is an increased risk of propylene/polyethylene glycol toxicity with frequent or high doses Hepatic impairment: Caution in hepatic insufficiency

Comparison of the Benzodiazepines (cont.)

Drug	Approximate Equivalent Dose[*]	Time to Peak Plasma Level PO (T_{max})	Lipid Solubility[**]	Onset of Action	Protein Binding (PB) Volume of Distribution (Vd)	Elimination Half-life (Parent and Active Metabolite)	Metabolic Pathway Active Metabolite(s)	Dosage for Approved Indications
Nitrazepam[(C)]	10 mg Potency: Medium	2–3 h	Low	30–60 min	PB: 85% Vd: 2.4 L/kg	Parent: 24–29 h	Reduction (CYP2E1) Active metabolite(s): No Excreted as amino and acetamide analogs; metabolism impaired in the elderly; accumulates with chronic use	*Insomnia*: 5–10 mg at bedtime Renal impairment: Avoid in patients with severe renal failure Hepatic impairment: No information
Oxazepam	20 mg Potency: Low	2–4 h	Low	30–60 min	PB: 86–99% Vd: 0.6 L/kg	Parent: 5–20 h; longer half-life in women; prolonged half-life in renal impairment	Conjugation (glucuronidation) Active metabolite(s): No	*Anxiety*: 10–30 mg tid-qid *Insomnia*: 15–30 mg 60 min before bedtime *Alcohol withdrawal*: 15–30 mg tid-qid Renal impairment: No dosage adjustment necessary Hepatic impairment: No information
Temazepam	20 mg Potency: Low	2–3 h Variable rate of absorption depending on formulation	Moderate	30–60 min	PB: 96% Vd: 1.4 L/kg	Parent: 10–20 h; longer elimination half-life in women	Conjugation (glucuronidation) Active metabolite(s): None 5% excreted as oxazepam in urine; plasma concentration too low to detect	*Insomnia*: 7.5–30 mg at bedtime Renal impairment: No dosage adjustment necessary Hepatic impairment: No information
Triazolam	0.5 mg Potency: High	1–2 h Well absorbed sublingually	Moderate	15–30 min	PB: 89–94% Vd: 0.8–1.8 L/kg	Parent: 1.5–5 h	Oxidation: (CYP3A4) Active metabolite(s): None Clearance in the elderly only 50–80% that of young adults	*Insomnia*: 0.125–0.25 mg at bedtime Renal impairment: No dosage adjustment necessary Hepatic impairment: Start at 0.125 mg qhs

[*] Based on Dr. Heather Ashton's "benzodiazepine equivalency table," which provides the approximate equivalent dose to 10 mg of diazepam. See https://www.benzo.org.uk/bzequiv.htm; the site states that "these equivalents do not agree with those used by some authors and are firmly based on clinical experience during switch-over to diazepam at start of withdrawal programs but may vary between individuals", [**] Lipid solubility positively correlates with enhancing benzodiazepines' (1) affinity for peripheral adipose tissue, resulting in redistribution from the vascular compartment (this increases volume of distribution), and (2) passage across the blood/brain barrier, facilitating their CNS activity. The higher the lipid solubility the more rapid the onset of activity and the greater the risk of memory impairment.

[(B)] Not marketed in Canada,   [(C)] Not marketed in the USA

Buspirone

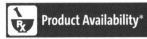

Product Availability*

Generic Name	Chemical Class	Neuroscience-based Nomenclature˙ (Pharmacological Target/Mode of Action)	Trade Name(A)	Dosage Forms and Strengths
Buspirone	Azaspirone	Serotonin/Partial agonist	Buspar	Tablets: 5 mg(B), 7.5 mg(B), 10 mg, 15 mg(B), 30 mg(B)

* Refer to Health Canada's Drug Product Database or the FDA's Drugs@FDA for the most current availability information ˙ Developed by a taskforce consisting of representatives from the American College of Neuropsychopharmacology (ACNP), the Asian College of Neuropsychopharmacology (AsCNP), the European College of Neuropsychopharmacology (ECNP), the International College of Neuropsychopharmacology (CINP), and the International Union of Basic and Clinical Pharmacology (IUPHAR) (see https://nbn2r.com),
(A) Generic preparations may be available,   (B) Not marketed in Canada

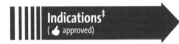

Indications‡ (👍 approved)

- 👍 Generalized anxiety disorder (GAD): Short-term symptomatic relief of excessive anxiety
- As an alternative to benzodiazepines in situations where sedation or psychomotor impairment may be dangerous
- Obsessive-compulsive disorder (OCD); may reduce symptoms of anxiety
- Depression – to augment effect of antidepressants
- Social phobia – contradictory evidence as to efficacy; may be useful as an augmenting agent in partial responders to SSRIs
- Premenstrual syndrome – may help reduce premenstrual irritability
- Bruxism caused by SSRI/SNRI antidepressants – may be useful in alleviation (case reports)
- Behavioral symptoms (aggression) related to dementia (case series)
- Adjunctive medication for opioid withdrawal. In a double-blind, randomized, placebo-controlled, pilot clinical trial, buspirone 45 mg/day adjunctive to buprenorphine mitigated opioid withdrawal during a supervised opioid taper[4]

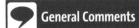

General Comments

- Buspirone is a selective anxiolytic of the azaspirone class; unlike the benzodiazepines, it has no anticonvulsant or muscle-relaxant properties
- Tolerance to effects of buspirone has not been reported
- Lack of effect on respiration may make it useful in patients with pulmonary disease or sleep apnea; may actually stimulate respiration
- Minimal effect on cognition, memory or driving performance
- May have a preferential effect for symptoms of anxiety, irritability, and aggression, with little effect on behavioral manifestations
- Eight 3-way (buspirone, diazepam, placebo) controlled trials have been conducted evaluating buspirone as an anxiolytic agent. Buspirone was significantly better than placebo in 4 trials, not better than placebo in the other trials

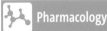

Pharmacology

- Unlike the benzodiazepines, buspirone does not bind to the "benzodiazepine"-GABA$_A$ receptor complex
- Buspirone pharmacology is not fully understood; it has affinity for central D$_2$ receptors (antagonist and agonist) and 5-HT$_{1A}$ receptors (partial agonist)
- Buspirone does not block transporters of monoamines
- Buspirone's major metabolite (1-(2-pyrimidinyl)-piperazine) is an α_2-adrenergic receptor antagonist, thus enhancing norepinephrine release

Dosing

- Initial dose: 5 mg bid-tid; may be increased in increments of 5 mg/day every 2–3 days to a maximum of 60 mg/day
- Usual therapeutic dose for most patients is 20–30 mg/day (10–15 mg bid)
- Doses up to 90 mg/day have been used in patients with major depressive disorder and significant associated anxiety symptoms
- Slow onset of action, may take as long as 2–4 weeks for anxiolytic effect to occur
- ☞ **Not effective on a prn basis**

‡ Indications listed here do not necessarily apply to all countries. Please refer to a country's regulatory database (e.g., US Food and Drug Administration, Health Canada Drug Product Database) for the most current availability information and indications

Buspirone (cont.)

Pharmacokinetics	• Absorption is virtually complete; first-pass effect reduces bioavailability to about 4% • Food may reduce rate of absorption (95%), decrease extent of first-pass effect, and therefore increase oral bioavailability; C_{max} increased up to 116% (8 participants) • Highly bound to plasma proteins (86%) • T_{max}: 0.7–1.5 h • Elimination half-life: 2–3 h. Parent drug metabolized by CYP3A4; metabolite (1-(2-pyrimidinyl) piperazine) is active and metabolized by 2D6 • Clearance reduced in renal and hepatic impairment
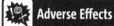 **Adverse Effects**	• Causes little sedation; does not impair psychomotor or cognitive functions • Headache (up to 6%), dizziness (up to 12%), lightheadedness (3%), nervousness (5%), excitement (2%), fatigue, paresthesia, numbness, and GI upset seen in less than 10% of patients • A literature review found 65 cases of buspirone-associated movement disorders: 14 dyskinesia, 10 akathisia, 8 myoclonus, 6 parkinsonism, 6 dystonia; others not clearly defined included 7 tension, 14 incoordination, and undefined cases of dyskinesia, tics, and parkinsonism. Time to onset was one month or less in 76% of the cases • Has been reported to precipitate hypomania or mania (primarily in the elderly); high doses may worsen psychosis • Dose-dependent increase in prolactin and growth hormone levels reported
D/C Discontinuation Syndrome	• Withdrawal effects have not been reported
Precautions	• Has no cross-tolerance with benzodiazepines and will not alleviate benzodiazepine withdrawal; when switching, taper benzodiazepine dose while adding buspirone to the regimen • Buspirone does not have anticonvulsant activity and has not been evaluated in patients with a history of seizures; not recommended for patients with seizures
Toxicity	• Excessive doses produce extension of pharmacological effects including dizziness, nausea, and vomiting; monitor respiration, blood pressure, and pulse, and give symptomatic and supportive therapy
Pediatric Considerations	• For detailed information on the use of buspirone in this population, please see the *Clinical Handbook of Psychotropic Drugs for Children and Adolescents*[1] • Buspirone used in ADHD, aggression, autism, and to augment SSRIs in obsessive-compulsive disorder (10–30 mg/day) • Dizziness, behavior activation, euphoria, increased aggression, and psychosis reported
Geriatric Considerations	• Buspirone is not known to cause sedation, cognitive impairment, disinhibition or motor impairment in the elderly • Dosage should be decreased in patients with reduced hepatic or renal function
Use in Pregnancy◊	• No fetal adverse effects reported in animal studies; inadequate human data, safety in pregnancy has not yet been determined
Breast Milk	• In animals, buspirone is excreted into milk; unknown excretion into human milk; unknown effects on nursing infants. Consider alternative anti-anxiety agent

◊ See p. 473 for further information on drug use in pregnancy and effects on breast milk

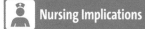 **Nursing Implications**

- The effect of buspirone is gradual; improvement may be seen 7–10 days (but may take as long as 2–4 weeks) after starting therapy
- When switching from a benzodiazepine to buspirone, it is important to gradually taper the benzodiazepine to avoid precipitating a withdrawal reaction
- Buspirone should be taken consistently, not on an as needed basis

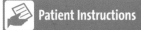 **Patient Instructions**

- For detailed patient instructions on buspirone, see the Patient Information Sheet (details on p. 474)

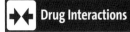 **Drug Interactions**

- Clinically significant interactions are listed below
- For more interaction information on any given combination, also see the corresponding chapter for the second agent

Class of Drug	Example	Interaction Effect
Antibiotic	Clarithromycin, erythromycin	Increased plasma level of buspirone (5-fold increase in C_{max}) due to inhibited metabolism via CYP3A4
	Linezolid	Linezolid reversibly inhibits MAO and can potentially lead to amplification of serotonergic effects of buspirone
Antidepressant		
SSRI	Fluoxetine, fluvoxamine	Concomitant use of serotonergic agents increases the risk of serotonin syndrome
		Increased plasma level of buspirone (3-fold increase in AUC) with fluvoxamine
		Case reports of serotonin syndrome, euphoria, seizures or dystonia with combination
SARI	Trazodone	Concomitant use of serotonergic agents increases the risk of serotonin syndrome
TCA	Amitriptyline, clomipramine	Concomitant use of serotonergic agents increases the risk of serotonin syndrome
Irreversible MAOI	Phenelzine, tranylcypromine	MAOIs may potentiate the activity of serotonergic agents like buspirone via inhibition of serotonin metabolism. The result is an increased risk of serotonin syndrome
		MAOIs combined with buspirone can increase blood pressure
Antifungal	Itraconazole, ketoconazole	Increased plasma level and/or effect of buspirone, due to inhibited metabolism via CYP3A4
Antipsychotic	Haloperidol	Increased plasma level of haloperidol (by 26%) perhaps due to competitive metabolism via CYP3A4
Antiretroviral		
Protease inhibitor	Indinavir, ritonavir	Increased plasma level of buspirone due to CYP3A4 inhibition
Antitubercular drug	Rifampin	Decreased peak plasma concentration and half-life of buspirone due to induced metabolism via CYP3A4
Benzodiazepine	Diazepam	Prior treatment with benzodiazepines for generalized anxiety disorder (GAD) may reduce response to buspirone
Calcium channel blocker	Diltiazem, verapamil	Increased peak plasma level of buspirone (3.4- and 4-fold increase in C_{max}, respectively) due to inhibited metabolism via CYP3A4
Grapefruit juice		Increased peak plasma level of buspirone (up to 15-fold), AUC (up to 20-fold), and half-life (1.5-fold) due to inhibited metabolism via CYP3A4
Immunosuppressant	Cyclosporine A	Increased serum level of cyclosporine A with possible renal adverse effects
St. John's wort		Concomitant use of serotonergic agents increases the risk of serotonin syndrome
		Decreased level of buspirone due induction of CYP3A4

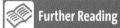 **Further Reading**

References

1. Elbe D, Black TR, McGrane IR, et al. Clinical handbook of psychotropic drugs for children and adolescents. (4th ed.). Boston, MA: Hogrefe Publishing, 2019.
2. Lee H, Koh J-W, Kim Y-A, et al. Pregnancy and neonatal outcomes after exposure to alprazolam in pregnancy. Front Pharmacol. 2022;13:854562. doi:10.3389/fphar.2022.854562
3. Schoretsanitis G, Ruan C-J, Rohde C, et al. An update on the complex relationship between clozapine and pneumonia. Expert Rev Clin Pharmacol. 2021;14(2):145–149. doi:10.1080/17512433.2021.1877135
4. Bergeria CL, Tan H, Antoine D, et al. A double-blind, randomized, placebo-controlled, pilot clinical trial examining buspirone as an adjunctive medication during buprenorphine-assisted supervised opioid withdrawal. Exp Clin Psychopharmacol. 2022. doi:10.1037/pha0000550

Additional Suggested Reading

- Baldwin DS, Anderson IM, Nutt DJ, et al. Evidence-based pharmacological treatment of anxiety disorders, post-traumatic stress disorder and obsessive-compulsive disorder: A revision of the 2005 guidelines from the British Association for Psychopharmacology. J Psychopharmacol. 2014;28(5):403–439. doi:10.1177/0269881114525674
- Bandelow B, Reitt M, Rover C, et al. Efficacy of treatments for anxiety disorders: A meta-analysis. Int Clin Psychopharmacol. 2015;30(4):183–192. doi:10.1097/YIC.0000000000000078
- Bachhuber MA, Hennessy S, Cunningham CO, et al. Increasing benzodiazepine prescriptions and overdose mortality in the United States, 1996–2013. Am J Public Health. 2016;106(4):686–688. doi:10.2105/AJPH.2016.303061
- Canadian Agency for Drugs and Technologies in Health. Discontinuation strategies for patients with long-term benzodiazepine use: A review of clinical evidence and guidelines. [Rapid Response Report: Summary with critical appraisal; July 29, 2015]. Retrieved from http://www.ncbi.nlm.nih.gov/books/NBK310990/
- Canadian Agency for Drugs and Technologies in Health. Use of antipsychotics and/or benzodiazepines as rapid tranquilization in in-patients of mental facilities and emergency departments: A review of the clinical effectiveness and guidelines. [Rapid Response Report: Summary with critical appraisal; October 29, 2015]. Retrieved from http://www.ncbi.nlm.nih.gov/books/NBK350030/
- Canadian Agency for Drugs and Technologies in Health. Treatment of older adults with insomnia, agitation, or delirium with benzodiazepines: A review of the clinical effectiveness and guidelines [Rapid Response Report: Summary with critical appraisal; January 14, 2016]. Retrieved from http://www.ncbi.nlm.nih.gov/books/NBK343886/
- Chen SJ, Yeh CM, Chao TF, et al. The use of benzodiazepine receptor agonists and risk of respiratory failure in patients with chronic obstructive pulmonary disease: A nationwide population-based case-control study. Sleep. 2015;38(7):1045–1050. doi:10.5665/sleep.4808
- Gerlach LB, Wiechers IR, Maust DT. Prescription benzodiazepine use among older adults: A critical review. Harv Rev Psychiatry. 2018;26(5):264–273. doi:10.1097/HRP.0000000000000190
- Haas DM, McHugh KW, Durst PJ, et al. Psychotropic medications in pregnancy and the postpartum period. Clinical Medicine Insights: Therapeutics. 2015;7. doi:10.4137/CMT.S18902
- Hirschtritt ME, Olfson M, Kroenke K. Balancing the risks and benefits of benzodiazepines. JAMA. 2021;325(4):347–348. doi:10.1001/jama.2020.22106
- Hoge EA, Ivkovic A, Fricchione GL. Generalized anxiety disorder: Diagnosis and treatment. BMJ. 2012;345:e7500. doi:10.1136/bmj.e7500
- Katzman MA, Bleau P, Blier P, et al. Canadian clinical practice guidelines for the management of anxiety, posttraumatic stress and obsessive-compulsive disorders. BMC Psychiatry. 2014;14 Suppl 1:S1. doi:10.1186/1471-244X-14-S1-S1
- Pariente A, de Gage SB, Moore N, et al. The benzodiazepine-dementia disorders link: Current state of knowledge. CNS drugs. 2016;30(1):1–7. doi:10.1007/s40263-015-0305-4
- Park TW, Saitz R, Ilgen MA, et al. Benzodiazepine prescribing patterns and deaths from drug overdose among US veterans receiving opioid analgesics: Case-cohort study. BMJ. 2015;350:h2698. doi:10.1136/bmj.h2698
- Richardson K, Mattishent K, Loke YK, et al. History of benzodiazepine prescriptions and risk of dementia: Possible bias due to prevalent users and covariate measurement timing in a nested case-control study. Am J Epidemiol. 2019;188(7):1228–1236. doi:10.1093/aje/kwz073

Product Availability*

Generic Name	Chemical Class	Neuroscience-based Nomenclature* (Pharmacological Target/Mode of Action)	Trade Name[(A)]	Dosage Forms and Strengths
	Benzodiazepines	GABA/Benzodiazepine receptor agonist (GABA$_A$ receptor positive allosteric modulator)		See pp. 240–248
Chloral hydrate[(C)]	Chloral derivative	GABA/Benzodiazepine receptor agonist (GABA$_A$ receptor positive allosteric modulator)		Oral solution: 100 mg/mL
Daridorexant[(B)]	Dual orexin receptor antagonist	Orexin/Antagonist	Quviviq	Tablets: 25 mg, 50 mg
Diphenhydramine	Antihistamine	Histamine/Antagonist	Benadryl, Compoz[(B)], Insomnal, Nytol, Simply Sleep, Sominex, Unisom	Tablets: 12.5 mg, 25 mg, 50 mg Caplets: 25 mg, 50 mg Capsules: 25 mg, 50 mg Chewable tablets: 25 mg Oral solution: 6.25 mg/5 mL[(C)], 12.5 mg/5 mL Injection: 50 mg/mL
Doxepin	Antidepressant	Norepinephrine, serotonin/Multimodal	Silenor	See pp. 54–63
Doxylamine	Antihistamine	Histamine/Antagonist	Unisom[(B)]	Tablets: 25 mg
Eszopiclone[(D)]	Cyclopyrrolone	GABA/Benzodiazepine receptor agonist (GABA$_A$ receptor positive allosteric modulator)	Lunesta	Tablets: 1 mg, 2 mg, 3 mg
Hydroxyzine	Antihistamine	Histamine/Antagonist	Atarax[(C)], Vistaril[(B)]	Tablets[(B)]: 10 mg, 25 mg, 50 mg Capsules[(C)]: 10 mg, 25 mg, 50 mg Oral syrup: 10 mg/5 mL Injection: 25 mg/mL[(B)], 50 mg/mL
Lemborexant	Dual orexin receptor antagonist	Orexin/Antagonist	Dayvigo	Tablets: 5 mg, 10 mg
Mirtazapine (off label)	Antidepressant	Norepinephrine, serotonin/Multimodal	Remeron	See pp. 49–53
Pentobarbital**	Barbiturate	Not listed	Nembutal	Injection: 50 mg/mL[(B)]
Promethazine	Antihistamine	Histamine, dopamine/Antagonist	Phenergan	Tablets: 12.5 mg[(B)], 25 mg[(B)], 50 mg Oral Solution[(B)]: 6.25 mg/5 mL Suppositories[(B)]: 12.5 mg, 25 mg Injection[(B)]: 25 mg/mL, 50 mg/mL
Ramelteon[(B)]	Selective melatonin agonist	Melatonin/Agonist	Rozerem	Tablets: 8 mg
Secobarbital**[(B)]	Barbiturate	Not listed	Seconal	Capsules: 50 mg, 100 mg
Suvorexant[(B)]	Dual orexin receptor antagonist	Orexin/Antagonist	Belsomra	Tablets: 5 mg, 10 mg, 15 mg, 20 mg
Tasimelteon[(B)]	Selective melatonin agonist	Melatonin/Agonist	Hetlioz	Capsules: 20 mg
Zaleplon[(B)]	Pyrazolopyrimidine	GABA/Benzodiazepine receptor agonist (GABA$_A$ receptor positive allosteric modulator)	Sonata	Capsules: 5 mg, 10 mg

Hypnotics/Sedatives (cont.)

Generic Name	Chemical Class	Neuroscience-based Nomenclature* (Pharmacological Target/Mode of Action)	Trade Name[A]	Dosage Forms and Strengths
Zolpidem	Imidazopyridine derivative	GABA/Benzodiazepine receptor agonist (GABA_A receptor positive allosteric modulator)	Ambien Ambien CR Edluar[B], Sublinox [C] Zolpimist[B]	Tablets: 5 mg, 10 mg Extended-release tablets[B]: 6.25 mg, 12.5 mg Sublingual tablets: 1.75 mg[B], 3.5 mg[B], 5 mg[C], 10 mg[C] Metered oral spray[B]: 5 mg/spray
Zopiclone[C]	Cyclopyrrolone		Imovane	Tablets: 3.75 mg, 5 mg, 7.5 mg

* Refer to Health Canada's Drug Product Database or the FDA's Drugs@FDA for the most current availability information.   * Developed by a taskforce consisting of representatives from the American College of Neuropsychopharmacology (ACNP), the Asian College of Neuropsychopharmacology (AsCNP), the European College of Neuropsychopharmacology (ECNP), the International College of Neuropsychopharmacology (CINP), and the International Union of Basic and Clinical Pharmacology (IUPHAR) (see https://nbn2r.com), [A] Generic preparations may be available,   [B] Not marketed in Canada,   [C] Not marketed in the USA,   [D] S-isomer of zopiclone   ** These drugs are not recommended for use as hypnotics/sedatives because they are habit forming, causing physical dependence and relatively more adverse effects than other options. Furthermore, they can have severe withdrawal symptoms; tolerance develops quickly, requiring increased dosage; they have a low margin of safety (therapeutic dose close to toxic dose); they are involved in many drug interactions (induce metabolizing enzymes); they can evoke behavioral complications in children and depression in adults

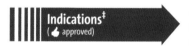

Indications‡ (👍 approved)

- 🛌 Nocturnal sedation; short-term management of insomnia
- 🛌 Preoperative/procedural sedation (chloral hydrate, hydroxyzine, promethazine)
- 🛌 Chronic insomnia management (ramelteon, eszopiclone, suvorexant – USA)
- 🛌 Non-24-hour sleep-wake disorders (tasimelteon – USA)

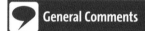

General Comments

- Prior to treatment of insomnia, determine if sleep disturbance is secondary to:
  - Psychiatric disorder (e.g., depression, mania, anxiety, psychosis, Alzheimer's disease, ADHD)
  - Medical disorder (e.g., thyroid, peptic ulcer, pain)
  - Drug-induced (e.g., theophylline, sympathomimetics, some antidepressants, decongestants, diuretics, etc.)
  - Breathing disorders during sleep (e.g., sleep apnea, sleep-related asthma, hypoventilation)
  - Lifestyle (e.g., shift work, poor sleep hygiene)
  - Excessive use/abuse of psychoactive drugs (e.g., caffeine, alcohol, cocaine, amphetamines)
  - Other sleep disorders (e.g., periodic limb movement disorder, restless legs syndrome, circadian rhythm disorders, narcolepsy)
- Insomnia is an important risk factor for neurodegenerative diseases such as Alzheimer's disease and Parkinson's disease. Chronic insomnia leads to neurodegenerative changes in Alzheimer's disease brains through the accumulation of β-amyloid and tau proteins
- Treat the underlying cause whenever possible (e.g., precipitating factors, perpetuating factors)
- Psychological therapies are as efficacious as pharmacological therapies for primary insomnia, and psychological therapies provide more durable response. Non-pharmacological methods (e.g., cognitive-behavioral therapy, relaxation therapies) should be tried prior to, or concurrently with, pharmacological therapy - see nursing section p. 261
- The goals of pharmacological therapy are to (a) prevent the progression from transient to chronic insomnia, (b) reverse sleep disruption to prevent deterioration of daytime performance, (c) resolve or mitigate underlying conditions that may be contributing to insomnia, promote a sound and satisfying sleep (sleep initiation, quality, quantity, and continuity), (d) prevent dependence on drug therapy, (e) reinstate a normal sleep pattern without the need for medication, and (f) promote healthy sleep hygiene practices
- Use of hypnotics is only recommended for short periods; long-term, continuous treatment is not recommended (though may be required in cases of severe, chronic insomnia)
- Eszopiclone, zaleplon, zolpidem, and zopiclone are frequently referred to as "Z-drugs"
- In a network meta-analysis comparing the efficacy and safety of lemborexant with other insomnia treatments (i.e., suvorexant, benzodiazepines, Z-drugs, trazodone, and ramelteon), lemborexant was ranked as the best treatment based on polysomnography-total sleep time, latency to persistent sleep, and sleep efficiency, and was ranked second to suvorexant on wake after sleep onset. In this study, eszopiclone was highly ranked for subjectively measured sleep onset latency and Insomnia Severity Index at 4 weeks, 3 months, and 6 months

‡ Indications listed here do not necessarily apply to all hypnotics/sedatives or all countries. Please refer to a country's regulatory database (e.g., US Food and Drug Administration, Health Canada Drug Product Database) for the most current availability information and indications

- In a network meta-analysis[1] of 154 double-blind, randomized controlled trials (30 interventions and 44,089 participants), the following was reported:
  - Eszopiclone and lemborexant had the best profile for acute and long-term treatment in terms of efficacy, acceptability, and tolerability; however, eszopiclone might cause substantial adverse events and safety data on lemborexant were inconclusive
  - Benzodiazepines were very effective in the acute treatment, but their tolerability and safety profiles were not favorable. There were no data available for benzodiazepines from long-term trials
  - Doxepin, seltorexant, and zaleplon were well tolerated, but data on efficacy were scarce and do not allow firm conclusions
  - Melatonergic interventions had poor efficacy, with no long-term data

 Pharmacology

- Sedating antihistamines antagonize histamine (subtype 1) receptors in the brain and disrupt cortical neurotransmission associated with the arousal action of histamine
- Benzodiazepines bind nonselectively to various subtypes of "benzodiazepine"-GABA$_A$-chloride ionotropic receptors in the brain; GABA$_A$ receptor subtypes containing an α_1 subunit are associated with sedation and ataxia; GABA$_A$ receptor subtypes containing α_2 and/or α_3 subunits generally have greater anxiolytic activity
- Zolpidem, zopiclone, eszopiclone, and zaleplon bind selectively to GABA$_A$ receptor subtypes containing α_1 subunits (and less so α_2 or α_3) and thus do not have anxiolytic properties like benzodiazepines
- Ramelteon has high binding affinity for MT$_1$ and MT$_2$ melatonin receptors (in the suprachiasmatic nucleus) and enhances the effect of endogenous melatonin; it has no anxiolytic or muscle relaxant properties, and has no tolerance or abuse potential. It has not been shown to cause significant respiratory depression
- Tasimelteon is an agonist for MT$_1$ and MT$_2$ melatonin receptors (greater affinity for MT$_2$ receptor than MT$_1$ receptor). MT$_2$ melatonin receptor is thought to preferentially influence regulation of circadian rhythms
- Daridorexant, suvorexant, and lemborexant are dual orexin receptor antagonists that blocks both OX1R and OX2R. They block binding of orexin A and B, which are neuropeptides that promote wakefulness

 Dosing

- See pp. 264–267 for individual agents
- Dosage should be adjusted in the elderly and in patients with hepatic impairment
- Zolpidem's starting and maximum dose are lower for females compared to males, due to pharmacokinetic differences between sexes

Pharmacokinetics

- See pp. 264–267
- Daridorexant: Age, sex, race, body size, and mild to severe renal impairment does not have a clinically significant effect on the pharmacokinetics
- Eszopiclone: T_{max} delayed after high-fat meal; increased AUC by 41% and $T_{1/2}$ to 9 h in the elderly; AUC increased 2-fold in moderate to severe liver impairment
- Lemborexant: High-fat, high-calorie meal delays T_{max} by 2 h
- Ramelteon: High inter-patient variability in C_{max} and AUC; high-fat meal delays T_{max} and increases AUC by 31%. Drug exposure increased 4-fold in mild hepatic impairment; 4 active metabolites; 84% of metabolites are eliminated in urine
- Suvorexant: Food delays T_{max} by approximately 90 min
- Tasimelteon: High-fat meal delays T_{max} by 1.75 h and decreases C_{max} by 44%. Smokers have 40% decrease in tasimelteon exposure
- Zaleplon: Absorption and peak plasma level may decrease with high-fat meal (C_{max} and T_{max} decreased by 35%). In one study, Japanese patients showed increased C_{max} and AUC by 37% and 64%, respectively; differences in body weight or hepatic enzyme activity may explain this difference
- Zolpidem: C_{max}, T_{max}, and AUC increased by 50%, 32%, and 64%, respectively, in the elderly (over 70 years) compared to young adults (20–40 years) following a single 20 mg dose. The CR preparation is formulated with an immediate-release layer and a slow-release layer; C_{max} occurs later and is higher than with regular-release product. Women attain significantly higher serum zolpidem concentrations than men. Due to high protein binding, patients with low serum albumin attain higher levels of free zolpidem
- Zopiclone: Half-life can double in the elderly and patients with hepatic impairment

 Onset & Duration of Action

- See pp. 264–267

Hypnotics/Sedatives (cont.)

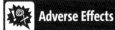 **Adverse Effects**

- See chart pp. 267–269
- Daytime sedation and impairment: Dependent on drug dosage, half-life, and patient tolerance; higher rates of motor vehicle accidents and other unintentional injuries reported
- Anterograde amnesia is dependent on drug, potency, and dose
- Rebound insomnia is dependent on drug, dose, half-life, and duration of use
- High dose may result in respiratory depression and reduce blood pressure
- Ramelteon has been associated with an effect on reproductive hormones (decreased testosterone and increased prolactin) in adults; long-term effects unknown
- Priapism reported with hydroxyzine (rare) – the metabolite of hydroxyzine (norchlorcyclizine) has structural and conformational similarities to trazodone's metabolite (m-chlorophenylpiperazine) and may suggest common underlying pharmacologic mechanism
- Nightmares and abnormal dreams reported with zaleplon and lemborexant upon initiation
- Falls and related injuries (e.g., fractures)
- A study (120 participants) that examined cognitive impairment found that long-term use of benzodiazepines was an independent risk factor for cognitive impairment in middle-aged and older patients with chronic insomnia. No correlation was found between Z-drug use and cognitive impairment

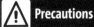 **Discontinuation Syndrome**

- Can occur with chronic use of all hypnotics (exceptions: daridorexant, lemborexant, ramelteon, suvorexant, and tasimelteon)
- Discontinuation of hypnotics can produce:
  - Withdrawal: Occurs within 1–2 days (with short-acting agents) to 3–7 days (with long-acting agents) following discontinuation of regular use of most hypnotics (for more than 2 weeks); suggested to occur less frequently with zopiclone and zolpidem. Common symptoms include insomnia, agitation, dizziness, nausea/vomiting, anxiety, perceptual disturbances (e.g., photophobia), malaise, and anorexia. Abrupt withdrawal of high doses may result in twitching, hyperthermia, tremors, seizures and/or psychosis, and possibly death
  - Rebound: Occurs hours to days after drug withdrawal; described as worsening of insomnia beyond pretreatment levels, nightmares (due to REM rebound). More likely to occur with short-acting agents
  - Relapse: Recurrence of the insomnia, to pretreatment levels, when the hypnotic is discontinued

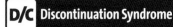 **Management**

- Withdrawal of a hypnotic (after chronic use) should be tailored to each patient; consider switching medications (if on a short-acting agent) to a comparable dose of a long-acting agent and gradually tapering the dose over several weeks. For benzodiazepines examples, see p. 245
- Concomitant cognitive-behavioral therapy may be helpful in facilitating taper and discontinuation of a hypnotic

⚠ **Precautions**

- Abrupt withdrawal of hypnotics (excluding lemborexant, ramelteon, suvorexant, and tasimelteon) may produce a significant discontinuation syndrome. See preceding section for symptoms and consequences of abrupt discontinuation
- Caution regarding drug interactions
- Concomitant use of CNS depressants (e.g., zolpidem, zopiclone) with opioids may result in profound respiratory depression, coma, and death. Consider other alternatives. Limit dosages and durations to the minimum if required. A population-based cohort study of 510,529 patients prescribed opioids alone or with concomitant Z-drugs found the combination of medications was associated with a substantial relative increase in the risk of overdose after controlling for all confounding factors
- Long-term use (for years) of hypnotics occurs as patients report unsuccessful efforts to decrease use (due to withdrawal effects); can result in memory impairment, motor vehicle accidents or falls/fractures
- Sedatives are associated with an increased risk of unintentional injuries
- Recreational abuse can occur; avoid use in individuals with high risk of substance misuse (no abuse potential reported with ramelteon and tasimelteon)
- Abuse may result in clouding of consciousness and visual hallucinations
- Use in individuals with sleep apnea is contraindicated
- Complex sleep-related behaviors (e.g., incidents of sleepwalking, driving while "asleep," and food binging while "asleep") have been reported with short acting benzodiazepine receptor agonists (i.e., eszopiclone, zaleplon, zolpidem, zopiclone)
- Due to reports of next-day impairment, zolpidem maximum dose has been reduced based on sex. See pp. 267 for dosing information

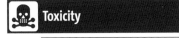 **Toxicity**	• Symptoms of overdose include varying degrees of drowsiness, mental confusion, and lethargy; in more serious cases, symptoms may include ataxia, hypotonia, hypotension, respiratory depression, rarely coma, and very rarely death
Management	• Symptomatic and supportive treatment along with immediate gastric lavage where appropriate. Intravenous fluids as needed • As in all cases of drug overdose, respiration, pulse, blood pressure, and other appropriate vital signs should be monitored and general supportive measures employed

Pediatric Considerations	• For detailed information on the use of hypnotics in this population, please see the *Clinical Handbook of Psychotropic Drugs for Children and Adolescents*[2] • Antihistamines: Paradoxical CNS excitation can occur

Geriatric Considerations	• Lowest effective dose should be utilized in the elderly for the least amount of time • The elderly have increased sensitivity to sedatives and are more susceptible to falls and related injuries. Systematic reviews and meta-analyses suggest an increased risk for falls and fractures with Z-drugs (especially zolpidem) in the elderly • Caution when using drugs that have long half-lives and are extensively metabolized via Phase I pathways (oxidation, reduction, hydrolysis) as they can accumulate in the elderly or in persons with liver disease • Caution when combined with other drugs that have CNS properties; additive effects can increase risk of confusion, disorientation, and delirium • Antihistamine hypnotics, including diphenhydramine, are not recommended in the elderly because of anticholinergic as well as CNS properties (see table pp. 268) • Anterograde amnesia reported with higher doses • Ramelteon: AUC and C_{max} increased 97% and 86%, respectively, and half-life increased in elderly subjects • Eszopiclone, zolpidem, and zopiclone levels are increased in the elderly (see pharmacokinetics section pp. 259–259) • The elderly have approximately 2-fold increased tasimelteon exposure compared to non-elderly adults • A meta-analysis of 18 studies reported that both benzodiazepine and Z-drug use were significantly associated with an increased risk of hip fracture • Early data suggests that ramelteon and/or suvorexant may prevent delirium in high-risk elderly patients • A retrospective cohort study of 268,170 subjects over age 50 showed a higher risk of Alzheimer's disease in those exposed to sedative hypnotics for more than 5 years (especially benzodiazepines and zolpidem) than in those not exposed • A 4-week controlled trial in patients with Alzheimer's disease found that treatment with suvorexant with 142 patients, compared to placebo including 143 patients, resulted in significantly longer sleep times and reduced awakening after sleep onset

Use in Pregnancy◇	• See pp. 267–269 for individual agents. For benzodiazepines, see p. 246
Breast Milk	• The American Academy of Pediatrics considers many hypnotics/sedatives compatible with breastfeeding – see table pp. 267–269

Nursing Implications	• Assess personal sleep habits and underlying factors that may be contributing to insomnia (e.g., medical disorders, use/abuse of psychoactive drugs, lifestyle, etc.) • Provide all patients with general sleep hygiene tips such as avoiding daytime naps and avoiding caffeine 6 h before bedtime • Inform patient not to operate vehicles or machinery, or engage in any potentially hazardous activities while under the influence of sedating medications • Suggest non-pharmacological methods of treating insomnia (e.g., cognitive-behavioral therapy, relaxation techniques, regular sleep/wake cycle 7 days/week, sleep restriction) • Assess whether medications/substances (e.g., nicotine, stimulants, alcohol) may be contributing to insomnia • Counsel patient regarding chronic use of hypnotics, risk of dependence, and potential for cognitive side effects • Patients on ramelteon should avoid taking the drug with or immediately after a high-fat meal because fat increases the drug's absorption from the intestine • Food significantly delays the peak plasma level of suvorexant, tasimelteon, and zolpidem

◇ See p. 473 for further information on drug use in pregnancy and effects on breast milk

Hypnotics/Sedatives (cont.)

- Abrupt withdrawal after chronic use of most hypnotics may result in serious adverse events and rebound symptoms (see Discontinuation Syndrome, p. 260); drugs should be tapered over time
- Patients taking zolpidem CR or ramelteon should not split, crush or chew the tablet

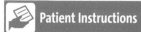 **Patient Instructions**

- For detailed patient instructions on hypnotics/sedatives, see the Patient Information Sheet (details p. 474)

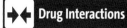 **Drug Interactions**

- Only clinically significant interactions are listed below
- For more interaction information on any given combination, also see the corresponding chapter for the second agent

Class of Drug	Example	Interaction Effects
Antibiotic	Ciprofloxacin	*Ramelteon:* Increased plasma level of ramelteon, possibly due to inhibited metabolism via CYP1A2
	Clarithromycin, doxycycline	*Eszopiclone, lemborexant, zaleplon, zolpidem, and zopiclone:* Increased plasma level of hypnotic due to inhibited metabolism via CYP3A4
		Daridorexant, lemborexant, and suvorexant: Increased plasma level due to inhibited metabolism via CYP3A4. Avoid combination
Anticoagulant	Warfarin	*Chloral hydrate* will displace drugs from plasma proteins and temporarily enhance hypoprothrombinemic response; increased or decreased PT ratio or INR response
Anticonvulsant	Carbamazepine, phenytoin	*Daridorexant, eszopiclone, lemborexant, suvorexant, zolpidem, zopiclone:* Decreased plasma level due to induced metabolism via CYP3A4
Antidepressant		
SSRI	Fluoxetine, fluvoxamine	*Chloral hydrate:* Increased sedation and side effects of *chloral hydrate* due to inhibited metabolism
	Fluvoxamine	*Ramelteon:* DO NOT COMBINE; increased C_{max} (70-fold) and AUC (190-fold) of ramelteon due to inhibited metabolism via CYP1A2
		Tasimelteon: Increased C_{max} (2-fold) and AUC (7-fold)
SSRI/NDRI	Fluoxetine, paroxetine, sertraline, bupropion	*Zolpidem:* Case reports of hallucinations and delirium with sertraline, fluoxetine, paroxetine, and bupropion
SNRI	Venlafaxine	*Diphenhydramine:* Decreased metabolism of venlafaxine via CYP2D6
Tricyclic	Desipramine	*Diphenhydramine:* May increase plasma level of antidepressants metabolized primarily by CYP2D6 due to inhibited metabolism
Antifungal	Itraconazole, ketoconazole	*Daridorexant:* Increased AUC by more than 400% due to inhibited metabolism by itraconazole via CYP3A4
		Eszopiclone: Increased C_{max} (1.4-fold) and $T_{½}$ (1.3-fold) of eszopiclone with ketoconazole due to decreased metabolism via CYP3A4
		Lemborexant: Increased C_{max} (36%) and AUC (270%) due to decreased metabolism via CYP3A4
		Ramelteon: Increased C_{max} (36%) and AUC (84%) due to inhibited metabolism by ketoconazole via CYP3A4
		Suvorexant: Increased AUC (approximately two-fold) due to inhibition via CYP3A4
		Tasimelteon: Increased tasimelteon AUC by approximately 50%
		Zaleplon: Increased plasma level of zaleplon due to decreased metabolism via CYP3A4
		Zolpidem: Decreased clearance of zolpidem (by 41%); half-life increased (by 26%) with ketoconazole
		Zopiclone: Increased AUC and elimination half-life of zopiclone due to inhibited metabolism via CYP3A4
	Fluconazole	*Lemborexant:* Increased C_{max} of lemborexant by 62% due to inhibited metabolism via CYP3A4
		Ramelteon: Increased AUC and C_{max} of ramelteon by 150% due to inhibited metabolism via CYP2C9
Antipsychotic	Aripiprazole, chlorpromazine, fluphenazine, perphenazine, quetiapine, risperidone, thiothixene	*Diphenhydramine:* May increase plasma level of antipsychotic metabolized via CYP2D6 due to inhibited metabolism
		Additive CNS depression and psychomotor impairment

Class of Drug	Example	Interaction Effects
Antiretroviral		
Combination	Stribild (Elvitegravir + cobicistat + emtricitabine + tenofovir)	*Ramelteon:* Cobicistat may increase ramelteon concentrations. Use with caution and monitor for toxicity *Zolpidem:* A 50% zolpidem dose reduction may be warranted when used with potent CYP3A4 inhibitors such as cobicistat
Protease inhibitor	Atazanavir, darunavir, indinavir,lopinavir, ritonavir, saquinavir	*Daridorexant, eszopiclone, lemborexant, suvorexant, zolpidem, zopiclone:* Increased plasma level of hypnotic due to inhibited metabolism via CYP3A4 *Ramelteon:* Ritonavir may decrease ramelteon plasma level via CYP1A2, 2C9 induction. Use with caution and monitor for efficacy
Antitubercular drug	Rifampin	*Daridorexant:* Decreased AUC by more than 50% due to induced metabolism via CYP3A4 *Eszopiclone:* Decreased AUC of eszopiclone due to induced metabolism via CYP3A4 *Lemborexant:* Decreased C_{max} and AUC (by 90%) due to induced metabolism via CYP3A4 *Ramelteon:* Decreased C_{max} and AUC of ramelteon (by 40–90%) due to induced metabolism *Suvorexant:* Decreased AUC (by 88%) due to induced metabolism via CYP3A4 *Tasimelteon:* Decreased plasma concentration of tasimelteon (by 90%) via CYP2C9 and CYP3A4 *Zaleplon:* Decreased AUC of zaleplon (by 80%) due to induced metabolism via CYP3A4 *Zolpidem:* Decreased peak plasma level of zolpidem (by 60%) and decreased elimination half-life (by 36%) due to induced metabolism via CYP2C9, CYP2C19, CYP2D6, and CYP3A4 *Zopiclone:* Decreased AUC of zopiclone (by 80%) due to induced metabolism via CYP3A4
Anxiolytic	General	Additive CNS effects and psychomotor impairment
	Lorazepam	*Eszopiclone:* C_{max} of both drugs increased by 22%
Barbiturates		Barbiturates are potent inducers of several CYP450 enzymes (see p. 264). Since these agents are rarely utilized as hypnotic agents, many important drug interactions have not been included in this handbook. Please refer to a drug interaction text for a list of drugs interacting with barbiturates
β-blocker	Metoprolol	*Diphenhydramine:* Decreased clearance of metoprolol (2-fold) due to inhibited metabolism via CYP2D6
Caffeine	Tea, coffee, colas, "energy drinks"	May counteract sedation and increase insomnia
CNS depressant	Alcohol	Increased CNS depression and psychomotor impairment; in "high" doses coma and respiratory depression can occur *Chloral hydrate:* Disulfiram-like reaction may occur
CNS stimulant	Dextroamphetamine, methylphenidate	May counteract sedation and increase insomnia
Flumazenil		*Zaleplon* and *zolpidem:* Antagonism of hypnotic effects
Grapefruit juice		*Daridorexant, eszopiclone, lemborexant, suvorexant, zaleplon, zolpidem, zopiclone:* Increased plasma level of hypnotic due to inhibited metabolism via CYP3A4 in gut wall; may result in increased bioavailability
H₂ antagonist	Cimetidine	*Diphenhydramine:* Increased AUC and half-life, and decreased clearance *Eszopiclone, zopiclone:* Increased plasma level of hypnotic due to inhibited metabolism via CYP3A4 *Zaleplon:* Increased peak plasma level and AUC of zaleplon by 85% due to inhibited metabolism via CYP3A4 and aldehyde oxidase
Opioid	General	Increased risk of serious side effects, including slowed or difficult breathing and death, when used with other CNS depressants
	Codeine	*Diphenhydramine:* Inhibited conversion of codeine to its active moiety morphine, via CYP2D6, resulting in decreased analgesic efficacy
	Methadone	*Diphenhydramine:* Increased plasma levels of methadone, possibly due to inhibited metabolism via CYP2D6
St. John's wort		*Daridorexant, eszopiclone, suvorexant, zolpidem, zopiclone:* May reduce plasma level of hypnotic due to induced metabolism via CYP3A4

For drugs interacting with benzodiazepines see pp. 246–248

Comparison of Hypnotics/Sedatives

	Usual Oral Dose in Adults	Onset of Action	Time to Peak Plasma Level (T_{max})	Bio-availability	Protein Binding (PB) Volume of distribution (Vd)	Elimination Half-life ($T_{1/2}$)	Tolerance	Metabolizing Enzymes (CYP450)*	CYP450 Effect**	Indications
Chloral hydrate	0.5–1 g Renal impairment: Contraindicated Hepatic impairment: Contraindicated	15–30 min	?	> 95% (active metabolite trichloro-ethanol)	PB: 70–80% (trichloro-ethanol) 94% (trichloro-acetic acid metabolite) Vd: 0.61 L/kg	4–12 h (tri-chloroethanol) 100 h (trichloroacetic acid metabolite)	Loses effect after 2 weeks	2E1	?	Nocturnal and preoperative sedation, procedural sedation, alcohol withdrawal
Daridorexant (Quviviq)	25–50 mg Renal impairment: No adjustment Hepatic impairment: Maximum dose 25 mg in moderate impairment, use not recommended in severe impairment	15–30 min May be delayed if taken with or soon after a meal	1–2 h (delayed by 1.3 h after high-fat, high-calorie meal)	Absolute bioavailabil-ity 62%	PB: 99.7% (in vitro) Vd: 31 L	8 h	No tolerance reported	3A4	–	Insomnia
Diphenhydramine (Benadryl, Compoz[(B)], Nytol, Simply Sleep, Sominex, Unisom)	12.5–50 mg (as sleep aid) Renal impairment: No dosage adjustment necessary Hepatic impairment: No information	60–80 min	2–4 h	40–60%	PB: 98–99% Vd: 13–20 L/kg	2–10 h (13.5 h in the elderly)	Antihistamines lose hypnotic efficacy with time	3A4, 2D6[(D)]	Inhibitor of 2D6	Sedation, insomnia, motion sickness, allergic reactions
Doxylamine[(C)] (Unisom)	25 mg (as sleep aid) Renal impairment: Decrease dose by 50% in patients with CrCl less than 10 mL/min—Hepatic impairment: Caution advised	1–2 h	2–4 h	25%	PB: ? Vd: 2.5 L/kg	10–12 h (15.5 h in the elderly)		–	–	Insomnia, allergic rhinitis, common cold – symptom control
Eszopiclone (Lunesta)	1–3 mg (1–2 mg in the elderly) Renal impairment: No dosage adjustment necessary Hepatic impairment: If severe, start at 1 mg qhs, max. 2 mg/day	0.5–1 h	1 h (2 h after high-fat meal)	80%	PB: 52–59% Vd: 1.4 L/kg	6 h (9 h in the elderly)	No tolerance reported after 12 months	3A4, 2E1	–	Insomnia

	Usual Oral Dose in Adults	Onset of Action	Time to Peak Plasma Level (T_{max})	Bio-availability	Protein Binding (PB) Volume of distribution (Vd)	Elimination Half-life ($T_{1/2}$)	Tolerance	Metabolizing Enzymes (CYP450)*	CYP450 Effect**	Indications
Hydroxyzine (Atarax, Vistaril)	50–100 mg qid (anxiety) 50–100 mg (preoperative sedation) Renal impairment: Decrease dose by 50% in patients with CrCl less than 50 mL/min Hepatic impairment: No information	15–30 min	2 h	80%	PB: 93% Vd: 16 L/kg	3–7 h (shorter in children)		–	Inhibitor of 2D6 (weak)	Anxiety disorder, preoperative sedation, antipruritic
Lemborexant (Dayvigo)	5 mg Maximum dose: 10 mg Renal impairment: No adjustment Hepatic impairment: Maximum dose 5 mg in moderate impairment, use not recommended in severe impairment	15–30 min	1-3 h (delayed to 3-5 h after high-fat, high-calorie meal)	?	PB: 94% (in vitro) Vd: 1970 L	17–19 h	No tolerance reported	3A4	Weak inducer of 2B6	Insomnia
Pentobarbital (Nembutal)	100 mg (150–200 mg IM for preoperative sedation) Renal impairment: Reduce start dose, amount not defined Hepatic impairment: Reduce start dose, amount not defined	1 min	15 min	70–90%	PB: 35–55% Vd: 1 L/kg	35–50 h	Loses effect after 2 weeks	?	Inducer of 2A6, 2B6, 2C9, 3A4	Preoperative sedation for anxiety and tension, anesthesia, refractory status epilepticus
Promethazine (Phenergan)	25–50 mg (preoperative sedation) 12.5–25 mg every 4 h prn (nausea/vomiting)	15–60 min	2–3 h	Low (?)	PB: 76–93% Vd: 1970 L	5–14 h	?	2D6		Preoperative or obstetric sedation, prevention/control of nausea and vomiting associated with anesthesia and surgery, prophylactic treatment of motion sickness

Comparison of Hypnotics/Sedatives (cont.)

	Usual Oral Dose in Adults	Onset of Action	Time to Peak Plasma Level (T_{max})	Bio-availability	Protein Binding (PB) Volume of distribution (Vd)	Elimination Half-life ($T_{1/2}$)	Tolerance	Metabolizing Enzymes (CYP450)*	CYP450 Effect**	Indications
Ramelteon[(B)] (Rozerem)	8 mg Renal impairment: No dosage adjustment necessary Hepatic impairment: Caution in mild–moderate impairment. Contraindicated if severe	30 min	0.5–1.5 h (fasting); 2.6 h in the elderly; food delays T_{max} by 45 min	Absolute bioavailability 2% due to extensive first-pass metabolism	PB: 82% Vd: 1.05 L/kg	1–2.6 h (M-II metabolite = 2–5 h)	No tolerance reported	1A2[(D)], 2C9, 3A4	–	Insomnia
Secobarbital (Seconal)	100 mg (200–300 mg for preoperative sedation) Renal impairment: Decrease start dose, amount not defined Hepatic impairment: Decrease start dose, amount not defined. Contraindicated in patients with significant impairment	15 min	2–4 h	90%	PB: 30–45% Vd: 1.5 L/kg	15–40 h	Loses effect after 2 weeks	–	Inducer of 2A6, 2B6, 2C9, 3A4	Preanesthetic agent, dental procedures, short-term insomnia
Suvorexant[(B)] (Belsomra)	10–20 mg Renal impairment: No dosage adjustment necessary Hepatic impairment: No dosage adjustment in mild–moderate impairment. No data for severe impairment	30 min	2 h (food delays T_{max} by 90 min)	82%	> 99%	Approximately 12 h	No tolerance reported	2C19, 3A4[(D)]	–	Insomnia
Tasimelteon[(B)] (Hetlioz)	20 mg Renal impairment: No dosage adjustment necessary Hepatic impairment: No dosage adjustment in mild–moderate impairment. Contraindicated if severe	Weeks to months due to action on circadian rhythm	0.5–3 h	38%	PB: 90% Vd: 56–126 L/kg	1.3 h (Metabolites = 1.3–3.7 h)	No tolerance reported	1A2, 3A4	–	Non-24-hour sleep-wake disorder

	Usual Oral Dose in Adults	Onset of Action	Time to Peak Plasma Level (T_{max})	Bio-availability	Protein Binding (PB) Volume of distribution (Vd)	Elimination Half-life ($T_{1/2}$)	Tolerance	Metabolizing Enzymes (CYP450)[*]	CYP450 Effect[**]	Indications
Zaleplon (Sonata)	5–10 mg (5 mg in the elderly) Renal impairment: No dosage adjustment necessary for mild–moderate impairment. No data for severe impairment Hepatic impairment: In mild–moderate impairment, 5 mg qhs. Avoid in severe impairment	15–30 min	0.9–1.5 h (delayed up to 3 h after high-fat meal)	30%	PB: 60% Vd: 1.4 L/kg	0.9–1.1 h	No tolerance up to 12 months reported	3A4, aldehyde oxidase[(D)]	?	Insomnia – useful for nocturnal awakenings due to fast onset and short duration of action
Zolpidem (Ambien, Ambien CR)[(E)]	5 mg (female), 5–10 mg (male) (5 mg in the elderly) Extended-release: 6.25 mg (female), 6.25–12.5 mg (male) Sublingual tab for middle-of-night awakening: 1.75 mg (female), 3.5 mg (male) Renal impairment: No dosage adjustment necessary Mild hepatic impairment: 5 mg Severe hepatic impairment: Avoid use	15–30 min	1.6 h; 2.2 h with food CR: 1.5 h; 4 h with food SL: 0.5–3 h (delayed 28% with food) Spray: 0.9 h (mean; delayed with food)	70%	PB: 93% Vd: 0.54 L/kg	1.5–4.5 h CR: 2.8 h SL: 1.57–6.73 h (5 mg), 1.75–3.77 h (10 mg) Spray: 1.7–5 h (5 mg), 1.7–8.4 h (10 mg) (Increased significantly in the elderly and in hepatic impairment)	No tolerance after 50 weeks reported	1A2, 2C9, 2C19, 2D6, 3A4[(D)]		Insomnia (difficulty of sleep onset and/or maintenance)
Zopiclone[(C)] (Imovane)	5–7.5 mg (initial dose of 3.75 mg in the elderly) Renal impairment: Start treatment with 3.75 mg; maximum: 5 mg Hepatic impairment: Caution in mild–moderate impairment. Recommended dose is 3.75 mg; maximum: 5 mg. Contraindicated in severe impairment	30 min	< 2 h	> 75% (increased in the elderly to 94%)	PB: 45% Vd: 0.54 L/kg	3.8–6.5 h (5–10 h in the elderly)	No tolerance up to 4 weeks reported	2C8, 3A4[(D)]	?	Insomnia

[*] Cytochrome P-450 isoenzymes involved in drug metabolism, [**] Effect of drug on cytochrome enzymes, [(B)] Not marketed in Canada, [(C)] Not marketed in the USA, [(D)] Primary route of metabolism, [(E)] Sublingual and oral dissolving tablets have been formulated in two strengths and may have a faster onset of action

Comparison of Hypnotics/Sedatives (cont.)

	Effect on Sleep Architecture	Main Side Effects	Precautions	Pregnancy/Lactation ◊
Antihistamine (Diphenhydramine, doxylamine, hydroxyzine)	Decreased sleep onset latency	Residual daytime sedation, incoordination; anticholinergic effects at high doses (dry mouth, blurred vision, confusion, delirium, urinary retention, etc.); elderly patients more prone to CNS effects including inattention, disorganized speech, behavior disturbance, altered consciousness GI disturbances; paradoxical CNS excitation can occur; tolerance to effects occurs within days or weeks	Elderly patients more susceptible to adverse effects including increased sedation, cognitive impairment, and increased risk of falls May precipitate seizures in patients with focal lesions Diphenhydramine and hydroxyzine are inhibitors of CYP2D6 and may interact with a number of drugs (see pp. 262–263)	Diphenhydramine: Fetal risk: Considered safe for use in pregnancy Breastfeeding: Excreted into milk; limited human data; manufacturer states use contraindicated in nursing mother because of increased sensitivity in newborn Hydroxyzine: Fetal risk: One study reports increased risk of congenital malformations but risk not seen in other studies; consider alternative antihistamine Breastfeeding: Unknown effects on nursing infants Doxylamine: Approved for use in pregnancy-associated nausea and vomiting; excretion in breast milk unknown
Barbiturate (Pentobarbital, Secobarbital)	Suppresses REM sleep and delta sleep; REM rebound on withdrawal	Confusion, hangover, drowsiness, lethargy, nightmares, excitement if given to patients in severe pain, bradycardia, hypotension, syncope Can cause severe depression (risk of suicide) Skin rash (1–3%), nausea, vomiting Weight gain	AVOID barbiturates in: Severe hepatic impairment, porphyria, uncontrolled pain (delirium may result) pulmonary insufficiency, confused and restless elderly patients Watch for CNS depression, hypotension, paradoxical stimulatory response (agitation and hyperactivity), and respiratory depression Risk of tolerance; high potential for abuse and dependence	Fetal risk: Limited human data but barbiturates cross the placenta; an increase in congenital defects and hemorrhagic disease of newborns reported; withdrawal symptoms seen in neonate Breastfeeding: Excreted in breast milk; not recommended
Chloral hydrate	Decreases sleep onset latency and nighttime awakenings with minimal effects on REM sleep	Nausea, vomiting, unpleasant taste, flatulence, hangover, ataxia, nightmares, skin rash Does not accumulate with chronic use; will displace other highly protein-bound drugs from plasma proteins	CAUTION in hepatic and renal impairment, gastritis, peptic ulcer, and cardiac distress Doses above 2 g can impair respiration and decrease blood pressure Tolerance can occur with chronic use; withdrawal reactions reported	Fetal risk: Limited human data to assess risk Breastfeeding: Excreted into human breast milk; use by nursing mothers causes neonatal sedation. Considered compatible with breastfeeding by American Academy of Pediatrics
Daridorexant	Decreased sleep onset latency; increased total sleep time	Somnolence, fatigue, headache	Potential to impair performance of activities requiring mental alertness May increase risk for sleep paralysis, cataplexy, complex sleep behaviors	Fetal risk: No human data available Breastfeeding: Safety not established
Eszopiclone	Decreased sleep onset latency, decreased nighttime awakenings, increased total sleep time	> 10%: Unpleasant taste, headache > 5–10%: Dry mouth, dyspepsia, dizziness, somnolence, respiratory infection Withdrawal effects have been reported including rebound insomnia Memory impairment reported in the morning, often only in the first week of treatment	High doses (> 6 mg) can produce amnesia, euphoria, and hallucinations Caution in respiratory impairment, liver dysfunction, depression, elderly patients, and in combination with CYP3A4 inhibitors	Fetal risk: No evidence of teratogenicity in animal models (high dose). No adequate or well-controlled studies in pregnant women. Consider alternative agent Breastfeeding: Excretion in breast likely given pharmacokinetic parameters; effects on nursing infant unknown but potential for sedation
Lemborexant	Decreased sleep onset latency; increased total sleep time	Somnolence, fatigue, headache, abnormal dreams	Potential to impair performance of activities requiring mental alertness May increase risk for sleep paralysis, cataplexy, complex sleep behaviors	Fetal risk: No human data available Breastfeeding: Safety not established

	Effect on Sleep Architecture	Main Side Effects	Precautions	Pregnancy/Lactation $^\diamond$
Ramelteon	Decreased sleep onset latency; no effect on night waking; small decreases in stages 3 and 4	Drowsiness, dizziness, fatigue, headache, nausea No behavioral impairment reported	Case reports of decreased testosterone and increased prolactin levels; not known what effect chronic or even chronic intermittent use may have on the reproductive axis AUC and T_{max} increased 4-fold in mild hepatic impairment	Fetal risk: Animal data suggest low risk. No controlled data in human pregnancy Breastfeeding: Excretion into breast milk likely given drug properties. No human data available
Suvorexant	Increased total sleep time; decreased sleep onset latency; small reduction in REM latency. Study suggests sleep architecture appears to be preserved	Somnolence, fatigue, headache, abnormal dreams, muscle weakness, dry mouth	Higher doses (above 20 mg) may increase risk of impaired motor coordination, sleep paralysis, hallucinations, and daytime somnolence	Fetal risk: Animal data suggest low risk. No controlled studies in pregnant women Breastfeeding: Excretion into breast milk unknown; no human data
Tasimelteon	Entrains circadian rhythm in totally blind patients; increases night-time sleep duration; reduces daytime sleep	Headache, nightmares or abnormal dreams, increased serum ALT	Potential to impair performance of activities requiring mental alertness	Fetal risk: Animal data suggest low risk; no controlled data in human pregnancy Breastfeeding: Excretion into breast milk unknown; no human data
Zaleplon	Decreased sleep onset latency and increased slow-wave sleep	> 10%: Headache 1–10%: Dizziness, somnolence, amnesia, malaise, pruritus, dysmenorrhea, nausea, paresthesia, tremor < 1%: Alopecia, ALT & AST increased, anemia, angina, ataxia, bundle branch block, palpitation Case reports: Anaphylaxis, angioedema, complex sleep-related behavior (sleep-driving, cooking or eating food, making phone calls)	Due to rapid onset of action, should be taken immediately before bedtime Dependence, withdrawal, and rebound insomnia reported after prolonged use Moderate abuse potential Caution in liver dysfunction: 4-fold increase in C_{max} and 7-fold increase in AUC	Fetal risk: Animal data suggest low risk. Human studies did not identify increased risk of malformations. Consider risk and benefit before use. Restrict use to occasional and short term Breastfeeding: Excreted into breast milk; no data on breastfed infants; possibly compatible
Zolpidem	Increased total sleep time and decreased sleep onset latency Time spent in REM sleep decreased with higher doses No effect on stages 3 and 4	> 10%: Drowsiness, dizziness, somnolence 1–10%: Abnormal dreams, anxiety, apathy, amnesia, ataxia, attention disturbance, disinhibition, euphoria, constipation, diarrhea < 1%: Agitation, anorexia, bronchitis, diaphoresis, hepatic function abnormalities, postural hypotension Case reports: Anaphylaxis, angioedema, complex sleep-related behavior (sleep-driving, cooking or eating food, making phone calls) Residual sedation upon awakening reported, especially with CR preparation	CAUTION in liver dysfunction, respiratory impairment; elderly patients more prone to impaired motor and/or cognitive performance Due to higher exposure in females and reports of daytime impairment, maximum dose for females has been lowered Habituation reported Possible increase in epilepsy risk with typical or supratherapeutic doses	Fetal risk: Studies indicate increased risk for pre-term infant, low birth weight, small gestational age infant, and cesarean birth Breastfeeding: Excreted into breast milk; can cause sedation, lethargy, and changes in feeding habits in exposed infants; considered compatible with breastfeeding by American Academy of Pediatrics
Zopiclone	Little effect on slow-wave sleep REM delayed but duration the same; stage 1 shortened; stage 2 increased	Somnolence, dizziness, confusion, anterograde amnesia or memory impairment, agitation, nightmares, bitter taste, dry mouth, bad breath, dyspepsia, palpitations, tremor, rash, chills, sweating Severe drowsiness, confusion, and incoordination are signs of drug intolerance or excessive dosage Rarely hallucinations and behavioral disturbances	CAUTION. May lead to abuse, physical and psychological dependence, and withdrawal symptoms; rebound insomnia reported. Elderly patients more prone to adverse effects Caution in liver dysfunction: T_{max} and half-life increased Not recommended in children	Fetal risk: No increase of congenital malformations when used in 1st trimester. If used in 3rd trimester, monitor newborn for side effects Breastfeeding: Excreted into breast milk in small amounts. Monitor infant for side effects

$^\diamond$ See p. 473 for further information on drug use in pregnancy and effects on breast milk

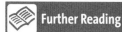 **Further Reading**

References

1 De Crescenzo F, D'Alò GL, Ostinelli EG, et al. Comparative effects of pharmacological interventions for the acute and long-term management of insomnia disorder in adults: A systematic review and network meta-analysis. Lancet. 2022;400(10347):170–184. doi:10.1016/S0140-6736(22)00878-9

2 Elbe D, Black TR, McGrane IR, et al. Clinical handbook of psychotropic drugs for children and adolescents. (5th ed.). Boston, MA: Hogrefe Publishing, 2023.

Additional Suggested Reading

- Brandt J, Leong C. Benzodiazepines and z-drugs: An updated review of major adverse outcomes reported on in epidemiologic research. Drugs R D. 2017;17(4):493–507. doi:10.1007/s40268-017-0207-7
- Buysse DJ. Insomnia. JAMA. 2013;309(7):706–716. doi:10.1001/jama.2013.193
- Harbourt K, Nevo ON, Zhang R, et al. Association of eszopiclone, zaleplon, or zolpidem with complex sleep behaviors resulting in serious injuries, including death. Pharmacoepidemiol Drug Saf. 2020;29(6):684–691. doi:10.1002/pds.5004
- Janto K, Prichard JR, Pusalavidyasagar S. An update on dual orexin receptor antagonists and their potential role in insomnia therapeutics. J Clin Sleep Med. 2018;14(8):1399–1408. doi:10.5664/jcsm.7282
- Kishi T, Nishida M, Koebis M, et al. Evidence-based insomnia treatment strategy using novel orexin antagonists: A review. Neuropsychopharmacol Rep. 2021;41(4):450–458. doi:10.1002/npr2.12205
- Pariente A, de Gage SB, Moore N, et al. The benzodiazepine-dementia disorders link: Current state of knowledge. CNS drugs. 2016;30(1):1–7. doi:10.1007/s40263-015-0305-4
- Pillai V, Roth T, Roehrs T, et al. Effectiveness of benzodiazepine receptor agonists in the treatment of insomnia: An examination of response and remission rates. Sleep. 2017;40(2):zsw044. doi:10.1093/sleep/zsw044
- Qaseem A, Kansagara D, Forciea MA, et al. Management of chronic insomnia disorder in adults: A clinical practice guidelines from the American College of Physicians. Ann Intern Med. 2016;165(2):125–133. doi:10.7326/M15-2175
- Roehrs TA, Randall S, Harris E, et al. Twelve months of nightly zolpidem does not lead to rebound insomnia or withdrawal symptoms: A prospective placebo-controlled study. J Psychopharmacol. 2012;26(8):1088–1095. doi:10.1177/0269881111424455
- Stranks EK, Crowe SF. The acute cognitive effects of zopiclone, zolpidem, zaleplon, and eszopiclone: A systematic review and meta-analysis. J Clin Exp Neuropsychol. 2014;36(7):691–700. doi:10.1080/13803395.2014.928268
- Willems IA, Gorgels WJ, Oude Voshaar RC, et al. Tolerance to benzodiazepines among long-term users in primary care. Fam Pract. 2013;30(4):404–410. doi:10.1093/fampra/cmt010
- Wilson S, Anderson K, Baldwin D, et al. British Association for Psychopharmacology consensus statement on evidence-based treatment of insomnia, parasomnias and circadian rhythm disorders: An update. J Psychopharmacol. 2019;33(8):923–947. doi:10.1177/0269881119855343

MOOD STABILIZERS

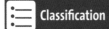 **Classification**

- Mood stabilizers can be classified as follows:

Drug Class	Agent	Page
Lithium	Lithium carbonate, lithium citrate	See p. 271
Anticonvulsants	Carbamazepine, gabapentin, lamotrigine, oxcarbazepine, topiramate, valproate	See p. 283
Antipsychotics		
Second-generation (SGA)	Asenapine, clozapine, lurasidone, olanzapine, paliperidone, quetiapine, risperidone, ziprasidone	See p. 146
Third-generation (TGA)	Aripiprazole, brexpiprazole, cariprazine	See p. 177
Antipsychotic/antidepressant combination	Olanzapine/fluoxetine[B] (Symbyax)	See p. 3

[B] Not marketed in Canada

Lithium

 Product Availability*

Generic Name	Chemical Class	Neuroscience-based Nomenclature* (Pharmacological Target/Mode of Action)	Trade Name[A]	Dosage Forms and Strengths
Lithium carbonate	Lithium salt	Lithium/Enzyme modulator	Lithane[C], Carbolith[C] Lithobid[B], Lithmax[C]	Capsules: 150 mg, 300 mg, 600 mg Tablets: 300 mg[B] Extended-release tablets: 300 mg, 450 mg[B]
Lithium citrate	Lithium salt	Lithium/Enzyme modulator	Lithium citrate oral solution[B]	Oral solution: 8 mEq/5 mL (equivalent to 300 mg lithium carbonate)

* Refer to Health Canada's Drug Product Database or the FDA's Drugs@FDA for the most current availability information.   * Developed by a taskforce consisting of representatives from the American College of Neuropsychopharmacology (ACNP), the Asian College of Neuropsychopharmacology (AsCNP), the European College of Neuropsychopharmacology (ECNP), the International College of Neuropsychopharmacology (CINP), and the International Union of Basic and Clinical Pharmacology (IUPHAR) (see https://nbn2r.com), [A] Generic preparations may be available,   [B] Not marketed in Canada,   [C] Not marketed in the USA

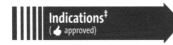 **Indications‡** (👍 approved)

- 🔥 Bipolar I disorder (monotherapy or combination therapy):
  - Management of acute manic or mixed episodes
  - Maintenance therapy to prevent subsequent manic or depressed episodes
    - Lithium more effective than placebo at reducing the number of suicides and deaths from any cause
    - Lithium may reduce intensity of subsequent episodes of mania or depression
    - Lithium has demonstrated to decrease relapse rates (vs. placebo) and prevent relapse
      - In a comparative real-world effectiveness study, lithium use for bipolar patients was associated with the lowest risk of all-cause rehospitalization
      - In a meta-analysis of bipolar treatment follow-up of > 6 months, lithium had significantly lower risk of relapse of any mood episode

‡ Indications listed here do not necessarily apply to all countries. Please refer to a country's regulatory database (e.g., US Food and Drug Administration, Health Canada Drug Product Database) for the most current availability information and indications

Lithium (cont.)

- Maintenance therapy of bipolar II disorder
- Acute depression associated with bipolar I and II disorder
  - Some treatment guidelines place lithium as a first-line treatment option; however, supporting controlled trial evidence is lacking and contradictory, especially for monotherapy. Poorer outcomes when lithium serum levels were less than 0.8 mmol/L[1]
- Unipolar treatment-resistant depression (adjunctive therapy)[2]
  - Lithium use was associated with a reduced risk of suicide and total number of deaths compared to placebo; wide confidence intervals
  - Response to lithium may be greater in patients with melancholic unipolar depression compared to non-melancholic depression
- Chronic aggression/antisocial behavior/impulsivity across a broad range of diagnoses; may be useful in patients with an affective component to symptoms (weak evidence for lithium in adult patients for this indication)
- Pathological gambling – double-blind and open studies suggest that lithium may reduce gambling behavior and affective instability (especially if comorbid bipolar)
- Prophylaxis of chronic cluster headaches
- Neuroprotection – evidence to suggest a neuroprotective effect on the central nervous system

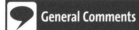

General Comments

- Predictors of positive response to lithium:
  - Index manic episode with euphoria (vs. dysphoria) and flight of ideas (i.e., "classic grandiose mania")
  - Mania–depression–interval sequence
  - Absence of psychotic features
  - Absence of comorbid substance use disorder
  - Shorter pre-lithium illness duration (especially if untreated); few prior episodes
  - Later illness onset
  - Family history of lithium response in first-degree relative
  - No neurological impairment
  - Predominant hypomania
- Severe mania – considered first-line therapy (in combination with an antipsychotic)
- Rapid cycling – as effective in reducing clinical symptoms as in non-rapid cycling persons with no evidence for superiority of any mood stabilizer; higher rates of recurrence in rapid cycling compared to non-rapid cycling, regardless of treatment used. Since lithium-induced hypothyroidism may contribute to some rapid cycling, it is important to regularly assess thyroid function and presence of other agents that may aggravate rapid cycling (such as concurrent antidepressant use, substance use)
- Adjunctive therapies may be required to manage acute symptoms (e.g., benzodiazepines, antidepressants)
- Risk of death from suicide shown to be lower with lithium than with valproate

Pharmacology

- Exact mechanism of action unknown
- Alters many signaling cascades with downstream effects on cell function, gene expression, neuronal plasticity. Collectively, these mechanisms are thought to reduce the responsiveness of neurons to stimuli from muscarinic, cholinergic, and α-adrenergic neurotransmitters. The overall effect of lithium is that it stimulates inhibitory neurotransmission (e.g., γ-aminobutyric acid, GABA) and reduces excitatory neurotransmission (e.g., dopamine and glutamate)
- Postulated actions of lithium:
  - Replaces sodium and alters calcium-mediated intracellular functions
  - Inhibits release of norepinephrine, serotonin, and dopamine
  - Regulates Na+/K+-ATPase pump (mania may be associated with an increase of calcium in the presynaptic compartment, while depression may be associated with a decrease in pump activity)
  - Stabilizes second messenger systems and calcium-dependent intracellular signaling cascades by regulating the levels of: cAMP-dependent phosphodiesterases, inositol monophosphatase, inositol bisphosphate nucleosidases
  - Prevents adrenergic and muscarinic coupling to G proteins by competing with magnesium (hyperfunction of G proteins, as well as changes in

the activity of protein kinase C (PKC) and protein kinase A (PKA) may contribute to an unstable nervous system and, ultimately, mood instability. Lithium attenuates G protein and helps create mental state stability

- Interaction at various sites with downstream signal transduction cascades (e.g., inhibition of glycogen synthase kinase 3 beta ($GSK_3\beta$) and PKC)
- Reduces oxidative stress, increases protective proteins (such as brain-derived neurotrophic factor (BDNF) and B-cell lymphoma 2), and reduces apoptotic processes through inhibition of $GSK_3\beta$ and autophagy
- Its efficacy may be related to its modulation of abnormal calcium activity at the NMDA ionotropic receptor
- Appears to increase neurogenesis and neuroprotective factors and, in patients with bipolar disorder, may preserve or increase cortical gray matter, white matter integrity, and limbic structures
- Lithium and valproic acid influence circadian rhythms in ways that may promote mood stability
- May exert its anti-suicidal effects though multiple mechanisms: reducing relapses, anti-aggression properties, reduced impulsivity, need for regular monitoring

 Dosing

- Lithium has a narrow therapeutic range; effective serum levels are close to toxic concentrations
- Dosing requires guidance of plasma levels (see pharmacokinetics); increase slowly to minimize side effects. Predictive dosing methods show inconsistent or poor results
- Healthy adults:
  - Starting dose: 600–900 mg/day
  - Acute treatment of mania: Dosage should be adjusted to obtain a trough serum level: 0.8–1.2 mmol/L; typically 900–2100 mg/day in three divided doses
  - Acute mania: Patients appear to have increased tolerance to lithium; control of mania may require lithium level of 0.9–1.4 mmol/L until patient settles
  - Maintenance: Dosage should be adjusted to obtain a trough serum level: 0.6–1.0 mmol/L); typically 900 mg/day with a range of 600–1800 mg/day in divided doses
- Relapse prevention: Concentrations below 0.6 mmol/L have been shown in controlled trials to be less effective in preventing relapse. However, lower lithium doses and serum trough target concentrations may be acceptable when using combinations of mood stabilizers or for other indications
- Elderly patients: Starting dose should not exceed 300 mg/day. Usual dose range 300–1200 mg/day. Aim for lower target trough levels for acute mania and for maintenance therapy (e.g., 0.4–0.8 mEq/L). The lithium dose found to achieve a given concentration between the ages of 49 and 95 decreased 3-fold in one study and was related to the decline in estimated glomerular filtration rate. See Geriatric Considerations p. 279
- Renal disease: If CrCl is 30–60 mL/min, start at 150–300 mg/day, CrCl < 30 mL/min avoid use. Patients undergoing dialysis should take their dose AFTER each dialysis treatment
- Once patient is stabilized, once-daily dosing is preferable (if patient can tolerate this), usually given at night for improved compliance. Some trials have shown a decrease in urine volume, lower daily dose required, and less renal toxicity; no trials of once daily dosing showed a reduction in efficacy and once daily dosing was generally well tolerated
- Patients sensitive to side effects that are related to high peak plasma levels, e.g., tremor, urinary frequency, and GI effects (i.e., nausea), may respond to slow-release preparations. Alternatively, continued splitting of the dose may be required to decrease adverse effects related to peak serum levels
- Missed doses or drug interactions may reduce the lithium level and precipitate relapse; however, the majority of drug interactions precipitate toxicity (see Drug Interactions p. 281)

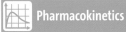 **Pharmacokinetics**

- Lithium is completely absorbed from the GI tract
- Peak plasma level: 1–2 h (slow-release preparation = 4–5 h)
- 12-hour trough levels are used for therapeutic monitoring. Measurement of serum levels should be approximately 12 h after the last dose. It is recommended that two consecutive serum levels be established in the therapeutic range during the acute phase. Thereafter, measurements can be repeated every 3–6 months, or more frequently if clinically indicated
- Half-life: approximately 24 h; half-life increases with duration of therapy (e.g., up to 58 h after 1 year of therapy)
- Lithium is excreted unchanged primarily (95%) by the kidney; therefore, adequate renal function is essential in order to avoid accumulation and intoxication (see Dosing, above); clearance is significantly correlated with total body weight. 80% of filtered lithium is reabsorbed in the proximal convoluted tubules; therefore, clearance approximates 20% of GFR or 20–40 mL/min
- Lithium is secreted in saliva, reaching concentrations 3 times that seen in plasma – saliva composition is altered (see GI Effects below)
- SR forms produce lower C_{max} but similar AUC

Lithium (cont.)

- Factors that reduce lithium clearance and increase lithium serum levels:
  - Reduced renal function
  - Reduced salt intake
  - Dehydration
  - Increased age
  - Cirrhosis
- Factors that increase lithium clearance and reduce lithium serum levels:
  - Pregnancy
  - Obesity
  - Increased salt intake
  - Caffeine
  - Burns

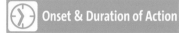 **Onset & Duration of Action**	• Steady state concentrations are reached in 4 days, with the onset of antimanic effect usually occurring in 5–7 days. Full therapeutic effect for mania may require 10–21 days, therefore acute mania symptoms are often treated with an antipsychotic in conjunction with lithium (or monotherapy, and lithium may subsequently be added) • Onset of therapeutic effect for depressive symptoms is around 4–6 weeks, with full effect possibly taking longer

 Adverse Effects

- See table p. 310

CNS Effects

- General weakness (up to 33%), fatigue, dysphoria, and restlessness are usually transient and may coincide with peaks in lithium concentration
- Drowsiness, tiredness
- Driving: Not generally considered sedating when used as a single agent, but reaction time may be impaired
- Dizziness and vertigo [Management: Administer with food, use slow-release preparation to avoid peak lithium levels, or reduce or split dosage]
- Cognition:
  - Lithium-induced cognitive impairment is common, distressing, and often leads to nonadherence. May overlap with symptoms of bipolar disorder (e.g., depressive symptoms) and can be aggravated by concurrent cognitive-dulling medications or by concurrent ECT
  - May be dose related; usually persists
  - A 2009 meta-analysis of cognitive performance found a small but significant impairment in immediate verbal learning, memory, and creativity. Delayed verbal memory, visual memory, attention, executive function, and processing speed were not significantly affected. Psychomotor performance was substantially impaired in patients on longer-term lithium (46.8 +/- 42.7 months)
  - RCT data suggests lithium monotherapy is less likely to contribute to cognitive dysfunction than quetiapine monotherapy
  - [Management: Dose reduction may help, eliminate other CNS-depressing medications where appropriate]
- Neuromuscular: Incoordination, muscle weakness. Note: persistent neurological (cerebellar and basal ganglia) dysfunction may remain after lithium toxicity
  - Cogwheel rigidity and choreoathetosis reported
  - Chronic treatment can affect the peripheral nervous system involving motor and sensory function
- Tremor:
  - Incidence reported to be about 27% (range of 4–65% in individual studies)
  - Can emerge at any time, usually earlier in treatment. Often dose related. Sometimes will spontaneously resolve
  - Considered to be an "action" tremor and subcategorized as a postural tremor that occurs when a specific posture, such as holding arms outstretched or while standing, is voluntarily maintained
  - Generally symmetric, related to dose and blood level, and non-progressive. Usually limited to hands or upper limbs, worsening with fine motor activities (e.g., writing)
  - Is at a higher frequency than with antipsychotics (8–13 Hz vs. 4–7 Hz)

- Coarse or severe tremor (especially if changed) may be a sign of lithium toxicity
- More frequent in combination with an antidepressant or antipsychotic, valproic acid, or carbamazepine, with excessive caffeine use, or alcoholism
- [Management: Reduce dose, eliminate dietary caffeine (caution, this can elevate lithium level); β-blocker (e.g., propranolol or atenolol) may be of benefit]
- Seizures rare, will also occur with severe toxicity
- Headaches; rarely, papilledema/elevated intracranial pressure (pseudotumor cerebri) reported
- Slurred speech, ataxia – evaluate for lithium toxicity
- Serotonin syndrome (see p. 10): lithium can precipitate a potentially life-threatening serotonin syndrome when used in combination with other serotonergic agents (e.g., SSRIs, SNRIs, triptans, tricyclic antidepressants, buspirone, fentanyl, tramadol, tryptophan, St. John's wort) or agents that impair metabolism of serotonin (e.g., MAOIs). Evidence from case reports suggests clinical significance likely low; monitor when serotonergic or interacting medications are started

Cardiovascular Effects

- Bradycardia, arrhythmias, hypotension have been reported
- ECG changes: 20–30% benign T-wave changes (flattening or inversion) and QRS widening at therapeutic doses; use lithium cautiously in patients with pre-existing cardiac disease; arrhythmias and sinus node dysfunction occur less frequently (sinus node dysfunction reported with lithium-carbamazepine combination, with high plasma levels of lithium, in the elderly, and in patients taking other drugs that may affect conduction)
- May unmask Brugada syndrome and should not be used in patients with this syndrome (a cardiac conduction disorder that has led to sudden cardiac death). [Assess patient who has syncopal episode]

Endocrine & Metabolic Effects

- Hypothyroidism: occurs in up to 34% of patients; risk increased 6-fold compared to non-lithium users. Often within the first year; usually reversible if lithium discontinued; does not appear to be dose-related. Risk factors include: female, older age, family history of hypothyroidism, presence of antithyroid antibodies, possibly rapid cyclers – may be more common in regions of high dietary iodine. Subclinical hypothyroidism (high TSH and normal free T_4) found in 25% of patients on lithium. Rare cases of hyperthyroidism reported [Management: Monitor TSH levels every 6–12 months, may require levothyroxine therapy; does not necessitate discontinuation]
- Goiter (not necessarily associated with hypothyroidism) – may be more common in regions of iodine deficiency
- Hyperparathyroidism with hypercalcemia: reported in 10–40% of patients on maintenance therapy, may predispose to decreased bone density or to cardiac conduction disturbances; case reports of parathyroid adenoma and hyperplasia; other symptoms include weakness, fatigue, abdominal pain, psychological disturbance [Management: Monitor calcium and PTH annually]. Clinical manifestations of hypercalcaemia may necessitate lithium discontinuation; weigh risks and benefits
- Hypermagnesemia also associated with lithium therapy, occurring in up to 30% of cases in one series
- Reports of irregular or prolonged menstrual cycles in up to 15% of females
- Weight gain: upwards of 70% incidence in several studies (20% of patients gained excessive weight of more than 10 kg; mean gain is around 4–7 kg). Often very distressing to patients; usually occurs in first 1–2 years). May be related to increased appetite, fluid retention, altered carbohydrate and fat metabolism, or hypothyroidism, or concurrent weight-gaining medications. Some studies have observed correlation with lithium levels; others not dose related [Management: Reduce caloric intake; lifestyle modifications; reduce polypharmacy where appropriate]
- Abnormal sugar and insulin metabolism: appear to relate less closely to lithium concentrations than to being overweight. In controlled studies, lithium did not directly influence glucose tolerance

GI Effects

- Usually coincide with peaks in lithium concentration and are probably due to rapid absorption of the lithium ion; most disappear after a few weeks; if they occur late in therapy, evaluate for lithium toxicity
- Nausea: up to 50% incidence, abdominal pain [Management: Administer with food, use slow-release preparation or lithium citrate liquid, temporary divided dosing]
- Vomiting: higher incidence with increased plasma level [Management: Use multiple daily dosing, change to a slow-release preparation or lower dose]
- Diarrhea, loose stools: up to 20% incidence; more common in first 6 months. Slow-release preparation may worsen this side effect in some patients [Management: If on a slow-release product, change to a regular lithium preparation; fewer problems noted with lithium citrate preparations; if diarrhea persists and cannot decrease the lithium dose, use loperamide prn]
- Metallic taste: composition of saliva altered (ions and proteins)
- Excessive thirst (up to 36% incidence), dry mouth, mucosal ulceration (rare); hypersalivation occasionally reported

Lithium (cont.)

Renal Effects	

- Polydipsia and polyuria are common (up to 70%) and usually transient [Management: Once daily dosing, sugarless gum or oral moisturizers]
- Lithium-induced nephrogenic diabetes insipidus (NDI):
  - Rates of 12–40% of patients taking long-term lithium (15 years)
  - Development of overt NDI is characterized by polydipsia, the production of excessive amounts of urine (more than 3000 mL/24 h) and a dilute urine osmolality (less than 300 mOsm/kg). The reduced ability to concentrate urine may be seen as early as 2–4 months after starting lithium but typically becomes more evident during prolonged exposure. This treatment-emergent effect is usually reversible on cessation of lithium but may become irreversible with prolonged therapy
  - Polyuria (19%) and impaired renal concentrating ability (59%), without full development of NDI, is more commonly reported and may be dose related. One study found polyuria strongly associated with concomitant serotonergic antidepressants
- NDI management strategies:
  - Usually reversible if lithium stopped (after medium-term treatment, i.e., up to 6 years, but often irreversible after 15 years); several cases of persistent diabetes insipidus reported up to 57 months after lithium stopped
  - Sustained-release preparations or single day dosing may cause less impairment of urine concentrating function
  - If NDI does not resolve with lithium discontinuation or if lithium must be continued, the following pharmacological strategies may be considered:
    - Amiloride (10–20 mg/day), a potassium-sparing diuretic that targets distal tubule epithelial sodium channels is the most established therapy for lithium-induced NDI
    - Thiazide diuretics (i.e., hydrochlorothiazide) can be added to amiloride if monotherapy is ineffective
    - Nonsteroid anti-inflammatory drugs, especially indomethacin, as adjunctive treatment can also be considered
    - DDAVP tablets 0.2 mg may be useful for persistent NDI, especially if non-responsive to lithium discontinuation, amiloride, thiazide diuretics, or NSAIDs
    - NOTE: if lithium is continued, monitor lithium levels closely as amiloride, thiazide diuretics, and NSAIDs can all contribute to lithium toxicity
- Lithium-induced nephropathy:
  - Consistent reports that polyuria may be an indication of underlying, irreversible, structural damage to kidney
  - Histological changes include: (a) interstitial fibrosis, tubular atrophy, and glomerulosclerosis (seen in 26% of patients after treatment beyond 2 years, primarily those with impaired urine concentrating ability); (b) distal tubular dilatation and macrocyst formation
  - Rare cases of nephrotic syndrome with proteinuria, glycosuria and oliguria, edema, and hypoalbuminemia
  - Polyuria and corresponding structural damage correlates weakly with reduced kidney function, but may be a risk factor for developing CKD
- Chronic kidney disease (CKD):
  - Some patients taking lithium for many years develop progressively declining kidney function. Studies report 20–30% have gradual decline in GFR over many years. Appears to be a slowly progressive disease. A recent meta-analysis concluded the risk of renal impairment is not clinically significant in most patients
  - Rate of eGFR decline has been suggested to average around 0.92%/year of lithium treatment
  - Renal failure may still progress after discontinuation of lithium and may depend on severity of renal disease. A retrospective cohort study found a hazard ratio of 2.5 for renal failure in bipolar patients who had ever used lithium. Absolute risk was age dependent, with patients over 50 at higher risk
  - Progression to end-stage renal disease (ESRD) is rare with high variability in incidence across studies. One meta-analysis reported absolute risk increase of 0.5%. Average latency period from lithium initiation to presence of ESRD is at least 20 years, and more than 80% of patients taking lithium and having ESRD have been taking lithium for more than 20 years
- Risk factors for lithium-induced CKD:
  - Using multivariate regression, risk for declining eGFR ranked as follows: longer lithium treatment, higher serum lithium concentration, older age, and medical comorbidity
  - Concomitant CKD risks (hypertension, diabetes, age, coronary artery disease)
  - Prior episodes of lithium toxicity
  - Concurrent medications that are nephrotoxic or reduce lithium excretion rate (e.g., NSAIDs, ACE inhibitors, ARBs, and thiazide diuretics)
  - Lower initial GFR, reduced nephron mass, background tubulointerstitial damage

- NDI – volume contraction leading to elevated lithium concentrations, may be surrogate marker for morphological changes occurring within kidney tubules
- Conditions that promote sodium retention (e.g., cirrhosis, congestive heart failure, lithium toxicity) [Management: Monitor renal function every 6–12 months, target lower end of therapeutic range; once daily dosing may help prevent. If significant rise in SCr (one study suggests 140 µmol/L), consult nephrologist and consider discontinuation of lithium by SLOW TAPER over 4–8 weeks]

Dermatological Effects	• Lithium may be associated with a variety of potentially distressing skin conditions including: dry skin, acne, eczema, hidradenitis suppurativa, mucosal lesions, and folliculitis. Most cases can be managed symptomatically and rarely require discontinuation of lithium • Skin rash, pruritus, exacerbation or new onset of psoriasis. Incidence of exacerbation has ranged widely (3.4–45%). A 2012 meta-analysis suggested there was no significant difference in prevalence of skin disorders in patients on lithium[4] • Dryness and thinning of hair (possibly related to hypothyroidism); alopecia reported in 12–19% of chronic lithium users • Case reports of nail pigmentation and nail dystrophy • May be dose related
Other Adverse Effects	• Blurred vision: may be related to peak plasma levels; reduction in retinal light sensitivity, nystagmus (can also be a sign of toxicity) • Changes in sexual function: up to 10% risk; includes decreased libido, erectile dysfunction, priapism, and decreased sperm motility; soreness and ulceration of genitalia (rare) • Edema, swelling of extremities: evaluate for sodium retention [use diuretics with caution – see Drug Interactions p. 282 – spironolactone may be preferred] • Blood dyscrasias: anemia, leukocytosis 1.5 times normal (common), leukopenia, albuminuria; rarely aplastic anemia, agranulocytosis, thrombocytopenia, occasional eosinophilia, and thrombocytosis

D/C Discontinuation Syndrome	• Anxiety, instability, and emotional lability have been reported following abrupt withdrawal. Withdrawal symptoms uncommon • Rapid discontinuation (over 1–14 days) led to a more rapid (5-fold) recurrence risk of mania or bipolar depression than did a more gradual discontinuation over 2–4 weeks • A few cases of hyperthyroidism developing after cessation or reduction of lithium therapy
⚠ Precautions	• Good kidney function, consistent salt and fluid intake are essential • Excessive loss of sodium (due to vomiting, diarrhea, heavy sweating, use of diuretics, etc.) causes increased lithium retention, possibly leading to toxicity; lower doses of lithium are necessary if patient is on a salt-restricted diet • Use cautiously and in reduced dosage in the elderly as the ability to excrete lithium decreases with age (see Geriatric Considerations p. 279) • **ECT** – concurrent ECT may increase the risk of developing cerebral toxicity from lithium – early case reports included cognitive disturbance, prolonged apnea, and prolonged seizures. More recent case reports and series of effective combined use reported. Average time to post-ECT recovery was directly correlated with serum lithium level. A recent regression analysis of a large US patient sample (64,728 patients) with ECT + lithium resulted in having 11.7-fold higher odds of delirium compared to ECT alone. In the ECT + lithium group, delirium prevalence was 0% for bipolar mania, 3.4% for bipolar depression, and 7.8% for unipolar depression.[6] Low to moderate serum lithium levels (< 0.7 mmol/L) may not be associated with longer reorientation time in patients undergoing right unilateral ultrabrief pulse and bilateral brief pulse ECT.[7] See also ECT chapter pp. 104–110 • Do not rapidly increase lithium and antipsychotic dosage at the same time, due to risk of neurotoxicity • Baseline thyroid dysfunction: patient may require more frequent monitoring and possible dose adjustments of thyroid medications. Treatment emergent hypothyroidism does not necessitate discontinuation if benefits of lithium have been established[8] • Lithium-induced hypothyroidism: Re-assess need for continued thyroid supplementation if it was started during lithium therapy as thyroid function may revert to normal with continued lithium; continued unnecessary thyroid treatment may increase risk for developing hyperthyroidism and increased mood cycling • Use extreme caution in people with traumatic brain injury due to risk of seizures and further cognitive impairment • High lethality risk in overdose
STOP Contraindications	• Significant renal disease – especially if low sodium diet required; absolute contraindication in severe insufficiency • Severe cardiovascular disease; lithium may unmask Brugada syndrome and should not be used in patients with this syndrome • Severe debilitation, dehydration, or sodium depletion

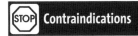

Lithium (cont.)

 Toxicity

- Three types of toxicity:
  - Acute overdose (lithium-naïve):
    - 10–20% of cases
    - Mainly CNS (confusion, tremor, dysarthria, ataxia, nystagmus) with fasciculations, fibrillations, myoclonia, and polyneuropathy seen occasionally; GI symptoms – frequent nausea, vomiting, and diarrhea; renal symptoms of polyuria, polydipsia or nephrogenic diabetes insipidus and cardiovascular signs of arrhythmia, Brugada syndrome, low blood pressure, and rarely shock may occur
    - Usually carries less risk and patients usually show only mild symptoms independent of lithium concentration, possibly due to delay between ingestion and clinical signs
  - Acute on chronic overdose (in the context of chronic lithium use): Largest group, more likely to develop clinical toxicity as brain concentration has already reached equilibrium with their plasma concentration. Even moderately high serum concentrations may be associated with severe symptoms. Elimination half-life of lithium may be prolonged
  - Chronic ingestion: Can occur at any time during lithium therapy. Contributing factors include change in daily dose, chronic excessive dosing, changes in sodium or water status, renal disease, drug interactions, infection, and surgery. This type of toxicity demonstrates closest correlation between clinical signs, lithium concentration, and prognosis
- Sustained-release preparations: Delayed onset of toxicity, may result in severe or prolonged symptoms. Repeated determinations of serum lithium levels should be performed due to sustained absorption
- Persistent sequelae, usually renal or CNS lesions, can result from episodes of lithium toxicity

Mild Toxicity

- At lithium levels of 1.5–2 mmol/L; occasionally occurs with levels in the normal range
- Develops gradually over several days
- Adverse effects such as diarrhea, vomiting, ataxia, coarse tremor, muscle weakness, fasciculation, confusion, drowsiness, and slurred speech may occur

Management
- Stop lithium or hold dose until serum level normalizes and symptoms of toxicity resolve

Moderate/Severe Toxicity

- At lithium levels in excess of 2 mmol/L
- Acute lithium toxicity can present as acute delirium with disorientation, fluctuating levels of consciousness, hallucinations, and extrapyramidal symptoms; may manifest as a catatonic stupor
- Severe poisoning may result in coma with hyperreflexia, muscle tremor, hyperextension of the limbs, pulse irregularities, hypertension or hypotension, ECG changes (T-wave depression or inversion), peripheral circulatory failure, neuroleptic malignant syndrome, and epileptic seizures; acute tubular necrosis (renal failure) can occur
- In some patients, lithium toxicity causes persistent neurological (cerebellar and basal ganglia) dysfunction
- At toxic levels, lithium may inhibit its own excretion, as can renal dysfunction, sodium depletion as well as certain drugs (e.g., NSAIDs)
- Note: The discrepancy between high serum levels and advanced symptoms of toxicity reflects delayed distribution of drug into susceptible tissues (see types of toxicity above); accumulation in the CNS explains persistent symptoms despite falling serum levels
- Deaths have been reported; when serum lithium level exceeds 4 mmol/L the prognosis is poor

Management
- Symptomatic: Reduce absorption, restore fluid and electrolyte balance, regulation of kidney function
- Severe cases: remove drug from body (vomiting, gastric lavage, hemodialysis); urea, mannitol, and aminophylline increase lithium excretion
- Blood lithium concentration may be reduced by forced alkaline diuresis, or by prolonged peritoneal dialysis which clears 15 mL/min, or hemodialysis which clears 50 mL/min and should be considered in severe cases. Severity of symptoms in additions to serum lithium concentrations should be taken into account when determining whether to use hemodialysis. May require repeating due to rebound increase in serum levels 6–12 h later
- Convulsions may be controlled by IV benzodiazepines

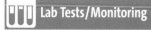 **Lab Tests/Monitoring**

- At beginning of treatment: Personal and family medical history, including previous heart disease, renal disease, thyroid disease, concurrent medications. Baseline:

1. Fasting blood glucose
2. CBC and differential
3. TSH
4. BUN, serum creatinine, electrolytes
5. Calcium
6. Urinalysis
7. ECG for patients over 40 or with a history of cardiac problems
8. Pregnancy test, if appropriate; ensure adequate contraception in place for women of child-bearing age

- Monitoring of renal function: Baseline testing (as outlined above), at 3 months, then minimally every 6–12 months thereafter (depending on stability and concurrent medications, e.g., NSAIDs, ACE inhibitors, diuretics). Patients require further investigation if creatinine levels consistently trend upwards. Urinalysis to evaluate for hematuria and proteinuria is required. Overt proteinuria should be quantified with a urine protein to creatinine ratio[5]
- On an outpatient basis, repeat tests: (1) and (2) if clinically indicated; (3) and (4) at 3 months, then every 6–12 months in stable patients; (5) at 6 months and annually, and consider parathormone to identify or rule out hyperparathyroidism; (6) and (7) as clinically indicated. Serum calcium is monitored annually
- Plasma level monitoring: Measure first plasma level 5 days after starting therapy (sooner if toxicity is suspected). Measure once weekly until levels stable at therapeutic concentration. Thereafter q 3–6 months and at clinical discretion, or whenever an interacting drug is prescribed, or if the lithium dose changes, or at emergence of adverse effects or toxicity symptoms. Test more frequently in the elderly or those with unstable renal function or physical illness
- Blood levels should be measured at 12 h after last dose. Note that morning levels will be higher if moving from bid or tid dosing to once daily at bedtime if serum levels are taken the following morning. In one study, serum levels were 17% higher when moving from bid dosing to hours when serum levels were taken 12 h later
- Symptoms of moderate toxicity are not always evident, so regular lithium levels are important for detection. In one study, 6.8% of patients had levels greater than 1.5 mmol/L, with only 28% showing toxic symptoms

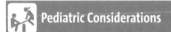 **Pediatric Considerations**

- For detailed information on the use of lithium in this population, please see the *Clinical Handbook of Psychotropic Drugs for Children and Adolescents*[9]
- Lithium has been used successfully in children with chronic aggressive conduct disorders, in bipolar disorder, in periodic mood and behavior disorders, and in pervasive developmental disorder (autism)
- Half-life shorter and clearance faster than in adults

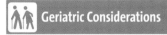 **Geriatric Considerations**

- Good kidney function, adequate salt and fluid intake are essential; ability to excrete lithium decreases with age, resulting in a longer elimination half-life
- Start therapy at lower doses (i.e., 300 mg once or twice daily) and monitor serum level frequently
- Dose required to achieve same serum levels estimated to decrease up to 3-fold between the ages of 40 and 95 due to decline in renal function
- Lower end of therapeutic range (i.e., 0.5–0.8 mmol/L) recommended for the elderly
- The elderly have lower volume of distribution secondary to increased body fat and decreased total body water
- Incidence of adverse effects may be greater and occur at lower plasma levels, including tremor, GI disturbances, polyuria, ataxia, myoclonus, and EPS
- Elderly patients may be more at risk for hypercalcemia and hyperparathyroidism
- Elderly patients are at increased risk for hyponatremia after an acute illness or if fluid intake is restricted
- Elderly patients are at higher risk for neurotoxicity and cognitive impairment, even at therapeutic plasma levels
- Slow-release preparation may decrease side effects that occur as a result of peak plasma levels; prolonged elimination half-life

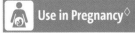 **Use in Pregnancy**◇

- If possible, lithium should be avoided during pregnancy, especially during the period of organogenesis (first trimester).[10] Risk of congenital anomalies varies in literature:

◇ See p. 473 for further information on drug use in pregnancy and effects on breast milk

Lithium (cont.)

- A 2017 retrospective cohort (663 cases, 1,322,955 controls) reported adjusted risk ratio for cardiac malformations in newborns with first trimester exposure to lithium of 1.65 compared to non-exposed. Risk ratios were greater with higher daily doses of lithium[11]
- Overall risk of fetal malformations is 4–12%; cardiovascular malformations risk ratio is 1.2–7.7 (level A evidence) (e.g., tricuspid valve malformations; 0.05–0.1% risk of Ebstein's anomaly). Fetal echocardiography may be considered if exposure in first trimester (level C evidence) and high-resolution ultrasound at 16–18 weeks gestation
- A 1994 review reported risk ratios of 1.5–3.0 for all congenital anomalies and 1.2–7.7 for cardiac malformations based on two cohort studies
- A statistically significant association noted between higher doses of lithium in the first trimester and premature deliveries; a higher rate of macrosomia reported in these premature infants
- One prospective cohort study found no difference between groups and concluded that lithium is not an important teratogen and could be continued due to risks of discontinuing therapy, provided fetal ultrasounds and echocardiograms are performed. Other studies have determined the risk of cardiac malformations may be lower than once thought. Similarly, a recent meta-analysis evaluated 62 studies assessing teratogenicity, 48 of which were case reports, and found no significant association between lithium and congenital abnormalities, although estimates were unstable due to low event rate and low cases of lithium exposure
- Other non-teratogenic adverse effects have been reported in the fetus or newborn and were usually self-limiting (cardiovascular, respiratory, hematologic abnormalities, etc.)
- In patients with bipolar disorder, the peripartum period is associated with a high risk of relapse. Relapse during this period may affect fetal and child development
- If lithium is continued, use at the lowest possible divided daily dose to avoid peak concentrations, and supplement with folic acid 5 mg daily
- Serum levels should be monitored more frequently (e.g., every 4 weeks, then weekly from 36th week gestation)
- Lithium clearance increases by 30–50% in third trimester secondary to an increase in plasma volume and greater glomerular filtration rate; rate returns to pre-pregnancy levels after delivery
- If patient/clinician deems risks to outweigh benefits, can consider withholding lithium during first trimester and restarting in second trimester
- Discontinuation of lithium therapy during pregnancy is associated with an increase in bipolar recurrences. Gradual cessation over 2–4 weeks is advised whenever the risk is considered in favour of discontinuing
- Dose should be decreased, or drug discontinued, 2–3 days prior to delivery
- Lithium should be discontinued during labor to avoid lithium toxicity in the infant
- Use of lithium near term may produce severe toxicity in the newborn, which is usually reversible, including nontoxic goiter, atrial flutter, T-wave inversion, nephrogenic diabetes insipidus, floppy baby syndrome, cyanosis, and seizures
- Postpartum period is associated with a definite increase in the recurrence of bipolar disorder by a factor of 3–8 times. Restart lithium immediately after birth
- Observe infant for lithium toxicity for first 10 days of life

Breast Milk

- In general, lithium is not recommended during breastfeeding due to toxicity risk to the baby
- Present in breast milk at a concentration of 30–80% of mother's serum (infant's serum concentration is approximately 10–50% of the mother's serum concentration). Reported symptoms in infant include lethargy, hypothermia, hypotonia, involuntary movements, dehydration, hypothyroidism, cyanosis, heart murmur, and T-wave changes
- Infants have decreased renal clearance (in general, so may retain lithium in their bodies); the American Academy of Pediatrics recommends that lithium should be given to nursing mothers only if benefits outweigh risks, and with caution. Due to high risk of relapsing mood episodes postpartum, consider using milk formula
- If breastfeeding is undertaken, the mother should be educated about signs and symptoms of lithium toxicity and risk of infant dehydration; monitor infant lithium levels and consider periodic thyroid evaluation

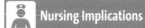 **Nursing Implications**

- Accurate observation and assessment of patient's behavior before and after lithium therapy is initiated is important
- Be alert for, observe, and report any signs of side effects or symptoms of toxicity; if signs or suspicions of lithium toxicity occur (see p. 278), withhold the next dose and call doctor immediately
- Lithium use requires regular blood monitoring for lithium levels, renal function, and electrolytes

- Advise patient to maintain consistent salt and water intake; adjust fluid and salt ingestion to compensate if excessive loss occurs through vomiting or diarrhea
- Expect nausea, thirst, frequent urination, and generalized discomfort during the first few days to weeks; therapeutic effects occur gradually and may take up to 3 weeks
- Lithium may be given with meals to avoid GI disturbances
- Caffeine intake should not be significantly altered while taking lithium
- Withhold morning dose of lithium until after the blood draw on mornings when blood is drawn for a lithium level
- Withhold lithium dose prior to ECT
- Avoid lithium with angiotensin-acting drugs, diuretics, and NSAIDs
- Patient and family should be educated regarding the drug's effects and toxicities and prevention of same. Involve families in treatment plan as they may be the first to notice early signs of toxicity
- Slow-release preparations should not be broken or crushed. The therapeutic benefit of intact slow-release preparations is reduction of side effects such as tremor and gastrointestinal symptoms that occur as a result of high peak plasma levels (i.e., 1–2 h post dose)
- Because lithium may cause drowsiness, caution patient to avoid activities requiring alertness until response to drug has been determined

 Patient Instructions

- For detailed patient instructions on lithium, see the Patient Information Sheet (details on p. 474)

 Drug Interactions

- Clinically significant interactions are listed below
- For more interaction information on any given combination, also see the corresponding chapter for the second agent

Class of Drug	Example	Interaction Effects
Alcohol		Increased tremor/shakiness with chronic alcohol use
Angiotensin-converting enzyme (ACE) inhibitor	Benazepril, captopril, cilazapril, enalapril, fosinopril, lisinopril, perindopril, quinapril, ramipril, trandolapril	Increased lithium toxicity – although mechanism not clearly established, it may involve angiotensin II and decreased aldosterone levels, resulting in sodium depletion; average increase in lithium level of 36% reported, with a significant delay in the manifestation of toxicity (3–5 weeks after introduction of ACE inhibitor); avoid combination, if possible
Angiotensin II receptor blocker (ARB)	Candesartan, eprosartan, irbesartan, losartan, olmesartan, telmisartan, valsartan	Reports of lithium toxicity (timing ranged from 11 days to 5 weeks after starting an ARB), possibly due to reduced renal elimination of lithium; avoid combination, if possible
Antibiotic	Doxycycline, metronidazole, moxifloxacin sulfamethoxazole-trimethoprim, tetracycline	Case reports of increased lithium effect and toxicity due to decreased renal clearance of lithium. Monitor lithium level, electrolytes, and creatinine if combination used
Anticonvulsant	Carbamazepine, fosphenytoin, phenytoin	Increased neurotoxicity of both drugs at therapeutic doses
	Topiramate	May increase the serum concentration of lithium
	Valproate	Valproate may aggravate action tremor
Antidepressant		
SSRI	Citalopram, escitalopram, fluoxetine, fluvoxamine, paroxetine, sertraline	Elevated lithium serum level with possible neurotoxicity; serotonin syndrome (see p. 10) reported
SNRI	Desvenlafaxine, duloxetine, levomilnacipran, venlafaxine	Elevated lithium serum level with possible neurotoxicity; serotonin syndrome (see p. 10) reported
		Not usually clinically significant
Cyclic, RIMA	Moclobemide, tricyclic antidepressants	May increase lithium tremor, neurotoxicity
Irreversible MAOI	Phenelzine, tranylcypromine	Avoid due to risk of malignant hyperthermia
Antihypertensive	Acetazolamide	Increased renal excretion of lithium, decreasing its effect
	Methyldopa	Increased lithium effects and toxicity due to decreased renal clearance of lithium
Antipsychotic	General	See Antipsychotics chapter for further information. Combinations used in practice
	Chlorpromazine	Lithium may decrease the serum concentration of chlorpromazine

Lithium (cont.)

Class of Drug	Example	Interaction Effects
	Clozapine	Possible increased risk of agranulocytosis with clozapine; may mask signs due to lithium increasing WBC. Case reports of seizures and diabetic ketoacidosis reported with combination
	Haloperidol, perphenazine, phenothiazines	Increased neurotoxicity possible at therapeutic doses; may increase EPS; cases of NMS reported
	Risperidone	Case report of severe neurotoxicity
Antiviral agent	Zidovudine	Reversal of zidovudine-induced neutropenia
β-blocker	Bisoprolol, carvedilol, metoprolol, oxprenolol, propranolol	Beneficial effect in treatment of lithium tremor; propranolol lowers glomerular filtration rate and has been associated with a 19% reduction in lithium clearance
Benzodiazepine	Clonazepam	Increased incidence of sexual dysfunction (up to 49%) reported with the combination
Caffeine		Increased renal excretion of lithium, resulting in decreased plasma level May increase lithium tremor
Calcium channel blocker	Diltiazem, verapamil (nondihydropyridines)	Increased neurotoxicity of both drugs; increased bradycardia and cardiotoxicity with verapamil due to combined calcium blockade. Does not appear to involve dihydropyridine class (e.g., nifedipine, felodipine)
Desmopressin (DDAVP)		Lithium may diminish the therapeutic effectiveness of desmopressin. Desmopressin may increase the serum concentration of lithium
Diuretic	Acetazolamide	May decrease serum concentration of lithium
	Amiloride	May be used to treat polyuria
	Eplerenone	May increase serum concentration of lithium
	Furosemide	Isolated reports of lithium toxicity with enhanced risk in older populations and those with comorbid medical conditions or sodium-restricted diets
	Mannitol	Increased renal excretion of lithium, decreasing its effect
	Spironolactone, triamterene	Monitor for increased effect of lithium
	Thiazides	Increased lithium effects and toxicity due to decreased renal clearance of lithium; combination should be avoided in patients already stabilized on lithium, but if thiazide diuretics must be added, a 25–50% decrease in lithium dose and obtaining plasma concentrations once a new steady-state concentration has been achieved (e.g., approximately 1 week after initiation of thiazide) is recommended
Herbal diuretic	Agrimony, dandelion, horsetail, juniper, licorice, uva ursi	Elevated lithium level possible due to decreased renal clearance
	Cola nut, guarana, maté	Increased excretion and decreased lithium level possible due to high content of caffeine in herbal preparations
Hormone	Calcitonin	May decrease lithium concentration
Immunostimulator	Sargramostim	May increase the myeloproliferative adverse effects of lithium
Iodide salt	Calcium, potassium iodate, potassium iodide	May act synergistically to produce hypothyroidism. AVOID
Lactulose		Case series of 3 acutely manic patients developing lithium toxicity when lactulose added for hyperammonemia or constipation, possibly due to volume depletion
L-tryptophan		Increased plasma level and efficacy and/or toxicity of lithium
Methylene blue		May enhance the serotonergic effect of lithium; may result in serotonin syndrome
Muscle relaxant	Baclofen	May cause hyperkinetic movements
	Metaxalone	May enhance the serotonergic effect of lithium; may result in serotonin syndrome

Class of Drug	Example	Interaction Effects
NSAID	Celecoxib, diclofenac, ibuprofen, indomethacin, ketorolac, mefenamic acid, naproxen, sulindac (no interaction with ASA)	Increased lithium level and possible toxicity due to decreased renal clearance of lithium (up to 133% increase reported with celecoxib, up to 300% with mefenamic acid); serum creatinine increased in several reports. Use caution and monitor lithium level every 4–5 days until stable
Neuromuscular blocker	Pancuronium, succinylcholine	Potentiation of muscle relaxation
Opioid	Fentanyl, meperidine, methadone	May enhance serotonergic effect of lithium; may result in serotonin syndrome
	Tramadol	Lithium may enhance the adverse/toxic effect of tramadol; the risk of seizures may be increased. Tramadol may enhance the serotonergic effect of lithium; may result in serotonin syndrome
Peripheral nerve blocker	Lidocaine with epinephrine	Cases of extremely prolonged anesthesia
Psychostimulant	Amphetamine, methylphenidate	May enhance the adverse/toxic effect of lithium. Specifically, risk of serotonin syndrome or serotonin toxicity may be increased. Lithium may diminish the stimulatory effect of amphetamines
Psyllium	Metamucil, Prodiem	Decreased lithium level if drugs taken at the same time. Increased water drawn into the colon by the bulk laxatives would increase the amount of ionized lithium, which would remain unabsorbed
Retinoid	Isotretinoin	One case report suggested adding isotretinoin to lithium carbonate caused mild lithium toxicity. Isotretinoin may be prescribed for lithium-induced acne, but there is strong evidence that demonstrates an association of isotretinoin to depression, probable clinical exacerbation of bipolar mood disorder, and possible links to psychosis
Sodium salt		Increased intake results in decreased lithium plasma level; decreased intake causes increased lithium plasma level
Theophylline	Aminophylline, oxtriphylline, theophylline	Enhanced renal lithium clearance and reduced plasma level (by approx. 20%) May increase lithium tremor
Urinary alkalizer	Potassium citrate, sodium bicarbonate	Enhanced renal lithium clearance and reduced plasma level

Anticonvulsants

℞ Product Availability*

Generic Name	Drug Class	Neuroscience-based Nomenclature* (Pharmacological Target/Mode of Action)	Trade Name[A]	Dosage Forms and Strengths
Carbamazepine	Second-generation anticonvulsant	Glutamate/Channel blocker	Epitol[B], Tegretol	Tablets: 100 mg[B], 200 mg (scored[B]), 300 mg[B], 400 mg[B] Chewable tablets: 100 mg, 200 mg
			Teril[B], Tegretol (liquid)	Oral suspension: 100 mg/5 mL
			Tegretol CR	Controlled-release tablets[C]: 200 mg, 400 mg
			Carbatrol[B], Equetro[B]	Extended-release capsules: 100 mg, 200 mg, 300 mg
			Tegretol XR[B]	Extended-release tablets: 100 mg, 200 mg, 400 mg

Anticonvulsants (cont.)

Generic Name	Drug Class	Neuroscience-based Nomenclature* (Pharmacological Target/Mode of Action)	Trade Name(A)	Dosage Forms and Strengths
Divalproex sodium(E)	Second-generation anticonvulsant	Glutamate/Unclear	Depakote(B), Epival(C)	Delayed-release tablets: 125 mg, 250 mg, 500 mg
			Depakote(B)	Delayed-release pellets: 125 mg(B)
			Depakote ER(B)	Extended-release tablets: 250 mg(B), 500 mg(B)
			Epival ECT(C)	Enteric-coated tablets: 125 mg, 250 mg, 500 mg
Gabapentin(D)	Third-generation anticonvulsant	Glutamate/Channel blocker	Neurontin	Capsules: 100 mg, 300 mg, 400 mg, 800 mg(B) Tablets: 600 mg, 800 mg Oral solution(B): 250 mg/5 mL
			Gralise(B)	Tablets: 300 mg, 600 mg
Gabapentin enacarbil(D)	Third-generation anticonvulsant	Glutamate/Channel blocker	Horizant(B)	Extended-release tablets: 300 mg, 600 mg
Lamotrigine	Third-generation anticonvulsant	Glutamate/Channel blocker	Lamictal	Tablets: 25 mg, 100 mg, 150 mg, 200 mg(B)
			Lamictal CD(B)	Chewable dispersible tablets: 2 mg, 5 mg, 25 mg(B)
			Lamictal ODT(B)	Oral disintegrating tablets: 25 mg, 50 mg, 100 mg, 200 mg
			Lamictal XR(B)	Extended-release tablets: 25 mg, 50 mg, 100 mg, 200 mg, 250 mg, 300 mg
Oxcarbazepine	Third-generation anticonvulsant	Glutamate/Channel blocker	Trileptal	Tablets: 150 mg(B), 300 mg, 600 mg Oral suspension: 300 mg/5 mL
			Oxtellar XR(B)	Extended-release tablets: 150 mg, 300 mg, 600 mg
Topiramate(D)	Third-generation anticonvulsant	GABA, Glutamate/Unclear	Topamax	Tablets: 25 mg, 50 mg(B), 100 mg, 200 mg
			Topamax Sprinkle	Sprinkle capsules: 15 mg, 25 mg
			Trokendi XR(B)	Extended-release capsules(B): 25 mg, 50 mg, 100 mg, 200 mg
			Qudexy XR(B)	Delayed-release capsules(B): 25 mg, 50 mg, 100 mg, 150 mg, 200 mg
Valproate sodium(E)	Second-generation anticonvulsant	Glutamate/Unclear	Depacon(B)	Injection: 100 mg/mL(B)
Valproic acid(E)	Second-generation anticonvulsant	Glutamate/Unclear	Depakene	Capsules: 250 mg Enteric-coated capsules: 500 mg(C) Oral syrup: 250 mg/5 mL

* Refer to Health Canada's Drug Product Database or the FDA's Drugs@FDA for the most current availability information.   * Developed by a taskforce consisting of representatives from the American College of Neuropsychopharmacology (ACNP), the Asian College of Neuropsychopharmacology (AsCNP), the European College of Neuropsychopharmacology (ECNP), the International College of Neuropsychopharmacology (CINP), and the International Union of Basic and Clinical Pharmacology (IUPHAR) (see https://nbn2r.com), (A) Generic preparations may be available,   (B) Not marketed in Canada,   (C) Not marketed in the USA,   (D) There is no reliable evidence favoring the use of gabapentin or topiramate either in acute mood episodes or to prevent relapse. They have been included here as they are anticonvulsants with some psychotherapeutic effect. Very limited evidence (one open label study) for pregabalin use in bipolar disorder; thus, it has been excluded here,   (E) Valproate derivates include: valproic acid which is a weak organic acid, valproate which is the conjugated base, divalproex which is a prodrug complex of sodium valproate and valproic acid

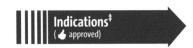

Indications‡
(👍 approved)

	SECOND-GENERATION AGENTS		THIRD-GENERATION AGENTS			
	Carbamazepine	**Valproate**	**Gabapentin**	**Lamotrigine**	**Oxcarbazepine**	**Topiramate**
Acute mania	👍 + (second-line agent as combination therapy)	👍 + (first-line agent as mono- or combination therapy; also effective in case series of corticosteroid-induced mania)	not recommended	not recommended	+/− (third-line agent as combination therapy)	not recommended
Acute bipolar I depression	+ (third-line agent)	+ (second-line agent)	−	+ (first-line agent) (− evidence in combination with folic acid)	?	?
Maintenance of bipolar I disorder	👍 + (second-line agent)	+ (first-line agent)	+ (third-line adjunctive agent)	👍 + (first-line agent; limited efficacy in preventing mania)	+/−	?
Acute bipolar II depression	?	?	?	+ (second-line agent)	?	?
Maintenance of bipolar II disorder	+ (third-line agent)	+ (third-line agent)	?	+ (first-line agent	?	?
Rapid-cycling bipolar disorder	👍 +/−	+	?/−	− (bipolar I) + (bipolar II)	−	?/−
Mixed states	+	+	?	not recommended	+ (adjunctive drug)	−
Anticonvulsant	👍 Partial and generalized tonic-clonic seizures. Not effective for absence, myoclonic or atonic seizures	👍 Complex partial seizures with and without other seizure types (monotherapy or adjunctive) 👍 Simple and complex absence seizures (monotherapy or adjunctive) 👍 Adjunctive agent in adults with multiple seizure types	👍 Partial seizures with and without secondary generalization (adjunctive) 👍 Epilepsy not satisfactorily controlled by conventional therapy (adjunctive)	👍 Partial onset seizures and primary generalized tonic-clonic seizures (adjunctive) 👍 Partial-onset seizures (monotherapy) 👍 Generalized seizures associated with Lennox-Gastaut (adjunctive)	👍 Partial seizures (monotherapy or adjunctive)	👍 Partial onset or primary generalized tonic-clonic seizures (monotherapy) 👍 Partial onset seizures, primary generalized tonic-clonic seizures, seizures associated with Lennox-Gastaut (adjunctive)
Paroxysmal pain syndromes	👍 + (Trigeminal neuralgia); glossopharyngeal neuralgia in some patients ? Fibromyalgia	+ (diabetic neuropathy, postherpetic neuralgia)	👍 Postherpetic neuralgia + (neuropathic pain) ? Complex regional pain syndrome/ fibromyalgia	+/− (central pain); Cochrane review: ineffective in neuropathic pain and fibromyalgia	+/− (neuropathic pain, trigeminal neuralgia)	− (neuropathic pain); Cochrane review: no separation from placebo

‡ Indications listed here do not necessarily apply to all anticonvulsants or all countries. Please refer to a country's regulatory database (e.g., US Food and Drug Administration, Health Canada Drug Product Database) for the most current availability information and indications

Anticonvulsants (cont.)

	SECOND-GENERATION AGENTS		THIRD-GENERATION AGENTS			
	Carbamazepine	**Valproate**	**Gabapentin**	**Lamotrigine**	**Oxcarbazepine**	**Topiramate**
Migraine headaches	+	👍 (prophylaxis) + (chronic daily headaches)	+/? + (chronic daily headaches)	+ (Basilar migraine)	−	👍 (prophylaxis) + (medication overuse headaches) + (post-ECT treatment headaches)
Behavior disturbances Explosive disorder, conduct disorder, developmental delay, brain damage	+ (alone or in combination with lithium, antipsychotics or β-blockers)	+	−	?	+	+/?
Dementia	+/−	−	+ (small case series)	+/? (case report)	−	?/−
Panic disorder	+	+ (third-line agent)	+ (third-line agent)	+	+ (case report)	− (may be associated with development of panic attacks)
Social anxiety disorder (SAD), generalized anxiety disorder (GAD)	−	+/− (open trials)	+ (social phobia)	?	?	?/(third-line agent for SAD)
Feeding and eating disorders	+/− bulimia nervosa	+/− bulimia nervosa	?	+ binge eating disorder	?	+/− bulimia nervosa and binge-eating disorder (Case report of abuse in anorexia nervosa)
Posttraumatic stress disorder (PTSD)	+ (open trials)	+/− (systematic review, open trials)	+ (adjunctive)	? (preliminary evidence/case report[12])	+ (case reports)	+/−[13]
Obsessive-compulsive disorder (OCD)	+/− (adjunctive drug − preliminary data)	+/− (adjunctive drug, case reports)	−	+/− (case report − adjunctive to SSRI in treatment-resistant OCD)	+ (case report − adjunctive drug)	+/− (trial as adjunct in treatment-resistant OCD)[14], + (trial as adjunct in bipolar) + (pathological gambling)
Core symptoms of borderline personality disorder	+	+ (preliminary data)	?	−	+ (preliminary data)	+
Paranoid ideation, hallucinations, and negative symptoms of schizophrenia	+/− (adjunctive drug)	+ (adjunctive drug)	−	+/− (adjunctive drug − benefit on positive symptoms)	+ (preliminary data − alone or as adjunctive drug)	+ (adjunctive drug)/?
Movement disorders	Dystonic disorder in children ? Restless legs syndrome	−	+/? Essential tremor; + restless legs syndrome	−	+ Essential tremor (case report) + Restless legs syndrome (case reports)	+ Essential tremor

	SECOND-GENERATION AGENTS		THIRD-GENERATION AGENTS			
	Carbamazepine	Valproate	Gabapentin	Lamotrigine	Oxcarbazepine	Topiramate
Drug dependence	Aid in alcohol or sedative/hypnotic withdrawal; may play a role in cocaine dependence (– systematic review)	Aid in alcohol withdrawal (open trials)	Alcohol use disorder and alcohol withdrawal (monotherapy) Adjunct in opioid, alcohol, or cannabis withdrawal. Studies have found gabapentin abuse associated with opioid addiction	Aid in alcohol withdrawal (open trials)	–	Treatment of alcohol use disorder Promotes smoking cessation in alcohol-dependent smokers Increases cocaine-free days Not efficacious for increasing cocaine abstinence in methadone patients

+ = positive data; – = negative data; ? = no data available or data of poor quality to guide therapy

 Dosing

- See table p. 303 for specific agents
- Carbamazepine and valproate: Plasma level monitoring (measured at trough/immediately prior to the next dose) can help guide dosing. However, levels are extrapolated from seizure/epilepsy treatment and patients with bipolar disorder may respond to doses outside of seizure therapeutic range
- Lamotrigine: Slow dosage titration (as per product monograph) required to decrease risk of Stevens-Johnson syndrome (SJS) and toxic epidermal necrolysis (TEN). Given a half-life of approximately 24 h, retitration is required if more than 5 days of treatment missed. Faster titrations not recommended even if patient previously exposed to lamotrigine
- Gabapentin: Dosing in renal dysfunction:
  - If CrCl 50–79 mL/min, no dose adjustment necessary, maximum dose 1800 mg/day
  - If CrCl 30–49 mL/min, give drug bid to tid to a maximum dose of 900 mg/day
  - If CrCl 15–29 mL/min, give drug once or twice daily to a maximum dose of 600 mg/day
  - If CrCl is less than 15 mL/min, give drug once daily to a maximum of 300 mg
- Topiramate: Dosing in renal dysfunction: If CrCl less than 70 mL/min, reduce dose to 50% of normal dose and titrate cautiously
- Reduced dosages recommended in the elderly and in hepatic or renal disorders

Pharmacokinetics

- See table p. 304 for specific agents

Carbamazepine

- Induces its own metabolism. Single-dose studies show half-life ranges of 30–40 h that decrease to 20 h after 3 weeks. During chronic monotherapy, half-life is 12 h, and during concurrent therapy with enzyme inducers may decrease to 8 h
- The epoxide (10,11) metabolite of carbamazepine can reach up to 50% of the plasma concentration of the parent drug; it is pharmacologically active and associated with neurological side effects

Valproate

- Pharmacokinetics show significant variation with changes in body weight. Valproate exhibits concentration-dependent protein binding, therefore at high doses and plasma concentrations a larger proportion may exist in unbound (free) form; the free fraction of drug increases from 10% at a concentration of 40 micrograms/mL to 18.5% at a concentration of 130 micrograms/mL. Increased age, low albumin levels, and/or concurrent use of highly protein-bound drugs will result in higher free fraction of valproate and patients may exhibit signs of toxicity within the therapeutic serum level range
- As binding sites become saturated and the free fraction increases, valproate clearance also increases, reducing total serum concentrations such that at higher dosing non-linear changes in serum concentrations occur
- Absorption of divalproex may be delayed such that levels taken in the morning after evening doses may more closely approximate a peak concentration; switching from divalproex to valproic acid liquid for compliance purposes may show a decline in serum levels. Pharmacokinetic differences also exist between divalproex formulations (i.e., divalproex delayed release vs. extended release)

Anticonvulsants (cont.)

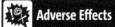

Gabapentin	• Gabapentin shows dose-dependent bioavailability as a result of a saturable transport mechanism. Absorbed from proximal small bowel by L-amino transport system. Improved bioavailability with more frequent dosing; plasma level is proportional to dose. Elimination is predominantly via kidneys and reduced in renal dysfunction (see Dosing p. 303)
Lamotrigine	• Large individual variation seen in plasma lamotrigine concentration in renal impairment; half-life is also prolonged in hepatic dysfunction
Oxcarbazepine	• Completely absorbed. Extensively metabolized to pharmacologically active 10-monohydroxy metabolite • A structural analogue of carbamazepine, but undergoes different metabolism pathway. Does not undergo autoinduction
Topiramate	• Good absorption, ingestion with high-fat meal may alter C_{max} and T_{max} of some formulations. Protein binding is inversely related to plasma concentrations • Excreted renally (70% as unchanged drug), may undergo renal tubular reabsorption

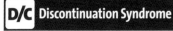

Adverse Effects

- See table pp. 304–307 for specific agents
- Many side effects can be minimized with slower dosage titration
- Common (for all anticonvulsants):
  - GI issues, e.g., nausea (especially with valproic acid liquid) [Management: Take with food, change to an enteric-coated preparation, change to lower doses at more frequent intervals, use ranitidine 150 mg/day or famotidine 20 mg/day]
  - Dose-related lethargy, sedation, behavior changes/deterioration, ataxia, reversible dementia/encephalopathy; cognitive effects are more prominent on drug initiation and are minimized with slow dosage increases. Sudden cognition/LOC changes for patients on valproate warrant a serum ammonia assessment (see Precautions)
  - Tremor: Dose related; tends to be rhythmic, rapid, symmetrical, and most prominent in upper extremities [Management: reduce dose (if possible); change to extended-release formulation; may respond to propranolol]
  - Weight: Changes in appetite, weight gain (except topiramate and lamotrigine) – more common in females; may be associated with features of insulin resistance, impaired glucose tolerance, hyperinsulinemia, and hyperlipidemia. Weight increases with duration of treatment. Obesity may increase risk of hyperandrogenism in females [Management: Can trial metformin 500 mg tid]
  - Menstrual disturbances (except gabapentin and topiramate; lamotrigine low risk), including: Prolonged cycles, oligomenorrhea, amenorrhea, polycystic ovaries, elevated testosterone – rates may be higher in females who begin taking valproate before age 20. Clinical features of polycystic ovary syndrome include hirsutism, alopecia, acne, menstrual irregularities, and obesity; lab indices show increased total and free testosterone, decreased FSH, increased serum prolactin and LH, and LH/FSH ratio greater than 2, incidence most common with valproate
- Occasional (for all anticonvulsants, often dose related):
  - Dysarthria, incoordination
  - Diplopia, nystagmus
- Rare: Anticonvulsant hypersensitivity syndrome with fever, rash, and internal organ involvement; cross-sensitivity (related to aromatic ring) reported between carbamazepine, eslicarbazepine, oxcarbazepine, phenytoin, barbiturates, lamotrigine, and possibly lacosamide. Valproate structure different (organic acid) and considered safe

D/C Discontinuation Syndrome

- No evidence of psychological or physical dependence to anticonvulsants (except for gabapentin)[15]
- Myoclonic jerks have been reported following the tapering of carbamazepine or valproate
- Case of anhedonia, tremor, tachycardia, and hyperhidrosis reported following rapid discontinuation of lamotrigine
- Abrupt discontinuation (especially in patients with a seizure disorder) may provoke rebound seizures – taper even in absence of seizure history
- Rare reports of psychiatric symptoms on withdrawal, including psychosis (exacerbation of schizophrenia)

 Precautions

- Monitoring: Prior to treatment, laboratory investigations should be performed (see p. 292)
- Contraception: Ensure adequate contraception in place for women of child-bearing age, especially prior to carbamazepine and valproate (contraception underutilized despite known risks[16]) (see Use in Pregnancy p. 308)

- Suicidal behavior or ideation: According to the FDA (February 2008), patients receiving antiepileptic drugs have a slightly increased risk of suicidal behavior or ideation (0.43%) compared to patients receiving placebo (0.22%). Increased risk observed as early as one week and continued through 24 weeks. Patients who were treated for epilepsy, psychiatric disorders, and other conditions were all at increased risk for suicidality but the relative risk for suicidality was higher in the patients with epilepsy than in those with psychiatric or other conditions.[15] Risk not consistently found with all antiepileptic drugs and has been questioned by experts

Carbamazepine	

- **Patients of Asian ancestry (particularly Han Chinese) and with a positive test for HLA-B*1502, and patients with HLA-A*3101 (particularly Japanese and Northern European) are at increased risk of serious, and possibly fatal, skin reactions (Stevens-Johnson syndrome, toxic epidermal necrolysis). Screen for testing eligibility prior to use and avoid if patient tests positive**
- **Hypersensitivity syndrome** with fever, skin eruptions, and internal organ involvement (i.e., DRESS) occurs rarely, cross-sensitivity with other aromatic anticonvulsants suggested; discontinue carbamazepine at first sign of drug-induced rash
- **Hepatoxicity** – between 1–22% have transient serum aminotransferase elevations which are usually benign, however, mixed or cholestatic injury can occur (usually associated with DRESS)
- **Hematologic concerns** – potentially fatal blood cell abnormalities have been reported. Mild degree of blood cell suppression can occur; stop therapy if WBC levels drop below 3,000 white cells/mm^3; erythrocytes less than 4×10^6/mm^3; platelets less than 100,000/mm^3
- Due to anticholinergic action, give cautiously to patients with increased intraocular pressure or urinary retention
- Hyponatremia (SIADH) occurs in 10–15% of patients; elderly patients at slightly increased risk. Risk of SIADH appears to be dose related
- Use cautiously in patients with history of coronary artery disease, organic heart disease, or congestive heart failure; may suppress ventricular automaticity
- Use with caution in patients with renal impairment (carbamazepine and active metabolite can accumulate)
- Tolerance to effects has been reported; efficacy not improved with dose increase
- Carbamazepine induces the metabolism of drugs metabolized by the CYP450 system (including metabolism of itself) (see pp. 294–298). Monitoring of clinical status and dosage adjustment of many drugs, including contraceptives (both oral and patches), in particular, may be required. De-induction following carbamazepine discontinuation estimated to take two weeks
- Do not administer carbamazepine suspension together with any other liquid preparation as formation of an insoluble precipitate can occur
- Can lead to false-positive tricyclic antidepressant drug screen results

Valproate	

- **Hepatic toxicity** – may show no relation to hepatic enzyme levels. Asymptomatic ALT elevations occur in 5–10% of treated patients and resolve with drug discontinuation. Three clinically distinct forms of hepatoxicity can occur: hyperammonemia with minimal evidence of hepatic injury, acute hepatocellular injury with jaundice, and Reye-like syndrome (in children). Monitor liver function prior to and at regular intervals after initiation of therapy. Stop drug if hepatic transaminase 2–3 times the upper limit of normal
- **Hyperammonemia and/or encephalopathy**, sometimes fatal, have been reported following initiation of valproic acid therapy and may be present with normal transaminase levels. One study found hyperammonemia encephalopathy in 2.52% of patients treated with valproate over 5 years. Ammonia levels should be measured in patients who develop unexplained lethargy and vomiting or changes in mental status, or in patients who present with hypothermia. Increased risk with extremes of age, higher dose, and concomitant phenytoin, phenobarbital, topiramate or carbamazepine use. Carnitine may be beneficial for acute valproic acid toxicity
- **Hyponatremia** – cases of hyponatremia/SIADH especially at high doses
- **Pancreatitis** – cases of life-threatening pancreatitis at start of therapy or following years of use. In patients with severe abdominal pain, lethargy, and weight loss, rule out pancreatitis – do serum amylase level
- **Thrombocytopenia** – platelet counts and bleeding time determinations are recommended prior to therapy and at periodic intervals; withdraw if hemorrhage, bruising, or coagulation disorder is detected
- Drug reaction with eosinophilia and systemic symptoms (DRESS)/multiorgan hypersensitivity reported in a few cases. Monitor for signs and symptoms and discontinue if confirmed. Increased risk when combined with lamotrigine
- Diabetic patients on valproic acid may show false-positive ketone results
- Polycystic ovary syndrome: Due to risk, consider monitoring for bioavailable androgens (free testosterone) as well as prolactin, LH, and TSH in females with menstrual irregularities, obesity, hirsutism, alopecia, and evidence of anovulation
- In patients with decreased or altered protein binding it may be more useful to monitor unbound (free) valproate concentrations rather than total concentrations

Anticonvulsants (cont.)

- Valproate will inhibit the metabolism of a number of drugs metabolized by CYP2C9, epoxide hydroxylase, UGT2B7 (see Drug Interactions, pp. 298–299). Rare case reports of valproate autoinduction
- Hyponatremia – cases of hyponatremia/SIADH, especially at high doeses

Gabapentin	

- Isolated cases of drug reaction with eosinophilia and systemic symptoms (DRESS)/multi-organ hypersensitivity reported, including fatal cases; evaluate early signs/symptoms and discontinue gabapentin if confirmed
- Risk of psychomotor impairment. Advise patients to avoid activities that require mental alertness and physical coordination until cognitive effects assessed
- Case report of gabapentin-induced cardiomyopathy
- Abuse potential (sedative-hypnotic and dissociative effects), especially in patients with pre-existing substance use disorder
- Requests from patients for high-dose gabapentin may signal opiate misuse
- Respiratory depression in those with pre-existing respiratory risk factors (concurrent use of opioids, benzodiazepines, COPD, elderly)
- Case reports of myoclonus in patient with renal failure

Lamotrigine	

- Severe, potentially life-threatening rashes, including Stevens-Johnson syndrome (SJS) and toxic epidermal necrolysis (TEN), have been reported – higher incidence in children, rapid dosage titration, and in combination with valproate. Most occur within first 8 weeks of starting lamotrigine. Patient should be educated to immediately report any rash or systemic symptoms (fever, malaise, pharyngitis, flu-like symptoms), sores or blisters on soles, palms or mucus membranes. Do not rechallenge
- Use cautiously in patients with renal dysfunction and in patients with moderate to severe hepatic impairment as elimination half-life of lamotrigine is increased
- Use cautiously in patients with structural (myocardial ischemia, heart failure, Brugada syndrome) or functional conduction (second- or third-degree heart block, ventricular arrhythmia, other sodium channelopathies) abnormalities. Lamotrigine has class IB antiarrhythmic activity at therapeutically relevant concentrations (may slow ventricular conduction (widen QRS), induce proarrhythmic, sudden cardiac death). Concomitant use of other sodium channel blockers may increase risk of proarrhythmic
- FDA warning (August 2010) of aseptic meningitis – more than 40 cases reported; patients should be advised to immediately report symptoms of headache, fever, stiff neck, nausea, vomiting, rash, and sensitivity to light

Oxcarbazepine	

- Monitor sodium levels with chronic use due to risk of hyponatremia – particularly in first 3 months
- Serious dermatological reactions, including Stevens-Johnson syndrome (SJS) and toxic epidermal necrolysis (TEN), have been reported in both children and adults; multi-organ hypersensitivity reactions have occurred in close temporal association (median time to detection 13 days, range: 4–60) to the initiation of therapy in adult and pediatric patients
- 25–30% of patients who exhibited hypersensitivity reactions to carbamazepine may also have these reactions with oxcarbazepine
- Patients of Asian ancestry (particularly Han Chinese) and with a positive test for HLA-B*1502 are at increased risk of serious skin reactions (Stevens-Johnson syndrome and toxic epidermal necrolysis). Avoid use if patient tests positive
- Rare reports of agranulocytosis, aplastic anemia, and pancytopenia

Topiramate	

- Topiramate alone or in combination with valproate can cause hyperammonemia with or without encephalopathy – monitor for acute alterations in level of consciousness with fatigue and/or vomiting; if suspected, order ammonia level
- Hypothermia (body core temperature below 35°C (95°F)) reported with concurrent valproate use
- Decreased sweating (oligohidrosis) and hyperthermia reported
- Acute myopia secondary to angle closure glaucoma reported; ophthalmological consult recommended for patients who complain of acute visual problems and/or painful/red eyes
- Ten-fold increased risk of renal stone (calcium phosphate) formation due to inhibition of renal tubular carbonic anhydrase leading to renal tubular acidosis and hypocitraturia. Ensure adequate fluid intake and avoid excessive antacid use and carbonic anhydrase inhibitors
- Chronic metabolic acidosis may increase risk for nephrolithiasis or nephrocalcinosis and may result in osteomalacia and/or osteoporosis with an increase in risk of fractures [reduce dose or taper and discontinue drug]
- Decrease in sodium bicarbonate (up to 30% incidence); symptoms include fatigue, stupor, anorexia, hyperventilation, and cardiac arrhythmia

- Cognitive side effects are dose related
- Use cautiously in patients with hepatic impairment due to reduced clearance

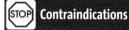 **Contraindications**

- Hypersensitivity to any tricyclic compound (carbamazepine), and demonstrated hypersensitivity to any of the other agents
- Patients with history of atrioventricular heart block, hepatic disease, history of hepatic porphyria, serious blood disorder (carbamazepine)
- Concurrent use with nefazodone, delavirdine or other non-nucleoside reverse transcriptase inhibitors that are substrates of CYP3A4 (carbamazepine)
- Conjunction with itraconazole and voriconazole or combined use with monoamine oxidase inhibitor (carbamazepine)
- Concurrent clozapine due to increased risk of agranulocytosis (carbamazepine, oxcarbazepine)
- Hepatic disease or significant impairment, urea cycle disorders, known mitochondrial disorder caused by mutations in mitochondrial DNA polymerase gamma, known porphyria
- Valproate contraindicated in females of childbearing potential unless conditions of Pregnancy Prevention Programme are met (CAD, UK)

 Toxicity

Carbamazepine

- Usually occurs with plasma levels above 50 mmol/L; children may be at risk for toxicity at lower serum concentrations due to increased production of toxic epoxide metabolite. Measurement of epoxide level may be beneficial if patient develops clinical signs of carbamazepine toxicity at therapeutic concentrations of the parent drug (however, many labs are unable to measure epoxide level)
- Maximum plasma concentration may be delayed for up to 70 h after an overdose; onset of symptoms begin 1–3 h after ingestion
- Signs:
  - Dizziness, blood pressure changes, sinus tachycardia, ECG changes
  - Drowsiness, stupor, agitation, disorientation, seizures, and coma
  - Nausea, vomiting, decreased intestinal motility, urinary retention
  - Tremor, involuntary movements, opisthotonos, abnormal reflexes, myoclonus, ataxia, rhabdomyolysis
  - Mydriasis, nystagmus
  - Flushing, respiratory depression, cyanosis
- No known antidote, treat symptomatically. Hemodialysis if refractory seizures, hemodynamic instability, life-threatening dysrhythmias

Valproate

- Maximum plasma concentration may not occur for up to 18 h following an overdose, and serum half-life may be prolonged
- Onset of CNS depression may be rapid (within 3 h); enteric-coated preparations may delay onset of symptoms
- Signs/symptoms: Severe dizziness, hypotension, supraventricular tachycardia, bradycardia; severe drowsiness; trembling; irregular, slow or shallow breathing, apnea, and coma; loss of tendon reflexes, generalized myoclonus, seizures; cerebral edema – evident 2–3 days after overdose and may last up to 15 days; hematological changes, electrolyte, and metabolic abnormalities; optic nerve damage reported
- Overdose can result in heart block, coma, or death; naloxone may reverse the CNS depressant effects, and may also reverse anti-epileptic effects
- Supportive treatment [L-carnitine supplementation 100 mg/kg/day (maximum 6 g) followed by 15 mg/kg every 4 h until clinical improvement recommended for patients with CNS depression, evidence of hepatic dysfunction, and hyperammonemia]. Hemodialysis may result in significant removal of drug during acute overdose as unbound valproic acid concentration is high

Gabapentin

- Signs and symptoms: Double vision, slurred speech, drowsiness, lethargy, unresponsiveness, and diarrhea. Most case reports of overdose are polyintoxications. Symptoms of acute overdose are generally mild and most recover. Fatalities reported in polyintoxications
- No known antidote. Removed by hemodialysis

Lamotrigine

- Overdose can result in ataxia, nystagmus, delirium, seizures, intraventricular conduction delay, and coma. Fatalities reported
- No known antidote – treat symptomatically

Oxcarbazepine

- No deaths reported following overdose of up to 24,000 mg; no known antidote – treat symptomatically. Carbamazepine levels not helpful
- Removal of the drug by gastric lavage and/or inactivation by administering activated charcoal should be considered

Topiramate

- Emesis and gastric lavage recommended; topiramate can be removed by hemodialysis
- Treat symptomatically
- Overdose can result in severe metabolic acidosis

Anticonvulsants (cont.)

Lab Tests/Monitoring

	Carbamazepine	Valproate	Gabapentin	Lamotrigine	Oxcarbazepine	Topiramate
Work-up	(1) CBC including platelets and differential (2) Serum electrolytes, urea, creatinine (3) Liver function (4) ECG (in patients over age 45 or with a cardiac history) (5) HLA-B*1502/HLA-A*3101 typing in patients with high-risk ancestry (6) Pregnancy test if appropriate	(1) CBC including platelets and differential (2) Liver function (3) Total and HDL cholesterol and triglycerides (4) Body weight/BMI (5) Menstrual history (6) Bone density (7) Pregnancy test if appropriate	BUN and serum creatinine	Liver function BUN and serum creatinine. ECG	Serum electrolytes Serum creatinine (dose needs to be adjusted with CrCl less than 30 mL/min)	Baseline serum bicarbonate, BUN, and serum creatinine
Follow-up	Repeat CBC, LFT, electrolytes, urea, creatinine monthly for 3 months, as clinically indicated or annually Bone density if risk factors for osteopenia are present	Repeat (1) and (2) monthly for 2 months, then 2–3 times a year (4) and (5) Q3 months for first year, then annually Ammonia level in event of lethargy, mental status changes (6) if risk factors for osteopenia are present	Renal function if suspect toxicity	None required; monitor for rash during titration. ECG if syncope or cardiac concerns	Sodium levels periodically and when patient has symptoms of hyponatremia	Periodic serum bicarbonate (to rule out metabolic acidosis) Renal function if suspect toxicity; ammonia levels in unexplained lethargy, vomiting or change in mental state
Plasma level monitoring	Levels for seizure disorders (17–51 μmol/L) are generally used as target range in bipolar disorder not established. Levels are suggested during initiation phase to establish non-toxic and reference levels for the individual patient. Carbamazepine induces its own hepatic metabolism; therefore, levels 4 weeks apart are suggested, after which dose adjustment may be required. Levels also suggested 5 days after change in dose or addition/deletion of possible interacting agent (see Drug Interactions pp. 294–298) or as clinically indicated. It may be necessary to check serum levels of other drugs if carbamazepine is added to the regimen	Two levels to establish therapeutic dose (at least 3–5 days after start of therapy) and 5 days after change in dose or addition/deletion of interacting drug (see Drug Interactions pp. 298–299 and Precautions p. 289) or as clinically indicated Response in mania usually seen with trough between 350 and 875 μmol/L, although individual response variable. Toxicity may occur at levels above 700 μmol/L	None required	None required although may be indicated if interacting drugs present. Therapeutic range not well established	None required	None required

Pediatric Considerations

- For detailed information on the use of anticonvulsants in this population, please see the *Clinical Handbook of Psychotropic Drugs for Children and Adolescents*[9]

Carbamazepine

- Used in episodic dyscontrol and assaultive behavior disorder
- Children may be at risk for major toxicities at lower serum concentrations due to increased production of toxic metabolite; case reports of behavior disturbances, mania, and worsening of tics
- Common side effects include: Unsteadiness, dizziness, diplopia, drowsiness, nausea, and vomiting

Valproate

- Efficacy reported in treatment of bipolar disorder, acute mania, migraine prophylaxis, temper/aggressive outbursts in adolescents and young adults
- Children ages 3–10 are at higher risk for hepatotoxicity compared to adults especially if taking other anticonvulsants

- Use in female children and adolescents may result in increased risk of hyperandrogenism, and polycystic ovary syndrome, delayed or prolonged puberty; excessive weight gain, hyperinsulinemia, and dyslipidemia; decreased bone mineral density reported (in up to 14%) – may conduce to osteoporosis

Gabapentin	• Incidence of side effects in children reported to be similar to that in adults. Case reports of behavioral problems including hyperactivity, aggression, and irritability
Lamotrigine	• Has been used in adolescents as add-on therapy in refractory bipolar depression. Common side effects included headache, tremor, somnolence, and dizziness • Risk of severe, life-threatening rash increased in children
Oxcarbazepine	• Used in children and adolescents as sole or add-on therapy for partial seizures
Topiramate	• Used as add-on therapy in seizure disorders and prophylaxis of migraine headaches • Side effects include sedation, cognitive and behavioral problems, and weight loss • Dose-related hyperammonemia reported • Oligohidrosis (decreased sweating), anhidrosis, and hyperthermia reported – most case reports in children • Persistent treatment-emergent decreases in serum bicarbonate and metabolic acidosis

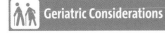 **Geriatric Considerations**

- Dosing should be instituted more gradually in the elderly and those with liver impairment
- May cause confusion, cognitive impairment, ataxia (may lead to falls)
- Dementia: Meta-analysis and 3 RCTs support the efficacy of carbamazepine in managing aggression and hostility in patients with dementia; meta-analysis and 5 RCTs do not strongly support the use of valproate. Open trials and case series suggest gabapentin, topiramate, and lamotrigine may show benefit; oxcarbazepine ineffective. Caution advised due to adverse effects and potential for drug interactions
- Caution when combining with other drugs with CNS or anticholinergic properties; additive effects can result in confusion, disorientation, delirium
- Hip fractures: Continuous anticonvulsant use in elderly women is associated with increased rates of bone loss at the calcaneus and hip. Increases risk of hip fracture by 29% over 5 years among women aged 65 and older
- Renal disease: Reduce dose of gabapentin if CrCl less than 60 mL/min; oxcarbazepine if CrCl less than 30 mL/min; topiramate if CrCl less than 70 mL/min
- Valproate: Due to reduced protein binding and hepatic oxidation, the elderly may have a higher proportion of unbound (free) valproate and a reduced clearance, resulting in elevated levels of unbound valproate (within therapeutic plasma levels of total drug); case report of acute parkinsonism with valproate in an elderly patient with dementia. Increased risk of thrombocytopenia
- Valproate: Similar tolerability and efficacy compared to lithium in treatment of mania in elderly patients while maintaining a mean daily dose of 1200 mg and serum concentration of 513 micromol/L
- Carbamazepine: Elderly patients with pre-existing cardiac disease should have a thorough cardiac evaluation prior to use
- Carbamazepine/oxcarbazepine: Higher risk of hyponatremia with carbamazepine and oxcarbazepine and increased risk of SIADH with carbamazepine
- Lamotrigine: Plasma level increased in elderly patients

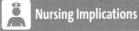 **Nursing Implications**

- Monitor patients starting drug treatment for behavioral changes that could indicate emergence or worsening of depression, or suicidal thoughts/behaviors
- Watch out for signs of fever, sore throat, and bruising or bleeding
- Close clinical and laboratory supervision should be maintained (see Adverse Effects pp. 304–307 and Monitoring p. 292) throughout treatment to detect signs of possible blood dyscrasias or liver involvement
- A rash, especially with carbamazepine, oxcarbazepine, or lamotrigine, may signal incipient blood dyscrasia; advise the physician
- Anorexia, nausea, vomiting, edema, malaise, and lethargy may signify hepatic toxicity
- Since drowsiness can occur, patients should exercise caution when performing tasks that require alertness especially during treatment initiation; will enhance the effects of alcohol and other CNS drugs
- Monitor patient's height, weight, and BMI
- In the elderly, monitor for ataxia, confusion, and cognitive impairment
- Advise patient to store medication away from heat and humidity as the drug may lose potency

Anticonvulsants (cont.)

- Enteric-coated, controlled-release, or delayed-release formulations should not be broken or crushed but should be swallowed whole; chewing capsules can cause local irritation in the mouth and throat
- Carbamazepine:
  - Check for urinary retention and constipation; increase fluids to lessen constipation
  - Liquid carbamazepine should not be mixed or taken at the same time as any other liquid medication
  - Grapefruit and grapefruit juice should be avoided as it can elevate the blood level of carbamazepine
  - A rash may signal incipient blood dyscrasia; advise the physician immediately
- Valproic acid:
  - Liquid valproate should not be administered with carbonated beverages as mouth irritation can occur
  - In females (particularly on valproate), obtain baseline body weight/BMI and measure periodically, monitor for menstrual disturbances, hirsutism, obesity, alopecia, and infertility – two or more of these symptoms may be associated with polycystic ovary syndrome
  - To treat occasional pain, avoid use of acetylsalicylic acid (ASA or aspirin) as it can affect the blood level of valproate – acetaminophen or ibuprofen (and related drugs) are safer alternatives
  - If sudden change in level of consciousness, ammonia level should be checked
- Lamotrigine: A rash, may signal incipient blood dyscrasia; advise the physician immediately
- Oxcarbazepine:
  - Monitor for symptoms of hyponatremia – i.e., nausea, malaise, headache, lethargy, confusion
  - Fever or rash may be a sign of serious skin reaction or organ involvement
- Topiramate:
  - Patients should drink plenty of fluids and avoid the regular use of antacids (e.g., Tums, Maalox, Rolaids, etc.) to reduce risk of renal stone formation
  - Patients should report eye pain or continued visual disturbances to the physician

 Patient Instructions

- For detailed patient instructions on Anticonvulsant Mood Stabilizers, see the Patient Information Sheet (details p. 474)

 Drug Interactions

- Clinically significant interactions are listed below
- For more interaction information on any given combination, also see the corresponding chapter for the second agent

DRUGS INTERACTING WITH CARBAMAZEPINE

Class of Drug	Example	Interaction Effects
Anesthetic	Halothane	Enzyme induction may result in hepatocellular damage
	Isoflurane, sevoflurane	Enzyme induction may result in renal damage
	Ketamine	Decreased serum concentration of ketamine due to CYP 2B6 induction
Antiarrhythmic	Disopyramide	Increased metabolism and decreased plasma level of disopyramide
	Propafenone	Decreased serum concentrations due to CYP 3A4 induction
	Quinidine	Increased metabolism and decreased plasma levels of quinidine
Antibiotic	Clarithromycin, erythromycin	Increased plasma levels of carbamazepine due to reduced clearance (by 5–41%)
	Dapsone	Decreased serum concentration of dapsone due to CYP 3A4 induction
	Doxycycline (no interaction with other tetracyclines)	Decreased serum level and half-life of doxycycline due to enhanced metabolism (alternatively, tetracycline can be used or doxycycline can be dosed q 12 h)
	Metronidazole	Increased plasma level of carbamazepine due to inhibited metabolism
	Quinupristin/dalfopristin	Increased plasma level of carbamazepine due to inhibited metabolism via CYP3A4

Class of Drug	Example	Interaction Effects
Anticoagulant	Apixaban, dabigatran, edoxaban	Increased metabolism of anticoagulant; combined use with carbamazepine not recommended
	Rivaroxaban	Case report of pulmonary embolism suspected due to increased clearance of rivaroxaban
	Warfarin	Enhanced metabolism of anticoagulant and impaired hypoprothombinemic response; decreased PT ratio or INR response. Average warfarin dose increased by 49% in one study
Anticonvulsant	Brivaracetam, levetiracetam	May increase serum concentrations of the active metabolite of carbamazepine. Carbamazepine may decrease the serum concentrations of brivaracetam
	Cenobamate	May decrease the serum concentration of carbamazepine
	Clobazam, clonazepam, eslicarbazepine, ethosuximide, oxcarbazepine, tiagabine, topiramate, zonisamide	Clearance of the anticonvulsants is increased by carbamazepine, with possible decrease in efficacy (40% decrease in concentration of topiramate and of oxcarbazepine metabolite)
	Ezogabine, tiagabine	Decreased serum concentration of ezogabine and tiagabine
	Felbamate	Decreased carbamazepine level by 50%, but increased level of epoxide metabolite Decreased felbamate level
	Fosphenytoin, phenobarbital, phenytoin, primidone	Decreased carbamazepine level due to increased metabolism via CYP3A4, but ratio of epoxide metabolite increased Altered plasma level of co-prescribed anticonvulsant
	Lacosamide	May enhance the adverse/toxic effects of lacosamide (especially bradycardia, ventricular tachyarrhythmias, and prolonged PR interval)
	Lamotrigine	Increased plasma level of epoxide metabolite of carbamazepine (by 10–45%), with resultant increased side effects Increased metabolism of lamotrigine; half-life and plasma level decreased by 30–50%
	Rufinamide, stiripentol	May decrease the serum concentration of carbamazepine
	Topiramate	Increased plasma level of carbamazepine by 20%
	Valproate, valproic acid	Increased plasma level of epoxide metabolite of carbamazepine; may result in toxicity even at therapeutic carbamazepine concentrations Effects on carbamazepine levels are variable and inconsistent Decreased valproate level due to increased clearance and displacement from protein binding
Antidepressant		
SSRI	Fluoxetine, fluvoxamine	Increased plasma level of carbamazepine and its active metabolite with fluoxetine; increased nausea with fluvoxamine
	Citalopram, sertraline	Decreased plasma level of sertraline or citalopram due to enzyme induction via CYP3A4 (case report)
NDRI	Bupropion	Decreased serum concentration of buproprion due to induction of CYP 2B6
SARI	Nefazodone	Increased plasma level of carbamazepine with nefazodone due to decreased metabolism via CYP3A4
	Trazodone	Decreased plasma level of trazodone
SPARI	Vilazodone	Up to 50% decreased plasma level of vilazodone
SMS	Vortioxetine	Decreased serum concentration of vortioxetine due to CYP 3A4 induction
NaSSA	Mirtazapine	Decreased serum concentration of mirtazapine due to CYP 3A4 induction
Cyclic (nonselective)	Amitriptyline, clomipramine, doxepin, imipramine, nortriptyline	Decreased plasma level of antidepressant (by up to 46%) due to enzyme induction
	Desipramine	Carbamazepine induces the production of hydroxymetabolites of desipramine which have been reported to cause ECG changes. Medically ill patients on a combination of a TCA and carbamazepine should have post-treatment ECGs
MAOI	Phenelzine, tranylcypromine	Possible decrease in metabolism and increased plasma level of carbamazepine

Anticonvulsants (cont.)

Class of Drug	Example	Interaction Effects
Antidiabetic	Gemigliptin, nateglinide	Decreased serum concentration due to CYP 3A4 induction
	Linagliptin, saxagliptin	Decreased serum concentration due to CYP 3A4 induction and p-glycoprotein/ABCB1 induction
Antifungal	Caspofungin	Decreased plasma level of antifungal. Consider using increased caspofungin dose
	Fluconazole, isavuconazonium sulfate, itraconazole, ketoconazole, voriconazole	Decreased plasma levels of antifungals
	Fluconazole, ketoconazole	Increased plasma level of carbamazepine with ketoconazole (by 29%) due to inhibited metabolism via CYP3A4; clearance decreased by 50% with fluconazole
Antineoplastic	Afatinib	Decreased serum concentration of afatinib due to P-glycoprotein/ABCB1 induction
	Cisplatin, dabrafenib	Decreased carbamazepine concentrations due to enzyme induction
	Cyclophosphamide	May increase serum concentrations of the active metabolite of cyclophosphamide due to CYP 2B6 induction
	Darolutamide, vincristine	Decreased serum concentration due to CYP 3A4 and P-glycoprotein induction
	Doxorubicin	Decreased cisplatin and doxorubicin concentrations due to enzyme induction
Antiplatelet	Ticagrelor	Decrease concentration of the active metabolite of ticagrelor
Antipsychotic	General	See Antipsychotics chapter for further information
	Aripiprazole, brexpiprazole, cariprazine, flupenthixol, haloperidol, lumateperone, lurasidone, olanzapine, paliperidone, phenothiazines, pimavanserin, quetiapine, risperidone, thiothixene, ziprasidone, zuclopenthixol	Decreased plasma levels of antipsychotics (64% with aripiprazole, up to 61% with haloperidol, 44% with olanzapine, 45–65% with paliperidone depending on carbamazepine dose, 70% with risperidone, 35% with ziprasidone). Quetiapine may also increase levels of the epoxide metabolite; olanzapine may increase carbamazepine levels Increased akathisia Increased neurotoxicity of both antipsychotic and carbamazepine at therapeutic doses
	Clozapine	Avoid combination due to possible potentiation of bone marrow suppression Decreased plasma level of clozapine by up to 63%
	Loxapine	May increase concentrations of active metabolites of carbamazepine
Antiretroviral	General	Decreased concentrations of antiretroviral regimens containing cobicistat (atazanavir/cobicistat, darunavir/cobicstat, elvitegravir/cobicistat); avoid combination
Integrase inhibitor	Bictegravir, dolutegravir, elvitegravir, raltegravir	Decreased antiviral concentrations due to increased metabolism; use with caution
Non-nucleoside reverse transcriptase inhibitor (NNRTI)	Delavirdine, doravirine, efavirenz, etravirine, nevirapine, rilpivirine	Decreased antiviral concentration and potential loss of virologic response; avoid combination
Protease inhibitor	Atazanavir, darunavir, indinavir, lopinavir, nelfinavir, ritonavir, saquinavir	Decreased protease inhibitor concentrations due to increased metabolism; avoid combination Increased plasma level of carbamazepine due to inhibited metabolism via CYP3A4, potentially resulting in toxicity
CCR5 antagonist	Maraviroc	Decreased serum concentration of maraviroc due to enzyme induction
Antitubercular drug	Bedaquiline, pretomanid	Decreased serum concentration due to enzyme induction
	Isoniazid	Increased plasma level of carbamazepine; clearance reduced by up to 45%

Class of Drug	Example	Interaction Effects
Antiviral (direct acting)	Asunnaprevir, daclatasvir, dasabuvir, elbasvir, gleca-previr, grazoprevir, ledipasvir, pibrentasvir, sime-previr, sofosbuvir, tenofovir, velpatasvir, voxilaprevir	Decreased plasma levels and efficacy of direct-acting antivirals due to enzyme induction via CYP3A4; avoid combination
	Letermovir	Decreased serum concentration of letermovir due to P-glycoprotein/ABCB1 induction. May increase the serum concentration of carbamazepine via UGT1A1 induction
	Rifampin	Decreased plasma level of carbamazepine
Anxiolytic	Alprazolam, clonazepam	Decreased plasma level of alprazolam (more than 50%) and clonazepam (19–37%) due to enzyme induction
	Buspirone	Decreased serum concentration of buspirone due to enzyme induction
β-blocker	Propranolol	Decreased plasma level of β-blocker due to enzyme induction
Calcium channel blocker	Diltiazem, verapamil	Increased plasma levels of carbamazepine due to decreased metabolism (total carbamazepine increased 46%, free carbamazepine increased 33%)
	Flunarizine, nifedipine, nimodipine	Decreased serum concentration due to CYP3A4 induction
Cannabis	Cannabidiol, cannabis, dronabinol	May decrease serum concentration due to CYP3A4 induction
Corticosteroids	Dexamethasone, methylprednisolone, prednisolone	Decreased plasma level of corticosteroid due to enzyme induction
Desmopressin (DDAVP)		Concurrent use may increase antidiuretic effect, resulting in decreased sodium concentration with resultant seizures
Diuretic	Acetazolamide, brinzolamide, dorzolamide	Increased plasma level of carbamazepine due to inhibited metabolism
	Hydrochlorothiazide	Concomitant use has been associated with hyponatremia, particularly in the elderly
	Thiazides	May enhance the adverse effects of carbamazepine (e.g., hyponatremia)
Folate supplement	Folic acid	Decreased plasma level of folic acid
	Methylfolate	May decrease serum concentration of carbamazepine
Grapefruit juice		Decreased metabolism of carbamazepine resulting in increased plasma level (by up to 40%)
H₂ antagonist	Cimetidine	Transient increase in carbamazepine levels and possible toxicity due to inhibited metabolism (no interaction with ranitidine, famotidine, and nizatidine)
Hormone-mediated agent	Oral contraceptive	Increased metabolism of oral contraceptive and increased binding of progestin and ethinyl estradiol to sex hormone binding globulin, may result in decreased contraceptive efficacy
	Bazedoxifene, dienogest, enzalutamide, exemestane, tamoxifen	Decreased serum concentration and potential loss of efficacy due to enzyme induction
	Danazol	Plasma levels of carbamazepine increased by 50–100%; half-life is doubled and clearance reduced by half
	Medroxyprogesterone acetate injection	Concomitant administration is expected to decrease medroxyprogesterone concentrations
	Ulipristal	Decreased plasma level and efficacy of ulipristal due to CYP3A4 induction
Hypnotic/Sedative	Zaleplon	Decreased serum concentration of zaleplon due to CYP 3A4 induction
	Zolpidem	May enhance the CNS depressant effect of carbamazepine. Carbamazepine may decrease the serum concentration of zolpidem
Immunosuppressant	Cyclosporine, sirolimus, tacrolimus	Decreased plasma level and efficacy of immunosuppressants due to CYP3A4 induction
	Everolimus	Decreased plasma level and efficacy of immunosuppressants due to CYP3A4 and p-glycoprotein induction
	Sarilumab	May decrease the concentration of carbamazepine
Influenza vaccine		Decreased elimination and increased half-life of carbamazepine
Isotretinoin		Decreased plasma level of carbamazepine and its metabolite
Lithium		Increased neurotoxicity of both drugs; sinus node dysfunction reported with combination

Anticonvulsants (cont.)

Class of Drug	Example	Interaction Effects
Muscle relaxant (non-depolarizing)	Pancuronium	Decreased duration of action and efficacy of muscle relaxant
NSAID	Diclofenac, ibuprofen	Increased plasma level of carbamazepine due to decreased metabolism
Opioid	Buprenorphine, hydrocodone, methadone, tramadol	Decreased effect of methadone (up to 60%) due to enhanced metabolism; buprenorphine, hydrocodone, and tramadol are metabolized by CYP3A4 and concomitant use is expected to decrease efficacy
	Codeine	Decreased serum concentrations of the active metabolite of codeine
	Fentanyl, sufentanil	Decreased serum concentration due to enzyme induction
Phosphodiesterase-4 inhibitor	Apremilast, roflumilast	Decreased serum concentration of apremilast due to CYP3A4 induction
Proton pump inhibitor	Omeprazole	Increased carbamazepine levels
Quinine		Increased plasma level of carbamazepine (by 37%) and AUC (by 51%) due to inhibited metabolism
Stimulant	Armodafinil	Carbamazepine may decrease the serum concentration of armodafinil and armodafinil may decrease serum concentration of carbamazepine
	Methylphenidate	Decreased plasma level of methylphenidate and its metabolite
	Modafinil	Decreased plasma level of modafinil due to enhanced metabolism
St. John's wort		Decreased carbamazepine plasma levels
Theophylline		Decreased theophylline level due to enzyme induction by carbamazepine; decreased carbamazepine level by up to 50%
Thyroid hormone		Decreased plasma level of thyroid hormone due to enzyme induction
VMAT2 inhibitor (for tardive dyskinesia)	Valbenazine	Decreased serum concentration of valbenazine due to CYP 3A4 induction

DRUGS INTERACTING WITH VALPROATE

Class of Drug	Example	Interaction Effects
Alcohol		Increased sedation, disorientation, hepatoxicity
Anesthetic	Propofol	Valproate reduces dose required to induce anesthesia for ECT
Antibiotic	Carbapenems	Significantly decreased valproate plasma concentrations
	Erythromycin	Increased valproate plasma level due to decreased metabolism; may also occur with clarithromycin
	Rifampin	May reduce valproate levels by up to 40%
Anticoagulant	Warfarin	Inhibition of secondary phase of platelet aggregation by valproate, thus affecting coagulation; increased PT ratio or INR response Displacement of protein binding of warfarin (free fraction increased by 33%)
Anticonvulsant	Carbamazepine	Decreased valproate levels due to increased clearance and displacement from protein binding Effects on carbamazepine levels are inconsistent
	Ethosuximide	Increased half-life of ethosuximide (by 25%)
	Felbamate	Increased plasma level of valproate (by 31–51%) due to decreased metabolism
	Lamotrigine	Increased lamotrigine plasma level (by up to 200%), half-life (by up to 50%), and decreased clearance (by up to 60%) Both decreases and increases in plasma level of valproate reported. This combination may be dangerous due to high incidence of Stevens-Johnson syndrome and toxic epidermal necrolysis

Class of Drug	Example	Interaction Effects
	Phenobarbital, primidone	Increased level of anticonvulsant (by 30–50%) due to decreased metabolism caused by valproate. Increased clearance of valproate. Additive CNS depression with concomitant administration (possibly severe)
	Phenytoin	Enhanced anticonvulsant effect due to displacement from protein binding (free fraction increased by 60%) and inhibited clearance (by 25%); toxicity can occur at therapeutic levels Possible decrease in valproate level
	Topiramate	Case reports of delirium and elevated ammonia levels; topiramate increases risk of valproate encephalopathy
Antidepressant SSRI SNRI Cyclic (nonselective)	Fluoxetine Venlafaxine Amitriptyline, doxepin, nortriptyline	Increased plasma level of valproate (up to 50%) Significantly increased levels of O-desmethylvenlafaxine Increased plasma level and adverse effects of antidepressant – consider therapeutic drug monitoring and monitor for adverse effects of increased antidepressant levels
Antihypertensive	Guanfacine	Increased level of valproate due to inhibited metabolism; monitor for potential CNS side effects
Antipsychotic	Clozapine	Both increased and decreased clozapine levels reported; changes in clozapine/norclozapine ratio Case report of hepatic encephalopathy Valproate may increase risk of clozapine myocarditis
	Haloperidol	Increased plasma level of haloperidol (by an average of 32%)
	Olanzapine	Combination associated with high incidence of weight gain Significantly lower levels of olanzapine in combination with valproic acid
	Phenothiazines	Increased neurotoxicity, sedation, and extrapyramidal side effects due to decreased clearance of valproate (by 14%)
	Risperidone	Case report of encephalopathy with initiation of risperidone
Antiretroviral Nucleoside reverse transcriptase inhibitor (NRTI) Protease inhibitor	Zidovudine Ritonavir Ritonavir and/or nevirapine[17]	Increased level of zidovudine (by 38%) due to decreased clearance Severe anemia reported with combination secondary to zidovudine; use combination with caution and monitor for zidovudine toxicity Decreased level of valproate due to increased metabolism; use with caution Case of hepatotoxicity with antiretroviral regimen containing ritonavir, saquinavir, stavudine, and nevirapine
Antitubercular drug	Isoniazid	Increased plasma level of valproate due to inhibited metabolism
	Rifampin	Increased clearance of valproate (by 40%)
Antiviral agent	Acyclovir	Decreased level of valproate
Anxiolytic	Chlordiazepoxide, clonazepam, lorazepam	Decreased metabolism and increased pharmacological effects of benzodiazepines resulting in increased sedation, disorientation (lorazepam clearance reduced by 41%)
	Clonazepam	Concomitant use may induce absence status in patients with a history of absence type seizures
	Diazepam	Increased plasma level of diazepam due to displacement from protein binding (free fraction increased by 90%)
H₂ antagonist	Cimetidine	Decreased metabolism and increased half-life of valproate
Hypnotic	Zolpidem	Case of somnambulism with combination
Lithium		Valproate may aggravate action tremor. Lithium may increase valproate levels (mechanism unknown)
Salicylate	Acetylsalicylic acid, bismuth subsalicylate	Displacement of valproate from protein binding and decreased clearance, leading to increased level of free drug (4-fold), with possible toxicity
Sulfonylurea	Tolbutamide	Increase in free fraction of tolbutamide from 20 to 50% due to displacement from protein binding
Thiopental		Displacement of thiopental from protein binding, resulting in an increased hypnotic/anesthetic effect

Anticonvulsants (cont.)

DRUGS INTERACTING WITH GABAPENTIN

Class of Drug	Example	Interaction Effects
Alcohol		Increased sedation, disorientation
Antacid	Al/Mg-containing antacids	Co-administration reduces gabapentin bioavailability by up to 24%. Administer gabapentin at least 2 h after antacid
Opioid	General	Increased sedation, disorientation Increased risk of opioid-related deaths due to additive respiratory depression and increased gabapentin concentrations (opioids slow GI transit time and gabapentin is absorbed in the upper small intestine, resulting in increased gabapentin bioavailability); monitor for CNS depression
	Hydrocodone	Decreased concentration of hydrocodone reported
	Morphine	Increased gabapentin concentrations; gabapentin has been shown to enhance the acute analgesic effects of morphine

DRUGS INTERACTING WITH LAMOTRIGINE

Class of Drug	Example	Interaction Effects
Alcohol		Increased sedation, disorientation
Analgesic	Acetaminophen	AUC of lamotrigine decreased by 20% when co-administered with 4 g of acetaminophen daily, due to induction of glucuronidation pathways
Antiarrhythmic	Procainamide	Increased procainamide concentrations
Anticonvulsant	Carbamazepine, phenobarbital, phenytoin, primidone	Plasma level and half-life of lamotrigine decreased due to increased metabolism (clearance increased 30–50% with carbamazepine; by 125% with phenytoin) Increased plasma level of epoxide metabolite of carbamazepine by 10–45% with resultant increased side effects
	Topiramate	Decreased plasma level of lamotrigine
	Valproate	Increased plasma level of lamotrigine (by up to 200%) and half-life (by up to 50%), and decreased clearance (by up to 60%), leading to an increased risk of lamotrigine toxicity and life-threatening rashes; both decreases and increases in valproate levels reported Increased risk of life-threatening rash with combination (Stevens-Johnson syndrome and toxic epidermal necrolysis)
Antidepressant SSRI	Escitalopram	Case reports of myoclonus
	Sertraline	Case reports of increased plasma level of lamotrigine resulting in toxicity
Antipsychotic	Olanzapine	AUC of lamotrigine decreased by 24%
Antiretroviral Non-nucleoside reverse transcriptase inhibitor (NNRTI)	Efavirenz, etravirine, nevirapine	Decreased lamotrigine concentrations due to increased metabolism; use with caution
Protease inhibitor	Atazanavir, lopinavir, ritonavir	Decreased plasma level of lamotrigine (by 50%) due to increased metabolism; use ritonavir-boosted regimens with caution
Antitubercular	Rifampin	Decreased lamotrigine levels and half-life
Herbal preparation	Ginseng	Case report of drug reaction with eosinophilia and systemic symptoms (DRESS)
Hormone	Oral contraceptive	Decreased plasma level of lamotrigine (by 27–64%) Reports of breakthrough bleeding and unexpected pregnancies
Opioid	General	Increased sedation, disorientation

DRUGS INTERACTING WITH OXCARBAZEPINE

Class of Drug	Example	Interaction Effects
Alcohol		Increased sedation, disorientation
Anticonvulsant	Carbamazepine, phenobarbital, phenytoin, valproate	Decreased plasma levels of oxcarbazepine MHD metabolite by 40% (carbamazepine); 30% (phenytoin); 25% (phenobarbital); 18% (valproate) Increased level of phenytoin (by 40%) and phenobarbital (by 14%) due to inhibited metabolism via CYP2C19
Antidepressant	Citalopram	May increase risk of QTc prolongation
	Sertraline	Case report of fatal serotonin syndrome in elderly patient when oxcarbazepine added, thought to be mediated through CYP2C19
Antiretroviral	General	Decreased concentrations of antiretroviral regimens containing cobicistat (atazanavir/cobicistat, darunavir/cobicistat, elvitegravir/cobicistat); avoid combination
Integrase inhibitor	Dolutegravir, elvitegravir, raltegravir	Decreased antiviral concentrations due to increased metabolism; use with caution
Non-nucleoside reverse transcriptase inhibitor (NNRTI)	Delavirdine, efavirenz, etravirine, nevirapine, rilpivirine	Decreased antiviral concentration and potential loss of virologic response; avoid combination
Protease inhibitor	Atazanavir, darunavir, indinavir, lopinavir, nelfinavir, ritonavir, saquinavir	Decreased protease inhibitor concentrations due to increased metabolism; avoid combination
Antiviral (direct acting)	Elbasvir, glecaprevir, grazoprevir, ledipasvir, pibrentasvir, sofosbuvir, velpatasvir, voxilaprevir	Decreased plasma levels and efficacy of direct-acting antivirals due to enzyme induction via CYP3A4; avoid combination
Calcium channel blocker	Felodipine	AUC of felodipine lowered by 28% – similar effect anticipated with other dihydropyridine calcium channel blockers
	Verapamil	Reduced oxcarbazepine MHD metabolite plasma level (by about 20%) – mechanism unknown
Diuretic	Furosemide	Increased risk of hyponatremia with oxcarbazepine
Hormone	Oral contraceptives	Increased metabolism of ethinyl estradiol and levonorgestrel through induction of CYP3A4

DRUGS INTERACTING WITH TOPIRAMATE

Class of Drug	Example	Interaction Effects
Alcohol		Increased sedation, disorientation
Antacid		Excessive use may increase renal stone (calcium phosphate) formation
Anticonvulsant	Carbamazepine, oxcarbazepine, phenobarbital, phenytoin, primidone	Decreased plasma levels of topiramate reported; by 40% with carbamazepine and 48% with phenytoin Increased plasma level of carbamazepine (by 20%) and of phenytoin
	Lamotrigine	Decreased plasma level of lamotrigine
	Valproate	Case reports of delirium and elevated ammonia levels; decreased clearance of topiramate by 25%
Biguanide	Metformin	May increase risk of lactic acidosis as topiramate may decrease sodium bicarbonate levels
Carbonic anhydrase inhibitor	Acetazolamide, zonisamide	Excessive use may increase renal stone (calcium phosphate) formation and/or hyperthermia
Cardiac glycoside	Digoxin	Decreased levels of digoxin by 12%
Diuretic	Furosemide, hydrochlorothiazide	Increased risk for hypokalemia
Hormone	Oral contraceptive	Possibly decreased levels of estrogen, resulting in decreased efficacy of oral contraceptive

Comparison of Anticonvulsants

	Carbamazepine	Gabapentin	Lamotrigine	Oxcarbazepine	Topiramate	Valproate
General Comments	Positive predictors of response include: Non-classic or secondary mania, early age at onset, negative family history of mood disorder, and patients with neurological abnormalities. Less response noted in patients with severe mania, dysphoric mania, and rapid cycling disorder	Not effective as a mood stabilizer. Not recommended for monotherapy in any phase of bipolar disorder	More effective in bipolar depression; suggested to have antidepressant properties. First-line agent for treatment of bipolar depression, acute and maintenance (limited efficacy/negative evidence in preventing mania): Does not induce switches to hypomania or mania. Prophylaxis of rapid cycling and bipolar II disorder	Pharmacological activity is exerted primarily through the 10-mono hydroxy metabolite (MHD) of oxcarbazepine. Less adverse effects and drug interactions compared to carbamazepine. Third-line option in bipolar disorder as monotherapy for acute mania and as adjunctive therapy in maintenance. Positive effects on verbal and visual memory, visuospatial function, naming ability, and frontal executive function in patients with epilepsy	Not recommended as monotherapy in any phase of bipolar disorder but may be useful as adjunctive therapy in maintenance	Positive predictors of response include: Pure mania, mixed or dysphoric mania, and patients with secondary or rapid cycling disorder. Recommended if multiple prior episodes, predominant irritable or dysphoric mood, comorbid substance abuse, or head trauma. Good response in adolescents (however, menstrual concerns for female patients). Less response noted in patients with comorbid personality disorder, severe mania, and those previously treated with antidepressants or stimulants. May be more effective in treating and preventing manic and mixed episodes
Pharmacology	Anticonvulsant, anti-kindling, and GABA-ergic activity. Blocks voltage-dependent sodium channels. May also act on other ion channels for calcium and potassium	Anticonvulsant, anti-kindling, and GABA-ergic activity. Blocks voltage-dependent sodium channels and calcium channels. Inhibits excitatory amino acids (glutamate)	Anticonvulsant and GABA-ergic activity. Blocks voltage-dependent sodium channels and calcium channels. Inhibits excitatory amino acids (glutamate)	MHD metabolite has anticonvulsant, anti-kindling, and GABA-ergic activity. Blocks voltage-dependent sodium channels and calcium channels	Anticonvulsant, anti-kindling, and GABA-ergic activity. Inhibits excitatory amino acids (glutamate). Inhibits carbonic anhydrase and blocks voltage-dependent sodium channels and calcium channels	Anticonvulsant, anti-kindling, and GABA-ergic activity. Indirectly blunts excitatory activity of glutaminergic system. Blocks calcium channels. Indirectly blocks voltage-dependent sodium channels. Increases serotonergic function

	Carbamazepine	Gabapentin	Lamotrigine	Oxcarbazepine	Topiramate	Valproate
Dosing	Begin at 200 mg daily and increase by 100 mg twice weekly, until either side effects limit dose, or therapeutic plasma level reached (auto-induction of metabolism complete by week 5 of stable dosing) Extended release: Begin at 200 mg bid and increase by 200 mg daily up to a maximum of 1600 mg/day (capsules can be opened and sprinkled on food)	Begin at 300–400 mg/day and increase by 300–400 mg a day Usual dose: 900–1800 mg/day Anxiety and neuropathic pain: Up to 3600 mg/day	Rapid titration associated with serious rash. Initial dose based on concomitant drugs prescribed; follow titration set out in product monograph	Begin at 150–300 mg/day and increase by 150 mg q 2 weeks When switching from carbamazepine, the equivalent dose is 50% higher	Begin at 25–50 mg/day and increase by 25–50 mg every 4–7 days up to 500 mg/day (a low initial dose and gradual increases minimize cognitive and behavioral side effects)	Begin at 250 mg bid and increase dose gradually, until either side effects limit dose, or therapeutic plasma level reached Once daily dosing has been used Loading dose strategy: *Oral:* Give stat dose of 20 mg/kg, then 12 h later initiate bid dosing at 10 mg/kg bid *IV:* 1200–1800 mg/day over 3 days then transition to oral *ER:* Only available in the USA, usually given once daily. Conversion from regular formulations may require 8–20% increase in total daily dose to maintain similar serum concentrations
	Dose range: 300–1600 mg/day in single or divided dose	Dose range: 900–3600 mg/day given as tid dosing (divide dosing tid due to saturable absorption) Gabapentin enacarbil dosed once daily	Dose range: 100–500 mg/day given in single or divided dose	Dose range: 600–1200 mg/day (divided doses)	Acute dose range: 200–600 mg/day Maintenance range: 50–400 mg/day	Dose range: 750–3000 mg/day in single or divided dose Maximum: 60 mg/kg/day
Renal impairment	No change	Decrease dose if CrCl less than 60 mL/min (see Precautions, p. 290)	Reduced clearance; half-life prolonged 63% in renal failure	Decrease dose by 50% if CrCl less than 30 mL/min. Start at 300 mg and increase slowly	Moderate: Clearance reduced by 42% Severe: Clearance reduced by 54% If CrCl less than 70 mL/min/1.73 m^2: Administer 50% dose and titrate more slowly	Decreased protein binding may double valproate level in renal impairment
Hepatic impairment	Reduced clearance – plasma concentrations increased by approximately 30% Do not use in active liver disease	Not hepatically metabolized	Reduce initial and maintenance doses by 25% in mild to moderate impairment and 50–75% in severe impairment	No dose adjustments required in mild to moderate impairment	Reduced clearance – plasma concentrations increased by approximately 30%; initiate same dose and titrate according to clinical outcome	See hepatic adverse effects (p. 306) and Precautions (p. 289) Hepatic disease is also associated with decreased albumin concentrations and 2- to 2.6-fold increase in unbound fraction. Free concentrations of valproate may be elevated while total concentrations appear normal. Use is contraindicated in severe impairment
Recommended plasma level	17–54 micromol/L (4–12 micrograms/mL)	2–20 mg/L reported for epilepsy (relationship between clinical efficacy and plasma concentration not clearly established)	2.5–15 mg/L reported for epilepsy (relationship between clinical efficacy and plasma concentration not clearly established)	15–35 micrograms/mL (MHD metabolite)	5–20 mg/L reported for epilepsy (relationship between clinical efficacy and plasma concentration not clearly established)	350–800 micromol/L (50–115 micrograms/mL). The higher end of the dosing range is recommended for acute mania

Comparison of Anticonvulsants (cont.)

	Carbamazepine	Gabapentin	Lamotrigine	Oxcarbazepine	Topiramate	Valproate
Pharmacokinetics						
Bioavailability	75–85%	Approx. 60% (dose dependent; higher with qid dosing)	100%	> 95%	80%	78–90%
Peak plasma level	1–6 h	2–3 h	1–5 h (rate may be reduced by food)	1–3 h (parent) 4–12 h (active MHD metabolite) and 2–4 h at steady state	2–4 h (delayed by food)	Oral valproic acid: 1–4 h (may be delayed by food) Divalproex and extended-release: 3–8 h
Protein binding	75–90%	Minimal	55%	40% (MHD)	15–41%	60–95% (concentration dependent); increased by low-fat diets. Decreased in elderly, hepatic or renal impairment, concurrent use of highly protein bound drugs
Half-life	15–35 h (acute use); 10–20 h (chronic use) – stimulates own metabolism	5–7 h	33 h mean (acute use) 26 h mean (chronic use)	Parent: 1–5 h MHD metabolite: 7–20 h	19–23 h	5–20 h
Metabolizing enzymes	CYP1A2, 3A4[(m)], 2C8, 2C9; P-gp	Not metabolized – eliminated by renal excretion	Metabolized primarily by glucuronic acid conjugation; also by UGT1A4, 2B7	Rapidly metabolized by cytosolic enzymes to active metabolite MHD	P-gp; 70% eliminated unchanged in urine	CYP2C9; UGT1A6, 1A9, 2B7
Metabolism effects	Inducer of CYP1A2[(p)], 3A4[(p)], 2C8[(p)], 2C9[(p)], 2C19[(p)], 2B6[(p)], 3A4[(p)] and UGT1A4 Induces own metabolism (auto-induction) Inducer of P-gp	–	–	Moderate inducer of CYP3A4 Inhibitor of CYP2C19[(w)] and UGT1A4 (does not induce own metabolism)	Weak inhibitor of CYP2C19; weak inducer of 3A4	Inhibitor of CYP2D6[(w)], 2C9, 2C19; UGT2B7[(p)], 2B15, 3A4[(w)]
Adverse Effects						
CNS	Sedation (11%), cognitive blunting, confusion (higher doses)	Sedation (19%), fatigue (11%), abnormal thinking, amnesia	Sedation (> 10%), asthenia, cognitive blunting, "spaced-out" feeling	Sedation (19%), lethargy	Sedation (6–15%), lethargy, fatigue (8–15%) Deficits in word finding, concentration, and memory (dose dependent, 1–11%)	Sedation (> 10%), lethargy, behavior changes/deterioration, cognitive blunting, encephalopathy
	Agitation, restlessness, irritability, insomnia May exacerbate schizophrenia on withdrawal	Nervousness, anxiety, hostility Rare switches to hypomania/mania Cases of depression	Agitation, activation, irritability, insomnia Switches to hypomania/mania		Anxiety, agitation, insomnia Increased panic attacks, worsening of depression or psychosis	Hyperactivity, aggression Case of delirium (following loading-dose strategy) Rare cases of psychosis

	Carbamazepine	Gabapentin	Lamotrigine	Oxcarbazepine	Topiramate	Valproate
	Headache		Headache (> 25%)	Headache (31%)	Headache	Headache (3%)
	Tremors, ataxia (up to 50%), paresthesias (3%), acute dystonic reactions, chronic dyskinesias	Tremors (7%), ataxia (13%), incoordination, dysarthria, myalgia Case report of acute dystonia; asterixis	Tremors, ataxia (22%), incoordination (14%), myalgia, arthralgia Case report of dystonia	Ataxia (> 25%), gait disturbances, tremor	Tremors, ataxia; paresthesias (19–51%)	Tremors (10% adults; 15% children – tend to be rhythmic, rapid, symmetrical, and most prominent in the upper extremities), ataxia, dysarthria, incoordination Association between prior use and dementia
Anticholinergic	Blurred vision (6%), mydriasis, cycloplegia, ophthalmoplegia, dry mouth, slurred speech Constipation	Dry mouth or throat (2%) Constipation	Blurred vision Constipation Dry mouth (> 5%)	Blurred vision	Blurred vision, sweating Acute angle closure reported (glaucoma)	
Gastrointestinal	Nausea (4%) Dry mouth	Nausea (4%), diarrhea (6%), dyspepsia (2%)	Nausea (19%), vomiting (9%), diarrhea (6%) Rarely esophagitis	Nausea (22%), vomiting (15%)	Nausea (4–13%), anorexia (4–15%) Change in taste of carbonated beverages	Nausea common, vomiting
Cardiovascular	Dizziness Vasculitis Cardiac conduction disorders – rare	Dizziness (17%), hypotension Occasionally hypertension Peripheral edema	Breathlessness, dizziness (38%) Conduction changes (prolongation of PR interval)	Dizziness (28%), peripheral edema, hypotension	Dizziness common	Rarely dizziness Vasculitis Case report of hyperkalemia
Dermatological	Rash (10–15%) – severe dermatological reactions may signify impending blood dyscrasias Hair loss (6%) Photosensitivity reactions Rarely: Fixed drug eruptions, lichenoid-like reactions, bullous reactions, exfoliative dermatitis Hypersensitivity syndrome – rare; with fever, skin eruptions, and internal organ involvement	Pruritus (1%), rash (1%)	Rash (up to 10%); in 2–3% require drug discontinuation – risk of severe rash increased with rapid dose titration, in children, and in combination with valproate Stevens-Johnson syndrome in 1–2% of children and 0.1% of adults (usually within first 8 weeks of therapy) Rarely, erythema multiforme, hypersensitivity syndrome Photosensitivity reactions	Rash less common than with carbamazepine; 25–30% of patients are cross-sensitive Stevens-Johnson syndrome and toxic epidermal necrolysis reported in adults and children	Rash	Rash Hair loss (up to 12% – higher incidence with higher doses); changes in texture or color of hair Case reports of nail pigmentation Rare cases of Stevens-Johnson syndrome (increased risk in combination with lamotrigine), toxic epidermal necrolysis, lupus, erythema multiforme, or skin pigmentation

Comparison of Anticonvulsants (cont.)

	Carbamazepine	Gabapentin	Lamotrigine	Oxcarbazepine	Topiramate	Valproate
Hematological	Transitory leukopenia (10%), persistent leukopenia (2%) Rarely, eosinophilia, aplastic anemia, thrombocytopenia, purpura, and agranulocytosis	Leukopenia (1%), purpura	Neutropenia Rarely, hematemesis, hemolytic anemia, thrombocytopenia, pancytopenia, aplastic anemia	Rare	Purpura	Reversible thrombocytopenia – may be related to high plasma levels; rare episodes of bleeding Macrocytic anemia, coagulopathies Case of pancytopenia (following loading-dose strategy)
Hepatic	Transient enzyme elevation (5–15%) – increased GGT due to hepatic enzyme induction common but not often clinically relevant – evaluate for hepatotoxicity if elevation > 3 times normal Rarely, hepatocellular and cholestatic jaundice, granulomatous hepatitis, and severe hepatic necrosis	Case reports of abnormal liver function	Rare	Rare Case report of increasing LFT in patient with elevated levels at baseline	Cases of severe liver damage	Asymptomatic hepatic transaminase elevation (44%) Cases of severe liver toxicity (all patients were also taking lamotrigine) Steatosis or nonalcoholic fatty liver disease (a symptom of insulin resistance)
Endocrine	Menstrual disturbances in females (up to 45%) Decreased libido in males Elevation of total cholesterol (primarily HDL) Can lower thyroxine levels and TSH response to TRH Polycystic ovaries reported in up to 22% of females; Hyperandrogenism in up to 17% Weight gain – may be independent of or secondary to peripheral edema/SIADH Occasional weight loss	Weight gain common with higher doses	Menstrual disturbances, dysmenorrhea, vaginitis No weight gain	Decreased T4 levels reported with normal T3 and TSH	Decreased sweating, hyperthermia resulting in hospitalization and some deaths; more common in children – caution with anticholinergic agents and carbonic anhydrase inhibitors Anorexia; weight loss (4–13%)	Menstrual disturbances (up to 60%) including prolonged cycles, oligomenorrhea, amenorrhea, polycystic ovaries (up to 67%) – higher incidence in obese women In females: Hyperandrogenism (increased testosterone in 33%), android obesity (in up to 53%), hirsutism, hyperinsulinemia Decreased levels of HDL, low HDL/cholesterol ratio, increased triglyceride levels Weight gain (59%) – mean gain of up to 21 kg reported; more common in females and with high plasma levels; may be associated with features of insulin resistance Weight loss (5%)
Hyponatremia	Hyponatremia and water intoxication (4–12%), more common in the elderly and with higher plasma levels			Hyponatremia (29%), higher risk in the elderly, with diuretics, and with other antiepileptic drug use	Hyponatremia (up to 25%)	

	Carbamazepine	Gabapentin	Lamotrigine	Oxcarbazepine	Topiramate	Valproate
Ocular	Diplopia (16%), nystagmus (up to 50%), visual hallucinations, lens abnormalities 2 cases of pigmentary retinopathy	Diplopia (6%), nystagmus (8%), amblyopia (4%)	Diplopia (28%) nystagmus, amblyopia	Diplopia (12%), nystagmus	Diplopia, nystagmus, visual field defects Cases of acute myopia and secondary angle closure glaucoma In patients under 50, 5-fold increased risk of angle closure glaucoma among current users of topiramate (RR = 1.23 [95% CI, 1.09–1.40]); new users (RR = 1.54 [95% CI, 1.09–2.17])	Diplopia, nystagmus, asterixis (spots before the eyes)
Osteoporosis	Can decrease vitamin D levels by increasing its metabolism, resulting in increased bone resorption, osteomalacia, osteoporosis, and fractures [bone density evaluation, supplement with calcium and vitamin D]			Conflicting reports on effects on bone mineral density	Osteomalacia and/or osteoporosis	Increased bone resorption with osteoporosis, osteopenia [bone density evaluation, supplement with calcium and vitamin D] Rarely osteomalacia
Other	Rarely: Acute renal failure, pancreatitis, splenomegaly, lymphadenopathy, systemic lupus erythematosus, and serum sickness	Rhinitis (4%), pharyngitis (3%)	Rhinitis, pharyngitis, flu-like syndrome (7%) Rarely: Apnea, pancreatitis	Upper respiratory tract infection (10%)	Nephrolithiasis (renal stone formation) in up to 1.5% with chronic use Decrease in sodium bicarbonate (in up to 30% of patients) usually mild but can be significant – see Precautions p. 290 Metabolic acidosis (may increase risk for nephrolithiasis or nephrocalcinosis Epistaxis Hyperammonemia and encephalopathy – rare reports Upper respiratory tract infection (13–26%)	Gingival hyperplasia Carnitine deficiency Rarely: Cholecystitis, pancreatitis and serum sickness Elevated ammonia levels common in valproate-treated patients, with risk of hyperammonemia encephalopathy. Consider in patients showing signs of lethargy, mental status changes

Comparison of Anticonvulsants (cont.)

	Carbamazepine	Gabapentin	Lamotrigine	Oxcarbazepine	Topiramate	Valproate
Use in Pregnancy◇	Avoid in first trimester (level A evidence). If necessary, use lowest amount possible in divided doses. Monitor drug levels throughout pregnancy, maternal α fetoprotein around week 16, and do fetal ultrasound around week 20 Concentration of drug in cord blood equals that in maternal serum Caution: Overall incidence of major malformations is 5.7%, with lower birth rates reported	Crosses placenta Fetotoxicity reported in animal studies; risk to humans is currently unknown	Crosses placenta; levels comparable to those in maternal plasma; considered a potential maintenance therapy option for pregnant women with mood disorders (level B evidence) 3.2% risk of malformations in first trimester; risk noted to increase to 5.4% when total daily dose > 200 mg	Crosses placenta; teratogenic effects reported in animals; likely to cause teratogenic effects in humans (folic acid supplementation recommended) Data on a limited number of pregnancies report cleft palate and other malformations. Case report of renal and cardiac malformations with hyponatremia and withdrawal symptoms at birth	Fetotoxicity reported in animal studies and evidence of increased risk of oral clefts NA Antiepileptic Drug Pregnancy Registry data suggests topiramate monotherapy in first trimester is associated with a 1.4% prevalence of oral clefts compared to 0.38–0.55% for infants exposed to other antiepileptic drugs	AVOID, especially in first trimester (level A evidence) Incidence of malformations is 11.1% – related to dose and drug plasma level. Fetal serum concentrations are 1.4 times that of the mother; half-life prolonged in infant If absolutely necessary, limit use to less than 1000 mg/day in 3 or more divided doses. Monitor plasma levels throughout pregnancy, maternal α fetoprotein around week 16, and do fetal ultrasound around week 20
	Risk of spina bifida up to 1%, congenital heart defects 2.9% One prospective study reported craniofacial defects in 11%, fingernail hyperplasia in 26%, and developmental delays in 20% of children exposed prenatally May cause vitamin K deficiency during latter half of gestation, resulting in bleeding [vitamin K and folic acid supplementation recommended] Clearance increased 2-fold during pregnancy; dose may need to be increased by 100%		Increased risk of cleft lip and/or cleft palate when used in first trimester (2–5%) Decreases fetal folate levels [folic acid supplementation recommended] Lamotrigine metabolism appears to be induced during pregnancy (decreased levels) and plasma levels increase rapidly after delivery	May cause vitamin K deficiency during latter half of gestation, resulting in bleeding [vitamin K and folic acid supplementation recommended]	Hypospadias in male infants [folic acid supplementation recommended] and anomalies involving various body systems	Risk of spina bifida 1–2%, neural tube defects up to 5%, neurological dysfunction and developmental deficits seen in up to 71% (FDA warning of lower cognitive test scores in children June 2011); musculoskeletal, cardiovascular, pulmonary, craniofacial, genital, and skin defects also reported May cause vitamin K deficiency during latter half of gestation, resulting in bleeding [vitamin K and folic acid supplementation recommended] Infants may be at higher risk for hypoglycemia Total plasma valproate concentration decreased during pregnancy as a result of increased volume of distribution and clearance; plasma protein binding decreased

	Carbamazepine	Gabapentin	Lamotrigine	Oxcarbazepine	Topiramate	Valproate
Breast Milk	American Academy of Pediatrics considers carbamazepine compatible with breastfeeding Breast milk contains 7–95% of maternal drug concentration; infant serum level is 6–65% of mother's Educate mother about signs and symptoms of hepatic dysfunction and CNS effects of drug in the infant Monitor liver enzymes and CBC of infant and mother No long-term cognitive or behavioral effects reported in infant	Gabapentin is excreted in breast milk. No long-term cognitive or behavioral effects reported in infant but data is limited Monitor infant for drowsiness, adequate weight gain, and developmental milestones	Excreted in breast milk; the milk/plasma ratio is about 0.6 Infant serum levels are up to 50% of those of mother Breastfeeding during lamotrigine monotherapy does not appear to adversely effect infant growth or development. Monitor for risk of life-threatening rash, drowsiness, poor sucking in infant. If lamotrigine required, not a reason to stop breastfeeding	Oxcarbazepine and active metabolite are excreted into breast milk at levels up to 50% of those in maternal plasma Effects on infant unknown Monitor for poor suckling, vomiting, and sedation. Breast feeding not recommended	Breastfeeding is not recommended due to possible psychomotor slowing and somnolence in infant; monitor infant for signs of toxicity including changes in alertness, behavior, and feeding habits	American Academy of Pediatrics considers valproate compatible with breastfeeding Infant plasma level of valproate is up to 40% of that of mother; half-life in infants is significantly longer than in adults Educate mother about the signs and symptoms of hepatic dysfunction and those of hematological abnormalities in the infant Monitor liver enzymes and CBC of infant and mother No long-term cognitive or behavioral effects reported in infant

$^{(m)}$ moderate, $^{(p)}$ potent, $^{(w)}$ weak; $\diamond$ See p. 473 for further information on drug use in pregnancy and effects on breast milk

P-gp = P-glycoprotein [*a transporter of hydrophobic substances across extra- and intra-cellular membranes that include the intestinal lumen and the blood-brain barrier*]; UGT = uridine diphosphate glucuronosyltransferase [*involved in Phase II reactions (conjugation)*]

Frequency of Adverse Reactions to Mood Stabilizers at Therapeutic Doses

Reaction	Lithium	Carbamazepine	Valproate	Gabapentin	Lamotrigine	Oxcarbazepine	Topiramate
CNS							
Drowsiness, sedation	< 2%[a]	> 10%	> 10%	> 10%	> 10%	> 10%	> 10%[b]
Headache	> 2%	> 2%	> 2%	> 10%	> 30%	> 10%	> 10%
Cognitive blunting, memory impairment	> 10%	> 2%	< 2%	> 2%	> 2%	> 2%	> 2%[b]
Weakness, fatigue	> 30%[a]	> 10%	> 10%	> 2%	> 10%	> 10%	> 10%
Insomnia, agitation	< 2%	< 2%	> 2%	> 2%	> 2%	> 2%	> 10%
Neurological							
Incoordination	< 2%[a]	> 10%	< 2%	> 2%	> 2%	> 2%	> 2%
Dizziness	–	> 10%	> 10%	> 30%	> 2%	> 10%	> 10%[b]
Ataxia	< 2%[a]	> 10%	> 10%	> 10%	> 2%	> 2%	> 2%[b]
Tremor	> 30%[a]	> 30%	> 2%	> 2%	> 10%	> 10%	> 2%
Paresthesias	–	> 2%	< 2%	< 2%	> 2%	> 2%	> 10%
Diplopia	–	> 10%	> 2%	> 10%	> 10%	> 10%	> 2%
Anticholinergic							
Blurred vision	> 2%[a]	> 2%	< 2%	> 10%	> 2	> 2%	> 2%
Cardiovascular							
ECG changes[c]	> 10%	> 2%	–	< 2%	< 2%	> 2%	–
Gastrointestinal							
Nausea, vomiting	> 30%	> 10%	> 2%	> 10%	> 10%	> 10%	> 2%
Diarrhea	> 10%[a]	> 2%	–	> 2%	> 2%	> 10%	> 2%
Weight gain	> 30%	> 2%	> 10%[b]	< 2%	> 2%	> 30%	–
Weight loss	< 2%	< 2%	< 2%	> 2%	< 2%	> 2%	> 10%[b]
Endocrine							
Hair loss, thinning	> 10%	> 2%	< 2%	–	< 2%	> 10%	< 2%
Menstrual disturbances	> 10%	> 30%	?	> 2%	< 2%	> 30%	–
Polycystic ovary syndrome	–	> 10%	> 2%	–	?	> 30%	–
Hypothyroidism	> 30%	< 2%	–	< 1%	?	< 2%	–
Polyuria, polydipsia	> 30%	> 2%	–	–	< 2%	–	–
Skin reactions, Rash	> 10%[d]	> 10%[e]	< 2%	> 10%[e]	> 2%	> 2%	< 2%
Sexual dysfunction	> 2%	< 2%	< 2%	–	–	> 2%	–
Blood dyscrasias							
Transient leukopenia	< 2%	> 10%	< 2%	< 2%	< 2%	< 2%	< 2%
Leukocytosis	> 10%	< 2%	–	–	< 2%	< 2%	–
Thrombocytopenia	–	> 2%	–	< 2%	–	> 30%[b]	–
Hepatic							
Transient enzyme elevation[f]	–	> 10%	< 2%	< 2%	< 2%	> 30%[b]	–

[a] Higher incidence and more pronounced symptoms with higher serum lithium concentration; may indicate early toxicity – monitor level   [b] Greater with higher doses;   [c] ECG abnormalities usually without cardiac injury, including ST segment depression, flattened T waves, and increased U wave amplitude;   [d] Worsening of psoriasis reported;   [e] May be first sign of impending blood dyscrasia;   [f] Evaluate for hepatotoxicity if elevation more than 3 times normal

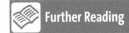**Further Reading**

References

1 Bahji A, Ermacora D, Stephenson C, et al. Comparative efficacy and tolerability of pharmacological treatments for the treatment of acute bipolar depression: A systematic review and network meta-analysis. J Affect Disord. 2020;269:154–184. doi:10.1016/j.jad.2020.03.030

2 Kennedy SH, Lam RW, McIntyre RS, et al. Canadian network for mood and anxiety treatments (CANMAT) 2016 clinical guidelines for the management of adults with major depressive disorder: Section 3. Pharmacological Treatments [published correction appears in Can J Psychiatry. 2017 May;62(5):356]. Can J Psychiatry. 2016;61(9):540–560. doi:10.1177/0706743716659417

3 Hui TP, Kandola A, Shen L, et al. A systematic review and meta-analysis of clinical predictors of lithium response in bipolar disorder. Acta Psychiatr Scand. 2019;140(2):94–115. doi:10.1111/acps.13062

4 McKnight RF, Adida M, Budge K, et al. Lithium toxicity profile: A systematic review and meta-analysis. Lancet. 2012; 379(9817):721–728. doi:10.1016/S0140-6736(11)61516-X

5 Davis J, Desmond M, Berk M. Lithium and nephrotoxicity: A literature review of approaches to clinical management and risk stratification. BMC Nephrol. 2018;19:305. doi:10.1186/s12882-018-1101-4

6 Patel RS, Bachu A, Youssef NA. Combination of lithium and electroconvulsive therapy (ECT) is associated with higher odds of delirium and cognitive problems in a large national sample across the United States. Brain Stimul. 2020;13(1):15–19. doi:10.1016/j.brs.2019.08.012

7 Martins-Ascencao R, Rodrigues-Silva N, Trovão N. Absence of longer reorientation times in patients undergoing electroconvulsive therapy and concomitant treatment with lithium. Clin Psychopharmacol Neurosci. 2021;19(4):695–704. doi:10.9758/cpn.2021.19.4.695

8 Gitlin M. Lithium side effects and toxicity: Prevalence and management strategies. Int J Bipolar Disord. 2016;4(1):27. doi:10.1186/s40345-016-0068-y

9 Elbe D, Black TR, McGrane IR, et al. Clinical handbook of psychotropic drugs for children and adolescents. (4th ed.). Boston, MA: Hogrefe Publishing, 2019.

10 Briggs GG, Freeman RK, Towers CV, et al. Drugs in pregnancy and lactation: A reference guide to fetal and neonatal risk. (11th ed.). Philadelphia, PA: Lippincott Williams & Wilkins, 2017.

11 Patorno E, Huybrechts KF, Bateman BT, et al. Lithium use in pregnancy and the risk of cardiac malformations. N Engl J Med. 2017;376(23):2245–2254. doi:10.1056/NEJMoa1612222

12 Thompson SI, El-Saden SM. Lamotrigine for treating anger in veterans with posttraumatic stress disorder. Clin Neuropharmacol. 2021;44(5):184–185. doi:10.1097/WNF.0000000000000477

13 Huang ZD, Zhao YF, Li S, et al. Comparative efficacy and acceptability of pharmaceutical management for adults with post-traumatic stress disorder: A systematic review and meta-analysis. Front Pharmacol. 2020;11:559. doi:10.3389/fphar.2020.00559

14 Zhou DD, Zhou XX, Li Y, et al. Augmentation agents to serotonin reuptake inhibitors for treatment-resistant obsessive-compulsive disorder: A network meta-analysis. Prog Neuropsychopharmacol Biol Psychiatry. 2019;90:277–287. doi:10.1016/j.pnpbp.2018.12.009

15 Mula M, Kanner AM, Schmitz B, et al. Antiepileptic drugs and suicidality: An expert consensus statement from the Task Force on Therapeutic Strategies of the ILAE Commission on Neuropsychobiology. Epilepsia. 2013;54(1):199–203. doi:10.1111/j.1528-1167.2012.03688.x

16 Gaudio M, Konstantara E, Joy M, et al. Valproate prescription to women of childbearing age in English primary care: Repeated cross-sectional analyses and retrospective cohort study. BMC Pregnancy Childbirth. 2022;22(1):73. doi:10.1186/s12884-021-04351-x

17 Goodlet KJ, Zmarlicka MT, Peckham AM. Drug-drug interactions and clinical considerations with co-administration of antiretrovirals and psychotropic drugs. CNS Spectr. 2019;24(3):287–312. doi:10.1017/S109285291800113X

Additional Suggested Reading

- Bauer MS, Miller CJ, Li M, et al. A population-based study of the comparative effectiveness of second-generation antipsychotics vs older antimanic agents in bipolar disorder. Bipolar Disord. 2016;18(6):481–489. doi:10.1111/bdi.12425

- Berlin RK, Butler PM, Perloff MD. Gabapentin therapy in psychiatric disorders: A systematic review. Prim Care Companion CNS Disord. 2015;17(5). doi:10.4088/PCC.15r01821

- Bowden CL, Mintz J, Tohen M. Multi-state outcome analysis of treatments (MOAT): Application of a new approach to evaluate outcomes in longitudinal studies of bipolar disorder. Mol Psychiatry. 2016; 21(2):237–242. doi:10.1038/mp.2015.21

- Feinn R, Curtis B, Kranzler HR. Balancing risk and benefit in heavy drinkers treated with topiramate: Implications for personalized care. J Clin Psychiatry. 2016;77(3):e278–e282. doi:10.4088/JCP.15m10053

- Smith RV, Havens JR, Walsh SL. Gabapentin misuse, abuse and diversion: A systematic review. Addiction. 2016;111(7):1160–1174. doi:10.1111/add.13324

- Yatham LN, Kennedy SH, Parikh SV, et al. Canadian Network for Mood and Anxiety Treatments (CANMAT) and International Society for Bipolar Disorders (ISBD) 2018 guidelines for the management of patients with bipolar disorder. Bipolar Disord. 2018;20(2):97–170. doi:10.1111/bdi.12609

- Zhang L, Li H, Li S, et al. Reproductive and metabolic abnormalities in women taking valproate for bipolar disorder: A meta-analysis. Eur J Obstet Gynecol Reprod Biol. 2016;202:26–31. doi:10.1016/j.ejogrb.2016.04.038

DRUGS FOR ADHD

Classification

- Drugs for ADHD can be classified as follows:

Drug Class	Agent[A]	Page
Psychostimulants	Amphetamine and related drugs (e.g., lisdexamfetamine)	See p. 312
	Methylphenidate, dexmethylphenidate[B]	
Selective norepinephrine reuptake inhibitors	Atomoxetine	See p. 323
	Viloxazine	
α_2 agonists	Clonidine	See p. 332
	Guanfacine	
Antidepressants	Bupropion	See p. 19
	Venlafaxine, desvenlafaxine	See p. 25
	Tricyclic agents	See p. 54
Dopaminergic agents	Modafinil	See p. 436
	Armodafinil[B]	

[A] Generic preparations may be available,   [B] Not marketed in Canada

Psychostimulants

Product Availability*

Generic Name	Neuroscience-based Nomenclature* (Pharmacological Target/Mode of Action)	Trade Name[A]	Dosage Forms and Strengths
Methylphenidate (MPH)	Dopamine, norepinephrine/Multimodal	ACT Methylphenidate ER[C], Apo-Methylphenidate ER[C]	Extended-release tablets: 18 mg, 27 mg, 36 mg, 54 mg
		Aptensio XR[B]	Extended-release capsules: 10 mg, 15 mg, 20 mg, 30 mg, 40 mg, 50 mg, 60 mg
		Biphentin[C]	Controlled-release capsules: 10 mg, 15 mg, 20 mg, 30 mg, 40 mg, 50 mg, 60 mg, 80 mg
		Concerta	Extended-release tablets: 18 mg, 27 mg, 36 mg, 54 mg
		Cotempla XR-ODT[B]	Extended-release orally disintegrating tablets: 8.6 mg, 17.3 mg, 25.9 mg
		Foquest[C]	Controlled-release capsules: 25 mg, 35 mg, 45 mg, 55 mg, 70 mg, 85 mg, 100 mg
		Jornay PM[B]	Delayed-release/Extended-release capsules: 20 mg, 40 mg, 60 mg, 80 mg, 100 mg

Generic Name	Neuroscience-based Nomenclature* (Pharmacological Target/Mode of Action)	Trade Name[A]	Dosage Forms and Strengths
		Metadate CD[B]	Extended-release capsules: 10 mg, 20 mg, 30 mg, 40 mg, 50 mg, 60 mg
		Methylin[B]	Oral solution: 5 mg/5 mL, 10 mg/5 mL
			Chewable tablets: 2.5 mg, 5 mg, 10 mg
		Methylin ER[B]	Extended-release tablets: 10 mg, 20 mg
		Quillichew ER[B]	Extended-release chewable tablets: 20 mg, 30 mg, 40 mg
		Quillivant XR[B]	Extended-release suspension: 5 mg/mL (after reconstitution)
		Ritalin	Tablets: 5 mg[B], 10 mg, 20 mg[B]
		Ritalin LA[B]	Extended-release capsules: 10 mg, 20 mg, 30 mg, 40 mg
		Ritalin SR[C]	Extended-release tablets: 20 mg
Methylphenidate transdermal patch[B]	Dopamine, norepinephrine/Multimodal	Daytrana	Transdermal patch: 10 mg/9 h, 15 mg/9 h, 20 mg/9 h, 30 mg/9 h
Dexmethylphenidate[B]	Dopamine, norepinephrine/Multimodal	Focalin	Tablets: 2.5 mg, 5 mg, 10 mg
		Focalin XR	Extended-release capsules 5 mg, 10 mg, 15 mg, 20 mg, 25 mg, 30 mg, 35 mg, 40 mg
Amphetamine	Dopamine, norepinephrine/Multimodal	Adzenys ER	Extended-release suspension: 1.25 mg/mL
		Adzenys XR-ODT	Extended-release orally disintegrating tablets: 3.1 mg, 6.3 mg, 9.4 mg, 12.5 mg, 15.7 mg, 18.8 mg
		Dyanavel XR	Extended-release suspension: 2.5 mg/mL
		Evekeo	Tablets: 5 mg, 10 mg
		Evekeo ODT	Orally disintegrating tablets: 5 mg, 10 mg, 15 mg, 20 mg
Dextroamphetamine/amphetamine salts (mixed amphetamine salts)	Dopamine, norepinephrine/Multimodal	Adderall[B]	Tablets: 5 mg, 7.5 mg, 10 mg, 12.5 mg, 15 mg, 20 mg, 30 mg
		Adderall XR	Extended-release capsules: 5 mg, 10 mg, 15 mg, 20 mg, 25 mg, 30 mg
		Mydayis[B]	Extended-release capsules: 12.5 mg, 25 mg, 37.5 mg, 50 mg
Dextroamphetamine	Dopamine, norepinephrine/Multimodal	Dexedrine	Tablets: 5 mg, 10 mg[B]
			Elixir: 5 mg/5 mL[B]
		Dexedrine Spansules	Extended-release capsules: 5 mg[B], 10 mg, 15 mg
		Xelstrym[B]	Transdermal system: 4.5 mg/9 h, 9 mg/9 h, 13.5 mg/9 h, 18 mg/9 h
		Zenzedi[B]	Tablets: 2.5 mg, 5 mg, 7.5 mg, 10 mg, 15 mg, 20 mg, 30 mg
Lisdexamfetamine	Dopamine, norepinephrine/Multimodal	Vyvanse	Capsules: 10 mg, 20 mg, 30 mg, 40 mg, 50 mg, 60 mg, 70 mg
			Chewable tablets: 10 mg, 20 mg, 30 mg, 40 mg, 50 mg, 60 mg
Methamphetamine[B] (desoxyephedrine)	Not listed	Desoxyn	Tablets: 5 mg

* Refer to Health Canada's Drug Product Database or the FDA's Drugs@FDA for the most current availability information. * Developed by a taskforce consisting of representatives from the American College of Neuropsychopharmacology (ACNP), the Asian College of Neuropsychopharmacology (AsCNP), the European College of Neuropsychopharmacology (ECNP), the International College of Neuropsychopharmacology (CINP), and the International Union of Basic and Clinical Pharmacology (IUPHAR) (see https://nbn2r.com), [A] Generic preparations may be available,   [B] Not marketed in Canada,   [C] Not marketed in the USA

Psychostimulants (cont.)

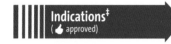

Indications‡ (👍 approved)

- 👍 Attention-deficit/hyperactivity disorder (ADHD)
- 👍 Parkinson's disease
- 👍 Narcolepsy
- 👍 Obesity (amphetamine, dextroamphetamine – USA only)
- 👍 Binge-eating disorder (lisdexamfetamine)
- Treatment-resistant depression
- Major depression in medically or surgically ill patients or in the elderly
- Augmentation of cyclic antidepressants, SSRIs, and RIMA
- ADHD in partial remission (ADHD-PR) in adults
- Chronic fatigue syndrome, neurasthenia
- Schizophrenia: Negative symptoms; some improvement noted in cognitive deficits, mood, and concentration with low doses of dextroamphetamine
- AIDS-related neuropsychiatric impairment: Improves fatigue and cognition
- Decreasing anger, irritability, and aggression in brain-injured patients, oppositional defiant disorder, conduct disorder, and ADHD – positive results with methylphenidate
- Inattention and hyperactivity in autism spectrum disorder and intellectual disability – controlled studies suggest methylphenidate has modest efficacy; adverse effects may be more problematic in this population

General Comments

- All psychostimulants, when dosed adequately, are considered to be equally effective at reducing symptoms of inattention, hyperactivity, and impulsivity
- Where possible, referral for parent behavioral management training (PBMT) should be made for children age 4 and up diagnosed with ADHD[1]
- General response occurs within the first week; response seen in approximately 75% of children and 25–78% of adults with ADHD (although individuals may respond better to one of the two stimulant classes)
- An untreated comorbid mood or anxiety disorder may diminish response to stimulants or decrease the ability to tolerate the medication – data contradictory
- Psychostimulants suggested to suppress physical and verbal aggression and reduce negative or antisocial interactions
- See Precautions (p. 319) and Contraindications (p. 319) regarding patient risks
- Careful monitoring necessary when using short-acting agents in patients with a propensity to abuse drugs or alcohol or who may be diverting for street use; when given to individuals with ADHD, they may help to decrease the risk of developing substance abuse disorder later in life
- Lisdexamfetamine is a prodrug which is converted to *d*-amphetamine following absorption. Considered to have less potential for abuse and diversion than short-acting stimulants

Pharmacology

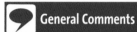

- Mechanism of action in treating ADHD is not well understood; methylphenidate blocks the reuptake of norepinephrine (NE) and dopamine (DA) into presynaptic nerve endings. In addition to blocking NE and DA reuptake, amphetamines also promote the release of DA and NE from presynaptic neurons. Increases in DA are suggested to improve attention, decrease distractibility, and modulate motivation, thus improving performance
- Release of DA and NE in subcortical limbic areas (e.g., nucleus accumbens) proposed as mechanism responsible for abuse potential of these drugs
- See chart p. 327

Dosing

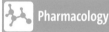

- See chart p. 328
- Treatment is often started at low doses (e.g., 5–10 mg of methylphenidate) in school-aged children and gradually increased over several days in 5 mg increments; initial improvement noted may plateau after 2–3 weeks of continuous use – this does not imply tolerance; patients, caregivers, and families should compare the plateau to baseline

‡ Indications listed here do not necessarily apply to all psychostimulants or all countries. Please refer to a country's regulatory database (e.g., US Food and Drug Administration, Health Canada Drug Product Database) for the most current availability information and indications

- Stimulant effect is not always associated with dose; methylphenidate doses above 1 mg/kg/day may not result in increased response, however, side effects can increase. Doses above 1 mg/kg/day may be tried in those who tolerate the stimulant and have had a moderate response. Some patients may be short-duration responders or high-dose responders[2]
- To minimize anorexia, give drug with or after meals; food can affect T_{max} and/or C_{max} of some formulations (see table p. 330)
- Patients who have problems swallowing pills may use one of several medications formulated as beads (Adderall XR, Aptensio XR/Biphentin, Dexedrine Spansules, Foquest, Jornay PM, Metadate CD, or Ritalin LA), by opening the capsule, sprinkling the beads on apple sauce or other soft food, and swallowing the mixture without chewing. Lisdexamfetamine capsules may be opened and the contents dispersed in a glass of plain water, orange juice or yogurt. This has the advantage of not only allowing for medication of children who cannot swallow the dose, but also of enabling fine tuning of the dose, and allowing parents to reduce the dose if necessary prior to seeing the physician. The orally disintegrating formulations of amphetamine (Evekeo ODT), mixed amphetamine salts (Adzenys XR-ODT) or methylphenidate (Cotempla XR-ODT) may be dissolved on the tongue and swallowed, and liquid suspensions of amphetamine (Dyanavel XR) and methylphenidate (Quillivant XR) are also available. There is also a methylphenidate immediate-release chewable tablet (Methylin), an extended-release chewable tablet (Quillichew ER) and a lisdexamfetamine chewable tablet (Vyvanse). Methylphenidate (Daytrana) and dextroamphetamine (Xelstrym) are also available as a transdermal skin patch that is applied in the morning and removed 9 h after application (see p. 315).
- Jornay PM is a delayed-release/extended-release methylphenidate formulation intended for evening administration, resulting in onset of stimulant action (approximately 10 h after administration) in the morning upon waking
- Divided doses required with immediate-release (IR) preparations of methylphenidate (dose approximately every 4 h). Important to document "wear-off" times (changes in behavior/attention, emergence of rebound symptoms) and adjust dosing interval accordingly
- Problems falling asleep occur most frequently when the medication is wearing off and the child experiences rebound irritability or return of symptoms. A small dose of methylphenidate at this time can minimize this effect. There is a group of children and adults who both find it easier to go to bed, and easier to fall asleep when given a low dose of stimulant before bedtime
- Methylphenidate SR has an erratic release in slightly less than half of patients and has been shown to be somewhat less effective. However, for patients who are methylphenidate SR responders, the duration of 5 h can carry them through transitions such as lunch or the bus ride home such that they get their next dose before they experience rebound. Methylphenidate IR in adequate doses usually lasts less than 3.5 h and so, if given after breakfast, may wear off before the next dose at lunchtime and, if given after lunch, may wear off before the child is home from school
- The extended-release, sustained-release, or controlled-release formulations may decrease interdose dysphoria or "wear off" phenomenon ("rebound" hyperactivity). Supplementation with short-acting preparations may be needed in the morning (to speed up onset) or in the afternoon (to extend duration of action) for some extended-release preparations with a relatively lower proportion of immediate-release stimulant such as Concerta (all others are active within 30–60 min)
- Methylphenidate transdermal patch (Daytrana): Total dose delivered is dependent on patch size and wear time. Dose delivered over 9 h: 10 mg for 27.5 mg patch, 15 mg for 41.3 mg patch, 20 mg for 55 mg patch, and 30 mg for 82.5 mg patch. Dose titration recommended on a weekly basis (9 h wear period/day), as required. Patch can be removed earlier than 9 h for shorter duration of effect or if late-day side effects are problematic
- Dextroamphetamine transdermal patch (Xelstrym): Total dose delivered is dependent on patch size and wear time. Dose delivered over 9 h: 4.05 mg for 4.5 mg patch, 8.1 mg for 9 mg patch, 12.2 mg for 13.5 mg patch, and 16.2 mg for 18 mg patch. Dose titration recommended on a weekly basis (9 h wear period/day), as required. Patch can be removed earlier than 9 h for shorter duration of effect or if late-day adverse effects are problematic
- Methylphenidate extended-release suspension (Quillivant XR): Reconstitution required prior to dispensing. Shake bottle vigorously for 10 sec prior to dose administration

Long-Acting Formulations

Drug	Drug[1]	Formulation	Duration of Effect	Usual Dosing[2]
Methylphenidate biphasic release	Aptensio XR, Biphentin	40% immediate-release beads + 60% delayed-release beads in a capsule	10–12 h	Once daily; can open and sprinkle on food
	Concerta	22% immediate-release coating + 78% delayed-release osmotic mechanism	10–12 h	Once daily
	Cotempla XR-ODT	25% immediate release + 75% delayed release formulated as an orally disintegrating tablet	12 h	Once daily; allow to disintegrate on tongue

Psychostimulants (cont.)

Drug	Drug[1]	Formulation	Duration of Effect	Usual Dosing[2]
	Foquest	20% immediate-release beads + 80% delayed-release beads in a capsule	16 h	Once daily; can open and sprinkle on food
	Metadate CD	30% immediate-release beads + 70% delayed-release beads in a capsule	8 h	Once daily
	Ritalin LA	50% immediate-release beads + 50% delayed-release beads in a capsule	6–8 h	Once daily; can open and sprinkle on food
Methylphenidate delayed release/extended release	Jornay PM	Beads coated with an extended-release layer and a delayed-release layer	10–14 h (onset delayed by 10 h)	Once daily in the evening; can open and sprinkle on food
Methylphenidate sustained/ slow release	Ritalin SR	Provides a slow continual release of drug from a wax matrix	4–6 h	Multiple daily dosing
	ACT Methylphenidate ER, Apo-Methylphenidate ER	Provides a slow continual release of drug from a polymer-coated tablet (though appearance and dosing similar to Concerta, these products do not deliver drug via an osmotic release mechanism)	10–12 h	Once daily
	Methylin ER	Provides a slow continual release of drug due to diffusion and erosion from a hydrophilic polymer	4–8 h	Multiple daily dosing
	Metadate ER	Provides a slow continual release of drug from a wax matrix	4–8 h	Multiple daily dosing
	Quillichew ER	30% immediate release + 70% delayed release formulated as a chewable tablet	8 h	Once daily
	Quillivant XR	20% immediate release + 80% delayed release formulated as a suspension for reconstitution	12 h	Once daily
Methylphenidate transdermal patch	Daytrana	Drug dispersed in an acrylic adhesive which is dispersed in a silicone adhesive. Total dose delivered is dependent on patch size and wear time (see Dosing p. 328)	Depends on length of time patch applied	Apply patch in a.m., remove after 9 h
Dexmethylphenidate extended-release	Focalin XR	50% immediate-release beads + 50% enteric-coated delayed-release beads in a capsule	10–12 h	Once daily; can open and sprinkle on food
Amphetamine	Adzenys XR-ODT	50% immediate release + 50% delayed release formulated as an orally disintegrating tablet	10–12 h	Once daily; allow to disintegrate on tongue
	Dyanavel XR	Extended-release suspension	up to 13 h	Once daily
Dextroamphetamine/ amphetamine salts	Adderall XR	50% immediate-release beads + 50% delayed-release beads in a capsule	10–12 h	Once daily; can open and sprinkle on food
	Mydayis	33.3% immediate-release beads + 33.3% each of two types of delayed-release beads (pH 5.5 release and pH 7 release) in a capsule	16 h	Once daily; can open and sprinkle on food
Dextroamphetamine	Dexedrine Spansules	50% immediate-release beads and 50% sustained-release beads in a capsule	4–9 h	Multiple daily dosing; can open and sprinkle on food
Dextroamphetamine transdermal patch	Xelstrym	Drug dispersed in an acrylic adhesive which is dispersed in a silicone adhesive. Total dose delivered dependent on patch size and wear time (see Dosing p. 315)	Depends on length of time patch applied	Apply in a.m., remove after 9 h

Drug	Drug[1]	Formulation	Duration of Effect	Usual Dosing[2]
Lisdexamfetamine	Vyvanse	Lisdexamfetamine is an inactive prodrug of *d*-amphetamine and L-lysine. The drug is converted to active dextroamphetamine as the prodrug molecule is hydrolyzed after absorption (cleaving off the amino acid)	10–13 h	Once daily (can open capsule and disperse contents in plain water, orange juice or yogurt). Chewable tablet should be chewed thoroughly before swallowing. The prolonged duration of action is from its properties as a prodrug and not due to a physical delayed-release formulation

[1] See available dosage forms in product availability table p. 312;   [2] "Usual" dosing implies: Most common dosing frequency. Note, some "once daily" stimulants are taken twice daily by some patients (e.g., adults looking for 18 h/day coverage) and some shorter-acting agents may be used once daily in some situations where a shorter daily duration of coverage is needed

Switching Formulations

- It is generally recommended to start treatment with a low dose of a long-acting preparation and titrate the dose slowly to a therapeutic level
- Conversions between dosage formulations are always approximations and are dependent on a number of factors
    - the pharmacokinetics of each preparation, including the duration of action of each product
    - the patient's age and weight (dosing recommendations are often based on weight)
    - the patient's response may vary between preparations of the same drug
- Check specific product labelling prior to attempting conversion. Due to differences in formulation and in drug base concentrations, many products are now considered non-interchangeable, with several product manufacturers recommending re-titration from starting dosages
- It is always important to monitor both response and adverse effects at each dosage level

Dosage Conversion

Immediate-Release Drug	Extended-Release Products (Daily Dose)
Methylphenidate	
5 mg bid-tid	Metadate/Methylin ER, Biphentin, or Ritalin LA 10–20 mg, or Metadate CD 10–20 mg, or Concerta 18 mg
10 mg bid-tid	Metadate/Methylin ER, Biphentin, or Ritalin LA 20–30 mg, or Ritalin SR 20 mg, or Metadate CD 30 mg, or Concerta 27–36 mg
15 mg bid-tid	Metadate/Methylin ER, Biphentin, or Ritalin LA 30–40 mg, or Ritalin SR 40 mg, or Metadate CD 30–40 mg, or Concerta 36–54 mg
20 mg bid-tid	Metadate/Methylin ER, Biphentin, or Ritalin LA 40–50 mg, or Ritalin SR 40–60 mg, or Concerta 54–72 mg
30 mg bid	Metadate/Methylin ER, Biphentin, or Ritalin LA 50–60 mg, or Ritalin SR 60 mg, or Concerta 72 mg[*]
Dexmethylphenidate	
Focalin 2.5 mg bid	Focalin XR 5 mg daily
Dextroamphetamine/amphetamine salts	
Adderall 5 mg bid	Adderall XR 10 mg daily
Dextroamphetamine	
5 mg bid	Dexedrine Spansules 10 mg daily (large inter-patient variance noted in conversion, from 1:1 to about 1:1.5)

[*] This amount comes from taking 2 × 36 mg tablets and roughly equates to about 15 mg a.m. and 45 mg after lunch of methylphenidate IR

Note: Conversion to methylphenidate transdermal patch (Daytrana) or dextroamphetamine transdermal patch (Xelstrym) from other formulations is currently unknown; individual patient titration recommended (see Dosing p. 315)

Conversion to lisdexamfetamine (Vyvanse) not recommended; start patient at 20–30 mg daily and titrate to effective dose

Conversion to methylphenidate extended-release suspension (Quillivant XR) and chewable tablets (Quillichew ER) is not recommended; start patients 6 years of age or older at 20 mg daily and titrate to effective dose.

Conversion to methylphenidate extended-release capsules (Aptensio XR/Biphentin or Foquest) is not recommended. Start patients 6 years of age or older at the smallest available dosage (10 mg daily for Aptensio XR/Biphentin or 25 mg daily for Foquest).

Conversion to methylphenidate extended-release orally disintegrating tablets (Cotempla XR-ODT) is not recommended; start patients 6 years of age or older at 17.3 mg daily and titrate in 10 mg increments to effective dose.

Conversion to Jornay PM is not recommended; start patients 6 years of age or older at 20 mg daily administered in the evening between 6:30 p.m. and 8:30 p.m. and titrate to effective dose, adjust administration based on response to achieve desired time of onset of action.

Conversion to amphetamine tablets (Evekeo) or suspension (Dyanavel XR) or amphetamine orally disintegrating tablets (Adzenys XR-ODT) or mixed amphetamine salts extended-release capsules (Mydayis) is not recommended. To avoid substitution errors and overdosage, do not substitute for other amphetamine products on a milligram-per-milligram basis because of different amphetamine base compositions and differing pharmacokinetic profiles

Psychostimulants (cont.)

 Pharmacokinetics

- See chart p. 329
- Large interindividual variation in absorption and bioavailability; food may affect T_{max} and C_{max} for some formulations (see table p. 330)
- Transdermal patches release drug at a steady rate per hour, related to dose. Absorption and C_{max} may increase with chronic dosing; rate and extent of absorption increase if patch applied to inflamed skin or if heat applied over patch
- Lisdexamfetamine is converted to d-amphetamine and L-lysine by enzymatic hydrolysis; peak plasma concentration of d-amphetamine after 50 mg dose of lisdexamfetamine is approximately equivalent to 15–30 mg of immediate-release d-amphetamine
- ACT Methylphenidate ER and Apo-Methylphenidate ER are similar in appearance and available dosage strengths to Concerta, and are marketed as generic forms of Concerta; however, these products are extended-release polymer-coated tablets and do not deliver drug via an osmotic-controlled release mechanism. While they meet Health Canada bioequivalence standards, in single-dose studies, time to peak methylphenidate blood level (T_{max}) is not an aspect of the bioequivalence definition; T_{max} may occur up to 3 h earlier with generic formulations compared to Concerta
- With the methylphenidate transdermal patch, it takes about 8 h after patch application for blood concentrations to reach maximum level. Substantial amounts of drug remain in the body for about 6 h after patch removal
- With the dextroamphetamine transdermal patch, it takes about 6 h after patch application for blood concentrations to reach maximum level. Substantial amounts of drug remain in the body for about 24 h after patch removal, with evidence of accumulation (104% increase in AUC) after repeated daily application compared to following a single patch application

 Onset & Duration of Action

- See chart p. 329

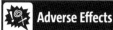 **Adverse Effects**

- See chart p. 331
- Common adverse effects include restlessness, irritability, anxiety, insomnia, anorexia, stomachache, tics, headaches, and worsening of aggressive behavior or hostility at start of therapy. Paradoxical psychiatric effects such as rebound, restlessness, irritability, anxiety, and increased aggression may be observed. The slower the rate of titration, the less severe the initial side effects. Many of these psychiatric and somatic side effects may endure throughout treatment, making drug holidays useful to assess impact of relative risk vs. benefit, and necessitating the regular monitoring of growth
- Drug-induced insomnia [can be managed by changing dose timing or formulation based on expected duration of action; addition of melatonin, sedating antihistamines or trazodone (25–50 mg) at bedtime or clonidine 100 micrograms given 2 h before bedtime]. When stimulants wear off at the end of the day, patient may experience rebound or a period of irritability and return of ADHD symptoms in excess of baseline – this may cause difficulty in falling asleep
- Anorexia, GI distress, and weight loss are common [can be minimized by taking medication with meals, eating smaller meals more frequently or drinking high-calorie fluids (e.g., Boost, Ensure, smoothies made with whole milk), drinking when thirsty and eating before bedtime]; if weight loss is evident (in patients who are not obese), despite attempts to increase caloric intake, and compromising the child's health or growth, consider switching to a shorter-acting agent that allows for return of appetite late in the day, or use of a non-stimulant such as atomoxetine or guanfacine
- Headache most common 2–3 h after a dose (tension-like or "achy"); tends to decrease over time [acetaminophen may be used as required]
- Hyperactive rebound can occur in the afternoon or evening [an earlier second dose, more frequent dosing or the use of extended-release preparations can be tried]
- Dysphoria or sadness has been noted to occur in patients taking stimulants, both during the day and when they are wearing off; more common with amphetamine-based products
- Recent FDA and Health Canada warning re: priapism with methylphenidate dose increase or discontinuation; case reports of priapism in patients taking amphetamine-based stimulants (though patients were also taking other medications and causality could not be established)
- Chemical leukoderma (permanent loss of skin color) with methylphenidate patch (Daytrana)
- Single case report of eosinophilic hepatitis with lisdexamfetamine
- Single case report of sudden, irreversible hearing loss following first dose of methylphenidate in a child

- Two cases of alopecia areata associated with Concerta, which resolved with dechallenge and did not recur with switch to an alternative extended-release methylphenidate formulation[3]
- Case report of hyperhidrosis, excessive thirst, polydipsia, hyponatremia, and status epilepticus following methylphenidate overdose (single 1.5 mg/kg dose) in an 8-year-old boy

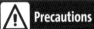 **D/C Discontinuation Syndrome**

- Abrupt withdrawal after prolonged use may result in dysphoria, irritability or a rebound in symptoms of ADHD; increase in sleep and appetite reported
- If a stimulant is taken in conjunction with an antipsychotic, sudden discontinuation of the stimulant may result in the emergence of extrapyramidal symptoms previously masked by the stimulant's anticholinergic properties and competition for D_2 receptors
- Case of priapism reported in 16-year-old each time he forgot to take his dose of extended-release methylphenidate (Concerta) 54 mg

⚠ Precautions

- Patients should be screened for cardiovascular risks by history[4] (early cardiac death in the family, syncope, chest pain on exertion, etc.) and given a physical exam. An ECG or cardiology consult should be considered[5] but, if not done, should not necessarily impede therapy if no evidence of cardiac concerns is present. If cardiac risk factors are present, the patient and/or parents should be informed of the relative risk and benefit of their treatment options, and treatment should only proceed with the consent of a cardiologist
- Canadian warning: ADHD drugs may increase risk of suicidal thoughts and behaviors in some people; benefits still outweigh risks. Suicidal thinking should be assessed at baseline prior to starting and periodically while on treatment
- Use cautiously in patients with anxiety, tension, agitation, restlessness, untreated psychosis, bipolar disorder, anorexia nervosa/disordered eating, renal impairment or peripheral vasculopathy (including Raynaud's phenomenon)
- May lower the seizure threshold (contradictory data); when starting stimulants in children with ADHD and seizures, ensure adequate seizure prophylaxis is employed and perform careful monitoring pre and post stimulant treatment for each individual. In the literature, there is more information regarding tolerability of methylphenidate compared to amphetamine-based treatments in regard to impact on seizure threshold
- May precipitate manic or hypomanic symptoms in a patient with undiagnosed bipolar disorder and exacerbate psychotic symptoms
- Some manufacturers advise periodic CBC monitoring in patients on long-term therapy due to rare reports of anemia and leukopenia secondary to nutritional deficiency
- Chronic abuse in patients can lead to tolerance and psychic dependence; drug dependence is rare; drug abuse or diversion is a risk, especially in children with comorbid conduct or substance use disorders. Stimulants can be abused orally, intravenously or nasally and may be combined with other drugs
- Tic disorders; research investigating increased risk of tics with the use of stimulants has yielded contradictory results. Tics tend to wax and wane, often independent of therapy, though clinicians have commented that stimulants can unmask tics
- Use with caution and with careful monitoring in patients with a history of alcohol and/or drug abuse
- Patients with structural cardiac abnormalities may benefit from treatment of ADHD but require close monitoring; coordination with cardiologist recommended[6]
- Some patients become tolerant to stimulant effects over time; may require an increased dosage or a drug holiday[2]
- Application of external heat (e.g., heating pad, sauna, etc.) over Daytrana or Xelstrym patch results in temperature-dependent increased drug release (Daytrana: 2.5-fold; Xelstrym: 50% increase)
- Caution when switching from Concerta to ACT Methylphenidate ER or Apo-Methylphenidate ER formulation as medication delivery system and pharmacokinetics are not the same; time to peak serum level (T_{max}) is several hours shorter with some generic formulations compared to Concerta; Health Canada has received numerous reports of shortened duration of action with loss of ADHD symptom control for patients following switch from Concerta to one of the generic formulations

🛑 Contraindications

- Patients with symptomatic cardiovascular disease, tachyarrhythmias, severe angina pectoris, moderate to severe hypertension
- Use cautiously and with careful monitoring in patients with a recent history of alcohol and/or drug abuse
- Anorexia nervosa
- Severe anxiety, tension, or agitation
- Uncontrolled hyperthyroidism, pheochromocytoma, narrow-angle glaucoma
- Within 14 days of taking MAOIs

Psychostimulants (cont.)

Toxicity	• See p. 332
Lab Tests/Monitoring	• Baseline: Height (children), weight, blood pressure, and pulse and repeat regularly throughout treatment. Patients with a prior or family history of cardiac disease should be further evaluated via ECG and cardiology consult, including echocardiogram as necessary. Cardiac evaluation recommended if patient experiences excessive increase in blood pressure or pulse, exertional chest pain, or unexplained syncope
Pediatric Considerations	• For detailed information on the use of psychostimulants in this population, please see the *Clinical Handbook of Psychotropic Drugs for Children and Adolescents*[7] • Psychostimulants used consistently in children and young teenagers over a period of years have been demonstrated to lead to reduction in adult height. Monitor height and weight (children) to ensure children are growing as per usual growth charts [if more than 10% of body weight is lost in a person of normal height and weight or if ongoing monitoring of the child indicates that they are no longer growing along their expected growth curve, consider dose reduction, periodic drug holidays, or switching treatment]. Recent data from long-term follow up of methylphenidate-treated children into young adulthood reported an association of decreased adult height with increasing exposure to methylphenidate. The pooled group of consistent and inconsistent stimulant users had a mean reduction in adult height of 2.55 cm compared to negligible stimulant users with ADHD[8] • May precipitate psychotic symptoms in children with a genetic predisposition or prior history of psychosis; risk of inducing hypomania, mania, depression or a combination (mixed features) in patients with a mood disorder. A recent meta-analysis does not support an association between new onset or worsening tics and psychostimulant use,[9] though data is contradictory. Clinicians may want to consider rechallenge of patients who report new onset or worsening of tics with psychostimulant treatment. With support, some of these patients may be able to be successfully established on psychostimulant treatment
Geriatric Considerations	• Useful in the treatment of elderly or medically ill patients with major depression (see Precautions p. 319 and Contraindications p. 319 with regard to cardiac status) • Dosing before breakfast and lunch may facilitate daytime activity • Initiate dosage gradually and increase in small increments every 2–3 days as tolerated
Use in Pregnancy◇	• See p. 332
Nursing Implications	• Ensure that beaded, sustained/extended-release, or osmotic-controlled release formulations are not chewed but opened and sprinkled on food or swallowed whole as appropriate for the dosage form (exception: Quillichew ER is intended to be chewed) • For patients who have difficulty swallowing medications whole, Adderall XR, Aptensio XR/Biphentin, Dexedrine Spansules, Foquest, Jornay PM, Metadate CD, Mydayis, or Ritalin LA can be prescribed; capsule can be opened and the beads sprinkled on applesauce, yogurt or other soft food and swallowed without chewing. Lisdexamfetamine (Vyvanse) capsules can be opened and the contents dispersed in a glass of plain water, orange juice or yogurt. Other alternatives include orally disintegrating tablets (Adzenys XR-ODT, Cotempla XR-ODT, Evekeo ODT), liquid suspension (Quillivant XR, Dyanavel XR), chewable tablets (Quillichew ER, Vyvanse Chewable), or transdermal patch (Daytrana or Xelstrym) • Monitor for adverse effects and changes in concentration, mood, and activity level; report any changes in behavior or in sleeping or eating habits • In patients with ADHD who drive, improvements in driving have been seen while on medication. Patients with a history of involvement in motor vehicle accidents should be cautioned about driving without first having taken medication or after medication effects have worn off (e.g., in the evening and night time) • Patients should be informed that abrupt discontinuation of treatment may lead to exacerbation of symptoms • Doses of psychostimulants in latter part of day (e.g., after noon for extended-release formulations or after 4 p.m. for immediate-release formulations) may cause insomnia

◇ See p. 473 for further information on drug use in pregnancy and effects on breast milk

- Monitor heart rate and BP prior to starting treatment and after dose increases
- Patients should be advised that the Concerta tablet shell does not dissolve and may be seen in the stool after a bowel movement; this is normal and the medication has still been absorbed
- Daytrana patch should be applied (immediately following removal from protective pouch) to clean, dry skin on the hip, 2 h before desired effect, and removed 9 h after application; advise patient not to apply patch to inflamed skin and to avoid exposing area of application to external heat (e.g., electric heating pads). Dispose patch by folding together the adhesive side – used patch can be disposed of in a lidded container or flushed down the toilet (do not flush in areas with septic tank service). NOTE: There have been several reports describing difficulties in removing the protective lining to expose the adhesive surface of Daytrana
- Xelstrym patch should be applied (immediately following removal from protective pouch) to clean, dry skin on hip, upper arm, chest, upper back or flank, 2 h before desired effect, and removed 9 h after application. Rotate application sites. Dispose patch by folding together the adhesive side – used patch should be disposed in a lidded container. Do not flush down the toilet
- Methylphenidate XR suspension: Reconstitution required prior to dispensing. Shake bottle vigorously for 10 sec prior to dose administration
- Amphetamine XR suspension: Shake bottle well prior to dispensing and prior to each use

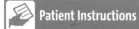 **Patient Instructions**

- For detailed patient instructions on psychostimulants, see the Patient Information Sheet (details p. 474)

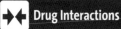 **Drug Interactions**

- Clinically significant interactions are listed below
- For more interaction information on any given combination, also see the corresponding chapter for the second agent

DRUGS INTERACTING WITH METHYLPHENIDATE AND DEXMETHYLPHENIDATE

Class of Drug	Example	Interaction Effects
Alcohol		*In vitro* studies show altered drug release characteristics with certain methylphenidate long-acting formulations (84–98% of total methylphenidate dose released within the first 30–60 min) when taken with alcohol (40% concentration). Interactions are formulation specific
α₂ agonist	Clonidine, guanfacine	Additive effect on sleep, hyperactivity, and aggression associated with ADHD. Consider ECG monitoring. Published case series of sudden death with combination clonidine and methylphenidate use. However, Kapvay (clonidine XR) is FDA approved and Intuniv/Intuniv XR (guanfacine XR) is FDA/Health Canada approved for combination use with stimulants in children and adolescents
Antibacterial	Linezolid	Linezolid inhibits MAO enzymes – AVOID combination (discontinue stimulant while linezolid used)
Anticoagulant	Warfarin	Decreased metabolism of anticoagulant Increased INR response
Anticonvulsant	Carbamazepine	Decreased plasma level of methylphenidate due to increased metabolism
	Phenobarbital, phenytoin, primidone	Possible increased level of phenytoin, phenobarbital, and primidone due to metabolism inhibition by methylphenidate
Antidepressant SSRI	Fluoxetine, sertraline	Potentiated effect in depression, dysthymia, and OCD, in patients with comorbid ADHD; may improve response in treatment-refractory paraphilias and paraphilia-related disorders Plasma level of antidepressant may be increased
SNRI	Desvenlafaxine, duloxetine, venlafaxine	Case report of serotonin syndrome with methylphenidate after one dose of venlafaxine given
NaSSA	Mirtazapine	May increase agitation and risk of mania, especially in patients with bipolar disorder
Tricyclic	Amitriptyline, desipramine	Used together to augment antidepressant effect Plasma level of tricyclic antidepressants may be increased due to metabolism inhibition by methylphenidate Cardiovascular effects increased, with combination, in children; monitor blood pressure and ECG Case reports of neurotoxic effects with imipramine, but considered rare; monitor

Psychostimulants (cont.)

Class of Drug	Example	Interaction Effects
RIMA	Moclobemide	Increased blood pressure and enhanced effect if used over prolonged period or in high doses
MAOI (Irreversible)	Phenelzine, tranylcypromine	Release of large amount of norepinephrine while ability to metabolize monoamines blocked by MAOI, leading to hypertensive reaction – AVOID; combination used very RARELY to augment antidepressant therapy with strict monitoring
Antihistamine	Diphenhydramine	Antagonism of sedative effects by stimulant
Antipsychotic	General	Antipsychotics can counteract many signs of stimulant toxicity (e.g., anxiety, aggression, visual or auditory hallucinations, psychosis), may impair the stimulatory effect of amphetamines, and have additive adverse effects (e.g., insomnia, restlessness, tremor) Methylphenidate may exacerbate or prolong withdrawal dyskinesia following antipsychotic discontinuation; conversely, following stimulant discontinuation, antipsychotic-related extrapyramidal side effects may emerge
	Olanzapine, quetiapine	Two case reports of priapism with concurrent use of stimulants
	Risperidone	Case reports of rebound dystonia when stimulant medication was withdrawn from patients taking risperidone. May be due to supersensitivity of dopamine receptors and/or removal of anticholinergic activity of stimulant
Disulfiram		Case of psychotic-like episode with concurrent use, possibly via disulfiram's action in blocking dopamine-beta-hydroxylase, whose low levels have been associated with ADHD and psychotic symptoms
Herbal preparation	Ephedra, St. John's wort, yohimbine	May cause hypertension, arrhythmias, and/or CNS stimulation
	Ginkgo biloba	Seizure threshold may be lowered with combination
Theophylline		Reports of increased tachycardia, palpitations, dizziness, weakness, and agitation

DRUGS INTERACTING WITH DEXTROAMPHETAMINE AND LISDEXAMFETAMINE

Class of Drug	Example	Interaction Effects
Alcohol		In vitro studies show altered drug release characteristics of certain formulations when taken with alcohol (40% concentration). Interactions are formulation specific
α_2 agonist	Clonidine, guanfacine	Additive effect on sleep, hyperactivity, and aggression associated with ADHD. Consider ECG monitoring. Published case series of sudden death with combination clonidine and methylphenidate use. However, Kapvay (clonidine XR) is FDA approved and Intuniv/Intuniv XR (guanfacine XR) is FDA/Health Canada approved for combination use with stimulants in children and adolescents
Acidifying agent	Ammonium chloride, ascorbic acid, fruit juices	Decreased absorption, increased elimination, and decreased plasma level of dextroamphetamine
Alkalinizing agent	Potassium citrate, sodium bicarbonate	Increased absorption, prolonged half-life, decreased elimination, and increased plasma level of dextroamphetamine
Antibiotic	Linezolid	Linezolid inhibits MAO enzymes – AVOID combination (discontinue stimulant while linezolid used)
Anticonvulsant	Valproic acid	Valproate may attenuate the effects of dextroamphetamine on mood changes, cognitive tasks, and blood pressure, possibly via opposing pharmacological actions on dopamine and norepinephrine release and uptake; clinical significance unclear
Antidepressant SSRI	Fluoxetine, sertraline	Potentiated effect in depression, dysthymia, and OCD, in patients with comorbid ADHD; may improve response in treatment-refractory paraphilias and paraphilia-related disorders Plasma level of antidepressant may be increased
NaSSA	Mirtazapine	May increase agitation and risk of mania, especially in patients with bipolar disorder

Class of Drug	Example	Interaction Effects
Tricyclic	Amitriptyline, desipramine	May enhance the stimulatory effect of amphetamines. Tricyclics may also potentiate the cardiovascular effects of amphetamines
RIMA	Moclobemide	Slightly enhanced effect if used over prolonged period or in high doses
MAOI (Irreversible)	Phenelzine, tranylcypromine	Hypertensive crisis due to increased norepinephrine release while ability to metabolize monoamines is blocked by MAOI; AVOID
Antipsychotic	Chlorpromazine	Dextroamphetamine can oppose the antipsychotic effects of chlorpromazine with detrimental effects on the control of schizophrenic symptoms; chlorpromazine may antagonize the effects of amphetamines and has been shown to treat amphetamine overdose
β-blocker	Propranolol	Increased blood pressure and tachycardia due to unopposed α stimulation
Urinary acidifier	Ammonium chloride	Increased excretion of dextroamphetamine
Urinary alkalinizer	Acetazolamide, sodium bicarbonate	Decreased excretion of dextroamphetamine; psychoses via amphetamine retention from alkaline urine has been described

Selective Norepinephrine Reuptake Inhibitors

 Product Availability*

Generic Name	Neuroscience-based Nomenclature* (Pharmacological Target/Mode of Action)	Trade Name[(A)]	Dosage Forms and Strengths
Atomoxetine	Norepinephrine/Reuptake inhibitor	Strattera	Capsules: 10 mg, 18 mg, 25 mg, 40 mg, 60 mg, 80 mg, 100 mg
Viloxazine	Norepinephrine/Reuptake inhibitor	Qelbree[(B)]	Extended-release capsules: 100 mg, 150 mg, 200 mg

* Refer to Health Canada's Drug Product Database or the FDA's Drugs@FDA for the most current availability information. • Developed by a taskforce consisting of representatives from the American College of Neuropsychopharmacology (ACNP), the Asian College of Neuropsychopharmacology (AsCNP), the European College of Neuropsychopharmacology (ECNP), the International College of Neuropsychopharmacology (CINP), and the International Union of Basic and Clinical Pharmacology (IUPHAR) (see https://nbn2r.com), (A) Generic preparations may be available, (B) Not marketed in Canada

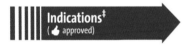 **Indications‡** (approved)

- 🔹 ADHD in children, adolescents, and adults (atomoxetine), in children and adolescents aged 6–17 years (viloxazine)
- Comorbid anxiety disorder: May reduce anxiety symptoms

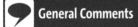 **General Comments**

- Most ADHD treatment guidelines list atomoxetine as a second-line agent. May be effective for some patients who have not responded to stimulant treatment, who have comorbid anxiety, or individuals who have an active comorbid substance use disorder. Benefits include a lack of euphoria, a lower risk of rebound, a lower risk of induction of tics or psychosis, low abuse potential, and increased somnolence
- Where possible, referral for parent behavioral management training (PBMT) should be made for children age 4 and up diagnosed with ADHD[1]
- Available evidence indicates that stimulants, atomoxetine, and viloxazine have been found to be superior to placebo for reducing the severity of ADHD symptoms on average in the short term
- Atomoxetine has a delayed onset of action and response may take up to 4 weeks – titrate dose gradually to help mitigate adverse effects (especially in patients who may be CYP2D6 poor metabolizers: ~10% of the population). Response is first seen at 4 weeks of full dose and full optimization of drug response requires at least 3 months
- Viloxazine response is first seen after 1 week of treatment. No dose adjustment required in CYP2D6 poor metabolizers
- Ultrarapid metabolizers of CYP2D6 (28% of North Africans, Ethiopians, and Arabs; 3% of African Americans; up to 2% of Caucasians; and up to 1% of Hispanics, Chinese, and Japanese) would be expected to have reduced efficacy of atomoxetine
- Selective NRIs reduce both the inattentive and hyperactive/impulsive symptom clusters of ADHD

‡ Indications listed here do not necessarily apply to all countries. Please refer to a country's regulatory database (e.g., US Food and Drug Administration, Health Canada Drug Product Database) for the most current availability information and indications

Selective Norepinephrine Reuptake Inhibitors (cont.)

- Head-to-head studies show greater reductions in ADHD symptoms (net effect size difference = 0.3) and a greater percentage of responders with stimulants when compared to atomoxetine. There are currently no published studies comparing viloxazine to other ADHD treatments
- A large head-to-head trial of OROS-methylphenidate (Concerta) vs. atomoxetine in over 600 children demonstrated that 40% of children who do not respond to methylphenidate are responders to atomoxetine, indicating selective response

Pharmacology

- Selectively block the reuptake of norepinephrine; increase dopamine and norepinephrine in the frontal cortex (without increasing dopamine in subcortical areas) – lead to cognitive enhancement without abuse liability; suggested to be important in regulating attention, impulsivity, and activity levels
- No stimulant or euphoriant activity – may be advantageous in patients with comorbid substance use disorder

Dosing

- See chart p. 328

Atomoxetine

- Dosing is based on body weight
- Children and adolescents up to 70 kg: See table p. 328; do not exceed 1.4 mg/kg or 100 mg/day, whichever is less
- Adults and children over 70 kg: See table p. 328; maximum of 100 mg/day. Doses greater than 100 mg/day have not been found to result in additional therapeutic benefit
- In patients with moderate hepatic dysfunction, reduce dose by 50%; in severe hepatic dysfunction, reduce dose to 25% of the usual recommended dosage
- No dose adjustment required in renal insufficiency; may exacerbate hypertension in patients with end-stage renal disease
- If atomoxetine is added to a regimen in combination with drugs that inhibit CYP2D6 or patient is a known CYP2D6 poor metabolizer (see Drug Interactions p. 327): Initiate atomoxetine at 0.5 mg/kg/day as above but do not increase to the usual target dose unless symptoms fail to improve *after 4 weeks* and the initial dose is well tolerated
- If a strong CYP2D6 inhibitor such as paroxetine, fluoxetine, or bupropion is added to a regimen containing atomoxetine, dosage reduction of atomoxetine should be considered (see Drug Interactions p. 327)
- For CYP2D6 ultrarapid metabolizers, be alert to reduced efficacy of atomoxetine – there are insufficient data to allow for an adjusted dose to be calculated, therefore an alternative drug may need to be prescribed

Viloxazine

- Children: 100 mg daily for 1 week, then may increase in 100 mg increments weekly to maximum of 400 mg/day depending on response and tolerability
- Adolescents: 200 mg daily for 1 week, then may increase to 400 mg/day depending on response and tolerability
- No dose adjustment required with mild or moderate renal insufficiency. In patients with severe renal dysfunction, starting dose of 100 mg/day, then may increase in 50–100 mg increments weekly to maximum of 200 mg/day depending on response and tolerability
- Avoid use with hepatic dysfunction
- Do not cut, crush or chew capsule. May open capsule and sprinkle contents on soft food (e.g., applesauce) prior to administration (consume within 2 h)

Pharmacokinetics

Atomoxetine

- Rapidly absorbed; may be taken with or without food – high-fat meal decreases rate but not extent of absorption (C_{max} delayed by 3 h and is 37% lower)
- Bioavailability: 63%; 94% in CYP2D6 poor metabolizers
- Protein binding: 98% for atomoxetine and 69% for the hydroxyatomoxetine metabolite
- Peak plasma level reached in 1–2 h; 3–4 h in CYP2D6 poor metabolizers
- Half-life is 5 h for atomoxetine and 6–8 h for hydroxyatomoxetine; in CYP2D6 poor metabolizers the values are 21.6 h and 34–40 h, respectively; metabolized primarily by CYP2D6, also by CYP2C19

- Hepatic dysfunction: 2-fold increase in atomoxetine AUC in moderate hepatic insufficiency and 4-fold increase in AUC in severe hepatic dysfunction (see Dosing above)

Viloxazine

- May be taken with or without food – high-fat meal decreases rate of absorption and slightly decreases extent of absorption (C_{max} delayed by 2 h and 9% lower, AUC 8% lower)
- Bioavailability: 88% (compared to (unmarketed) immediate-release formulation)
- Protein binding: 76–82%
- Peak plasma level reached in 5 h
- Half-life: 7 h

 Adverse Effects

- See table p. 331

Atomoxetine

- Common: Rhinitis, upper abdominal pain, nausea, vomiting, decreased appetite, weight loss (seen initially, especially if dose titrated too rapidly, but levels off with time), dizziness, headache, fatigue, emotional lability, insomnia is more common in adults, somnolence in children
- Less frequent: Irritability, aggression, sedation, depression, dry mouth, constipation, mydriasis, tremor, pruritus, tics, and urinary retention
- Small increases in blood pressure and pulse can occur at start of treatment; usually plateau with time
- Sexual dysfunction (2%) including erectile disturbance, impotence, and abnormal orgasm, case report of priapism
- Rare cases of elevated hepatic enzymes and bilirubin; severe hepatic injury reported; injury reversed when atomoxetine withdrawn (none required liver transplant); one adult died from hepatic and renal failure (the nature of the hepatic injury was considered to be idiosyncratic so that routine LFT monitoring is of little benefit)
- Increased risk of suicidal ideation in children and adolescents (see Precautions p. 325)
- Case report of atomoxetine-induced hypothermia in an 11-year-old boy

Viloxazine

- Common: Somnolence, decreased appetite, fatigue, nausea, vomiting, insomnia, irritability, increased blood pressure and pulse rate
- Less frequent: Fever, abdominal pain, weight loss, upper respiratory tract infection
- Increased risk of suicidal ideation in children and adolescents (see Precautions)

 Discontinuation Syndrome

- Evidence that no drug discontinuation or withdrawal syndrome exists for atomoxetine. Manufacturer states that atomoxetine may be discontinued without tapering of the dose. ADHD symptoms will return gradually following discontinuation. No information available with viloxazine

 Precautions

Atomoxetine

- Use with caution in patients with cardiovascular disease, including hypertension, arteriosclerosis, and tachyarrhythmias. Do a cardiac history and physical assessment prior to prescribing atomoxetine and evaluate symptoms suggestive of cardiac disease that develop during treatment
- Due to risk of hypertension, use cautiously in any condition that may predispose patients to hypertension
- Use caution in patients with liver dysfunction – see Dosing above
- Use with caution in patients with asthma being treated with oral or intravenous β_2 agonists (e.g., albuterol/salbutamol) (okay with inhaled β_2 agonist treatment)
- Use with caution in patients with peripheral vasculopathy (including Raynaud's phenomenon)
- Use with caution in known CYP2D6 poor metabolizers (see Dosing p. 324)
- Cases of liver injury reported (rare); discontinue drug in patients with jaundice or laboratory evidence of liver injury – rechallenge not advised
- Patients with structural cardiac abnormalities may benefit from treatment of ADHD but require close monitoring; coordination with cardiologist recommended[6]
- Atomoxetine has been associated with adverse psychiatric effects such as anger, hostility, irritability or suicidal ideation and that if these occur the drug dose should be lowered or discontinued. Suicidal thinking should be assessed at baseline prior to starting and periodically while on treatment

Viloxazine

- Use with caution in patients with personal/family history of suicide, bipolar disorder or depression. Suicidal thinking should be assessed at baseline prior to starting and periodically while on treatment

Selective Norepinephrine Reuptake Inhibitors (cont.)

 Contraindications

Atomoxetine
- Patients with symptomatic cardiovascular disease, tachyarrhythmias, moderate to severe hypertension, severe angina, or advanced ateriosclerosis
- Should not be administered together with a MAOI or within 2 weeks of discontinuing a MAOI
- Uncontrolled hyperthyroidism, pheochromocytoma, or narrow-angle glaucoma

Viloxazine
- Should not be administered together with a MAOI or within 2 weeks of discontinuing a MAOI
- Should not be administered together with a sensitive CYP1A2 substrate or a CYP1A2 substrate with a narrow therapeutic range

 Toxicity
- See p. 332
- Atomoxetine: Symptoms include anxiety, tremulousness, dry mouth, seizures, and prolonged QTc interval
- Viloxazine: Symptoms include drowsiness, impaired consciousness, diminished reflexes, increased heart rate

 Lab Tests/Monitoring
- Atomoxetine: Height, weight, suicidal thoughts or behaviors. Liver function tests with any symptoms or sign of liver dysfunction
- Viloxazine: Blood pressure, pulse, height, weight, suicidal thoughts or behaviors

 Pediatric Considerations
- For detailed information on the use of selective NRIs in this population, please see the *Clinical Handbook of Psychotropic Drugs for Children and Adolescents*[7]
- Safety and efficacy of atomoxetine and viloxazine have not been established in children less than 6 years of age
- Pharmacokinetics of atomoxetine in children are similar to those in adults

 Geriatric Considerations
- Use with caution in patients with cardiovascular disease, liver dysfunction, or urinary outflow obstruction

 Use in Pregnancy◇
- Effect of atomoxetine on humans unknown
- Discontinue viloxazine when pregnancy is recognized unless the benefits of therapy outweigh potential risk. Evidence of fetal toxicity in animal studies

Breast Milk
- Unknown if atomoxetine or viloxazine are excreted in human milk

 Nursing Implications

Atomoxetine
- Measure pulse and blood pressure at baseline and periodically during treatment
- Monitor for increased irritability, anger, depression or suicidal ideation
- Monitor growth and weight during treatment
- Monitor for signs of liver toxicity (pruritus, dark urine, jaundice, upper right quadrant tenderness, unexplained flu-like symptoms)
- Manufacturer recommends capsules of atomoxetine should not be opened (drug powder is an ocular irritant)
- Give atomoxetine with or after meals to minimize stomach ache, nausea, and vomiting

Viloxazine
- Measure pulse and blood pressure at baseline and periodically during treatment
- Monitor for increased irritability, anger, mood changes or suicidal ideation
- Monitor growth and weight during treatment
- Manufacturer recommends capsules of viloxazine should not be cut, crushed or chewed but may be opened and contents sprinkled on soft food (e.g., applesauce) prior to administration

◇ See p. 473 for further information on drug use in pregnancy and effects on breast milk

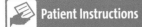 **Patient Instructions**

- For detailed patient instructions on atomoxetine and viloxazine, see the Patient Information Sheets (details p. 474)

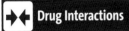 **Drug Interactions**

- Clinically significant interactions are listed below
- For more interaction information on any given combination, also see the corresponding chapter for the second agent

Class of Drug	Example	Interaction Effects
Antiarrhythmic	Quinidine	Increased plasma level and half-life of atomoxetine due to inhibited metabolism via CYP2D6
Antidepressant		
SSRI	Fluoxetine, paroxetine	Increased plasma level and half-life of atomoxetine due to inhibited metabolism via CYP2D6
NDRI	Bupropion	Increased plasma level and half-life of atomoxetine due to inhibited metabolism via CYP2D6
MAOI	Phenelzine, tranylcypromine	Do not administer concurrently or within 2 weeks of discontinuing a MAOI
Antiretroviral		
Non-nucleoside reverse transcriptase inhibitor (NNRTI)	Delavirdine	Increased atomoxetine level due to inhibited metabolism via CYP2D6
Protease inhibitor	Ritonavir	Increased atomoxetine level due to inhibited metabolism via CYP2D6
β-agonist	Albuterol/salbutamol, levalbuterol	Can potentiate cardiovascular effects, resulting in increased blood pressure and heart rate
CYP1A2 substrate	Clozapine, duloxetine, ramelteon, tizanidine	With viloxazine, sensitive CYP1A2 substrates with a narrow therapeutic range are contraindicated. Moderately sensitive CYP1A2 substrates should be avoided due to increased exposure
Dextromethorphan (DM)		Competitive inhibition of DM metabolism via CYP2D6 by atomoxetine, with potential for increased plasma level of either drug
QT-prolonging agent	Antiarrhythmics (e.g., amiodarone, sotalol), antimalarials (e.g., chloroquine, mefloquine), antipsychotics (quetiapine, thioridazine, ziprasidone), dolasetron, methadone, tacrolimus	Possible additive prolongation of QT interval with atomoxetine
Stimulant	Methylphenidate, amphetamine, and related products	Possible potentiation of therapeutic effects and adverse effects such as hypertension and tachycardia. However, combination use with atomoxetine recommended as an option by some ADHD treatment guidelines following monotherapy trials with each agent

Comparison of Drugs for ADHD

	Methylphenidate	Dexmethylphenidate	Amphetamine salts/Dextroamphetamine/Lisdexamfetamine/Methamphetamine	Atomoxetine	Viloxazine
Pharmacology	Selectively inhibits presynaptic transporters (i.e., reuptake) for DA and NE – dependent on normal neuronal activity Increases levels of synaptic DA and NE	Selectively inhibits presynaptic transporters (i.e., reuptake) for DA and NE – dependent on normal neuronal activity Increases levels of synaptic DA and NE	Competitive inhibitor and pseudosubstrate for presynaptic transporters (i.e., reuptake) for DA, NE, and 5-HT (though primarily DA). Main amphetamine effects are: 1) depletion of vesicular dopamine, 2) reversal of presynaptic DA transporters, and 3) presynaptic DA transporter inhibition	Selectively blocks reuptake of NE; increases NE and DA in prefrontal cortex	Selectively blocks reuptake of NE; increases NE and DA in prefrontal cortex

Comparison of Drugs for ADHD (cont.)

	Methylphenidate	Dexmethylphenidate	Amphetamine salts/Dextroamphetamine/Lisdexamfetamine/Methamphetamine	Atomoxetine	Viloxazine
Dosing ADHD	Start with 2.5–5 mg bid and increase by 2.5–5 mg weekly Usual dose: 10–60 mg/day or 0.25–1 mg/kg/day body weight (divided doses); up to 3 mg/kg/day has been used in children Aptensio XR/Biphentin: 10–20 mg q a.m.; can increase by 10 mg weekly to a maximum of 80 mg/day Concerta: 18–36 mg q a.m.; can increase by 18 mg weekly to a maximum of 72 mg/day (some references support a maximum of 108 mg/day) in adults and 90 mg/day in adolescents) Cotempla XR-ODT: 17.3 mg q a.m.; may increase by 8.6–17.3 mg in weekly intervals, to maximum of 51.8 mg/day Daytrana transdermal patch: Week 1, apply 10 mg/9 h patch (for 9 h/day); increase dose in weekly intervals as necessary Foquest: 25 mg q a.m.; may increase at no less than 5-day intervals to maximum of 100 mg/day Quillivant XR/Quillichew ER: 20 mg q a.m.; may increase by 10–20 mg weekly to a maximum of 60 mg/day	Over age 6: Start with 2.5 mg bid and can increase weekly in 2.5–5 mg increments to a maximum of 20 mg/day (divided dose, given at least q 4 h) Usual dose: 5–20 mg daily divided bid When switching from methylphenidate, the starting dose of dexmethylphenidate should be half that of methylphenidate	*Amphetamine:* Adzenys XR-ODT: Children: 6.3 mg q a.m. Increase by 3.1 or 6.3 mg weekly to maximum of 18.8 mg/day for children or 12.5 mg/day for adolescents. Adults: 12.5 mg q a.m. Dyanavel XR: Over age 6: Start with 2.5–5 mg q a.m. May increase by 2.5–10 mg every 4–7 days to a maximum of 20 mg/day Evekeo/Evekeo ODT: Age 3–5: Start with 2.5 mg and increase by 2.5 mg weekly. Over age 6: Start with 5 mg and increase by 5 mg weekly. Usual maximum: 40 mg/day *Dextroamphetamine/amphetamine salts:* Adderall: 2.5–5 mg to start and increase by 2.5–5 mg every 3–7 days up to 30 mg/day (given every 4–7 h). In adults up to 40 mg/day (in divided doses) Adderall XR: 10–30 mg q a.m. Mydayis: 12.5 mg q a.m.; may increase by 12.5 mg at weekly intervals to maximum of 25 mg/day for adolescents or 50 mg/day for adults *Dextroamphetamine:* Age 3–5: Start with 2.5 mg and increase by 2.5 mg weekly. Over age 6: Start with 5 mg and increase by 5 mg weekly. Usual dose: 2.5–40 mg/day or 0.1–0.8 mg/kg (in divided doses) Xelstrym transdermal patch: Week 1, apply 4.5 mg patch (for 9 h/day); increase dose in weekly intervals as necessary *Lisdexamfetamine:* Children age 6 and up, adolescents, and adults: 20–30 mg q a.m. and can increase by 10–20 mg every 7 days to a maximum of 60 mg/day (Canada) or 70 mg/day (USA) *Methamphetamine:* Start with 5 mg daily bid and increase by 5 mg/week. Usual dose: 20–25 mg/day – in divided doses; Gradumet given once daily	Dosing is based on body weight *Children up to 70 kg:* Canadian labeling: Initiate at 0.5 mg/kg/day for 7–14 days. Based on tolerability, increase to 0.8 mg/kg/day for 7–14 days, and then to 1.2 mg/kg/day, given once daily or bid in the morning and late afternoon. Do not exceed 1.4 mg/kg or 100 mg/day, whichever is less US labeling: 0.5 mg/kg/day for 3 days, then increase to 1.2 mg/kg/day if tolerated *Adolescents and adults over 70 kg:* Canadian labeling: Initiate at 40 mg/day for 7–14 days. Based on tolerability, increase to 60 mg/day for 7–14 days, and then to 80 mg/day, given once daily or divided bid in the morning and late afternoon. If response is inadequate after 2–4 weeks, the dose can be increased to a maximum of 100 mg/day US labeling: 40 mg/day for 3 days, then increase to 80 mg/day. May increase to maximum of 100 mg/day in 2-4 weeks to achieve optimal response	Children: 100 mg daily for 1 week, then may increase in 100 mg increments weekly to maximum of 400 mg/day depending on response and tolerability Adolescents: 200 mg daily for 1 week, then may increase to 400 mg/day depending on response and tolerability

	Methylphenidate	Dexmethylphenidate	Amphetamine salts/Dextroamphetamine/ Lisdexamfetamine/Methamphetamine	Atomoxetine	Viloxazine
Depression	10–30 mg/day	–	*Dextroamphetamine:* 5–60 mg/day	–	–
Narcolepsy	10–60 mg/day (usual dose: 10 mg 2–3 times/day)	–	*Dextroamphetamine:* 5–60 mg/day	–	–
Pharmacokinetics					
Bioavailability	30% (range 11–52%)	22–25%	*Amphetamine/ Dextroamphetamine:* > 90% *Lisdexamfetamine:* 96.4% *Methamphetamine:* 65–70%	63–94%	88% (compared to immediate-release formulation)
Peak plasma level	IR tabs: 0.3–4 h Slow-release tabs: 1 h Apo-Methylphenidate-ER: 4.63 h Aptensio XR/Biphentin: 2 h first peak, 7 h second peak Concerta: 1 h initial peak, 6.8 h second peak Cotempla XR-ODT: 5 h Foquest: 2 h first peak, 12 h second peak Metadate CD: 1.5 h first peak, 4.5 h second peak Quillichew ER: 5 h Quillivant XR: 5 h	1–1.5 h (fasting)	*Amphetamine:* Dyanavel XR: 4 h Evekeo: within 4 h *Dextroamphetamine/amphetamine salts:* Adderall: 1–2 h Adderall XR: 7 h Adzenys XR-ODT: d-amphetamine: 5 h (7 h with food) Mydayis: 8 h *Dextroamphetamine:* Tablets 1–4 h, Spansules: 6–10 h *Lisdexamfetamine:* 1 h, d-amphetamine: 3.5 h	1–2 h CYP2D6 poor metabolizers: 3–4 h	5 h
Protein binding	8–15%	12–15%	12–15%	Atomoxetine: 98% hydroxyatomoxetine metabolite: 69%	76–82%
Onset of effects	0.5–2 h Absorption from GI tract is slow and incomplete	0.5–2 h	0.5–2 h Readily absorbed from the GI tract Adderall: Saccharate and aspartate salts have a delayed onset	Delayed by up to 4 weeks, but then effective continuously with ongoing administration	1 week
Plasma half-life	IR (regular) tabs: 2.9 h mean (range: 2–4 h) SR and Concerta: 3.4 h mean Daytrana: 3–4 h after removal of patch Metadate CD: 6.8 h mean Quillichew ER: 5.2 h Quillivant XR: 5.6 h	2.2 h	*Amphetamine:* Dyanavel XR: Contains d-amphetamine and l-amphetamine with half-lives of 12.4 h and 15.1 h, respectively Evekeo: 11 h *Dextroamphetamine/amphetamine salts:* Adderall: 6–8 h *Dextroamphetamine:* 6–8 h in acidic pH, 18.6–33.6 h in alkaline pH *Lisdexamfetamine:* < 1 h; d-amphetamine (after conversion): 10–13 h Xelstrym: 6.4–11.5 h after removal of patch *Methamphetamine:* 6.5–15 h	Atomoxetine = 5 h (CYP2D6 poor metabolizers = 21.6 h) hydroxyatomoxetine = 6–8 h (CYP2D6 poor metabolizers = 34–40 h)	7 h

Comparison of Drugs for ADHD (cont.)

	Methylphenidate	Dexmethylphenidate	Amphetamine salts/Dextroamphetamine/ Lisdexamfetamine/Methamphetamine	Atomoxetine	Viloxazine
Duration of action	IR (regular) tablets: 3–5 h SR: Theoretically 5–8 h, but 3–5 h practically Extended-release formulations: 8–12 h Foquest: 16 h	6–7 h	*Amphetamine:* Dyanavel XR: Up to 13 h Evekeo: 4–6 h *Dextroamphetamine/amphetamine salts:* Adderall: 5–7 h Adderall XR: 12 h Mydayis: 16 h *Dextroamphetamine:* Tablets 4–5 h, Spansules: 7–8 h *Lisdexamfetamine:* Up to 13 h *Methamphetamine:* 6–12 h; effects may continue up to 24 h following administration of large doses	Approx. 24 h	24 h
Metabolism	Hepatic via carboxylesterase CES1A1 to minimally active metabolite Weak CYP2D6 inhibitor		Minor CYP2D6 substrate (*lisdexamfetamine* enzymatically converted to active d-amphetamine by hydrolytic enzymes on erythrocytes)	Metabolized primarily by CYP2D6; also by CYP2C19	CYP2D6, UGT1A9, UGT2B15
Hepatic impairment	No change	No change	No change	Moderate: Reduce dose by 50% Severe: Reduce dose by 75%	Not recommended
Renal impairment	No adjustment	?	Decreased excretion	No adjustment	Severe: Reduce dose by 50%
Effect of Food	Concerta: Delayed T_{max} by 1 h and reduced C_{max} by 10–30% Metadate CD: Delayed T_{max} by 1 h	–	Decreased extent of absorption Adzenys XR-ODT: T_{max} increased by 2–2.5 h, C_{max} reduced by 19% Mydayis: T_{max} increased 5 h for d-amphetamine and 4.5 h for l-amphetamine *Lisdexamfetamine:* No change	T_{max} delayed by 3 h	
High-fat meal	Aptensio XR/Biphentin: diminished second peak level, C_{max} increased by 28%, AUC by 19% Cotempla XR-ODT: C_{max} decreased by 24%, AUC increased by 16%, T_{max} decreased by 0.5 h Foquest: No change Metadate CD: C_{max} increased by 30% Quillichew ER: T_{max} unchanged, C_{max} increased by 20%, AUC by 4% Quillivant XR: T_{max} increased by 1 h, C_{max} by 28%, AUC by 19% Ritalin and Ritalin LA: T_{max} delayed	Delayed T_{max}	Dyanavel XR: T_{max} increased by 1 h, C_{max} by 2%, AUC by 6%	C_{max} 37% lower	T_{max} delayed by 2 h, C_{max} 9% lower, AUC 8% lower

	Methylphenidate	Dexmethylphenidate	Amphetamine salts/Dextroamphetamine/ Lisdexamfetamine/Methamphetamine	Atomoxetine	Viloxazine
Adverse Effects (Dose related)					
CNS	Nervousness (16%), anxiety, insomnia (up to 28%), restlessness, activation, irritability (up to 26%), headache (up to 14%), tearfulness, drowsiness (10%), rebound depression, may exacerbate mania or psychosis (See Precautions p. 319) Cases of suicidal thoughts, hallucinations, and psychotic or violent behavior reported with Concerta Tourette's syndrome, tics (up to 10%, mostly with higher doses) Social withdrawal, dullness, sadness, and irritability reported in children with autism	Drowsiness, headache Fever (5%) Arthralgia, dyskinesias (See Precautions p. 319)	Nervousness, insomnia, activation, restlessness, anxiety, emotional lability, mania (with high doses), dysphoria, irritability, headache, confusion, delusions, rebound depression; may exacerbate mania or psychosis (See Precautions p. 319) Headache Tremor, Tourette's syndrome, tics – usually with higher doses	Insomnia, dizziness, fatigue, headache, emotional lability Less common: Drowsiness, irritability, depression, tremor, aggression Reports of psychotic/manic symptoms (hallucinations, delusions, and mania) in children and adolescents with no prior history of psychotic illness Case reports of tics; however, patients in clinical trials with baseline tics showed some improvement in tic frequency	Somnolence, headache, fatigue, insomnia, fever, irritability, suicidal thoughts and behaviors
GI	Abdominal pain (up to 23%), nausea, vomiting, and diarrhea (more than 10%), anorexia (up to 41%, dose-related)	Abdominal pain (15%), nausea, anorexia (6%)	Abdominal pain common; nausea, vomiting, anorexia	Upper abdominal pain, nausea, vomiting, anorexia	Nausea, vomiting, abdominal pain, decreased appetite, weight loss
Cardiovascular	Increased heart rate and blood pressure at start of therapy, dizziness (13%), hypotension, palpitations (See Precautions p. 319)	Increased heart rate and blood pressure at start of therapy (See Precautions p. 319)	Increased heart rate and blood pressure at start of therapy, dizziness, palpitations (See Precautions p. 319)	Small increases in heart rate and blood pressure at start of treatment (See Precautions p. 325)	Increases in heart rate and blood pressure
Anticholinergic	Dry mouth, blurred vision	Blurred vision	Dry mouth, dysgeusia, blurred vision	Dry mouth, constipation, mydriasis, urinary retention	–
Endocrine	Growth delay (height and weight), may occur initially but tends to normalize over time (unless high chronic doses used), weight loss	Growth delay, weight loss	Growth delay (height and weight), may occur initially but tends to normalize over time (unless high chronic doses used), weight loss, impotence, changes in libido	Sexual dysfunction, weight loss	–
Other	Upper respiratory infections (pharyngitis (4%), sinusitis (3%), rhinitis (13%), cough (4%)), fever, rash, contact sensitization/dermatitis Daytrana transdermal patch application site reactions: redness, itching, blistering, chemical leukoderma Leukopenia, blood dyscrasias, anemia, hair loss, priapism	Cough, upper respiratory infections, priapism	Urticaria, anemia Xelstrym transdermal patch: application site reactions: discomfort, edema, erythema, pain, pruritus, rash, burning sensation, swelling	Cases of liver damage with elevated AST/ALT and bilirubin in adults and children Pruritus, rhinitis, priapism	Upper respiratory tract infection

Comparison of Drugs for ADHD (cont.)

	Methylphenidate	Dexmethylphenidate	Amphetamine salts/Dextroamphetamine/Lisdexamfetamine/Methamphetamine	Atomoxetine	Viloxazine
Toxicity	CNS overstimulation with vomiting, agitation, tremors, hyperreflexia, convulsions, confusion, hallucinations, delirium, cardiovascular effects (e.g., hypertension, tachycardia); seizures reported	CNS overstimulation with vomiting, agitation, tremors, hyperreflexia, convulsions, confusion, hallucinations, delirium, cardiovascular effects (e.g., hypertension, tachycardia)	Restlessness, dizziness, increased reflexes, tremor, insomnia, irritability, assaultiveness, hallucinations, panic, cardiovascular effects, circulatory collapse, convulsions, and coma	Anxiety, tremulousness, dry mouth; case of seizures & QTc prolongation	Drowsiness, impaired consciousness, diminished reflexes, increased heart rate
	Supportive therapy should be given	Supportive therapy should be given	Supportive therapy should be given	Supportive therapy should be given	Supportive therapy should be given
Use in Pregnancy◊	No evidence of teratogenicity reported	Safety not established	High doses have embryotoxic and teratogenic potential; use of amphetamine in pregnant animals has been associated with permanent alterations in the central noradrenergic system of the neonate Increased risk of premature delivery and low birth weight; withdrawal reactions in newborn reported	Safety not established	Discontinue when pregnancy is recognized unless benefits of therapy outweigh potential risk. Evidence of fetal toxicity in animal studies
Breastfeeding	No data	No data	Excreted into breast milk; recommended not to breastfeed	No published experience with this drug during breastfeeding; however, there have been reports of no serious adverse effects in 2 breastfed infants	No data

◊ See p. 473 for further information on drug use in pregnancy and effects on breast milk

α_2 agonists

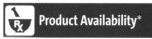 **Product Availability***

Generic Name	Neuroscience-based Nomenclature* (Pharmacological Target/Mode of Action)	Trade Name(A)	Dosage Forms and Strengths
Clonidine	Norepinephrine/Agonist	Catapres, Dixarit(C)	Tablets: 0.025 mg(C), 0.1 mg, 0.2 mg, 0.3 mg(B)

Generic Name	Neuroscience-based Nomenclature* (Pharmacological Target/Mode of Action)	Trade Name(A)	Dosage Forms and Strengths
		Kapvay(B)	Extended-release tablets: 0.1 mg
		Catapres TTS(B)	Transdermal patch: 0.1 mg/24 h, 0.2 mg/24 h, 0.3 mg/24 h
Guanfacine	Norepinephrine/Agonist	Tenex(B)	Tablets: 1 mg, 2 mg
		Intuniv(B), Intuniv XR(C)	Extended-release tablets: 1 mg, 2 mg, 3 mg, 4 mg

* Refer to Health Canada's Drug Product Database or the FDA's Drugs@FDA for the most current availability information.   • Developed by a taskforce consisting of representatives from the American College of Neuropsychopharmacology (ACNP), the Asian College of Neuropsychopharmacology (AsCNP), the European College of Neuropsychopharmacology (ECNP), the International College of Neuropsychopharmacology (CINP), and the International Union of Basic and Clinical Pharmacology (IUPHAR) (see https://nbn2r.com), (A) Generic preparations may be available,   (B) Not marketed in Canada,   (C) Not marketed in the USA

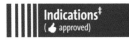

Indications‡
(👍 approved)

- 🖐 ADHD (long-acting formulations of clonidine (Kapvay) and guanfacine (Intuniv/Intuniv XR) in children 6 years of age and older) – meta-analysis of studies suggests a moderate effect size in children and adolescents; reduced hyperarousal, agitation, aggression, impulsivity, and sleep disturbances; useful in patients with concurrent tic disorders or conduct disorder; minimal benefit on inattentive symptoms
- 🖐 Hypertension (IR formulations; guanfacine – USA only)
- 🖐 Vascular stabilizer for treatment of menopausal flushing (clonidine)
- Some benefit apparent in combination with stimulants; may help ameliorate sleep disturbances caused by psychostimulants (Caution – see Drug Interactions p. 336)
- May improve behavior or impulsivity when used alone or in combination with methylphenidate (Caution – see Drug Interactions p. 336)
- Autism – reported to be effective for reducing hyperarousal and controlling some problematic behaviors in children and adults
- Generalized anxiety disorder (GAD), panic attacks, phobic disorders, and obsessive-compulsive disorders: Of some benefit; may augment effects of SSRIs and cyclic antidepressants in social phobia; helpful for symptoms of hyperarousal, hypervigilance, aggression, and irritability of PTSD
- May relieve antipsychotic-induced asthenia and improve symptoms of tardive dyskinesia
- May help decrease clozapine-induced sialorrhea
- Heroin, cocaine, and nicotine withdrawal: Used to reduce agitation, tremor, and diaphoresis, and to increase patient comfort. Opioid antagonists (e.g., naltrexone) as well as dicyclomine (for stomach cramps) and cyclobenzaprine (for muscle cramps) often given concomitantly

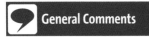

General Comments

- Reduce the hyperactive/impulsive and aggressive symptoms of ADHD but may be less effective for inattention problems; considered generally less effective than psychostimulants and thus second-line or adjunctive treatments, though may be beneficial for some patients who have not responded to stimulant treatment or those with comorbid tic disorder
- Where possible, referral for parent behavioral management training (PBMT) should be made for children age 4 and up diagnosed with ADHD[1]
- In anxiety disorders, psychological symptoms respond better than somatic symptoms; anxiolytic effects may be short-lived

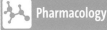

Pharmacology

- Mechanism of action for the treatment of ADHD is unknown; agonizing α_{2A} receptors in the prefrontal cortex appears to improve "signal-to-noise ratio"
- Clonidine is a relatively nonselective α_2-adrenergic agonist (α_{2A}, α_{2B}, and α_{2C} receptors). It also has affinity for imidazoline receptors, which may be responsible for some of its sedating and hypotensive action
- Guanfacine is a more selective agonist for postsynaptic α_{2A} receptors in the prefrontal cortex. It has less sedating and hypotensive effects compared to clonidine
- Both clonidine and guanfacine stimulate α_2-adrenergic receptors in the brain stem. This reduces sympathetic outflow from the CNS and decreases peripheral resistance, renal vascular resistance, heart rate, and blood pressure

Dosing

- ADHD:
  - Clonidine IR: 3–10 micrograms/kg body weight per day (0.05–0.4 mg/day) in 3–4 divided doses
  - Clonidine XR: initially 0.1 mg/day, may adjust by increments no larger than 0.1 mg/day every week to maximum of 0.4 mg/day based on clinical response. Doses above 0.1 mg/day should be divided twice daily, split equally or with the larger portion of the split dose given at bedtime

‡ Indications listed here do not necessarily apply to all countries. Please refer to a country's regulatory database (e.g., US Food and Drug Administration, Health Canada Drug Product Database) for the most current availability information and indications

α₂ agonists (cont.)

- – Guanfacine IR: 0.5–4 mg/day divided bid
- – Guanfacine XR: initially 1 mg once daily; may adjust by increments no larger than 1 mg at weekly intervals based on clinical response, to a maximum of 4 mg/day in children (as monotherapy or in combination with stimulant) or adolescents (in combination with stimulant) and 7 mg/day in adolescents (as monotherapy). Clinical response is associated with weight-based doses of 0.05–0.08 mg/kg/day. Doses up to 0.12 mg/kg/day may provide additional benefit
- Antisocial behavior/aggression: Clonidine: Children: 0.1–0.4 mg/day as tablets (IR: in 3–4 divided doses) or transdermal patch; adults: 0.4–0.6 mg/day
- Anxiety disorders: Clonidine: 0.15–0.5 mg/day (IR: in 3–4 divided doses)
- Drug dependence: Clonidine IR: 0.1–0.3 mg tid to qid for up to 7 days; nicotine withdrawal: 0.1 mg bid to 0.4 mg/day for 3–4 weeks
- Tic disorders: Clonidine IR: 3–5 micrograms/kg body weight per day in 2–4 divided doses; guanfacine IR: 0.5 mg tid to maximum of 4 mg/day in 3 divided doses

 Pharmacokinetics

- Clonidine is well absorbed orally and percutaneously (when patch applied to the arm or chest)
- Peak plasma level of oral clonidine occurs in 1–3 h (IR) or 7–8 h (XR); therapeutic plasma concentration of clonidine transdermal patch occur within 2–3 days
- Clonidine plasma half-life is 8–12 h in children and 12–20 h in adults; in patients with impaired renal function, half-life range is 18–41 h. Elimination half-life is dose dependent
- Guanfacine is metabolized via CYP3A4; peak plasma level of oral guanfacine occurs in 1–4 h (IR) or 5 h (XR) in children and adolescents, 4–8 h in adults; half-life is 14–18 h in children and adolescents, 10–30 h in adults
- Bioavailability is reduced with guanfacine XR tablets compared to IR tablets, therefore IR and XR forms and their respective dosing guidelines are not considered interchangeable

 Onset & Duration of Action

- Oral clonidine IR tablets: Onset of effects occurs in 30–60 min and effects last about 6–10 h (except for XR formulations)
- Clonidine transdermal patch: Therapeutic plasma concentrations are attained within 2–3 days and effects last for 7 days

 Adverse Effects

- With clonidine and guanfacine, sedation, dizziness, bradycardia, and hypotension common on initiation (monitor BP and heart rate) – these effects are lessened with use of extended-release formulations
- Less common with both drugs: anxiety, irritability, decreased memory, headache, dry mouth, and lack of energy
- Dermatological reactions reported in up to 50% of patients using transdermal clonidine patch
- Clonidine and guanfacine may increase agitation and produce depressive symptoms
- Case reports of mania induced by guanfacine

 D/C Discontinuation Syndrome

- Withdrawal reactions may occur after abrupt cessation of long-term clonidine or guanfacine therapy (over 1–2 months)
- Taper clonidine and guanfacine (e.g., reduce dose by approximately 25% [round to nearest tablet size] every 3–7 days) on drug discontinuation to prevent rebound hypertension and insomnia, as well as tic rebound in patients with Tourette's syndrome
- Cases of rebound psychotic symptoms reported with both drugs

 Precautions

- Case reports (4) of sudden death with combination of methylphenidate and clonidine but causal relationship not established; FDA recommended removal of drug interaction statement regarding methylphenidate and clonidine. Long-acting formulations are FDA/Health Canada approved for adjunctive use with stimulants
- Use with caution in patients with or at risk of CVD, cerebrovascular disease, chronic hepatic or renal impairment or any condition that may predispose to syncope
- Use with caution when prescribing/transcribing clonidine doses: high potential for 10-fold dosing errors due to inadvertent decimal misplacement when converting doses between units of micrograms and milligrams
- Do not use clonidine drug powder for compounding suspensions. 1000-fold overdoses reported when preparing compounded clonidine suspensions from drug powder due to confusion when converting between units of micrograms and milligrams

Contraindications	• Patient/caregiver inability to ensure regular administration without missing doses (due to risk of rebound hypertension if stopped abruptly)
Toxicity	• Signs and symptoms of clonidine or guanfacine overdose occur within 60 min of drug ingestion (with IR tablets; may be delayed with XR tablets) and may persist for up to 48 h or longer • Symptoms include transient hypertension followed by hypotension, bradycardia, weakness, pallor, sedation, vomiting, hypothermia; can progress to CNS depression, diminished or absent reflexes, apnea, respiratory depression, cardiac conduction defects, seizures, and coma
Treatment	• Supportive and symptomatic
Lab Tests/Monitoring	• Baseline: blood pressure and pulse, repeat regularly throughout treatment and following discontinuation (α_2 agonists should not be stopped abruptly due to risk of rebound hypertension) • EKG/QTc interval if known underlying condition or taken concurrently with medications known to increase QTc interval
Pediatric Considerations	• For detailed information on the use of clonidine and guanfacine in this population, please see the *Clinical Handbook of Psychotropic Drugs for Children and Adolescents*[7] • Children metabolize clonidine faster than adults and may require more frequent dosing (usually 3–4 divided doses/day for IR formulation) • Children metabolize guanfacine faster than adults and may require more frequent dosing (2–3 divided doses/day for IR formulation)
Geriatric Considerations	• Use with caution in patients with cardiovascular disease or chronic renal failure
Use in Pregnancy◊	• Clonidine: Animal studies suggest teratogenic effects; no adequate well-controlled studies of clonidine in pregnant women. Clonidine passes the placental barrier and may lower fetus heart rate. Transient rise in blood pressure in the newborn cannot be excluded postpartum • Clonidine crosses the placenta and may lower the heart rate of the fetus • Guanfacine: No adequate well-controlled studies of guanfacine in pregnant women
Breast Milk	• Clonidine is distributed into breast milk; effects on infant unknown • It is unknown whether guanfacine is distributed into breast milk • If used by nursing mothers, observe milk-fed infants for somnolence and sedation
Nursing Implications	• Clonidine and guanfacine should not be discontinued suddenly due to risk of rebound hypertension and insomnia • Advise patient to swallow XR formulations whole, and not to break, chew, or crush XR tablets • Should be taken with a full glass of water. Advise patient to maintain adequate hydration (unless instructed to restrict fluid intake) • Handle used transdermal patches carefully (fold in half with sticky sides together for disposal) • Should the transdermal patch begin to loosen from the skin, apply adhesive overlay over the system to ensure good adhesion over the period of application • Monitor for skin reactions around area when transdermal patch is applied • Monitor for dizziness/lightheadedness and possibly blood pressure (sitting/standing) after initiation or dose increase • Assess potential for interactions with other CNS depressants. Do not discontinue abruptly; taper, decreasing dose gradually to prevent rebound hypertension • Bioavailability is reduced with XR tablets compared to IR tablets, therefore IR and XR products and their respective dosing guidelines are not interchangeable
Patient Instructions	• For detailed patient instructions, see the Patient Information Sheet (details p. 474)

◊ See p. 473 for further information on drug use in pregnancy and effects on breast milk

α₂ agonists (cont.)

◆▶◀ **Drug Interactions**	• Clinically significant interactions are listed below
	• For more interaction information on any given combination, also see the corresponding chapter for the second agent

Class of Drug	Example	Interaction Effects
Antibiotic	Clarithromycin, erythromycin	Decreased clearance and increased plasma level of guanfacine due to inhibition of CYP3A4 metabolism
	Rifampin	Decreased guanfacine levels due to CYP3A4 induction; monitor for signs and symptoms of altered response. With the XR formulation, higher dosages (up to 8 mg/day) and dose increments (2 mg/week) may be required
Anticonvulsant	Carbamazepine	Decreased guanfacine levels due to CYP3A4 induction; monitor for signs and symptoms of altered response. With the guanfacine XR formulation, higher dosages (up to 8 mg/day) and dose increments (2 mg/week) may be required
	Divalproex, valproic acid	Increased valproate levels; may be due to competition between valproate and guanfacine metabolite (3-hydroxy guanfacine) for glucuronidation enzymes
Antidepressant	Bupropion, desipramine	Clonidine withdrawal may result in excess circulating catecholamines; use caution in combination with noradrenergic or dopaminergic antidepressants
	Desipramine, imipramine, SNRIs	Inhibition of antihypertensive effect of α₂ agonist by the antidepressant
Antifungal	Itraconazole, ketoconazole	Decreased clearance and increased plasma level of guanfacine due to inhibition of CYP3A4 metabolism
Antihypertensive	Hydrochlorothiazide, ramipril	Additive hypotensive effects
β-blocker	Propranolol	Additive bradycardia; increased risk for rebound hypertension with abrupt discontinuation of α₂ agonist
CNS depressant	Alcohol, antihistamines, benzodiazepines, suvorexant, zolpidem, zopiclone	Additive CNS depressant effects
Stimulant	Dextroamphetamine, methylphenidate	Additive effect on hyperactivity and aggression associated with ADHD Kapvay (clonidine XR) is FDA approved and Intuniv/Intuniv XR (guanfacine XR) is FDA/Health Canada approved for adjunctive use with stimulant medications in children and adolescents

Augmentation Strategies in ADHD

Nonresponse in ADHD	• Ascertain whether diagnosis is correct
	• Ascertain if patient is adherent with therapy (speak with caregivers, check with pharmacy for late refills, count remaining pills in container and compare to prescription fill date)
	• Ensure dosage prescribed is therapeutically appropriate and tailor regimen to have peak serum levels occur at those times of the day that symptoms are most prominent
	• Consider trying a stimulant from an alternate class (methylphenidate class or amphetamine class) if the first stimulant trial was ineffective and the patient was adhering to therapy recommendations

Factors Complicating Response	• Concurrent medical or psychiatric condition, e.g., anxiety disorder, bipolar disorder, conduct disorder, autism spectrum disorder, learning disability
	• Concurrent prescription drugs may interfere with efficacy, e.g., antipsychotics (see Drug Interactions pp. 321–323, 327, 336)
	• Metabolic inducers (e.g., carbamazepine) may decrease the plasma level of methylphenidate or guanfacine
	• High intake of acidifying agents (e.g., fruit juices, vitamin C) may decrease the efficacy of amphetamine preparations

- Substance use, including alcohol and marijuana, may complicate management and treatment selection; need to discontinue substance use to optimize treatment outcomes
- High level of adverse effects with atomoxetine may be due to patient being a CYP2D6 poor metabolizer
- Poor efficacy with atomoxetine may be due to patient being a CYP2D6 ultrarapid metabolizer
- Side effects to medication
- Psychosocial factors may affect response; nonpharmacological treatment approaches (e.g., behavior modification, psychotherapy, and education) can increase the probability of response

 Augmentation Strategies

Methylphenidate/ Dexmethylphenidate/ Dextroamphetamine + α₂ agonist	• Additive effect on hyperactivity, aggression, mood lability, and sleep problems; studies indicate efficacy in 50–80% of patients. Has been found helpful in patients with concomitant tic disorders, conduct disorder or oppositional defiant disorder [monitor ECG, heart rate, and blood pressure with combination] • Kapvay (clonidine XR) is FDA approved and Intuniv/Intuniv XR (guanfacine XR) is FDA/Health Canada approved for adjunctive use with stimulant medications in children and adolescents
Psychostimulants + Antidepressants	• Tricyclics (imipramine, nortriptyline, and desipramine) useful in refractory patients or those with concomitant enuresis or bulimia; they may reduce abnormal movements in patients with tic disorders. There is an increase in the incidence of adverse effects, including cardiovascular, GI, anticholinergic effects, and weight gain; use caution and limit quantities prescribed in patients at risk of overdose • SSRIs or SNRIs may be effective in adult patients with concomitant mood or anxiety disorders (e.g., PTSD) • Bupropion used to augment effects of psychostimulants and in patients with concomitant mood disorder, substance abuse, or conduct disorder. May cause dermatological reactions, exacerbate tics, and increase seizure risk
Atomoxetine + Stimulants	• Use in patients who have partial relief of symptoms with maximally tolerated doses of stimulants and atomoxetine as monotherapy. Combination may permit lower stimulant doses and allows robust coverage as well as coverage early and late in the day • Monitor for increased blood pressure, tachycardia, weight loss, and reduced growth velocity
Psychostimulants + Antipsychotics	• Second- and third-generation antipsychotics (low doses of risperidone, aripiprazole) have been found useful in patients with comorbid symptoms of dyscontrol, aggression, hyperactivity, and tics. Ensure appropriate metabolic monitoring of antipsychotic therapy completed and discontinue antipsychotic treatment if excessive increases in blood pressure, weight, cholesterol, triglycerides or fasting glucose occur. Stimulants do not mitigate the effects of antipsychotics on weight and metabolic parameters
Psychostimulants + Mood Stabilizers	• Combination used in patients with comorbid bipolar disorder, conduct disorder, impulsivity, and aggression; infrequent case reports in children include the use of lithium, carbamazepine , and valproate – the possibility of drug interactions should be considered (see Drug Interactions pp. 321–323); limited likelihood of benefit
Psychostimulants + Buspirone	• Open studies suggest buspirone may improve rage attacks, impulsivity, inattention, and disruptive behavior at doses of 15–30 mg daily

 Further Reading

References
1. Wolraich ML, Hagan JF Jr, Allan C, et al. Clinical practice guideline for the diagnosis, evaluation, and treatment of attention-deficit/hyperactivity disorder in children and adolescents. Pediatrics 2019;144(4):e20192528. doi:10.1542/peds.2019-2528
2. Weiss MG, Surman CBH, Elbe D. Stimulant 'rapid metabolizers': Wrong label, real phenomena. Atten Def Hyperact Disord. 2018;10(2):113–118. doi:10.1007/s12402-017-0242-9
3. Ardic UA, Ercan ES. Resolution of methylphenidate osmotic release oral system-induced hair loss in two siblings after dose escalation. Pediatr Int. 2017;59(11):1217–1218. doi:10.1111/ped.13414
4. Warren AE, Hamilton RM, Bélanger SA, et al. Cardiac risk assessment before the use of stimulant medications in children and youth: A joint position statement by the Canadian Paediatric Society, the Canadian Cardiovascular Society, and the Canadian Academy of Child and Adolescent Psychiatry. Can J Cardiol. 2009;25(11):625–630. Retrieved from https://www.ncbi.nlm.nih.gov/pmc/articles/PMC2776560/
5. Vetter VL, Elia J., Erickson C, et al. Cardiovascular monitoring of children and adolescents with heart disease receiving medications for attention deficit/hyperactivity disorder [corrected]: A scientific statement from the American Heart Association Council on Cardiovascular Disease in the Young Congenital Cardiac Defects Committee and the Council on Cardiovascular Nursing. Circulation. 2008;117(18):2407–2423. doi:10.1161/CIRCULATIONAHA.107.189473

6   Hamilton RM, Rosenthal E, Hulpke-Wette M, et al. Cardiovascular considerations of attention deficit hyperactivity disorder medications: A report of the European Network on Hyperactivity Disorders work group, European Attention Deficit Hyperactivity Disorder Guidelines Group on attention deficit hyperactivity disorder drug safety meeting. Cardiol Young. 2012;22(1):63–70. doi:10.1017/S1047951111000928

7   Elbe D, Black TR, McGrane IR, et al. Clinical handbook of psychotropic drugs for children and adolescents. (5th ed.). Boston, MA: Hogrefe Publishing, 2023.

8   Swanson JM, Arnold LE, Molina BSG, et al. Young adult outcomes in the follow-up of the multimodal treatment study of attention-deficit/hyperactivity disorder: Symptom persistence, source discrepancy, and height suppression. J Child Psychol Psychiatry. 2017;58(6):663–678. doi:10.1111/jcpp.12684

9   Cohen SC, Mulqueen JM, Ferracioli-Oda E, et al. Meta-analysis: Risk of tics associated with psychostimulant use in randomized, placebo-controlled trials. J Am Acad Child Adolesc Psychiatry. 2015; 54(9):728–736. doi:10.1177/0269881108093841

Additional Suggested Reading

• Andrade C. Risk of major congenital malformations associated with the use of methylphenidate or amphetamines in pregnancy. J Clin Psychiatry. 2018;79(1):18f12108. doi:10.4088/JCP.18f12108

• Bangs ME, Tauscher-Wisniewski S, Polzer J, et al. Meta-analysis of suicide-related behavior events in patients treated with atomoxetine. J Am Acad Child Adolesc Psychiatry. 2008;47(2):209–218. doi:10.1097/chi.0b013e31815d88b2

• Canadian ADHD Resource Alliance. Canadian ADHD Practice Guidelines (4.1 ed.). Toronto, ON: CADDRA, 2020. Retrieved from https://www.caddra.ca/download-guidelines/

• Childress AC, Berry SA. Pharmacotherapy of attention-deficit hyperactivity disorder in adolescents. Drugs. 2012;72(3):309–325. doi:10.2165/11599580-000000000-00000

• Childress AC, Sallee FR. Attention-deficit/hyperactivity disorder with inadequate response to stimulants: Approaches to management. CNS Drugs. 2014;28(2):121–129. doi:10.1007/s40263-013-0130-6

• Cortese S, Brown TE, Corkum P, et al. Assessment and management of sleep problems in youths with attention-deficit/hyperactivity disorder. J Am Acad Child Adolesc Psychiatry. 2013;52(8):784–796. doi:10.1016/j.jaac.2013.06.001

• Elbe D, MacBride A, Reddy D. Focus on lisdexamfetamine: A review of its use in child and adolescent psychiatry. J Can Acad Child Adolesc Psychiatry. 2010;19(4):303–314. Retrieved from http://www.ncbi.nlm.nih.gov/pmc/articles/PMC2962544/

• Elbe D, Reddy D. Focus on guanfacine extended-release: A review of its use in child and adolescent psychiatry. J Can Acad Child Adolesc Psychiatry. 2014;23(1):48–60. Retrieved from http://www.ncbi.nlm.nih.gov/pmc/articles/PMC3917669/

• Findling RL, McBurnett K, White C, et al. Guanfacine extended release adjunctive to a psychostimulant in the treatment of comorbid oppositional symptoms in children and adolescents with attention-deficit/hyperactivity disorder. J Child Adolesc Psychopharmacol. 2014;24(5):245–252. doi:10.1089/cap.2013.0103

• Greenhill LL, Swanson JM, Hechtman L, et al. Trajectories of growth associated with long-term stimulant medication in the multimodal treatment study of attention-deficit/hyperactivity disorder. J Am Acad Child Adolesc Psychiatry. 2020;59(8):978–989. doi:10.1016/j.jaac.2019.06.019

• Lopez PL, Torrente FM, Ciapponi A. Cognitive-behavioural interventions for attention deficit hyperactivity disorder (ADHD) in adults. Cochrane Database Syst Rev. 2018;(3):CD010840. doi:10.1002/14651858.CD010840.pub2

• Man KKC, Ip P, Chan EW, et al. Effectiveness of pharmacological treatment for attention-deficit/hyperactivity disorder on physical injuries: A systematic review and meta-analysis of observational studies. CNS Drugs. 2017;31(12):1043–1055. doi:10.1007/s40263-017-0485-1

• Padilha SCOS, Virtuoso S, Tonin FS, et al. Efficacy and safety of drugs for attention deficit hyperactivity disorder in children and adolescents: A network meta-analysis. Eur Child Adolesc Psychiatry. 2018;27(10):1335–1345. doi:10.1007/s00787-018-1125-0

• Pérez-Lescure Picarzo J, Centeno Malfaz F, Collell Hernández R, et al. Recommendations of the Spanish Society of Paediatric Cardiology and Congenital Heart Disease as regards the use of drugs in attention deficit hyperactivity disorder in children and adolescents with a known heart disease, as well as in the general paediatric population: Position statement by the Spanish Paediatric Association. Pediatr (Barc). 2020;92:109.e1–109.e7. doi:10.1016/j.anpedi.2019.09.002[Article in Spanish]

• Royal College of Psychiatrists in Scotland. ADHD in adults: Good practice guidelines. Retrieved from https://www.rcpsych.ac.uk/docs/default-source/members/divisions/scotland/adhd_in_adultsfinal_guidelines_june2017.pdf?sfvrsn=40650449_2

• Steingard R, Taskiran S, Connor DF, et al. New formulations of stimulants: An update for clinicians. J Child Adolesc Psychopharmacol. 2019;29:324–339. doi:10.1089/cap.2019.0043

• Storebø OJ, Ramstad E, Krogh HB, et al. Methylphenidate for children and adolescents with attention deficit hyperactivity disorder (ADHD). Cochrane Database Syst Rev. 2015; 11:CD009885. doi:10.1002/14651858.CD009885.pub2

• Torgersen T, Gjervan B, Lensing MB, et al. Optimal management of ADHD in older adults. Neuropsychiatr Dis Treat. 2016;12:79–87. doi:10.2147/NDT.S59271

• Williams AE, Giust JM, Kronenberger, WG et al. Epilepsy and attention-deficit hyperactivity disorder: Links, risks, and challenges. Neuropsychiatr Dis Treat. 2016;12:287–296. doi:10.2147/NDT.S81549

DRUGS FOR TREATMENT OF DEMENTIA

Classification	• Drugs for treatment of dementia can be classified as follows:	

Chemical Class	Agent	Page
Cholinesterase inhibitors	Donepezil Rivastigmine Galantamine	See p. 339
Aminoadamantane	Memantine	See p. 346
Amyloid beta-directed antibody	Lecanemab	See p. 349

Cholinesterase Inhibitors

Product Availability*

Generic Name	Chemical Class	Neuroscience-based Nomenclature* (Pharmacological Target/Mode of Action)	Trade Name[A]	Dosage Forms and Strengths
Donepezil	Piperidine	Acetylcholine/Enzyme inhibitor	Aricept	Tablets: 5 mg, 10 mg, 23 mg[B] Orally disintegrating tablets: 5 mg, 10 mg
Galantamine (Galanthamine)	Phenanthrene alkaloid	Acetylcholine/Multimodal	Razadyne[B] Reminyl ER[C], Razadyne ER[B]	Tablets: 4 mg, 8 mg, 12 mg Liquid: 4 mg/mL Extended-release capsules: 8 mg, 16 mg, 24 mg
Rivastigmine	Carbamate	Acetylcholine/Enzyme inhibitor	Exelon Exelon Patch	Capsules: 1.5 mg, 3 mg, 4.5 mg, 6 mg Oral solution: 2 mg/mL Patch: 5 (4.6 mg/24 h), 10 (9.5 mg/24 h), 15 (13.3 mg/24 h)

* Refer to Health Canada's Drug Product Database or the FDA's Drugs@FDA for the most current availability information.   * Developed by a taskforce consisting of representatives from the American College of Neuropsychopharmacology (ACNP), the Asian College of Neuropsychopharmacology (AsCNP), the European College of Neuropsychopharmacology (ECNP), the International College of Neuropsychopharmacology (CINP), and the International Union of Basic and Clinical Pharmacology (IUPHAR) (see https://nbn2r.com).
[A] Generic preparations may be available,   [B] Not marketed in Canada,   [C] Not marketed in the USA

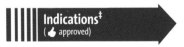

Indications‡
(👍 approved)

- 🔥 Dementia of Alzheimer's type – mild, moderate (donepezil, galantamine, rivastigmine), and severe (donepezil, memantine, rivastigmine patch (USA)): Symptomatic treatment of mild to moderate disease; no proof of a beneficial effect on the underlying neurodegenerative process but some disease markers may be positively affected (e.g., hippocampal volume loss)
- 🔥 Dementia of Parkinson's disease – mild to moderate (rivastigmine)
- 🔥 Alzheimer's disease: Treatment of severe disease (donepezil, memantine)
- • Galantamine in conjunction with memantine have shown efficacy for the treatment of cognitive impairment post traumatic brain injury
- • Galantamine and donepezil suggested to improve cognition and behaviors and to stabilize or improve activities of daily living

‡ Indications listed here do not necessarily apply to all cholinesterase inhibitors or all countries. Please refer to a country's regulatory database (e.g., US Food and Drug Administration, Health Canada Drug Product Database) for the most current availability information and indications

Cholinesterase Inhibitors (cont.)

- Schizophrenia – galantamine (alone, and in combination with memantine) has been shown to improve selective cognitive impairment in patients with schizophrenia. Galantamine increases dopaminergic activity and release in the prefrontal cortex in a dose-dependent manner, such benefits not seen with either donepezil or rivastigmine
- Dementia with Lewy bodies: Rivastigmine and other cholinesterase inhibitors have shown to improve cognition
- Reversion of neuromuscular blocking effects of curare-type muscle relaxants (galantamine)
- Substance use disorders - early data suggests that galantamine (as an allosteric potentiator of the nicotinic acetylcholine receptor, especially α_7 and $\alpha_4\beta_2$ subtypes) may be beneficial in the treatment of cocaine, opioid, and nicotine addiction
- Autism spectrum disorder: Double-blind studies report improvements in behaviors, attention, communication, and interactions
- Donepezil reportedly decreased in-hospital mortality (as a result of pneumonia) among older Japanese patients with dementia
- Rivastigmine and other cholinesterase inhibitors

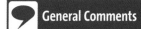 **General Comments**

- These drugs are suggested to ameliorate behavioral disturbances (such as apathy, depression, anxiety, disinhibition, aberrant motor behavior, delusions, and hallucinations) as well as enhance cognition. Benefits are lost after drug withdrawal. Therapeutic response following re-initiation of therapy shown to be less than that obtained with initial therapy
- Double-blind placebo-controlled studies involving patients with mild to moderate Alzheimer's disease showed improvement (i.e., less decline in cognitive ability). Approximately 25% of patients had significantly improved attention, interest, orientation, communication, and memory (controversy exists over whether cognition enhancers should be used routinely for dementia given their modest efficacy)
- A systematic review of the evidence from randomized, placebo-controlled trials showed a statistically significant though modest benefit of donepezil, galantamine, and rivastigmine in the treatment of behavioral and psychological symptoms of Alzheimer's disease
- Significant treatment benefits of donepezil demonstrated in early-stage Alzheimer's disease support initiating treatment early to improve daily cognitive functioning; shown to have additive effects with memantine in patients with moderate to severe Alzheimer's disease
- The improvement, on average, is modest and benefits may not be evident until 6–12 weeks of continuous treatment. In long-term studies, patients receiving treatment with cholinesterase inhibitors show improvement in cognitive ability after 6 months of therapy but then decline thereafter
- Drugs should not be stopped just because dementia severity increases
- A double-blind study conducted in over 2,000 patients with mild to moderate Alzheimer's disease established that galantamine treatment resulted in a significantly decreased mortality rate and showed benefits in cognition and activities of daily living that persisted for 2 years
- In an RCT with 130 patients, those treated with rivastigmine had improved gait stability, compared with placebo
- Economic analyses suggest that treatment initiated in early stages of Alzheimer's disease may be cost neutral as a result of patients remaining in a less severe state of disease for a longer time and delayed institutionalization
- Failure to respond to one agent does not preclude response to another; open-label studies suggest that approximately 50% of patients experiencing loss of efficacy with one drug respond to subsequent treatment with another agent
- Cholinesterase inhibitors promote lucid dreaming and out-of-body experiences
- Vascular dementia: No benefit of donepezil or galantamine on cognitive function. Efficacy on cognitive function and activities of daily living of cholinesterase inhibitors is unclear in people with Huntington's disease, cerebral autosomal dominant arteriopathy with subcortical infarcts and leukoencephalopathy (CADASIL), multiple sclerosis, and progressive supranuclear palsy or frontotemporal dementia (FTD). However, cholinesterase inhibitors are associated with more gastrointestinal side effects compared with placebo. Worsening of FTD has been reported
- No benefit in mild cognitive impairment (MCI)
- A meta-analysis of 15 trials on use of cholinesterase inhibitors or memantine as treatments for cognitive impairment in Parkinson's disease, Parkinson's disease with dementia, and dementia with Lewy bodies reported improvements, not only in global cognitive function and motor function, but also in attention, processing speed, executive function, memory, and language

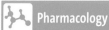 **Pharmacology**

- See chart on p. 353
- The precise mechanism of action is unknown. It is postulated that these compounds exert their therapeutic effect by enhancing cholinergic function. This is accomplished by increasing the concentration of acetylcholine through reversible inhibition of its hydrolysis by cholinesterase. If this mechanism is correct, the effect of these compounds may lessen as the disease process advances and fewer cholinergic neurons remain functionally intact

- Nicotinic cholinergic receptors may regulate cognitive functions, such as attention, and may increase the release of neurotransmitters throughout the brain
- Galantamine is also a positive allosteric modulator of the $\alpha_4\beta_2$ and α_7 nicotinic receptors that could lead directly to increased release of acetylcholine and activation of postsynaptic nicotinic receptors, or act indirectly through its effects on the release of other neurotransmitters, especially glutamate and dopamine. Galantamine increases dopaminergic activity and release in the prefrontal cortex and hippocampus in a dose-dependent manner
- Cholinesterase inhibitors with less specificity (e.g., rivastigmine) may be more efficacious in more advanced stages of dementia

Dosing

- See chart on p. 353
- With galantamine and rivastigmine, treatment is started at lower doses with gradual dose escalation to minimize side effects
- Effects on cognition and functional activities are dose dependent, while effects on behavioral disturbances are not
- Rivastigmine Patch 5 releases drug at a rate of 4.6 mg/24 h; Patch 10 releases drug at a rate of 9.5 mg/24 h. When switching from oral drug, Patch 5 is recommended for patients on less than 6 mg/day and Patch 10 can be used for patients on higher doses; apply patch the day following the last oral dose
- Donepezil 23 mg dose is recommended for patients with moderate to severe disease who have been stabilized on donepezil 10 mg for at least 3 months
- Patients who discontinue galantamine or rivastigmine for longer than several days should be restarted at the lowest daily dose (i.e., 4 mg bid for galantamine and 1.5 mg od or bid for rivastigmine) to reduce the possibility of severe vomiting; dosage should be titrated over a period of 2 months to the maintenance dose
- For dosing in patients with renal and/or hepatic insufficiency, see chart p. 353

Pharmacokinetics

- See chart, p. 354
- Duration of cholinesterase inhibition does not reflect plasma half-life of drug (e.g., rivastigmine half-life is 1–2 h, but cholinesterase inhibition lasts up to 10 h)
- Donepezil and galantamine are substrates for CYP2D6 and CYP3A4
- Plasma rivastigmine levels are approximately 30% higher in elderly male patients than in young adults
- Rivastigmine Patch produces lower peak levels but maintains steadier plasma levels than the oral formulation
- Exposure to galantamine in patients with moderate and severe renal impairment is significantly higher than in healthy subjects, and is approximately 30% higher in patients with moderate hepatic impairment

Pharmacogenetics

- Many patients with dementia take more than 6–10 drugs/day for the treatment of comorbidities, resulting in a significant risk for drug–drug interactions and adverse drug reactions (ADRs, more than 80%); adverse drug reactions that may accelerate cognitive decline can be mitigated with the implementation of pharmacogenetics (PGx)
- APOE-4 carriers are the worst responders to cholinesterase inhibitors and other conventional treatments
- Donepezil
  - Donepezil is a major substrate of ACHE, CYP2D6, CYP3A4, and UGTs, inhibits ACHE and BCHE, and is transported by ABCB1. Variants of BCHE-K* and CHRNA7 also affect donepezil efficacy and safety
  - Presence of CYP2D6 variants conferring decreased or absent CYP2D6 enzyme activity (intermediate or poor metabolizers) has been associated with greater response to donepezil treatment compared to rapid metabolizers. Analysis of CYP2D6 allele variants may be useful in identifying patients with Alzheimer's disease who are more likely to respond to donepezil[1]
  - In APOE-ε4 allele carriers, a single nucleotide polymorphism rs1080985 in the CYP2D6 gene, G allele carriers were found to be approximately 3 times less likely to respond to donepezil
  - Patients with the G allele have approximately 3 times greater risk of a poor response to donepezil treatment
- Galantamine
  - Galantamine is a major substrate of ABCB1, CYP2D6, CYP3A4, and UGT1A1, and an inhibitor of ACHE and BCHE. Variants of ACHE, APOE, APP, BCHE, CHRNA4, CHRNA7, and CHRNB2 may also modify the effects of galantamine
  - The FDA recommends, but does not require, genetic testing prior to initiating or reinitiating treatment with galantamine. Approximately 7% of the general population have reduced activity levels of CYP2D6 isozyme. Such individuals have been referred to as poor metabolizers. Galantamine

Cholinesterase Inhibitors (cont.)

levels are higher in poor metabolizers compared to extensive metabolizers (i.e., AUC of unchanged galantamine increased by 35% and median clearance decreased by 25%)
- Dosage adjustment is usually not necessary in patients identified as poor metabolizers as the drug dose is individually titrated to tolerability
- Rivastigmine metabolism is mediated by esterases in the liver and in the intestine. ACHE, APOE, APP, BCHE, CHAT, CHRNA4, CHRNB2, and MAPT variants may affect rivastigmine pharmacokinetics and pharmacodynamics, with special relevance in UGT2B7 poor metabolizers. CYP enzymes are not involved in rivastigmine metabolism

EFFECTS OF GENETIC POLYMORPHISMS[2]

Gene	rsID	Genotype	Drug effect
CHAT	rs2177370	AA vs. GG	Increased effect of ACHE inhibitors
CHAT	rs2177370	AA vs. GG	Increased effect of galantamine
CHAT	rs3793790	AA vs. GG	Decreased effect of ACHE inhibitors
CHRNA7	rs6494223	TT vs. CC	Increased effect of ACHE inhibitors

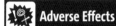 **Adverse Effects**

- See chart on pp. 355–356
- Increased risk of adverse effects when cholinesterase inhibitors used in combination with antipsychotics, antihypertensives or drugs acting on the GI tract
- Most common adverse effects are due to cholinomimetic activity: nausea, vomiting, diarrhea, constipation (rivastigmine), and anorexia – occur early in treatment and are associated with rapid dose titration
- Occur more often in patients over 85 years of age and in females
- Gastrointestinal symptoms (e.g., cramping, nausea, vomiting, and diarrhea) are dose dependent, occur more often during dose escalation, and tend to resolve with time; they are associated more frequently with the nonselective inhibitor rivastigmine than with donepezil or galantamine [reported to respond to short-term use of propantheline (7.5–15 mg) or domperidone (10 mg tid) – caution due to anticholinergic effects]; fewer side effects reported with the lower-dose rivastigmine patch than with the capsules or higher-dose patch – efficacy remains comparable; incidence reported to be 5% higher with donepezil 23 mg vs. 10 mg
- Rivastigmine has been associated with hepatitis
- A cohort study on the use of cholinesterase inhibitors in older adults with dementia showed higher rates of syncope, bradycardia, fall-related injuries, and hip fractures; dizziness and falls reported in 3–7%
- Other side effects (e.g., CNS, respiratory) occur more often during the maintenance phase and have no clear dose dependence; confusion (more than 4%) with rivastigmine and galantamine
- Aggression and hallucinations have been reported in association with rivastigmine. Truncal purpuric rash reported with donepezil
- Disseminated cutaneous hypersensitivity reactions have been reported in association with rivastigmine
- Skin reactions (redness, itching, irritation, swelling) can occur at application site of rivastigmine patch
- Weight loss. More likely to occur at higher doses. Increased risk of weight loss in patients taking 23 mg vs. 10 mg/day of donepezil
- Donepezil is more likely than rivastigmine to be associated with extrapyramidal symptoms, sleep disturbances, and muscle cramps

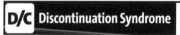 **D/C Discontinuation Syndrome**

- Sudden worsening of cognitive function and behavior reported following drug withdrawal – suggest that dose be reduced by 25–50% every 1–2 weeks, with close monitoring

 Precautions

- Caution should be exercised if any of the following exists:
  - Known hypersensitivity to above compounds

- History of or genetic predisposition to syncope, bradycardia, bradyarrhythmia, sick sinus syndrome, history of hepatic or renal disease, obstructive urinary disease, conduction disturbances, congestive heart failure, coronary artery disease, asthma, COPD, ulcers or increased risk of ulcers or GI bleeding (concomitant use of NSAIDS or higher doses of ASA)
  - Patient is taking drugs that significantly slow heart rate
  - Patients with acquired long QTc syndrome
- Cholinomimetics may cause bladder outflow obstruction
- Cholinesterase inhibitors may have vagotonic effects on the sinoatrial and atrioventricular nodes. May clinically manifest as bradycardia, heart block, and syncopal episodes in patients with and without known cardiac abnormalities
- With galantamine: monitor for respiratory adverse events in patients with a history of severe asthma or obstructive pulmonary disease
- With rivastigmine: isolated postmarketing reports of patients experiencing disseminated cutaneous hypersensitivity reactions, irrespective of the route of administration (oral or transdermal). Treatment should be discontinued if such skin reactions occur. Instruct patients and caregivers accordingly
- In patients who develop application site reactions suggestive of allergic contact dermatitis to rivastigmine patch and who still require rivastigmine, treatment should be switched to oral rivastigmine only after negative allergy testing and under close medical supervision. Some patients sensitized to rivastigmine by exposure to patch may not be able to take rivastigmine in any form
- Nausea and vomiting. Observe patients closely at initiation of treatment and after dose increases
- Peptic ulcer disease and GI bleeding. Monitor patients closely for symptoms of active or occult gastrointestinal bleeding, especially those at increased risk for developing ulcers. Increased incidence of peptic ulcer disease in a cohort taking 23 mg vs. 10 g/day of donepezil
- Anesthesia. Exaggeration of muscle relaxation induced by succinylcholine-type drugs
- Epilepsy, seizure disorders. Cholinesterase inhibitors are believed to have some potential to cause generalized convulsions. Patients with Alzheimer's disease should be monitored closely for seizures due to reduced seizure threshold
- Pulmonary conditions. Cholinesterase inhibitors should be prescribed with care to patients with a history of asthma or obstructive pulmonary disease
- Increased risk of death in patients with mild cognitive impairment (MCI) (galantamine)
- Significantly reduced clearance of donepezil when taken with a known CYP2D6 inhibitor

 Contraindications

- Donepezil is contraindicated in patients with known hypersensitivity to donepezil hydrochloride or to piperidine derivatives
- Galantamine is contraindicated in patients with severe hepatic and/or renal impairment (CrCl less than 9 mL/min)
- Previous application site reaction with rivastigmine transdermal patch suggestive of allergic contact dermatitis, in the absence of negative allergy testing

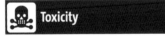 **Toxicity**

- Overdose can result in cholinergic crisis characterized by severe nausea, vomiting, salivation, sweating, hypotension, hallucinations, bradycardia, and syncope followed by respiratory depression and convulsions; increasing muscle weakness is a possibility and may result in death if respiratory muscles are involved. Atypical responses in blood pressure and heart rate have been reported
- Hospitalization and (rarely) death have been reported due to application of multiple patches at the same time. Ensure patients or caregivers receive instruction on proper dosing and administration

Management

- Institute general supportive measures
- Treatment: Atropine sulfate 1 mg to 2 mg IV with subsequent doses depending on clinical response. The value of dialysis in overdosage is not known
- In asymptomatic rivastigmine overdose, hold drug for 24 h, then resume treatment. Because of the short half-life of rivastigmine (plasma half-life of about 3.4 h after patch administration and a duration of acetylcholinesterase inhibition of about 9 h), the value of dialysis in treatment of cholinergic crisis is unknown

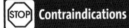 **Pediatric Considerations**

- There are no adequate and well-controlled trials to document the safety and efficacy of donepezil hydrochloride in any illness occurring in children

 Geriatric Considerations

- Caution should be exercised and adverse events closely monitored when using donepezil in doses over 5 mg/day
- Galantamine plasma concentrations are 30–40% higher in the elderly than in healthy young subjects
- Galantamine reported to increase mortality in patients with mild cognitive impairment and should not be used

Cholinesterase Inhibitors (cont.)

Use in Pregnancy◊

- Based on animal data, may cause fetal harm. Adequate, well-controlled human studies are lacking, and animal studies have shown risk to the fetus or are lacking as well

Breast Milk

- Not recommended for nursing women

Nursing Implications

- Advise patients to take the drug as directed; increasing the dose will increase adverse effects while skipping doses will decrease the benefit of the drug
- Advise patients not to stop the medication abruptly, as changes in behavior and/or concentration can occur
- Anticholinergic agents (including over-the-counter drugs, e.g., antinauseants) will reduce the effects of these drugs and should be avoided
- Rivastigmine patches should be kept sealed until use. Apply the first rivastigmine patch the day following the last oral dose. The location of the patch should be rotated and the patch applied to the upper or lower back, upper arm, or chest; if there is potential for the patient to remove the patch, apply it onto an inaccessible area. **Remove patch after 24 h, prior to applying the next dose** – fold it in half with the adhesive sides on the inside and dispose of in waste container; wash hands after handling
- Advise patient that rivastigmine patch may compromise driving ability
- Advise patient to stop taking rivastigmine and inform doctor if a rash develops
- The 23 mg donepezil tablet should not be split, crushed or chewed because this may increase the rate of absorption

Patient Instructions

- For detailed patient instructions on cognition enhancers, see the Patient Information Sheet (details p. 474)

Drug Interactions

- Clinically significant interactions are listed below
- For more interaction information on any given combination, also see the corresponding chapter for the second agent

DRUGS INTERACTING WITH DONEPEZIL

Class of Drug	Example	Interaction Effects
Antiarrhythmic	Quinidine	Inhibited metabolism of donepezil via CYP2D6
Antibiotic	Clarithromycin, erythromycin	Inhibited metabolism of donepezil via CYP2D6
Anticholinergic	Benztropine, diphenhydramine	Antagonism of effects
Anticonvulsant	Carbamazepine, phenytoin, phenobarbital	Increased metabolism of donepezil, resulting in decreased efficacy
Antidepressant	SSRI – fluoxetine, paroxetine	May increase plasma level of donepezil by inhibiting metabolism via CYP2D6. Fulminant hepatitis reported in combination with a high dose of sertraline Case reports of increased GI and CNS adverse effects as well as extrapyramidal symptoms with paroxetine and donepezil
	Nefazodone	Inhibited metabolism of donepezil via CYP3A4
Antifungal	Itraconazole, ketoconazole	Inhibited metabolism of donepezil via CYP3A4
Antipsychotic	Risperidone	Exacerbation of EPS; worsening of Parkinson's disease
Antitubercular drug	Rifampin	Increased metabolism of donepezil, resulting in decreased efficacy
β-blocker	Propranolol	May potentiate bradycardia; may increase risk of bronchospasm
Cholinergic agonist	Bethanechol	Synergistic effects: Increased nausea, vomiting, and diarrhea
Neuromuscular blocker	Succinylcholine, suxamethonium	Prolonged neuromuscular blockade

◊ See p. 473 for further information on drug use in pregnancy and effects on breast milk

DRUGS INTERACTING WITH GALANTAMINE

Class of Drug	Example	Interaction Effects
Antiarrhythmic	Quinidine	Decreased clearance of galantamine (by 25–30%) due to inhibited metabolism via CYP2D6
Antibiotic	Clarithromycin, erythromycin	Increased AUC of galantamine (by 10%) due to inhibited metabolism via CYP3A4
Anticholinergic	Benztropine, chlorpheniramine	Antagonism of effects
Antidepressant	Bupropion	Increased galantamine level possible, due to inhibited metabolism; may increase risk of seizures
	Fluvoxamine, nefazodone	Decreased clearance of galantamine (by 25–30%) due to inhibited metabolism via CYP2D6
	Paroxetine	Increased AUC of galantamine (by 40%) due to inhibited metabolism via CYP2D6
Antifungal	Ketoconazole	Increased AUC of galantamine (by 30%) due to inhibited metabolism via CYP3A4
Antiretroviral Protease inhibitor	Nelfinavir, ritonavir	May increase galantamine level due to inhibited metabolism via CYP3A4 Risk of cholinergic adverse effects
β-blocker	Propranolol	May potentiate bradycardia; may increase risk of bronchospasm
H$_2$ antagonist	Cimetidine	Increased AUC of galantamine (by 16%)
Neuromuscular blocker	Succinylcholine, suxamethonium	Prolonged neuromuscular blockade
NSAID	Ibuprofen, ketoprofen	Increased risk of bleeding

DRUGS INTERACTING WITH RIVASTIGMINE

Class of Drug	Example	Interaction Effects
Anticholinergic	Benztropine, diphenhydramine	Antagonism of effects
Antipsychotic	Haloperidol	Exacerbation of EPS
β-blocker	Propranolol	May potentiate bradycardia; may increase risk of bronchospasm
Neuromuscular blocker	Succinylcholine, suxamethonium	Prolonged neuromuscular blockade
Smoking (tobacco)		Increased clearance of rivastigmine by 23%

Memantine

 Product Availability*

Generic Name	Chemical Class	Neuroscience-based Nomenclature* (Pharmacological Target/Mode of Action)	Trade Name	Dosage Forms and Strengths
Memantine	Aminoadamantane	Glutamate/Antagonist (NMDA)	Ebixa(C), Namenda(B) Namenda XR	Tablets: 5 mg, 10 mg Solution(B): 2 mg/mL Extended-release capsules(B): 7 mg, 14 mg, 21 mg, 28 mg
Memantine extended release/donepezil	Aminoadamantane/ Piperidine	Glutamate/Antagonist (NMDA) Acetylcholine/Enzyme inhibitor	Namzaric(B)	Capsules (memantine extended release/donepezil): 7/10 mg, 14/10 mg, 21/10 mg, 28/10 mg

* Refer to Health Canada's Drug Product Database or the FDA's Drugs@FDA for the most current availability information. * Developed by a taskforce consisting of representatives from the American College of Neuropsychopharmacology (ACNP), the Asian College of Neuropsychopharmacology (AsCNP), the European College of Neuropsychopharmacology (ECNP), the International College of Neuropsychopharmacology (CINP), and the International Union of Basic and Clinical Pharmacology (IUPHAR) (see https://nbn2r.com), (B) Not marketed in Canada,   (C) Not marketed in the USA

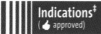 **Indications‡**
(👍 approved)

- 🔸 Dementia of Alzheimer's type: Symptomatic treatment of moderate to severe disease (memantine shows some efficacy in mild AD)
- 🔸 Memantine extended release/donepezil is indicated for treatment of moderate–severe dementia of Alzheimer's type in patients stabilized on 10 mg of donepezil hydrochloride once daily. Only FDA approved for the treatment of dementia of Alzheimer's type. All other indications are non-FDA approved
- Vascular dementia: Double-blind studies report benefit on cognitive function
- Alzheimer's disease: Reported to decrease delusions, agitation/aggression, and psychosis in patients with moderate to severe disease and improve behavioral and psychological symptoms of dementia (BPSD)[3]
- Dementia with Lewy bodies: Shown to improve global clinical status and behavioral symptoms in patients with mild to moderate disease in double-blind studies
- Pain: Memantine has demonstrated benefits in decreasing neuropathic pain, including fibromyalgia, in double-blind studies
- OCD: Contradictory results reported when memantine used as an augmenting agent with an SSRI in OCD treatment
- Bipolar disorder, treatment resistant: add-on memantine may show antimanic and mood-stabilizing effects
- Schizophrenia: Several RCTs and meta-analysis suggest that augmentation with 20 mg/day may improve persistent negative symptoms and cognitive impairment and benefit general psychopathology of schizophrenia
- Autism spectrum disorder: Double-blind and open studies report improvements in behaviors, attention, communication, and interactions

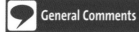 **General Comments**

- Memantine has additive effects, with cholinesterase inhibitors, in patients with moderate to severe Alzheimer's disease; reported to significantly delay time to nursing home admission
- Shown to modify the progressive symptomatic decline in global status, cognition, function, and behavior in patients with moderate to severe Alzheimer's disease over 28-week trial
- Fewer viral infections reported with memantine in clinical trials (as compared to comparator drugs) due to its antiviral properties (it belongs to the same chemical class as amantadine)
- Memantine treatment is associated with an increased life-expectancy relative to donepezil treatment
- Fronto-temporal dementia: No benefit of memantine on cognition or behavior
- A meta-analysis of 15 trials on use of cholinesterase inhibitors or memantine as treatments for cognitive impairment in Parkinson's disease, Parkinson's disease with dementia, and dementia with Lewy bodies reported improvements, not only in global cognitive function and motor function, but also in attention, processing speed, executive function, memory, and language

‡ Indications listed here do not necessarily apply to all countries. Please refer to a country's regulatory database (e.g., US Food and Drug Administration, Health Canada Drug Product Database) for the most current availability information and indications

- A meta-analysis of 8 studies with 125 participants showed OCD subjects receiving memantine augmentation were 3.61 times more likely to respond to treatment than those receiving placebo. A dose of 20 mg/day augmentation to first-line pharmacological treatment for at least 8 weeks was found to be a safe and effective intervention for moderate to severe OCD

 Pharmacology

- Memantine has N-methyl-D-aspartate (NMDA) inhibitory properties thought to contribute to its clinical effectiveness, and preserves neuronal function by selectively blocking the excitotoxic effects associated with abnormal glutamate transmission (blocks excessive extrasynaptic activity of the NDMA subtype of glutamate receptors, while largely sparing normal synaptic activity)
- Increases dopamine levels and reported to have antidyskinetic (antiparkinsonian) and antiviral properties

 Dosing

- See chart, p. 353
- Bid administration recommended for doses above 10 mg; usual daily dose is 20 mg (see table p. 353)
- As memantine is excreted predominantly by the kidneys, the following dosage adjustments are recommended in renal impairment:
  - In mildly impaired renal function (CrCl 50–80 mL/min), no dosage adjustment is required
  - In moderate renal impairment (CrCl 30–49 mL/min), a target dose of 5 mg bid is recommended. If well tolerated after at least 7 days of treatment, and based on clinical response, dose may be increased up to 10 mg bid according to standard titration scheme
  - In severe renal impairment (CrCl 15–29 mL/min), a target dose of 5 mg bid is recommended
- Please see dosing recommendations of memantine extended-release capsules p. 353
- Memantine extended release/donepezil recommended dosing is once a day. The capsules can be opened and sprinkled on food for patients who have difficulty swallowing
  - For patients stabilized on 10 mg donepezil and not currently on memantine, the recommended starting dose is 7 mg/10 mg, taken once a day in the evening. Increase dose in 7 mg increments of the memantine component to the recommended maintenance dose/maximum dose of 28 mg/10 mg once daily. The minimum recommended interval between dose increases is one week. Only increase dose if the previous dose has been well tolerated
  - Patients stabilized on both memantine (10 mg twice daily or 28 mg XR once daily) and donepezil 10 mg once daily can be switched to memantine extended release/donepezil 28 mg/10 mg, taken once a day in the evening. Patients should start taking the combination product the day following the last dose of memantine and donepezil administered separately. If a patient misses a single dose of memantine extended release/donepezil, the next dose should be taken as scheduled, without doubling the dose
  - Severe renal impairment (CrCl 5–29 mL/min, based on the Cockcroft-Gault equation): For patients stabilized on donepezil 10 mg once daily and not currently on memantine, starting dose is 7 mg/10 mg once a day in the evening. Increase to the maintenance dose of 14 mg/10 mg once daily after a minimum of one week. Patients stabilized on memantine (5 mg twice daily or 14 mg XR once daily) and donepezil 10 mg once daily can be switched to memantine extended release/donepezil 14 mg/10 mg, taken once daily in the evening

 Pharmacokinetics

- See chart, p. 354
- Alkalinization of urine (e.g., high antacid use or drastic diet change) can reduce renal elimination of memantine – monitor urine pH
- The CYP450 enzyme system does not play a significant role in the metabolism of memantine
- In a study comparing 28 mg once daily memantine XR to 10 mg twice daily memantine immediate release, C_{max} and AUC_{0-24} values were 48% and 33% higher for the XR dosage regimen, respectively
- The terminal elimination half-life increased by 18%, 41%, and 95% in subjects with mild, moderate, and severe renal impairment, respectively, compared to healthy subjects
- Immediate release:
  - Crosses blood/brain barrier readily and is detectable in cerebrospinal fluid within 30 min of administration
- Extended release:
  - Food has no effect on overall absorption, however, peak plasma concentrations occur early when administered with food
  - No difference in the absorption of memantine extended release when the capsule is taken intact or when the contents are sprinkled on applesauce

Adverse Effects

- See chart, pp. 355–356
- Most common: Confusion, agitation, insomnia, paranoia, mild to moderate dizziness, and headaches

Memantine (cont.)

- Urinary incontinence and urinary tract infections reported
- Blood and lymphatic system disorders (agranulocytosis, pancytopenia, thrombotic thrombocytopenic purpura, blood clots) reported
- Increased incidence of cardiac failure, angina, and hypertension occurred in clinical trials

 D/C Discontinuation Syndrome

- Cases of discontinuation syndrome following abrupt cessation of memantine have been documented
- Discontinuation syndrome consisted of insomnia, aggressive behavior, disinhibited behavior, and delusions
- Emergence of symptoms as early as 2 days after discontinuation

 Precautions

- Memantine should be used with caution under conditions that raise urine pH (including alterations by diet, drugs, and the clinical state of the patient). Alkaline urine conditions may decrease the urinary elimination of memantine, resulting in increased plasma levels and a possible increase in adverse effects
- Memantine has not been systematically evaluated in patients with a seizure disorder
- The combined use of memantine with other NMDA antagonists (amantadine, ketamine, or dextromethorphan) has not been systematically evaluated and such use should be approached with caution

 Contraindications

- Not recommended in patients with severe renal impairment

 Toxicity

- Overdose (up to 400 mg) resulted in CNS effects including restlessness, somnolence, stupor, visual hallucinations, seizures, and unconsciousness

Management

- Treatment: Elimination of memantine can be enhanced by acidification of urine

 Pediatric Considerations

- Beneficial effects have been reported in children and adolescents with autism spectrum disorder (ASD) and in treatment-resistant OCD

 Geriatric Considerations

- Caution in patients with decreased renal function
- Monitor adverse effects closely

 Use in Pregnancy◊

- Not teratogenic in animals; effects in humans unknown

Breast Milk

- Effect unknown

 Nursing Implications

- Minimize the use of antacids (e.g., Milk of Magnesia, Al/Mg products) as alkalinization of urine (pH higher than 8) will reduce elimination and increase the effects of the drug – monitoring urine pH is recommended by some
- Capsules of memantine extended release and of memantine extended release/donepezil combination can be opened and sprinkled on food for patients who have difficulties swallowing

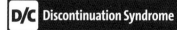 **Patient Instructions**

- For detailed patient instructions on memantine, see Patient Information Sheet (details on p. 474)

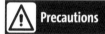 **Drug Interactions**

- Clinically significant interactions are listed below
- For more interaction information on any given combination, also see the corresponding chapter for the second agent

◊ See p. 473 for further information on drug use in pregnancy and effects on breast milk

Class of Drug	Example	Interaction Effects
Alkaline agent	Antacids, sodium bicarbonate, carbonic anhydrase inhibitors	Increased levels of memantine possible as elimination rate decreased significantly (by 80%) if pH higher than 8
Aminoadamantane	Amantadine, rimantadine	Do not combine as adverse effects may be enhanced
Anesthetic	Ketamine	Do not combine as adverse effects may be enhanced (additive effects of NMDA receptor blockade)
Antiarrhythmic	Procainamide, quinidine	Increased plasma levels of memantine possible due to competition for excretion via organic cation transporter-2 in the renal tubule
Antibiotic	Trimethoprim	Increased level of memantine due to competition for excretion via organic cation transporter-2 in the renal tubule
Anticoagulant	Warfarin	Monitor patients for increases in INR or prothrombin times
Anticonvulsant	Valproate	Synergistic effect in seizure suppression reported in animal studies
Antimalarial	Quinine	Increased level of memantine due to competition for excretion via organic cation transporter-2 in the renal tubule
Dextromethorphan		Do not combine as adverse effects may be enhanced (additive effects of NMDA receptor blockade)
Diuretic	Hydrochlorothiazide	Reduced excretion of hydrochlorothiazide possible; bioavailability of hydrochlorothiazide reduced by 20%
H₂ antagonist	Cimetidine, ranitidine	Increased plasma levels of memantine possible due to competition for excretion via organic cation transporter-2 in the renal tubule
Hypoglycemic agent	Metformin	Theoretical increased level of memantine due to competition for excretion via organic cation transporter-2 in the renal tubule, but one study showed administration of memantine had no effect on the pharmacodynamics activities of glyburide or metformin
Smoking (tobacco)		Increased plasma levels of memantine possible due to competition for excretion via organic cation transporter-2 in the renal tubule
N-methyl-d-aspartate (NMDA) receptor antagonist	Amantadine, dextromethorphan, ketamine	Combined use with other NMDA antagonists has not been systematically evaluated and should be approached with caution

Lecanemab

Rx Product Availability*

Generic Name	Chemical Class	Neuroscience-based Nomenclature* (Pharmacological Target/Mode of Action)	Trade Name	Dosage Forms and Strengths
Lecanemab	Amyloid beta-directed antibody	Not available	Leqembi[B]	500 mg/5 mL (100 mg/mL) solution in a single-dose vial 200 mg/2 mL (100 mg/mL) solution in a single-dose vial

* Refer to Health Canada's Drug Product Database or the FDA's Drugs@FDA for the most current availability information. * Developed by a taskforce consisting of representatives from the American College of Neuropsychopharmacology (ACNP), the Asian College of Neuropsychopharmacology (AsCNP), the European College of Neuropsychopharmacology (ECNP), the International College of Neuropsychopharmacology (CINP), and the International Union of Basic and Clinical Pharmacology (IUPHAR) (see https://nbn2r.com), [B] Not marketed in Canada

Indications‡ (👍 approved) ➤ 👍 Alzheimer's disease

‡ Please refer to a country's regulatory database (e.g., US Food and Drug Administration, Health Canada Drug Product Database) for the most current availability information and indications

Lecanemab (cont.)

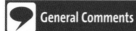 **General Comments**

- Confirmation of presence of amyloid beta pathology is necessary prior to initiating treatment
- Should be initiated in patients with mild cognitive impairment or mild dementia stage of disease
- There are no safety or effectiveness data on initiating treatment at earlier or later stages of the disease
- Approved for this indication by FDA via accelerated approval pathway based on reduction in amyloid beta plaques observed in patients treated with lecanemab
- Brief description of clinical trial (referred to as Study 1 in product monograph)[4, 5] that resulted in lecanemab's accelerated approval by the FDA:
  - Lecanemab efficacy was evaluated in participants with Alzheimer's disease (Stage 3 or 4) in a 79-week double-blind, placebo-controlled, parallel-group, dose-finding study with 856 subjects. The study was followed by an open-label extension period for up to 260 weeks, initiated after a gap period (range 9–59 months; mean of 24 months) off treatment. All participants had confirmed presence of amyloid pathology
  - Of the 856 participants, 609 were randomized to lecanemab and 245 were randomized to placebo. Of the participants randomized to receive one of 5 doses of lecanemab, 161 participants received the currently recommended dosing regimen of 10 mg/kg every 2 weeks
  - Participants were enrolled with or without concomitant approved therapies for Alzheimer's disease (i.e., cholinesterase inhibitors and memantine)
  - Primary endpoint: At 12 months, participants randomized to the 10 mg/kg biweekly dose of lecanemab showed a 64% probability to be better than placebo by 25% on Alzheimer's Disease Composite Score (ADCOMS), which missed the 80% threshold for the primary outcome
  - Secondary endpoints:
    - At 18 months, participants randomized to the 10 gm/kg biweekly lecanemab showed a reduction in brain amyloid (-0.306 SUVr units) while showing a drug–placebo difference in favor of active treatment vs. placebo on ADCOMS, Alzheimer's Disease Assessment Scale-Cognitive Subscale (ADAS-COG14), and Clinical Dementia Rating-Sum of Boxes (CDR-SB)
    - In the double-blind, placebo-controlled (DBPC) period of the study, an increase in plasma Aβ42/40 ratio was observed in participants randomized to lecanemab 10 mg/kg every two weeks compared to placebo
    - A reduction in plasma p-tau181 was observed with lecanemab 10 mg/kg every two weeks compared to placebo in the DBPC period of the study
    - During the gap period off treatment, rates of clinical progression were similar in lecanemab and placebo participants. Furthermore, plasma Aβ42/40 ratio and p-tau181 levels began to return towards pre-randomization levels more quickly than amyloid as measured by positron emission tomography (PET)

 Pharmacology

- Lecanemab is a humanized immunoglobulin gamma 1 (IgG1) monoclonal antibody directed against aggregated soluble and insoluble forms of amyloid beta. The accumulation of amyloid beta plaques in the brain is a defining pathophysiological feature of Alzheimer's disease

 Dosing

- The recommended dosage of lecanemab is 10 mg/kg that must be diluted then administered as an intravenous infusion over approximately 1 h, once every 2 weeks
- If an infusion is missed, administer the next dose as soon as possible
- Lecanemab can cause amyloid-related imaging abnormalities-edema (ARIA-E) and -hemosiderin deposition (ARIA-H)
- Monitoring for ARIA:
  - Obtain a recent (within one year) brain MRI prior to initiating treatment with lecanemab. Obtain an MRI prior to 5th, 7th, and 14th infusions
- Recommendations for dosing interruptions in patients with ARIA-E:

Clinical Symptom Severity[1]	ARIA-E Severity of MRI		
	Mild	Moderate	Severe
Asymptomatic	May continue dosing	Suspend dosing[2]	Suspend dosing[2]
Mild	May continue dosing based on clinical judgment	Suspend dosing[2]	Suspend dosing[2]
Moderate or severe	Suspend dosing[2]	Suspend dosing[2]	Suspend dosing[2]

[1] Mild: discomfort noticed, but no disruption of normal daily activity; Moderate: discomfort sufficient to reduce or affect normal daily activity; Severe: incapacitating, with inability to work or to perform normal daily activity,   [2] Suspend until MRI demonstrates radiographic resolution and symptoms, if present, resolve; consider a follow-up MRI to assess for resolution 2–4 months after initial identification. Resumption of dosing should be guided by clinical judgment

- Recommendations for dosing interruptions in patients with ARIA-H:

Clinical Symptom Severity	ARIA-H Severity of MRI		
	Mild	Moderate	Severe
Asymptomatic	May continue dosing	Suspend dosing[1]	Suspend dosing[2]
Symptomatic	Suspend dosing[1]	Suspend dosing[1]	Suspend dosing[2]

[1] Suspend until MRI demonstrates radiographic stabilization and symptoms, if present, resolve; resumption of dosing should be guided by clinical judgment; consider a follow-up MRI to assess for stabilization 2–4 months after initial identification, [2] Suspend until MRI demonstrates radiographic stabilization and symptoms, if present, resolve; use clinical judgment in considering whether to continue treatment or permanently discontinue lecanemab

- In patients who develop intracerebral hemorrhage greater than 1 cm in diameter during treatment with lecanemab, suspend dosing until MRI demonstrates radiographic stabilization and symptoms, if present, resolve. Use clinical judgment in considering whether to continue treatment after radiographic stabilization and resolution of symptoms or permanently discontinue lecanemab

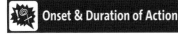

Pharmacokinetics

- Steady-state concentrations of lecanemab were reached after 6 weeks of 10 mg/kg administration every 2 weeks and systemic accumulation was 1.4-fold
- Peak concentration (C_{max}) and area under the plasma concentration vs. time curve (AUC) of lecanemab increased dose proportionally in the dose range of 0.3–15 mg/kg following single dose
- Mean value for central volume of distribution at steady state is 3.22 L
- Lecanemab is degraded by proteolytic enzymes in the same manner as endogenous IgGs. Lecanemab clearance is 0.434 L/day
- Terminal half-life is 5–7 days
- No clinical studies conducted to evaluate the pharmacokinetics of lecanemab in patients with renal or hepatic impairment. Lecanemab is degraded by proteolytic enzyme and is not expected to undergo renal elimination or metabolism by hepatic enzymes

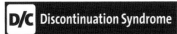

Onset & Duration of Action

- In the DBPC period of Study 1, treatment with lecanemab 10 mg/kg every two weeks reduced amyloid beta plaque levels in the brain, as evaluated using PET and quantified using the standard uptake value ratio (SUVr), compared to placebo at both Weeks 53 and 79. Magnitude of reduction was time and dose dependent
- During an off-treatment period, SUVr and Centiloid values began to increase with a mean rate of increase of 2.6 Centiloids/year; however, treatment difference relative to placebo at the end of the DBPC period in Study 1 was maintained

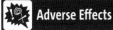

Adverse Effects

- The safety of lecanemab has been evaluated in 763 patients who received at least one dose of lecanemab
- In the DBPC period of Study 1, 15% of participants treated with lecanemab, compared to 6% of participants on placebo, stopped study treatment because of an adverse reaction
- Most common adverse reactions:
  - The most common adverse reaction leading to discontinuation of lecanemab was infusion-related reactions in 2% (4 of 161) of participants treated with lecanemab compared to 1% (2 of 245) of participants on placebo
  - Adverse reactions reported in at least 5% of participants treated with lecanemab included infusion-related reactions (20% vs. 3% for placebo), headache (14% vs. 10% for placebo), ARIA-E (10% vs. 1% for placebo), cough (9% vs. 5% for placebo), and diarrhea (8% vs. 5% for placebo)
  - Less common adverse reactions included atrial fibrillation (4% vs. 1% in participants on placebo). Lymphopenia or decreased lymphocyte count was reported in 4% of participants treated with lecanemab, all after the first dose, compared to less than 1% of participants on placebo

Discontinuation Syndrome

- No information is currently available regarding symptoms associated with the discontinuation of lecanemab

Precautions

- **Amyloid Related Imaging Abnormalities (ARIA):** Enhanced clinical vigilance for ARIA recommended during first 14 weeks of treatment with lecanemab. Risk of ARIA, including symptomatic ARIA, was increased in ApoE ε4 homozygotes compared to heterozygotes and noncarriers. Symptomatic ARIA occurred in 3% (5 of 161) of participants treated with lecanemab in Study 1. Of these 5 participants, 4 were ApoE ε4 homozygotes, 2 of whom experienced severe symptoms. (Note: In participants randomized to receive lecanemab in Study 1, 10 participants

Lecanemab (cont.)

were ApoE ε4 homozygotes.) If a participant experiences symptoms suggestive of ARIA, clinical evaluation should be performed, including MRI scan if indicated. Consider testing for ApoE ε4 status to inform the risk of developing ARIA when deciding to initiate treatment with lecanemab

- **Infusion-Related Reactions:** Observed in 20% (32 of 161) of participants treated with lecanemab compared to 3% (8 of 245) of participants on placebo; 88% (28 of 32) occurred with the first infusion. Symptoms of infusion-related reactions included fever and flu-like symptoms (chills, generalized aches, feeling shaky, and joint pain), nausea, vomiting, hypotension, hypertension, and oxygen desaturation. Infusion rate may be reduced, or infusion may be discontinued, and appropriated therapy administered as clinically indicated. Prophylactic treatment with antihistamines, acetaminophen, non-steroidal anti-inflammatory drugs, or corticosteroids prior to future infusions may be considered
- Because intracerebral hemorrhages greater than 1 cm in diameter have been observed in patients receiving lecanemab, additional caution should be exercised when considering the administration of antithrombotics or a thrombolytic agent (e.g., tissue plasminogen activator) to a patient already being treated with lecanemab

 Geriatric Considerations

- Confirm the presence of amyloid beta pathology prior to initiating treatment with lecanemab

 Nursing Implications

Dilution Instructions

- Prior to administration, lecanemab must be diluted in 250 mL of 0.9% sodium chloride injection, USP
- Use aseptic technique when preparing the lecanemab diluted solution for IV infusion
- Calculate dose (mg) and total volume (mL) of lecanemab solution required, and the number of vials needed based on the patient's actual body weight and the recommended dose of 10 mg/kg. Each vial contains a lecanemab concentration of 100 mg/mL
- Visually inspect for particulate matter and discoloration prior to administration. Check that the lecanemab solution is clear to opalescent and colorless to pale yellow. Do not use if opaque particles, discoloration, or other foreign particles are present
- Withdraw the required volume of lecanemab from the vial(s) and add to an infusion bag containing 250 mL of 0.9% sodium chloride injection, USP
- Each vial is for one-time use only. Discard any unused portion
- Gently invert the infusion bag containing the lecanemab diluted solution to mix completely. Do not shake
- After dilution, immediate use is recommended. If not administered immediately, store refrigerated at 2–8 degrees Celsius for up to 4 h, or at room temperature up to 30 degrees Celsius for up to 4 h. Do not freeze

Administration Instructions

- Visually inspect the lecanemab diluted solution for particles or discoloration prior to administration. Do not use if it is discolored or opaque, or foreign particles are seen
- Prior to infusion, allow the lecanemab diluted solution to warm to room temperature
- Infuse the entire volume of the lecanemab diluted solution IV over approximately one hour through an IV line containing a terminal low-protein binding 0.2 micron in-line filter. Flush infusion line to ensure all lecanemab is administered
- Monitor for any signs or symptoms of an infusion-related reaction. Infusion rate may be reduced, or infusion may be discontinued, and appropriate therapy administered as clinically indicated. Consider premedication at subsequent dosing with antihistamines, non-steroidal anti-inflammatory drugs, or corticosteroids

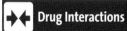 **Drug Interactions**

- None reported

	Donepezil	Galantamine	Rivastigmine	Memantine
Pharmacology	Piperidine-based Reversible inhibitor of AChE AChE > BuChE Binds to acetylcholinesterase in the brain and has little effect on cholinesterase in serum, heart or small intestine	Phenanthrene alkaloid Reversible inhibitor of AChE AChE > BuChE Allosteric modulator of central nicotinic receptors (may increase release of acetylcholine presynaptically)	A parasympathomimetic and a reversible cholinesterase inhibitor. Postulated to exert its therapeutic effect by enhancing cholinergic function. This is accomplished by increasing the concentration of acetylcholine through reversible inhibition of its hydrolysis by cholinesterase	Acts through uncompetitive NMDA receptor antagonism, binding more effectively than Mg^{2+} ions at the NMDA receptor. Thus protects against chronically elevated concentrations of glutamate. Also has antagonistic activity at the subtype 3 serotonergic ($5\text{-}HT_3$) receptor with a potency similar to that at the NMDA receptor, and lower antagonistic activity at the nicotinic acetylcholine receptor
Dosing	*Mild to moderate Alzheimer's disease:* 5 or 10 mg once daily *Moderate or severe Alzheimer's disease:* 10–23 mg once daily *Titration:* Recommended starting dose: 5 mg once daily at bedtime. A dose of 10 mg should not be administered until patient has been on a daily dose of 5 mg for 4–6 weeks. A dose of 23 mg once daily can be administered once patient has been on a dose of 10 mg once daily for at least 3 months	*Immediate-release tablets:* Initial dose is 4 mg bid with meals; after a minimum of 4 weeks, increase to initial maintenance dose of 8 mg bid; after a minimum of another 4 weeks, a further increase to 12 mg bid should be attempted, based on clinical benefit and tolerability *ER capsules:* Initial dose is 8 mg/day in a.m.; after a minimum of 4 weeks, increase to initial maintenance dose of 16 mg/day in a.m.; after a minimum of another 4 weeks, a further increase to 24 mg/day in a.m. should be attempted, based on clinical benefit and tolerability	*Alzheimer's disease Oral:* Initial dose is 1.5 mg bid, given with meals; after a minimum of 2 weeks, if tolerated, increase dose to 3 mg bid and further to 4.5 mg bid and 6 mg bid, if tolerated, with a minimum of 2 weeks at each dose *Parkinson's disease dementia:* Initial dose is 1.5 mg bid, given with meals; after a minimum of 4 weeks, if tolerated, increase dose to 3 mg bid and further to 4.5 mg bid and 6 mg bid, if tolerated, with a minimum of 4 weeks at each dose *Patch:* Apply patch on intact skin for a 24 h period; replace with a new patch every 24 h Initiate treatment with Patch 5 (4.6 mg/24 h) *Mild to moderate Alzheimer's disease and Parkinson's disease dementia:* After a minimum of 4 weeks of Patch 5 (4.6 mg/24 h), if tolerated, increase dose to Patch 10 (9.5 mg/24 h) for as long as therapeutic benefit persists. Can then be increased to a maximum of Patch 15 (13.3 mg/24 h) *Severe Alzheimer's disease:* Follow titration as above. Patch 15 (13.3 mg/24 h) is the effective dose After treatment interruption longer than 3 days, retitrate dosage starting with Patch 5 (4.6 mg/24 h) Consider dose adjustments in patients with low body weight (less than 50 kg)	*IR:* Recommended maintenance dose: 20 mg/day Dose escalation (over 1 month): 5 mg od for 7 days, 5 mg bid for 7 days, 10 mg a.m. and 5 mg p.m. for 7 days, then 10 mg bid; can be taken with or without food *XR capsules:* Initial dose is 7 mg once daily; increase in 7 mg increments after minimum of one week, if well tolerated, up to recommended maintenance dose of 28 mg once daily

Comparison of Drugs for Treatment of Dementia (cont.)

	Donepezil	Galantamine	Rivastigmine	Memantine
Renal impairment		If CrCl 9–59 mL/min, dose should not exceed 16 mg/day Not recommended if CrCl less than 9 mL/min		In renal insufficiency, see dosing recommendations p. 347 Severe renal impairment (CrCl 5-29 mL/min, based on the Cockcroft-Gault equation): Recommended that patient on 5 mg tablets twice daily be switched to XR capsules 14 mg once daily on the day following the last dose of a 5 mg tablet
Hepatic impairment		In patients with moderate impairment (Child-Pugh score of 7–9), dose should not exceed 16 mg/day Not recommended in patients with severe hepatic impairment (Child-Pugh score of 10–15)	Consider dose adjustments in patients with mild to moderate (Child-Pugh score of 5–6 to 7–9) hepatic impairment. Patch 5 (2.6 mg/24 h) is recommended	Use with caution in severe hepatic impairment
Switching		Conversion from tablets/oral solution to ER capsules should occur at the same daily dosage, with the last oral dose taken in the evening and ER capsules once daily started the next a.m.	When switching from oral drug, Patch 5 (4.6 mg/24 h) is recommended for patients on oral doses of less than 6 mg/day. Patch 10 (9.5 mg/24 h) is recommended for patients on oral doses above 6 mg/day; apply patch on the day following the last oral dose	Switching from tablets to XR capsules requires no titration Recommended that patient on tablets 10 mg twice daily be switched to XR capsules 28 mg once daily on the day following the last dose of a 10 mg tablet Patients stabilized on donepezil (with or without memantine) can be switched to the memantine extended release/donepezil combination. For dosing details, see p. 347
Pharmacokinetics Bioavailability	100%; is independent of food	90% (immediate release); food lowers C_{max} by 25% and delays T_{max} by 1.5 h ER: Not affected by food	Oral: 36%; food delays absorption, lowers C_{max}, and increases AUC by 25%	100%; food has no effect on absorption of memantine
Time to peak plasma level (T_{max})	3–4 h (10 mg tablets), 8 h (23 mg tablets)	Immediate release: 1 h ER: 4.5–5 h	Oral = 1 h Patch = 10–16 h after first dose	IR: 3–8 h XR: 9–12 h; peak level occurs earlier when given with food

	Donepezil	Galantamine	Rivastigmine	Memantine
Plasma protein binding	96%, predominantly to albumin (75%), and α_1-acid glycoprotein (21%). Interaction with drugs that are highly bound to plasma proteins (e.g., warfarin, digoxin) is unlikely	18%	40%	Approx. 45%. Interaction with drugs that are highly bound to plasma proteins (e.g., warfarin, digoxin) is unlikely
Plasma half-life	70–80 h in healthy adults; increases after multiple dose administration	IR: 7–8 h, ER: 7 h	Oral = 1–2 h (in both young and elderly patients) Patch = 3 h after patch removal	IR and XR: 60–80 h
Liver disease	Clearance decreased by 20% in patients with liver cirrhosis	Clearance decreased by 25–30% with liver disease	Clearance decreased by 60% in patients with liver disease	No dosage adjustment needed in mild or moderate hepatic impairment
Renal disease	Renal impairment has no effect on clearance	In moderate and severe renal impairment, AUC increased by 37% and 67%, respectively Clearance about 20% lower in females	Clearance decreased by 65% in moderate renal impairment	Clearance dependent on renal function (see Dosing, p. 347)
Metabolism	Metabolized via CYP2D6 and 3A4 and undergoes glucuronidation. Effects of CYP2D6 genotype: 31.5% slower clearance in poor metabolizers, 24% faster clearance in ultrarapid metabolizers 4 major metabolites, of which 2 are active	Metabolized via CYP2D6 and 3A4 (inhibitors of both pathways increase oral bioavailability of galantamine modestly)	Metabolized by esterase enzymes – low risk of drug interactions Phenolic metabolite has approximately 10% of the activity of parent drug	Excreted renally (60–80%). The hepatic microsomal CYP450 enzyme system does not play a significant role Renal elimination rate decreased significantly in alkaline pH (higher than 8) No pharmacokinetic interactions with drugs metabolized by CYP isozymes expected
Adverse Effects				
GI	5–10%: Nausea, vomiting, diarrhea, gastric upset, constipation; > 2%: Anorexia and weight loss (GI effects 5% higher with 23 mg vs. 10 mg dose)	10–30%: Nausea, vomiting; 5–10%: Diarrhea; 5–10%: Anorexia; > 1%: Flatulence	10–30%: Nausea, vomiting, diarrhea, abdominal pain; > 30%: Anorexia (with weight loss, especially in females)	> 5%: Diarrhea; 2–10%: Constipation
CNS	5–10%: Fatigue, headache; up to 18%: Insomnia; 2–5%: Abnormal dreams, nightmares, somnolence, agitation, activation, depression; < 2%: Restlessness, aggression, irritability; < 1%: Transient ischemic attack, hypokinesia, seizures Nightmares reported; manageable by switching from nighttime to morning dosing	5–10%: Insomnia, headache, depression, fatigue, agitation; 2–5%: Sedation, tremor; < 1%: Paranoia, delirium, ataxia, vertigo, hypertonia, seizures Reports of enhanced REM sleep, "lucid dreaming"	2–10%: Headache; > 5%: Sedation, asthenia; > 2%: Anxiety, insomnia, aggression, hallucinations; > 1%: Tremor, ataxia, abnormal gait Cases of seizures Case report of Pisa syndrome	5–20%: Insomnia, agitation; > 2%: Headache, confusion; < 2%: Lethargy Reports of vivid dreams, nightmares, and hallucinations

Comparison of Drugs for Treatment of Dementia (cont.)

	Donepezil	Galantamine	Rivastigmine	Memantine
Cardiovascular	Rapid onset of manic symptoms in patients with a history of BD reported Case report of delirium Worsening of parkinsonism and abnormal movements (restless legs, stuttering) reported Case reports of Pisa syndrome 2–10%: Dizziness; < 2%: Syncope, atrial fibrillation, hypotension; < 1%: Arrhythmia, first degree AV block, torsades de pointes, congestive heart failure, symptomatic sinus bradycardia, supraventricular tachycardia, deep vein thromboses	5–10%: Dizziness; > 2%: Bradycardia, syncope (dose-related); > 1%: Chest pain; < 1%: Edema, atrial fibrillation Case report of QTc prolongation	10–20%: Dizziness; 2–5%: Syncope	2–10%: Dizziness; 2–5%: Syncope
Respiratory	> 5%: Nasal congestion; < 2%: Dyspnea; < 1%: Pulmonary congestion, pneumonia, sleep apnea	> 2%: Nasal congestion	> 2%: Nasal congestion; < 2%: Dyspnea; < 1%: Upper respiratory tract infections	> 2%: Cough
Special senses	< 2%: Blurred vision; < 1%: Dry eyes, glaucoma		> 2%: Tinnitus	
Skin	2–10%: Flushing		> 5%: Increased sweating Flushing, skin reactions (e.g., rash, redness, inflammation at site of patch application) Disseminated cutaneous hypersensitivity reactions reported irrespective of administration route (oral or transdermal)	Cases of epidermal necrolysis
Urogenital	< 2%: Pruritus and urticaria; < 2%: Frequent urination, nocturia; < 1%: Prostatic hypertrophy; > 5%: Incontinence	> 5%: Urinary tract infection; > 2%: Hematuria; > 1%: Incontinence; < 1%: Urinary retention	> 5%: Urinary tract infection > 2%: Frequent urination, incontinence	> 5%: Incontinence; > 2%: Urinary tract infections; < 1%: Increased libido
Musculoskeletal	5–10%: Muscle cramps, pain; < 2%: Arthritis	5–10%: Muscle cramps	< 1%: Arthralgia, myalgia, pain	< 1%: hypertonia
Liver			Has been associated with hepatitis	Elevated ALT/SGPT Case of liver failure
Other	< 2%: Dehydration; < 1%: Blood dyscrasias, jaundice, renal failure	2–5%: Anemia; < 1%: Blood dyscrasias	< 1%: Dehydration, hypokalemia; < 1%: Nose bleeds	Case of aplastic anemia Cases of pancreatitis and renal failure

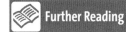

References

1. Seripa D, Bizzarro A, Pilotto A, et al., Role of cytochrome P4502D6 functional polymorphisms in the efficacy of donepezil in patients with Alzheimer's disease. Pharmacogenet Genomics. 2011;21(4):225–230. doi:10.1097/FPC.0b013e32833f984c
2. Whirl-Carrillo M, McDonagh EM, Hebert JM, et al. Pharmacogenomics knowledge for personalized medicine. Clin Pharmacol Ther. 2012;92(4):414–417. doi:10.1038/clpt.2012.96
3. Kishi T, Matsunaga S, Iwata N. The effects of memantine on behavioral disturbances in patients with Alzheimer's disease: A meta-analysis. Neuropsychiatr Dis Treat. 2017;13:1909–1928. doi:10.2147/NDT.S142839
4. Swanson CJ, Zhang Y, Dhadda S, et al. A randomized, double-blind, phase 2b proof-of-concept clinical trial in early Alzheimer's disease with lecanemab, an anti-Aβ protofibril antibody. Alzheimers Res Ther. 2021;13(1):80. doi:10.1186/s13195-021-00813-8
5. McDade E, Cummings JL, Dhadda S, et al. Lecanemab in patients with early Alzheimer's disease: Detailed results on biomarker, cognitive, and clinical effects from the randomized and open-label extension of the phase 2 proof-of-concept study. Alzheimers Res Ther. 2022;14(1):191. doi:10.1186/s13195-022-01124-2

Additional Suggested Reading

- Abe Y, Shimokado K, Fushimi K. Donepezil is associated with decreased in-hospital mortality as a result of pneumonia among older patients with dementia: A retrospective cohort study. Geriatr Gerontol Int. 2018;18(2):269–275. doi:10.1111/ggi.13177
- Baskys A, Cheng JX. Pharmacological prevention and treatment of vascular dementia: Approaches and perspectives. Exp Gerontol. 2012;47(11):887–891. doi:10.1016/j.exger.2012.07.002
- Cacabelos R. Pharmacogenetic considerations when prescribing cholinesterase inhibitors for the treatment of Alzheimer's disease. Expert Opin Drug Metab Toxicol. 2020;16(8):673–701. doi:10.1080/17425255.2020.1779700
- Deardorff WJ, Feen E, Grossberg GT. The use of cholinesterase inhibitors across all stages of Alzheimer's disease. Drugs Aging. 2015;32(7):537–547. doi:10.1007/s40266-015-0273-x. doi:10.1007/s40266-015-0273-x
- Herrmann N, Lanctot K, Hogan DB. Pharmacological recommendations for the symptomatic treatment of dementia: The Canadian Consensus Conference on the Diagnosis and Treatment of Dementia 2012. Alzheimers Res Ther. 2013;5(Suppl 1):S5. doi:10.1186/alzrt201
- Lane CA, Hard J, Schott JM. Alzheimer's disease. Eur J Neurol. 2018;25(1):59–70. doi:10.1111/ene.13439
- Li Y, Hai S, Zhou Y, et al. Cholinesterase inhibitors for rarer dementias associated with neurological conditions. Cochrane Database Syst Rev. 2015;(3):CD009444. doi:10.1002/14651858.CD009444.pub3
- McGuinness B, O'Hare J, Craig D, et al. Cochrane review on 'Statins for the treatment of dementia'. Int J Geriatr Psychiatry. 2013;28(2):119–126. doi:10.1002/gps.3797
- O'Brien JT, Holmes C, Jones M, et al. Clinical practice with anti-dementia drugs: A revised (third) consensus statement from the British Association for Psychopharmacology. J Psychopharmacol. 2017;31(2):147–168. doi:10.1177/0269881116680924
- Pasqualetti G, Tognini S, Calsolaro V, et al. Potential drug–drug interactions in Alzheimer patients with behavioral symptoms. Clin Interv Aging. 2015;10:1457–1466. doi:10.2147/CIA.S87466
- Sharma K. Cholinesterase inhibitors as Alzheimer's therapeutics (review). Mol Med Rep. 2019;20(2):1479–1487. doi:10.3892/mmr.2019.10374

SEX-DRIVE DEPRESSANTS

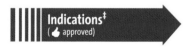 **Product Availability***

Generic Name	Chemical Class	Trade Name(A)	Dosage Forms and Strengths
Cyproterone	Antiandrogen	Androcur(C)	Tablets: 50 mg
		Androcur Depot(C)	Injection (IM depot): 100 mg/mL
Degarelix	GnRH/LHRH** antagonist	Firmagon	Injection (SC depot): 80 mg/vial, 120 mg/vial
Finasteride	Type II 5-α reductase inhibitor	Propecia	Tablets: 1 mg
		Proscar	Tablets: 5 mg
Goserelin	GnRH/LHRH agonist	Zoladex, Zoladex LA	Implant (SC depot): 3.6 mg/syringe [1-month implant], 10.8 mg/syringe [3-month implant]
Leuprolide	GnRH/LHRH agonist	Lupron	Injection (SC depot): 5 mg/mL(C)
		Lupron Depot	Injection (IM depot): 3.75 mg/syringe [1-month slow release], 7.5 mg/syringe [1-month slow release], 11.25 mg/syringe [3-month slow release], 11.25 mg/vial [3-month slow release], 15 mg/vial [1-month slow release](B), 22.5 mg/syringe [3-month slow release], 30 mg/syringe [4-month slow release], 45 mg/vial [6-month slow release](B)
		Eligard	Injection (SC depot): 7.5 mg/syringe [1-month slow release], 22.5 mg/syringe [3-month slow release], 30 mg/syringe [4-month slow release], 45 mg/syringe [6-month slow release]
Medroxyprogesterone	Progestogen	Provera	Tablets: 2.5 mg, 5 mg, 10 mg, 100 mg
		DepoProvera	Injection (depot): 150 mg/mL, 400 mg/mL(B)
Triptorelin	GnRH/LHRH agonist	Trelstar	Injection (IM depot): 3.75 mg/vial [1-month slow release], 11.25 mg/vial [3-month slow release], 22.5 mg/vial [6-month slow release]

* Refer to Health Canada's Drug Product Database or the FDA's Drugs@FDA for the most current availability information, (A) Generic preparations may be available, (B) Not marketed in Canada, (C) Not marketed in the USA
** GnRH = gonadotropin-releasing hormone, LHRH = Luteinizing hormone-releasing hormone; GnRH and LHRH are used interchangeably

Indications‡
(👍 approved)

- Reduction of sexual arousal and libido (usually for sexual offenders)
- Inappropriate or disruptive sexual behavior in patients with dementia

‡ Indications listed here do not necessarily apply to all sex-drive depressants or all countries. Please refer to a country's regulatory database (e.g., US Food and Drug Administration, Health Canada Drug Product Database) for the most current availability information and to know which drugs are indicated in which country

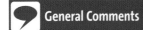	

💬 **General Comments**	• The goals of pharmacologic treatment of sex offenders include: – 1. reduce sexual offending and victimization, – 2. suppress sexual drive to a controllable level, – 3. possibly preferentially eliminate deviant arousal/thoughts, – 4. allow normal sexual relationships • Although controlled double-blind studies are lacking, given the nature of the difficulties suffered by the individuals being treated, and the seriousness of the condition, virtually all of the uncontrolled studies show a significant effect in the same direction, which would be unlikely if this effect were truly spurious • In an RCT that compared degarelix to placebo (26 patients in each group) in men with pedophilic disorder, a significant decrease in the Sexual Desire Inventory scores was reported at 2 and 10 weeks for participants assigned degarelix, compared to placebo. Fifteen (58%) of the participants in the degarelix group and 3 (12%) of the participants in the placebo group reported no further sexual interest in children at 10 weeks[1] • A group of 25 sex offenders[2] receiving both leuprolide acetate and CBT were compared with a group of 22 sex offenders receiving only CBT. Both groups recidivated at substantially lower rates than predicted by the Static-99R (a validated tool that positions offenders in terms of their relative degree of risk for sexual recidivism based on commonly available demographic and criminal history information that has been found to correlate with sexual recidivism in adult male sex offenders) • A systematic review reported the following findings: 1) that current studies suggest LHRH-agonists might be the most effective drugs to decrease paraphilic sexual fantasies, urges, and behaviors, 2) LHRH-agonists should be reserved for those with the highest risk of sexual offending because of their extensive side effects, 3) psychotherapy should always be carried out alongside pharmacotherapy[3] • Pharmacotherapy may be combined with intensive psychotherapy to possibly improve compliance and outcomes[4]. Treatment of any comorbid psychiatric conditions is recommended • Evidence for efficacy of serotonergic agents (e.g., SSRIs) is controversial and limited. Most studies showed response rates of 50–90%. Positive effects included decreases in: (1) paraphiliac fantasies, urges, and sexual acts, (2) masturbation, (3) hypersexual activity. SSRIs should NOT be used alone in serious offenders • The opioid antagonist naltrexone (100–200 mg per day) may provide a safe first step in treating adolescent sexual offenders • There is no evidence supporting finasteride use in sex offenders. Consider using only on an individual basis or as an adjunctive treatment • While medroxyprogesterone and cyproterone are effective for partial sex drive reduction in non-violent offenders, serious paraphilias in which ablation of testosterone of testicular origin is indicated require treatment with GnRH/LHRH agonists/analogs or antagonists; GnRH analogues have demonstrated a very high efficacy, notably where subjects have failed treatment with psychotherapy and other anti-androgens • Goserelin, leuprolide, and triptorelin (GnRH/LHRH agonists) may cause a transient increase (over 3 weeks or more) in luteinizing hormone and testosterone, followed by a dramatic decrease and suppression of the hormones. This transient increase does not occur with degarelix, a GnRH/LHRH antagonist • Longer-acting depot injections (e.g., leuprolide 30 mg q 4 months) have demonstrated efficacy in trials with high-risk sex offenders • Rarely, serious offenders partly refractory to GnRH/LHRH agents may require additional peripheral testosterone blockade with agents such as finasteride or other peripheral receptor blockers • The GnRH/LHRH agonists and antagonists are used for several other (nonpsychiatric) indications such as treatment and prevention of various types of prostate cancers (except medroxyprogesterone) • Seek consultation with an internist/endocrinologist prior to initiation of therapy; thereafter, yearly consultation and bone density monitoring is recommended (see Lab Tests/Monitoring, p. 364)

⚛️ **Pharmacology**	• See p. 361

Dosing	• See p. 362 • GnRH/LHRH agonists are relatively non-titratable in terms of testosterone suppression effects • Depot injections of medroxyprogesterone and cyproterone may initially be prescribed every 2 weeks with monitoring of serum testosterone and sexual self-report. Often, weekly injection schedule is necessary to achieve good behavioral control and testosterone suppression. Depot injections of GnRH/LHRH agonists are available in 1-month, 3-month, 4-month, and 6-month preparations • Anaphylaxis, while reported in the literature with leuprolide, has rarely been observed in clinical practice; however, some clinicians feel that a test dose of short-acting leuprolide acetate is indicated

Sex-Drive Depressants (cont.)

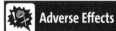

Adverse Effects

- See p. 363
- The main serious long-term side effect of GnRH/LHRH agonists and antagonists is decreased bone density mediated by testosterone depletion. Treatment with bisphosphonates, calcium, or vitamin D has been found to arrest or even reverse this side effect. Clear evidence of fractures caused by this treatment has not been reported (it should be remembered that "fracture risk" in densitometry readings is not standardized on this gender/age group).
- Androgen deprivation may also result in weight gain with increased visceral adiposity, mild anemia, impaired glucose tolerance, dyslipidemia, and rarely emotional disturbances[5]
- Often impotence or rarely gynecomastia
- Medroxyprogesterone and cyproterone carry risk of thromboembolism – risk increased with age and smoking
- QTc prolongation has been reported with GnRH/LHRH agonists, combined androgen blockade or a GnRH/LHRH antagonist in the treatment of prostate cancer, with 9–21 millisecond increases in QTc. Hypogonadism rather than a direct drug effect appears to account for the observed QTc prolongation

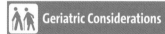

Geriatric Considerations

- Inappropriate sexual behaviors may occur in patients with dementia. Treatment must be individualized based on the medical status of the individual, including current drug therapy, as well as the risk this behavior poses to others
- SSRIs are considered first choice for nonthreatening, nonviolent patients with dementia and problematic sexual behaviors[6]. If refractory to these agents, GnRH/LHRH agonists are preferred due to a more favorable side effect profile, including fewer thromboembolic effects

Nursing Implications

- Degarelix is supplied as a powder to be reconstituted with sterile water for injection, prior to injecting; the solution should be clear. The drug is administered subcutaneously in the abdominal region that is not exposed to pressure (e.g., from a belt)
- Goserelin pellet requires administration by deep subcutaneous injection. Caution should be taken while injecting into the anterior abdominal wall due to the proximity of underlying inferior epigastric artery and its branches
- Leuprolide:
  - Lupron pre-filled dual-chamber syringe: Reconstitute drug with 1 mL of diluent provided. Shake well. Suspension is stable for 24 h and can be stored at room temperature. Inject using 23-gauge needle (or larger). Injection may rarely cause irritation (burning, itching, and swelling)
  - Eligard two-syringe system: Allow to reach room temperature by removing from refrigerator at least 30 min before mixing. Reconstitute with provided diluent. Once mixed, product must be administered within 30 min, as the viscosity of the solution increases with time
- Triptorelin: The lyophilized microgranules are to be reconstituted with 2 mL of sterile water for injection utilizing either a 21-gauge needle or the single-dose delivery system (Mixject)
- Medroxyprogesterone: Shake sterile aqueous suspension vigorously just before use to ensure that the dose being given represents a uniform suspension. Inject intramuscularly, preferably to the gluteus maximus, but other muscle tissue such as the deltoid may be used
- **CAUTION:** Women who are, or may be, pregnant should not handle crushed or broken tablets of cyproterone, medroxyprogesterone or finasteride because of risk of absorption and subsequent potential risk to a male fetus
- Drug must be taken consistently to maintain effect

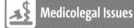

Medicolegal Issues

- As sex drive reduction is not an approved indication for these agents, good documentation of consent is essential
- Use of these drugs involves complex issues in regard to consent, as the patients are often involved with the legal system
- Some of the agents (GnRH/LHRH agonist/antagonist) have sex drive reduction as a formally approved indication in some European jurisdictions

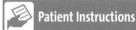

Patient Instructions

- For detailed patient instructions on sex-drive-depressants, see the Patient Information Sheet (details p. 474)

▶◀ Drug Interactions

- Clinically significant interactions are listed below
- For more interaction information on any given combination, also see the corresponding chapter for the second agent
- Leuprolide is considered to have few drug interactions since it is primarily degraded by peptidase enzymes (not CYP450 enzymes) and has a low degree of protein binding
- Finasteride is a minor CYP3A4 substrate and hence its levels can be altered by other drugs that induce or inhibit CYP3A4 enzymes

Class of Drug	Example	Interaction Effects
Alcohol		Alcohol may reduce the antiandrogenic effect of cyproterone when used for hypersexuality
Anti-androgen agent	Finasteride	Additive effects on testosterone reduction if utilized with goserelin, leuprolide or triptorelin
Antibiotic	Clarithromycin, erythromycin	May increase plasma levels of cyproterone, finasteride, and medroxyprogesterone due to inhibition of CYP3A4
	Rifampin	Decreased plasma levels of cyproterone, finasteride, and medroxyprogesterone due to induction of CYP3A4
Anticonvulsant	Carbamazepine, phenytoin	May decrease plasma level of cyproterone, finasteride, and medroxyprogesterone due to inhibition of CYP3A4
Antifibrinolytic	Tranexamic acid	Medroxyprogesterone and cyproterone may enhance the thrombogenic effect of tranexamic acid
Antifungal	Itraconazole, ketoconazole	May increase plasma levels of cyproterone, finasteride, and medroxyprogesterone due to inhibition of CYP3A4
Antiretroviral	Antivirals containing cobicistat	May increase plasma levels of cyproterone, finasteride, and medroxyprogesterone due to inhibition of CYP3A4
Protease inhibitor	Indinavir, nelfinavir, ritonavir, saquinavir	May increase plasma levels of cyproterone, finasteride, and medroxyprogesterone due to inhibition of CYP3A4
Herbs (with progestogenic properties)	Bloodroot, yucca	May enhance the adverse/toxic effect of progestins
Hypoglycemic	Glyburide, metformin	Diminished therapeutic effect of antidiabetic agent with leuprolide
QT-prolonging agent	Ciprofloxacin, pimozide, tetrabenazine, thioridazine, ziprasidone	Androgen deprivation can prolong the QT effect of the drug, leading to severe arrhythmia
St. John's wort		May decrease plasmas level of cyproterone, finasteride, and medroxyprogesterone due to induction of CYP3A4

Comparison of Sex-Drive Depressants

	Cyproterone	Degarelix	Finasteride	Goserelin	Leuprolide	Medroxyprogesterone	Triptorelin
Pharmacology	A potent progestogen, has antigonadotrophic effect. Intervenes with the hypothalamo-pituitary pathway, causing inhibition of increased secretion of LH, and decrease in gonadal testicular androgens	GnRH antagonist, competitively reversibly binds to GnRH receptors in the anterior pituitary gland. This reduces LH and FSH secretion, decreasing testosterone production. Note: Testosterone levels DO NOT have an initial flare as typically seen with GnRH agonists	Synthetic 5α-reductase inhibitor, prevents the conversion of testosterone to dihydrotestos-terone, a potent androgen	High-potency synthetic analog of GnRH that causes an initial surge in LH, FSH, and testosterone. Chronic administration results in decreased LH and FSH and suppression of testicular steroidogenesis	High-potency synthetic analog of GnRH that causes an initial surge in LH, FSH, and testosterone. Chronic administration results in decreased LH and FSH and suppression of testicular steroidogenesis	Inhibits secretion of pituitary gonadotropins by progestational feedback	High-potency synthetic analog of GnRH that causes an initial surge in LH, FSH, and testosterone. Chronic administration results in decreased LH and FSH and suppression of testicular steroidogenesis

Comparison of Sex-Drive Depressants (cont.)

	Cyproterone	Degarelix	Finasteride	Goserelin	Leuprolide	Medroxyprogesterone	Triptorelin
Dosing	Oral: 200–300 mg/day Depot: 300 mg/week	Depot: Initial dose = 240 mg given as two SC injections of 120 mg at a concentration of 40 mg/mL. Maintenance dose = 80 mg given as one SC injection at a concentration of 20 mg/mL	5 mg/day	3.6 mg/month; or 10.8 mg q 3 months	Depot: 7.5 mg/month; 22.5 mg q 3 months; 30 mg q 4 months; 45 mg q 6 months Lupron given IM Eligard given SC	Oral: 100–600 mg/day Depot: 100–700 mg/week IM	Depot: 3.75 mg/month IM; 11.25 mg/3 months IM; 22.5 mg/6 months IM
Pharmacokinetics							
Time to Peak Plasma Level (T_{max})	Oral: 3–4 h Depot: 3 days	2 days	1–2 h	3.6 mg implant: 12–15 days (males); 8–22 days (females)	Depot: Within 4 h of injection Metabolite: 2–6 h	Oral: 2–4 h Depot: Few days	3.75 mg: 1–2 h 11.25 mg: 2–4 h 22.25 mg: 3–12 h
Protein Binding	> 95%	90%	90%	27%	43-49%	90%	Does not bind to plasma proteins at clinically relevant concentrations
Metabolism	Via CYP3A4	Via peptidase	Primarily via CYP3A4	Via hydrolysis	Via peptidase	Via CYP3A4	Metabolism in humans is not well understood
Elimination Half-life ($T_{1/2}$)	Oral: 33–42 h Depot: 4 days	53 days	5-6 h (age 16–60), 8 h (over age 70)	3.6 mg implant: 4.2 h (males); 2–3 h (females)	2.9 h	Oral: 12–17 h Depot: 50 days	2.81 h (healthy males) 6.56 h (males with moderate renal impairment) 7.65 h (males with severe renal impairment) 7.65 h (males with liver disease)
Renal Impairment	Not determined	Clearance reduced by 23% if CrCl less than 50 mL/min; dose reduction not recommended in mild to moderate renal impairment. No data in severe renal insufficiency	Clearance of metabolites decreased; no adjustment in renal impairment	Half-life increased to 12 h in renal impairment	Not determined	No change in dosage	Decrease in total clearance of triptorelin and increase in elimination half-life

	Cyproterone	Degarelix	Finasteride	Goserelin	Leuprolide	Medroxyprogesterone	Triptorelin
Adverse Effects	Atrophy of seminiferous tubules with chronic use (possibly reversible if drug stopped) Gynecomastia (15–20%) Decrease in body hair and sebum production, weight gain Liver injury Thromboembolism Decreased bone density Vitamin B12 deficiency Cardiovascular disease	Decreased sperm count, hot flashes, sweating, impotence QT prolongation Dizziness Osteoporosis Increased appetite and weight gain Pain, erythema, swelling at injection site Increase in transaminase and GGT	Decreased sperm count, impotence, breast tenderness Male breast cancer Dizziness, postural hypotension, edema Decreased libido even after discontinuation of treatment	Decreased sperm count, atrophy of seminiferous tubules, impotence Hot flashes Sweating, rash, edema (3%), nausea, other GI effects, loss of body hair, myalgia, anemia, spasms, dyspnea Decreased bone density Although there has been speculation that the flare-up or increase in testosterone after the initial administration of GnRH agonists is significant and possibly associated with risk for increased sexual drive and deviant behavior, this observed flare-up has not been noted to be clinically significant Prostatic carcinoma, stage B2-C prostatic carcinoma	Decreased sperm count, atrophy of seminiferous tubules, impotence Hot flashes (60%) Sweating, rash, edema (3%), nausea, other GI effects, loss of body hair, myalgia, anemia, spasms, lethargy, dyspnea Decreased bone density Although there has been speculation that the flare-up or increase in testosterone after the initial administration of GnRH agonists is significant and possibly associated with risk for increased sexual drive and deviant behavior, this observed flare-up has not been noted to be clinically significant	Decreased sperm count, hot flashes, sweating, impotence Increased appetite and weight gain Dyspnea, hypertension, edema, muscle cramps, GI upset Thromboembolism (smoking may increase risk) Excess salivation	Asthenia, allergic reaction, hypertension, palpitations, dizziness, chest pain, skeletal pain, arthralgia, myalgia, leg pain, leg cramps, peripheral edema, breast pain, male gynecomastia, constipation, nausea, diarrhea, abdominal pain, dyspepsia, abnormal hepatic function, diabetes mellitus, anorexia, coughing, dyspnea, pharyngitis, rash, pruritus, testicular atrophy, impotence, urinary tract infection, dysuria, urinary retention, eye pain, conjunctivitis
CNS	Fatigue, depression (5–10%), irritability, suicidal ideation	Fatigue, headache, insomnia	Lethargy, headache, depression	Lethargy	Anxiety, insomnia	Mild depression, lethargy, nervousness, insomnia, nightmares, headaches	Lethargy, fatigue, headache, depression, insomnia
Precautions	May impair carbohydrate metabolism Fasting blood glucose and glucose tolerance tests recommended Hypercalcemia and changes in plasma lipids can occur Alcohol use may reduce the antiandrogenic effect Deep vein thrombosis and thromboembolism (smoking may increase risk)	Decreased bone density reported Anti-degarelix antibody development observed in 10% of patients after 1 year; efficacy and safety appears not affected Long-term androgen deprivation prolongs the QT interval; incidence of QTc interval greater than 450 ms is 20% Severe hepatic impairment Severe renal impairment	Patients with large residual urine volume and/or severely diminished urinary flow should be carefully monitored for obstructive uropathy Increased risk of high-grade prostate cancer	Transient elevation of BUN, creatinine, testosterone, and acid phosphatase reported (rarely seen) Hyperglycemia and diabetes, cardiovascular diseases, hypercalcemia Effect on QT/QTc interval	Long-term androgen deprivation prolongs the QT interval; incidence of QTc interval greater than 450 ms is 20% Hyperglycemia and diabetes, convulsions, allergies to benzyl alcohol (an ingredient of the drug's vehicle)	May decrease glucose tolerance Monitor patients with conditions aggravated by fluid retention, e.g., asthma, migraine Deep vein thrombosis and thromboembolism (smoking may increase risk) Depression	May cause worsening of prostate cancer symptoms at the beginning of treatment, clinical testosterone flare reaction in men with prostate cancer, bone thinning (osteoporosis)

Comparison of Sex-Drive Depressants (cont.)

	Cyproterone	Degarelix	Finasteride	Goserelin	Leuprolide	Medroxyprogesterone	Triptorelin
Contraindications	Liver disease, thromboembolic disorders Active pituitary pathology Dubin Johnson syndrome, Rotor syndrome Previous or existing liver tumors (only if these are not due to metastases from carcinoma of the prostate), history of meningioma, wasting diseases (except inoperable carcinoma of the prostate) Severe chronic depression	Hypersensitivity to drug Women who are or who may become pregnant	Liver disease, thromboembolic disorders Active pituitary pathology	Hypersensitivity to drug (rare) Active pituitary pathology Disorders of bone demineralization (relative contraindication)	Hypersensitivity to drug (rare) Active pituitary pathology Disorders of bone demineralization (relative contraindication)	Liver disease; thromboembolic disorders Active pituitary pathology History of or actual myocardial infarction or coronary artery disease Any ocular lesion arising from ophthalmic vascular disease Current or history of migraine with focal aura	Hypersensitivity to drug
Toxicity	No reports	No reports	No reports	No reports	No reports	No reports	No reports
Lab Tests/Monitoring Pretreatment	Serum testosterone, prolactin, LH, FSH, liver function, Hb, WBC, glucose, blood pressure, weight	ECG, Serum testosterone, prolactin, LH, FSH, liver function, Hb, WBC, glucose, baseline serum potassium, calcium and magnesium, blood pressure, weight	Serum testosterone, prolactin, LH, FSH, liver function, Hb, WBC, glucose, blood pressure, weight	Serum testosterone, prolactin, LH, FSH, ECG, BUN, creatinine, CBC, liver function, bone density scan	Serum testosterone, prolactin, LH, FSH, ECG, BUN, creatinine, CBC, liver function, bone density scan	Serum testosterone, prolactin, LH, FSH, liver function, Hb, WBC, glucose, blood pressure, weight	ECG, serum electrolytes, Hb, blood glucose and/or glycosylated hemoglobin (HbA1c), serum concentrations of testosterone and PSA
Chronic	Testosterone: q 6 months LH, FSH, and prolactin: q 6 months Blood pressure, weight: q 3 months	Testosterone: q 6 months LH, FSH, and prolactin: q 6 months Blood pressure, weight: q 3 months PSA periodically	Testosterone: q 6 months LH, FSH, and prolactin: q 6 months Blood pressure, weight: q 6 months PSA periodically	Testosterone: q 1 month for 4 months, then q 6 months BUN, creatinine, LH, FSH, and prolactin: q 6 months Bone density: q 1–2 years	Testosterone: q 1 month for 4 months, then q 6 months BUN, creatinine, LH, FSH, and prolactin: q 6 months Bone density: q 1–2 years PSA periodically	Testosterone: q 6 months LH, FSH, and prolactin: q 6 months Blood pressure, weight: q 6 months	Testosterone and PSA, bone and prostatic lesions, Hb, blood glucose levels and/or HbA1c, ECG, and electrolytes

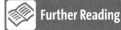
Further Reading

References

[1] Landgren V, Olsson P, Briken P, et al. Effects of testosterone suppression on desire, hypersexuality, and sexual interest in children in men with pedophilic disorder. World J Biol Psychiatry. 2022:1–12. doi:10.1080/15622975.2021.2014683

[2] Gallo A, Abracen J, Looman J, et al. The use of leuprolide acetate in the management of high-risk sex offenders. Sex Abuse. 2019;31(8):930–951. doi:10.1177/1079063218791176

[3] Turner D, Briken P. Treatment of paraphilic disorders in sexual offenders or men with a risk of sexual offending with luteinizing hormone-releasing hormone agonists: An updated systematic review. J Sex Med. 2018;15(1):77–93. doi:10.1016/j.jsxm.2017.11.013

[4] Khan O, Ferriter M, Huband N, et al. Pharmacological interventions for those who have sexually offended or are at risk of offending. Cochrane Database Syst Rev. 2015;(2):CD007989. doi:10.1002/14651858.CD007989.pub2

[5] Nguyen PL, Alibhai SM, Basaria S, et al. Adverse effects of androgen deprivation therapy and strategies to mitigate them. Eur Urol. 2015;67(5):825–836. doi:10.1016/j.eururo.2014.07.010

[6] De Giorgi R, Series H. Treatment of inappropriate sexual behavior in dementia. Curr Treat Options Neurol. 2016;18(9):41. doi:10.1007/s11940-016-0425-2

Additional Suggested Reading

- Assumpção AA, Garcia FD, Garcia HD, et al. Pharmacologic treatment of paraphilias. Psychiatr Clin North Am. 2014;37(2):173–181. doi:10.1016/j.psc.2014.03.002
- Carter NJ, Keam SJ. Degarelix: A review of its use in patients with prostate cancer. Drugs. 2014;74(6):699–712. doi:10.1007/s40265-014-0211-y
- Choi JH, Lee JW, Lee JK, et al. Therapeutic effects of leuprorelin (euprolide acetate) in sexual offenders with paraphilia. J Korean Med Sci. 2018;33(37):e231. doi:10.3346/jkms.2018.33.e231
- Holoyda BJ, Kellaher DC. The biological treatment of paraphilic disorders: An updated review. Curr Psychiatry Rep. 2016;18(2):19. doi:10.1007/s11920-015-0649-y
- Houts FW, Taller I, Tucker DE et al. Androgen deprivation treatment of sexual behavior. Adv Psychosom Med. 2011;31:149–163. doi:10.1159/000330196
- International Association for the Treatment of Sexual Offenders (IATSO). IATSO standards of care for the treatment of adult sex offenders. Vienna, Austria: IATSO. Retrieved from https://www.iatso.org/images/stories/pdfs/iatso_standardsofcare_adult_so.pdf
- Lippi G, van Staden PJ. The use of cyproterone acetate in a forensic psychiatric cohort of male sex offenders and its associations with sexual activity and sexual functioning. S Afr J Psychiatr. 2017;23:982. doi:10.4102/sajpsychiatry.v23i0.982
- Phillips EA, Rajender A, Douglas T, et al. Sex offenders seeking treatment for sexual dysfunction – Ethics, medicine, and the law. J Sex Med. 2015;12(7):1591–1600. doi:10.1111/jsm.12920
- Tan MHE, Li J, Xu HE, et al. Androgen receptor: Structure, role in prostate cancer and drug discovery. Acta Pharmacol Sin. 2015;36(1):3–23. doi:10.1038/aps.2014.18
- Turner D, Petermann J, Harrison K, et al. Pharmacological treatment of patients with paraphilic disorders and risk of sexual offending: An international perspective. World J Biol Psychiatry. 2019;20(8):616–625. doi:10.1080/15622975.2017.1395069

DRUGS OF ABUSE

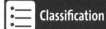 **Classification**

- This chapter gives a general overview of common drugs of abuse and is not intended to deal in detail with all drugs of abuse or to be a complete guide to treatment
- Slang names of street drugs change frequently and vary with country, region, and drug subculture. A list of common drug names is available from the NIH-sponsored website https://nida.nih.gov/research-topics/commonly-used-drugs-charts
- Drugs of abuse can be classified as follows:

Drug Class	Agent*	Page
Alcohol	(Ethyl) Alcohol	See p. 368
Stimulants	Examples: Amphetamine, cocaine, ephedrine, methamphetamine	See p. 372
Hallucinogens and Cannabinoids	Examples: Cannabis, lysergic acid diethylamide, mescaline, psilocybin	See p. 377
Opioids	Examples: Heroin, hydromorphone, morphine, oxycodone	See p. 386
Inhalants/Aerosols	Examples: Glue, paint thinner	See p. 390
Gamma-hydroxybutyrate		See p. 392
Sedatives/Hypnotics	Barbiturates**	See p. 257
	Benzodiazepines**	See p. 240
	Examples: Flunitrazepam	See p. 394
Nicotine	Examples: Cigarettes, cigars	See p. 395

* Only includes examples of commonly used substances; ** Not dealt with specifically in this chapter

 Definitions

- While DSM-5 combines substance abuse and substance dependence into a single disorder called substance use disorder, the following terms are still commonly used and their definitions have been retained here for readers' convenience

Drug Abuse

- Acute or chronic intake of any substance that: (a) has no recognized medical use, (b) is used inappropriately in terms of its medical indications or its dose. Drug abuse (sometimes referred to as substance misuse) is commonly associated with harm to the individual or others

Drug Dependence

a) Behavioral aspects
- Craving or desire for repeated administration of a drug to provide a desired effect or to avoid discomfort

b) Physical aspects
- A physiological state of adaptation to a drug which usually results in development of tolerance to drug effects and withdrawal symptoms when the drug is stopped

Addiction
- Intense persistent drug use associated with a strong desire to continue use, with disregard to consequences or personal harm

Tolerance
- Phenomenon in which increasing doses of a drug are needed to produce a desired effect or effect intensity decreases with repeated use

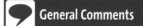 **General Comments**

- The effect which any drug of abuse has on an individual depends on a large number of variables:
  1. Dose (amount consumed)
  2. Potency and purity of drug
  3. Route of administration
  4. Past experience of the user (this will affect both physiological and psychological response to drug)
  5. Environmental factors, including other people present and concurrent drug use
  6. Personality and genetic profile of user

7. Age of user

8. Clinical status of user (e.g., psychiatric illness, recent stress, user's expectations, and present feelings)

- Some users may have different experiences with the same drug on different occasions. They may encounter both pleasant and unpleasant effects during the same drug experience
- Many street drugs are adulterated with other chemicals and may not be what the individual thinks they are; potency and purity of street drugs vary greatly
- It remains unclear whether drugs of abuse cause persistent psychiatric disorders in otherwise healthy individuals, or whether they precipitate latent psychiatric illness in predisposed individuals. Overall, in non-treatment community samples, it is estimated that over 50% of drug users have at least one other psychiatric disorder and those with certain psychiatric disorders (e.g., bipolar disorder, schizophrenia) are more likely to abuse substances than the general population
- Dual diagnosis or concurrent disorders refer to the co-occurrence of substance use disorder in a patient with a severe psychiatric illness. Substance abuse can occur during any phase of the psychiatric illness; it is associated with a variety of physical/psychosocial problems, can destabilize treatment, and lead to relapse
- Substance abuse has been associated with earlier onset of schizophrenia, decreased treatment responsiveness of positive symptoms of psychosis, and poor clinical functioning; similarly decreased treatment responsiveness in bipolar disorder can occur

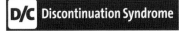 **Detection of Drugs of Abuse**

- Factors affecting detection of a drug in urine depend on dose and route of administration, drug metabolism, and characteristics of screening and confirmation assays; for instance:
  - Amphetamines in urine can be positive for up to 5 days
  - Cannabis (delta-9-THC) in urine can be positive 2–4 days after acute use and for up to 1–3 months after chronic use. Note that it is the major metabolite tetrahydrocannabinol carboxylic acid (THC-COOH) which is detected in most urine drug screens
  - Cocaine can be positive, as its metabolite, in urine for up to 1.5 days after IV use, for up to 1 week with street doses used by different routes, and for up to 3 weeks after use of very high doses
  - Heroin can be positive, as its metabolite, in urine for up to 1.5 days when administered parenterally or intranasally
  - Prescription drugs can sometimes cause unexpected positive results due to interference with lab assays (e.g., quetiapine for methadone)

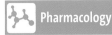 **Pharmacology**

- Research data have demonstrated that most drugs of abuse (except the hallucinogens) increase dopamine levels in the nucleus accumbens of the brain; the increased dopamine is suggested to be associated with the reinforcing effects of the drug and contributes to drug craving

 Adverse Effects

- See pharmacological/psychiatric effects under specific drugs
- Reactions are unpredictable and depend on the potency and purity of drug taken
- Psychiatric reactions secondary to drug abuse may occur more readily in individuals already at risk
- Renal, hepatic, cardiorespiratory, neurological, and gastrointestinal complications as well as encephalopathies can occur with chronic abuse of specific agents
- Intravenous drug users are at risk for infection, including cellulitis, endocarditis, hepatitis, and HIV
- Impurities in street drugs (especially if inhaled or injected) can cause tissue and organ damage (blood vessels, heart valves, kidney, lungs, and liver)
- Psychological dependence can occur; the drug becomes central to a person's thoughts, emotions, and activities, resulting in craving
- Physical dependence can occur; the body adapts to the presence of the drug and withdrawal symptoms occur when the drug is stopped abruptly

D/C Discontinuation Syndrome

- See specific agents
- Identification of drug(s) abused is important; some drug withdrawals have the potential to produce life-threatening withdrawal syndromes (e.g., alcohol, barbiturates), whereas others are less likely (e.g., opioids, stimulants, cannabis); toxicology may help in identification whenever multiple or combination drug use is suspected

 Treatment

Acute

- Treatment of substance use disorder presents challenges in patients with a diagnosed psychiatric disorder and is best done with an integrated treatment program that combines pharmacotherapy with psychosocial intervention

Drugs of Abuse (cont.)

- See specific agents (refer to Treatment of Substance Use Disorders chapter pp. 398–424
- Diagnosis must include mental status, physical and neurological examination, as well as a drug history: Whenever possible, collateral history should be sought
- In severe cases, monitor vitals and fluid intake
- Agitation can be treated conservatively by talking with the patient and providing reassurance until the drug wears off (i.e., "talking down"). When conservative approaches are inadequate or if symptoms persist, pharmacological intervention should be considered
- Despite drug effects on dopamine release, avoid low-potency antipsychotics due to anticholinergic effects, hypotension, and tachycardia

| Long-Term | • The presence of comorbid psychiatric disorders in substance abusers can adversely influence outcome in treatment of the substance use disorder as well as the psychiatric disorder |

 Further Reading

Additional Suggested Reading
- American Psychiatric Association. Practice guideline and resources for treatment of patients with substance use disorders, 2nd ed. Am J Psychiatry. 2006;163(8 Suppl):1–276. Retrieved from http://www.psychiatryonline.com/pracGuide/pracGuideTopic_5.aspx
- Forray A, Foster D. Substance use in the perinatal period. Curr Psychiatry Rep. 2015;17(11):91. doi:10.1007/s11920-015-0626-5
- Khokhar HY, Dwiel LL, Henricks AM et al. The link between schizophrenia and substance use disorder: A unifying hypothesis. Schizophre Res. 2018;194:78–85. doi:10.1016/j.schres.2017.04.016
- Klein JW. Pharmacotherapy for substance use disorder. Med Clin North Am. 2016;100(4):891–910. doi:10.1016/j.mcna.2016.03.011
- Volkow ND. Personalizing the treatment of substance use disorders. Am J Psychiatry. 2020;177(2):113–116. doi:10.1176/appi.ajp.2019.19121284

Alcohol

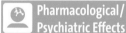 **General Comments**

- Slang: Booze, hooch, juice, brew
- Up to 50% of individuals with alcohol dependence meet the criteria for lifetime diagnosis of major depression
- Related problems include withdrawal symptoms, physical violence, loss of control when drinking, surreptitious drinking, change in tolerance to alcohol, deteriorating job performance, change in social interactions, increased risk for stroke, and injury or death from motor vehicle accidents
- Alcohol acts on numerous central neurotransmission pathways and has been labeled a CNS disorganizer

Pharmacological/ Psychiatric Effects

- Effects of alcohol have a close relationship with blood alcohol levels; impaired judgment and impulsivity can occur with levels of 4–6 mmol/L (20–30 mg/100 mL); levels of 17 mmol/ (80 mg/100 mL) are associated with slurred speech, incoordination, unsteady gait, and inattention. Higher levels can intensify cognitive deficits, aggressiveness, and cause anterograde amnesia (blackouts)
- Effects of a single drink occur within 15 min and peak at approximately 30–60 min, depending on amount taken; elimination is about 10 g alcohol per hour (about 30 mL (1 oz) whiskey or 1 bottle of regular beer). Blood alcohol level declines by 3–7 mmol/L per hour (~ 15 mg/100 mL)

| Acute | • Disinhibition, relaxation, euphoria, agitation, drowsiness, impaired cognition, judgment, and memory, perceptual and motor dysfunction |

☞ **Acute alcohol intake decreases hepatic metabolism of co-administered drugs by competition for microsomal enzymes**

| Chronic | • Chronic use results in an increased capacity to metabolize alcohol and a concurrent CNS tolerance; psychological as well as physical dependence may occur; hepatic metabolism decreases with liver cirrhosis |

☞ **Chronic alcohol use increases hepatic metabolism of co-administered drugs**

| Physical | • Hand tremor, dyspepsia, diarrhea, morning nausea and vomiting, polyuria, impotence, pancreatitis, headache, hepatomegaly, peripheral neuropathy |
| Mental | • Memory blackouts, nightmares, insomnia, hallucinations, paranoia, intellectual impairment, dementia, Wernicke-Korsakoff syndrome, and other organic mental disorders |

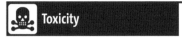 **Pharmacokinetics**	• Absorption occurs slowly from the stomach, and rapidly from the upper small intestine • Approximately 10% of ingested alcohol is eliminated by first-pass metabolism (less in females); percentage decreases as amount consumed increases • Alcohol is distributed in body fluids (is not fat soluble) and the blood alcohol level depends on gender, age, and body fluid volume/fat ratio • Metabolized in the liver primarily by alcohol dehydrogenase, CYP2E1, and CYP450 reductase (also by CYP3A4 and CYP1A2); activity of CYP2E1 is increased 10-fold in chronic heavy drinkers
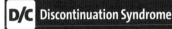 **Toxicity**	• Risk of injury or harm increases with more than 3 standard drinks for females and 4 for males on any single occasion (standard drink = approximately 5 oz or 140 mL wine, a 12 oz bottle of beer, 1.5 oz or 45 mL spirits)[1]; the legal blood alcohol concentration threshold for impaired driving in the Criminal Code of Canada is 80 mg in 100 mL blood (0.08) • Risk increases when combined with drugs with CNS depressant activity • Symptoms include: CNS depression, decreased or absent deep tendon reflexes, cardiac dysfunction, flushed skin progressing to cyanosis, hypoglycemia, hypothermia, peripheral vasodilation, shock, respiratory depression, and coma

D/C Discontinuation Syndrome	• Occurs after chronic use • Most effects seen within 5–7 days after stopping
Mild Withdrawal	• Insomnia, irritability, headache • Usually transient and self-limiting
Severe Reactions	• Phase I: Begins within hours of cessation and lasts 3–5 days. Symptoms: tremor, tachycardia, diaphoresis, labile BP, nausea, vomiting, anxiety • Phase II: Perceptual disturbances (usually visual or auditory) • Phase III: 10–15% untreated alcohol withdrawal patients reach this phase; seizures (usually tonic-clonic) last 0.5–4 min and can progress to status epilepticus • Phase IV: Delirium tremens (DTs) is usually a late complication of untreated alcohol withdrawal; includes autonomic hyperactivity and severe hyperthermia; mortality associated with alcohol withdrawal reduced due to early treatment preventing delirium tremens • Wernicke's encephalopathy can occur in patients with thiamine deficiency
Protracted Abstinence Syndrome	• Patients may experience subtle withdrawal symptoms that can last from weeks to months – include sleep dysregulation, anxiety, irritability, and mood instability • Cognitive impairment from chronic alcohol use will persist for several weeks after abstinence is achieved • Individuals are at high risk for relapse during this period • Hepatic metabolism of co-administered drugs may decrease following abstinence from chronic alcohol use

Precautions	• Increased risk of drug toxicity possible in patients with alcohol-induced liver impairment or cirrhosis • Risk and type of drug-drug interaction varies with acute and chronic alcohol consumption
Use in Pregnancy◇	• Drinking alcohol while pregnant increases the risk of problems in fetal development; fetal alcohol spectrum disorder (FASD) indicates full range of possible effects on the fetus; fetal alcohol syndrome (FAS) is characterized by severe effects of alcohol, including brain damage, facial deformities, and growth deficits. Infants should be reassessed and followed up regularly as early intervention improves long-term educational outcomes • Withdrawal reactions reported; seen 24–48 h after birth if mother is intoxicated at birth
Breast Milk	• Milk levels attain 90–95% of blood levels; prolonged intake can be detrimental

◇ See p. 473 for further information on drug use in pregnancy and effects on breast milk

Alcohol (cont.)

 Treatment

- In acute intoxication, minimize stimulation; effects will diminish as blood alcohol level declines (rate of 3–7 mmol/L per hour)
- Withdrawal reactions following chronic alcohol use may require
  a) vitamin supplementation (thiamine 50 mg orally or IM for at least 3 days) to prevent or treat Wernicke-Korsakoff syndrome (level of evidence 3)
  b) benzodiazepine for symptomatic relief (to control agitation) and to prevent seizures (chlordiazepoxide, lorazepam, diazepam, or oxazepam); these drugs reduce mortality, reduce the duration of symptoms, and are associated with fewer complications compared to antipsychotic drugs (level of evidence 1); risk of transferring dependence from alcohol to benzodiazepine is small; loading dose strategy used with diazepam (i.e., patient dosed until light somnolence is achieved (level of evidence 3); its long duration of action prevents breakthrough symptoms and possible withdrawal seizures)
  c) hydration and electrolyte correction
  d) high-potency antipsychotic (e.g., haloperidol, zuclopenthixol) to treat behavior disturbances and hallucinations (level of evidence 3)
  e) β-blockers may be considered for use in conjunction with benzodiazepines in select patients for control of persistent hypertension or tachycardia (level of evidence 3)
- SSRIs may be useful as treatment for late-onset alcoholics, or alcoholism complicated by comorbid major depression. Buspirone may have some utility for treating alcoholics with comorbid anxiety disorder
- Naltrexone and acamprosate reported to be effective adjuncts to treatment for relapse prevention following alcohol detoxification, see p. 400 and p. 405; the efficacy of each is increased significantly when combined with psychosocial treatments
- See p. 402 for use of disulfiram in treatment

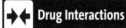 **Drug Interactions**

- Clinically significant interactions are listed below
- For more interaction information on any given combination, also see the corresponding chapter for the second agent

Class of Drug	Example	Interaction Effects
Analgesic	Acetaminophen	Chronic excessive alcohol use increases susceptibility to acetaminophen-induced hepatotoxicity due to enhanced formation of toxic metabolites through CYP2E1 induction
	Salicylates	Increased gastric bleeding with ASA; reduced peak plasma concentration of ASA reported ASA may increase blood alcohol concentration by reducing ethanol oxidation by gastric alcohol dehydrogenase
	NSAIDs	Increased risk of gastric hemorrhage
Anesthetic	Propofol	Chronic consumption increases the dose of propofol required to induce anesthesia
	Enflurane, halothane	Chronic consumption increases risk of liver damage
Antibiotic	Cephalosporins, metronidazole	Disulfiram-like reaction with nausea, hypotension, flushing, headache, tachycardia
	Doxycycline	Chronic alcohol use induces metabolism and decreases plasma level of doxycycline
Anticoagulant	Warfarin	Chronic alcohol use may increase or decrease international normalized ratio (INR) – close monitoring required
Anticonvulsant	Barbiturates, carbamazepine, phenytoin	Additive CNS effects Chronic ethanol use enhances metabolism of carbamazepine and phenytoin
Antidepressant	Tricyclic	Additive CNS effects, impairment in psychomotor performance Disrupted metabolism of antidepressant
	NaSSA	Additive CNS effects
	Irreversible MAOIs	Possible risk of hypertensive crisis with consumption of beer or wine, due to tyramine content (see p. 69)
Antifungal	Furazolidone, griseofulvin, ketoconazole	Disulfiram-like reaction

Class of Drug	Example	Interaction Effects
Antihypertensive		
α_1-blocker, β-blocker	Atenolol, metoprolol, prazosin	Acute alcohol ingestion may cause additive hypotensive effects, while chronic moderate–heavy drinking may raise blood pressure and reduce the effectiveness of antihypertensive medications
Calcium channel blocker	Verapamil	Verapamil may increase concentration of ethanol due to inhibited metabolism
Antipsychotic	Haloperidol, olanzapine, quetiapine	Additive CNS effects IM olanzapine given to alcohol-intoxicated patients for agitation was associated with a significant decrease in oxygen saturation Extrapyramidal side effects may be worsened by alcohol
Antitubercular	Isoniazid	Increased risk of hepatotoxicity Tyramine-containing alcoholic beverages may cause a hypertensive reaction (MAOI) Disulfiram-like reaction
Antiviral	Abacavir	Increased AUC of abacavir (by 41%)
Ascorbic acid		Increased ethanol clearance
Anxiolytic	Benzodiazepines (e.g., alprazolam, diazepam, lorazepam)	Potentiation of CNS effects. Use of lorazepam in intoxicated individuals has been reported to decrease respiration
	Buspirone	Combined use with alcohol can cause drowsiness faintness, fatigue, and/or weakness
Cannabis		Potentiation of CNS effects; additive detrimental effects on driving performance
Cardiovascular drug	Guanethidine, hydralazine, methyldopa, nitroglycerin	Increased dizziness or fainting upon standing up
CNS depressant	Sedating antihistamines, muscle relaxants, valerian	Potentiation of CNS effects. Caution with high doses due to risk of respiratory depression
Disulfiram		Flushing, sweating, palpitations, headache due to formation of acetaldehyde (see p. 402)
Hormone replacement therapy (HRT)	Premarin (conjugated estrogens)	Both chronic alcohol use and HRT increase the risk of breast cancer, it has been suggested that women on HRT limit their alcohol intake (e.g., less than 1 drink/day)
H$_2$ blocker	Cimetidine, ranitidine	Inhibit alcohol dehydrogenase in the stomach, reduce first-pass metabolism of alcohol, and increase gastric emptying – increased bioavailability of alcohol
Hypnotic	Chloral hydrate	Potentiation of CNS effects. Caution with high doses due to risk of respiratory depression Increased plasma level of metabolite of chloral hydrate (trichloroethanol), which inhibits the metabolism of alcohol and increases blood alcohol levels
Hypoglycemic	Chlorpropamide, glyburide, tolbutamide	Flushing, sweating, palpitations, headache due to formation of acetaldehyde; disulfiram-like reaction Acute alcohol use decreases metabolism of tolbutamide; chronic use increases it Increased risk of hypoglycemia
	Metformin	Possible increased levels of lactic acid in the blood after alcohol consumption
Immunosuppressive	Methotrexate	Increased risk of liver damage
	Pimecrolimus, tacrolimus	Facial flushing
Nitrate	Nitroglycerin	Increased risk of hypotension
Opioid	All opioids	Additive CNS effects; caution with excessive doses due to risk of respiratory depression
	Slow-release opioids (Morphine sustained-release: Kadian)	Alcohol can speed the release of opioids into the bloodstream by dissolving the slow-release system (not all products affected; no problems noted with Codeine Contin, Hydromorph Contin, and MS Contin). Use caution with other slow-release products
	Methadone	Additive CNS depression

Alcohol (cont.)

Class of Drug	Example	Interaction Effects
Prokinetic agent	Metoclopramide	Increases absorption rate of alcohol by speeding gastric emptying
Stimulant	Caffeine	While caffeine may oppose some of the CNS depressant effects of alcohol, it does not completely sober up those who have drunk too much, and could even make them more accident-prone
	Cocaine	Additive effects; increased heart rate; variable effect on blood pressure
	Methylphenidate	Alcohol may increase levels of methylphenidate (AUC by 25%, maximum serum level by 40%), and may exacerbate the CNS effects of methylphenidate

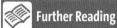 **Further Reading**

References

[1] Brenner DR, Haig TR, Poirier AE, et al. Alcohol consumption and low-risk drinking guidelines among adults: A cross-sectional analysis from Alberta's Tomorrow Project. Health Promot Chronic Dis Prev Can. 2017;37(12):413–424. doi:10.24095/hpcdp.37.12.03

Additional Suggested Reading

- Hasin DS. Alcohol use disorder and suicide risk: A fresh and closer look. Am J Psychiatry. 2020;177(7):572–573. doi:10.1176/appi.ajp.2020.20050628
- Korpi ER, den Hollander B, Farooq U, et al. Mechanisms of action and persistent neuroplasticity by drugs of abuse. Pharmacol Rev. 2015;67(4):872–1004. doi:10.1124/pr.115.010967
- Lev-Ran S, Balchand K, Lefebvre L, et al. Pharmacotherapy of alcohol use disorders and concurrent psychiatric disorders: A review. Can J Psychiatry. 2012;57(6):342–349. Retrieved from http://publications.cpa-apc.org/media.php?mid=1300
- Mirijello A, D'Angelo C, Ferrulli A, et al. Identification and management of alcohol withdrawal syndrome. Drugs. 2015;75(4):353–365. doi:10.1007/s40265-015-0358-1
- National Institute on Alcohol Abuse and Alcoholism. Alcohol's Effects on Health. Bethesda, MD: National Institute on Alcohol Abuse and Alcoholism. Retrieved from https://www.niaaa.nih.gov/alcohols-effects-health
- Patel AK, Balasanova AA. Treatment of alcohol use disorder. JAMA. 2021;325(6):596. doi:10.1001/jama.2020.2012
- Reus VI, Fochtmann LJ, Bukstein O, et al. The American Psychiatric Association Practice Guideline for the pharmacological treatment of patients with alcohol use disorder. Am J Psychiatry. 2018;175(1):86–90. doi:10.1176/appi.ajp.2017.1750101

Stimulants

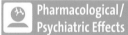 **Pharmacological/ Psychiatric Effects**

- Differ, depending on type of drug taken, dose, and route of administration
- Cause rapid and large increases in central and peripheral monoamines (dopamine, epinephrine, norepinephrine, serotonin)
- Effects occur rapidly, especially when drug used parenterally
- Acute toxicity reported with doses ranging from 5 to 630 mg of amphetamine; chronic users can ingest up to 1000 mg/day
- Following acute toxicity, psychiatric state usually clears within 1–4 weeks of amphetamine discontinuation

Physical

- Elevated BP, tachycardia, increased respiration and temperature, sweating, pallor, tremors, decreased appetite, dilated pupils, reduced fatigue, wakefulness, insomnia, increased sensory awareness, increased or decreased sexual arousal/libido

Mental

- Euphoria, exhilaration, alertness, improved task performance, exacerbation of obsessive-compulsive symptoms
- Methamphetamine reported to induce paranoia and hallucinations when used in binge-like doses

High Doses

- Anxiety, excitation, panic attacks, grandiosity, delusions, visual, auditory and tactile hallucinations, paranoia, mania, delirium, increased sense of power, violence
- Fever, sweating, headache, flushing, pallor, hyperactivity, stereotypic behavior, cardiac arrhythmias, respiratory failure, loss of coordination, collapse, cerebral hemorrhage, convulsions, and death

| Chronic Use | • Decreased appetite and weight, abdominal pain, vomiting, difficulty urinating, skin rash, increased risk of stroke, high blood pressure, irregular heart rate, impotence, headache, anxiety, delusions of persecution, violence, dental caries
• Tolerance to physical effects occurs but vulnerability to psychosis remains
• Chronic high-dose use causes physical dependence; psychological dependence can occur even with regular low-dose use
• Recovery occurs rapidly after amphetamine withdrawal, but psychosis may be lasting |

 Complications
- Exacerbation of hypertension or arrhythmias
- Strokes and retinal damage due to intense vasospasm, especially with "crack" and "ice"
- With methamphetamine, cerebral side effects reported include: vasculopathy with or without parenchymal infarction, hypertensive encephalopathy, and hemorrhage
- Can exacerbate harmful effects of co-occurring infections, such as neurological damage in HIV infection

D/C Discontinuation Syndrome
- Symptoms are very similar to those of major depressive disorder. Include depressed mood, anhedonia, anxiety, hypersomnia, fatigue, irritability, difficulty concentrating, craving, and suicidal or homicidal ideation

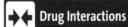 **Treatment**
- Use calming techniques, reassurance, and supportive measures
- Supportive care of excess sympathomimetic stimulation may be required (e.g., BP, temperature); monitor hydration, electrolytes, and for possible serotonin syndrome
- For severe agitation and to prevent seizures, sedate with benzodiazepine (e.g., diazepam, lorazepam)
- For psychosis, use a high-potency antipsychotic (e.g., haloperidol); avoid low-potency antipsychotics
- Non-pharmacological treatment approaches are the current mainstay for the treatment of stimulant addiction
- Agents under investigation with mixed results include GABAergic medications (e.g., vigabatrin, baclofen, topiramate), modafinil, drug vaccines, disulfiram, and cannabidiol

Drug Interactions
- Clinically significant interactions are listed below
- For more interaction information on any given combination, also see the corresponding chapter for the second agent

GENERAL

Class of Drug	Example	Interaction Effects
Antipsychotic		Diminished pharmacological effects of stimulants
Irreversible MAOI	Phenelzine	Severe palpitations, tachycardia, hypertension, headache, cerebral hemorrhage, agitation, seizures; AVOID. Serotonin syndrome reported with MDA, MDMA

AMPHETAMINES

Class of Drug	Example	Interaction Effects
Antidepressant	General	Enhanced antidepressant effect Increased blood pressure
	Tricyclics	Enhanced stimulant effects. Increased plasma level of amphetamine Cardiovascular effects increased
	MAOI (irreversible)	Release of large amount of norepinephrine while ability to metabolize monoamines blocked by MAOI, leading to hypertensive reaction
Antihypertensive	Guanethidine	Reversal of hypotensive effects
Antipsychotic	Chlorpromazine	Decreased effects of both agents Antipsychotics can counteract many signs of stimulant toxicity (e.g., anxiety, aggression, visual or auditory hallucinations, psychosis, hyperkinetic movements) and have additive adverse effects (e.g., insomnia, restlessness, tremor)

Stimulants (cont.)

Class of Drug	Example	Interaction Effects
CNS depressant	Triazolam	Decreased sedation and amnesia
NMDA receptor antagonist	Ketamine	Increased hallucinatory behavior
Opioid	Morphine	Decreased morphine dose required for analgesia
Smoking cessation medication	Varenicline	Decreased effectiveness of varenicline
Urinary acidifier	Ammonium chloride	Increased elimination of amphetamine due to decreased renal tubular reabsorption and increased elimination
Urinary alkalizer	Sodium bicarbonate	Prolonged pharmacological effects of amphetamine due to decreased urinary elimination of unchanged drug

COCAINE

Class of Drug	Example	Interaction Effects
Alcohol		Additive effects; increased heart rate; variable effect on blood pressure
Anorectic	Mazindol	May decrease craving for cocaine Increased lethality and convulsant activity reported
Antibiotic	Clarithromycin, erythromycin	Combination could result in cocaine overdose, due to inhibition of metabolism via CYP3A4, with rhabdomyolysis, arrhythmia, and cardiovascular collapse[1]
Antidepressant	Cyclic, SSRI Tricyclic: desipramine	Decreased craving Decreased seizure threshold Elevated heart rate and diastolic pressure (by 20–30%); increased risk of arrhythmia
Antifungal	Ketoconazole	Combination could result in cocaine overdose, due to inhibition of metabolism via CYP3A4, with rhabdomyolysis, arrhythmia, and cardiovascular collapse[1]
Antipsychotic	Clozapine, risperidone, ziprasidone	Case reports of EPS, particularly dystonia, with concurrent use of risperidone and ziprasidone, possibly via dopamine depletion from chronic use of cocaine; case report of clozapine causing a dose-dependent increase in plasma concentration of intranasal dose of cocaine, though the positive effects of cocaine were reduced

Antiretroviral
  Non-nucleoside reverse transcriptase inhibitor (NNRTI)
  Protease inhibitor
	Nevirapine
	
	Efavirenz, indinavir, ritonavir
		Potentially increased metabolism of cocaine to the hepatotoxic metabolite norcocaine, via CYP3A4[1]
		
		Combination could result in cocaine overdose, due to inhibition of metabolism via CYP3A4, with rhabdomyolysis, arrhythmia, and cardiovascular collapse

Barbiturate		Reports of enhanced hepatotoxicity
β-blocker	Propranolol	May increase the magnitude of cocaine-induced myocardial ischemia
Cannabis		Increased heart rate; blood pressure increased only with high doses of both drugs Increased plasma level of cocaine and increased subjective reports of euphoria
Catecholamine	Norepinephrine	Potentiation of vasoconstriction and cardiac stimulation
Disulfiram		Increased plasma level (3-fold) and half-life (60%) of cocaine with possible increased risk of cardiovascular effects
Opioid	Buprenorphine, methadone Heroin, morphine	Decreased trough methadone concentrations (effect more drastic for buprenorphine) May potentiate cocaine euphoria
Sympatholytic	Yohimbine	Enhanced effect of cocaine on blood pressure

Drug	Comments
AMPHETAMINE, DEXTROAMPHETAMINE (Dexedrine, Dexampex, Biphetamine) Taken orally as tablet, capsule, sniffed, smoked, injected Slang: Bennies, hearts, pep-pills, dex, beans, benn, truck-drivers, ice, jolly beans, black beauties, crank, pink football, dexies, crosses, hearts, LA turnaround	• Cause the release of monoamines (NE, 5-HT, DA) from central and peripheral neurons • Onset of action: 30 min after oral ingestion • Physical effects: Increased heart rate, BP, metabolism, decreased appetite, weight loss, rapid breathing, tremor, loss of coordination • CNS effects: Euphoria, increased energy and mental alertness, anxiety, insomnia, irritability, restlessness, panic, impulsive or aggressive behavior • Active drug use may be terminated by exhaustion with excessive sleeping • Tolerance and psychological dependence occur with chronic use • Excessive doses can lead to heart failure, delirium, psychosis, coma, convulsions, and death • Pregnancy: Increase in premature births; withdrawal symptoms and behavioral effects (hyperexcitability) noted in offspring • Breastfeeding: Irritability and poor sleeping pattern reported in infants
METHAMPHETAMINE (Desoxyephedrine) – Crystal Meth (Desoxyn, Methampex) Powder taken as tablets, capsules, liquid, injected, snorted, inhaled, smoked Slang: Speed, meth, uppers, crystal, shit, moth, crank, crosses, methlies quick, jib, fire, chalk, glass, go fast, tweak, yaba Crystal ("ice") is methamphetamine washed in a solvent to remove impurities – smoked in a glass pipe, "chased" on aluminium foil or injected	• Synthetic drug related chemically to amphetamine and ephedrine; can be manufactured in "home laboratories" from common household products • Enhances release of dopamine, norepinephrine, and serotonin[2] • Very rapid onset of action; can last 10–12 h • Powerful effects produced are referred to as a "rush". Used as a club drug at "raves" to increase alertness, energy, sociability, euphoria; has aphrodisiac effects and causes loss of inhibitions • A "run" refers to the use of the drug several times a day over a period of several days • "Ice" can be mixed with cannabis and smoked through a bong or injected • Physical effects: Tachycardia, tachypnea, diaphoresis, hyperthermia, mydriasis, hypertension; stroke reported • CNS effects: Anxiety, agitation, confusion, insomnia, delirium, delusions, hallucinations, paranoia, violence; powerful psychological dependence and addiction occurs, particularly with "ice" • Chronic use can result in weight loss, bruxism, cardiovascular problems, decreases in lung function, pulmonary hypertension, rapid tooth decay ("meth mouth"), mood disturbances, decreased cognitive functioning, anxiety, psychosis with suicidal or homicidal thoughts; may persist for months after drug use is stopped; has been associated with neuronal damage • Users are at high risk of sexually transmitted and blood-borne diseases due to disinhibitory high-risk behaviors that can occur (e.g., shared needles, multiple partners, unprotected sex) • Abuse of methamphetamine can produce impaired memory and learning, hyperawareness, hypervigilance, psychomotor agitation, movement abnormalities, irritability, aggression. Chronic intoxication (use) may result in a psychotic state with delusions, hallucinations, and delirium • Toxic effects: Arrhythmias, hypertension, heart failure, hyperthermia, seizures, encephalopathy, rhabdomyolysis (see Complications p. 373) • After abrupt discontinuation, withdrawal effects peak in 2–3 days and include GI distress, headache, depression, irritability, and poor concentration • Methamphetamine exposure during pregnancy is associated with decreased growth in infants; withdrawal effects reported in newborns and potentially developmental delays

Stimulants (cont.)

Drug	Comments
COCAINE Extract from leaves of coca plant Leaves chewed, applied to mucous membranes Powder taken orally, snorted, smoked, injected Slang: Coke, coca, snow, flake, lady, toot, blow, big C, candy, crack, joy dust, stardust, rock, nose, boulders, bump, bianca, perico, nieve, soda "Crack": Free base cocaine	• Inhibits dopamine, serotonin, and norepinephrine reuptake • Onset of action and plasma half-life varies depending on route of use (e.g., IV: Peaks in 30 sec, half-life 54 min; snorting: Peaks in 15–30 min, half-life 75 min) • Metabolized by hydrolysis to its major urinary metabolite, benzoylecgonine • Crack is a free-based and more potent form of cocaine (volatilized and inhaled) • Often adulterated with amphetamine, ephedrine, procaine, xylocaine or lidocaine • Used with heroin, morphine or cannabis for increased intensity • Used with flunitrazepam to moderate stimulatory effect • CNS effects: Rapid euphoria, increased energy and mental alertness, insomnia, anxiety, agitation, delusions, hallucinations, choreoathetosis ("crack dancing") • Physical effects: Nausea, vomiting, headaches, tachycardia, hypertension, chest pain, pyrexia, diaphoresis, mydriasis, ataxia, anorexia; tactile hallucinations occur • Tolerance develops to some effects (appetite), but increased sensitivity (reverse tolerance) develops to others (convulsions, psychosis) • Powerful psychological dependence occurs; dysphoria can last for weeks • Depression-like symptoms commonly occur after drug use; dysphoria promotes repetitive use • Chronic users can develop panic disorder, paranoia, dysphoria, irritability, assaultive behavior, paranoia, and delirium • Snorting can cause stuffy, runny nose, eczema around nostrils, atrophy of nasal mucosa, bleeding, and perforated septum • Smokers are susceptible to respiratory symptoms and pulmonary complications • Sexual dysfunction is common • Chronic users of "crack" can develop microvascular changes in the eyes, lungs, and brain; respiratory symptoms include asthma and pulmonary hemorrhage and edema • Dehydration can occur due to effect on temperature regulation, with possible hyperpyrexia • Toxic effects: Hypertension, paroxysmal atrial tachycardia, hyperreflexia, irregular respiration, hyperthermia, seizures, unconsciousness, death; fatalities more common with IV use • Pregnancy: Associated with spontaneous labor and abortion; increase in premature births; infants have lower weight, length, and head circumference, jitteriness, irritability, poor feeding, EEG abnormalities • Breastfeeding during cocaine intoxication reported to cause irritability, vomiting, diarrhea, tremulousness, and seizures in infants
KHAT (*Catha edulis*) Leaves chewed	• Grows in Africa and the Middle East • Cathinone is principal psychoactive agent • Symptoms occur within 3 h and last about 90 min • Acute symptoms include: euphoria, excitation, grandiosity, increased blood pressure, flushing • Chronic use can cause: anxiety, agitation, confusion, dysphoria, aggression, visual hallucinations, paranoia
METHYLPHENIDATE Tablets crushed and snorted, swallowed, injected Slang: Vitamin R, R-ball, skippy, the smart drug, JIF, MPH	• See p. 312 • Large doses can cause psychosis, seizures, stroke, and heart failure
SYMPATHOMIMETICS (Ephedrine, pseudoephedrine, phenylpropanolamine) Taken as capsules, tablets Slang: Look alikes, Herbal Bliss, Cloud 9, Herbal X	• Known as Herbal Ecstasy and sold as "natural" alternative to MDMA • Misrepresented as amphetamines and sold in capsules or tablets that resemble amphetamines • Doses of ingredients vary widely • Reports of hypertension and seizures; death due to stroke can occur after massive doses

Drug	Comments
SYNTHETIC CATHINONES **Mephedrone** (4-methylmethcathinone), **Methylone** (3,4-methylenedioxymethcathinone), **MDPV** (3,4-methylenedioxypyrovalerone), **flephedrone, ethylcathinone** Sold as capsules, tablets, or white crystalline powder that can be swallowed, snorted or injected Slang: "Bath salts", bath powder, plant food, plant fertilizer, Meph, drone, meow, rush, Ivory, Ivory Wave, Cloud 9, (9), Blizzard, Ocean Snow, Scarface, Hurricane Charlie, fine china, Silverback, Blue Magic, vanilla sky, Energy-1, bliss, Bolivian bath, MDPK, MTV, Magic, Maddie, Black Rob, Super Coke, PV and Peeve, Zoom, Bloom, insect repellant, potpourri,vacuum freshener, Heavenly Soak	• Mephedrone and methylone: Nonspecific substrates of transporters for dopamine, norepinephrine, and serotonin, preventing reuptake • MDPV: Specific inhibitor of dopamine and norepinephrine transporters • Effects similar to other stimulants such as cocaine, methamphetamine, including euphoria, excitement, anxiety, agitation, confusion, psychosis, and seizures • CNS effects last 3–4 h, while some physical effects (e.g., tachycardia, hypertension) can last 6–8 h • Higher doses can produce panic attacks, paranoia, confusion, psychotic delusions, extreme agitation, sometimes progressing to violent behavior, suicidal thoughts/actions • Physical effects: Tachycardia, hypertension, vasoconstriction, insomnia, hyper-reflexia, nausea, stomach cramps, and digestive problems, anorexia, bruxism, increased body temperature, chills, sweating, pupil dilation, headache, and tinnitus • Strong cravings and addiction reported • Withdrawal symptoms include: Depression, lethargy, headache, anxiety, postural hypotension, and severely bloodshot eyes – usually subside within 4–8 h

 Further Reading

References
1 Goodlet KJ, Zmarlicka MT, Peckham AM. Drug–drug interactions and clinical considerations with co-administration of antiretrovirals and psychotropic drugs. CNS Spectr. 2019;24(3):287–312. doi:10.1017/S109285291800113X
2 Panenka WJ, Procyshyn RM, Lecomte T, et al. Methamphetamine use: A comprehensive review of molecular, preclinical and clinical findings. Drug Alcohol Depend. 2013;129(3):167–179. doi:10.1016/j.drugalcdep.2012.11.016

Additional Suggested Reading
• Clemow DB. Misuse of methylphenidate. Curr Top Behav Neurosci. 2017;34:99–124. doi:10.1007/7854_2015_426
• Frazer KM, Richards Q, Keith DR. The long-term effects of cocaine use on cognitive functioning: A systematic critical review. Behav Brain Res. 2018;348:241–262. doi:10.1016/j.bbr.2018.04.005
• Horwitz H, Skanning P, Askaa B, et al. Amphetamine abuse and drug interactions [article in Danish]. Ugeskr Laeger. 2014;176(45):V01140042.
• Lindsey WT, Stewart D, Childress D. Drug interactions between common illicit drugs and prescription therapies. Am J Drug Alcohol Abuse. 2012;38(4):334–343. doi:10.3109/00952990.2011.643997
• McCance-Katz EF, Sullivan LE, Nallani S. Drug interactions of clinical importance among the opioids, methadone and buprenorphine, and other frequently prescribed medications: a review. Am J Addict. 2010;19(1):4–16. doi:10.1111/j.1521-0391.2009.00005.x
• Morley KC, Cornish JL, Faingold A, et al. Pharmacotherapeutic agents in the treatment of methamphetamine dependence. Expert Opin Investig Drugs. 2017;26(5):563–578. doi:10.1080/13543784.2017.1313229
• Smid MC, Metz TD, Gordon AJ. Stimulant use in pregnancy: An under-recognized epidemic among pregnant women. Clin Obstet Gynecol. 2019;62(1):168–184. doi:10.1097/GRF.0000000000000418

Hallucinogens and Cannabinoids

General Comments
• Cannabis is the most widely used illicit drug of abuse in the world; there have been recent increases in use in North America due to different constituencies allowing medical and legal recreational use
• The term medical cannabis refers to using the whole unprocessed cannabis plant or its basic extracts to treat a disease or symptom
• Typically provided by a legally approved supplier
• Dried cannabis and its oil are approved drugs/medicine in Canada. However, reasonable access to a legal source of cannabis is provided when authorized by a healthcare practitioner

 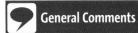

Hallucinogens and Cannabinoids (cont.)

- Medical cannabis has been used to treat chronic pain, muscle spasms, and nausea during chemotherapy, improve appetite in HIV/AIDS, improve sleep, and improve tics in Tourette's syndrome. More recent evidence indicates antipsychotic and anti-epileptic effects of cannabidiol
- Cannabis is legal in some jurisdictions of the USA for use in PTSD (literature suggests benefit for PTSD symptoms as well as worsening of symptoms)
- Increased recent interest in hallucinogens for the treatment of psychiatric disorders, such as psychotherapy-assisted psilocybin for depression

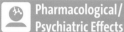 **Pharmacological/ Psychiatric Effects**

- Differ, depending on type of drug taken and route of administration (see specific agents below)
- Effects occur rapidly and last from 30 min (e.g., DMT) to several days (e.g., PCP)

Physical

- Increased BP, tachycardia, dilated pupils, nausea, sweating, flushing, chills, hyperventilation, incoordination, muscle weakness, trembling, numbness
- Cannabinoids may be effective for treating neuropathic pain (marketed in Canada under the name of Sativex or Cesamet [indicated for chemotherapy-induced nausea and vomiting, as adjunctive treatment for spasticity in multiple sclerosis, and as adjunctive treatment for neuropathic pain]); mixed effects found on multiple sclerosis symptoms; may have some benefit in Tourette's syndrome

Mental

- Alteration of perception and body awareness, impaired attention and short-term memory, disturbed sense of time, depersonalization, euphoria, mystical or religious experiences, grandiosity, anxiety, panic, visual distortions, hallucinations (primarily visual), erratic behavior, aggression

High Doses

- Confusion, restlessness, excitement, anxiety, emotional lability, panic, mania, paranoia, "bad trip"
- Cardiac depression and respiratory depression (mescaline), hypotension, convulsions and coma (PCP)

Chronic Use

- Anxiety, depression, personality changes
- Tolerance (tachyphylaxis) can occur with regular use (except with DMT); reverse tolerance (supersensitivity) has been described
- "Woolly" thinking, delusions, and hallucinations reported; may persist for months after drug discontinuation
- Flashbacks – recurrent psychotic symptoms, may occur years after discontinuation
- Cohort studies suggest that chronic use of cannabis by teenagers is associated with more than 5-fold increase in risk of later-life depression and anxiety as well as an increased risk of early-onset psychosis
- Regular (weekly) cannabis use has been associated with increased risk of tardive dyskinesia in schizophrenic patients on antipsychotics
- There is evidence that chronic cannabis users might experience sustained deficits in memory function

D/C Discontinuation Syndrome

- Withdrawal symptoms identified in frequent cannabis users consist of irritability, nervousness, anxiety, sleep disturbance, decreased appetite or weight loss, stomach pain, shakiness/tremors, sweating, fever, chills

 Treatment

- Provide reassurance and reduction of threatening external stimuli
- Supportive care for excess CNS stimulation may be required; monitor hydration, electrolytes, and for possible serotonin syndrome
- In severe cases, the "trip" should be aborted chemically as rapidly as possible. In mild cases, "talking down" may be appropriate
- Use high-potency antipsychotic (e.g., haloperidol) for psychotic symptoms
- Avoid low-potency antipsychotics with anticholinergic and α-adrenergic properties (e.g., chlorpromazine) to minimize hypotension, tachycardia, disorientation, and seizures
- Use benzodiazepines (diazepam, lorazepam) to control agitation and to sedate, if needed
- Propranolol and ascorbic acid may minimize effects of PCP and aid in its excretion

→← Drug Interactions

- Clinically significant interactions are listed below
- For more interaction information on any given combination, also see the corresponding chapter for the second agent

CANNABIS

Class of Drug	Example	Interaction Effects
Anticholinergic	Atropine, benztropine, oxybutynin	Increased heart rate and/or hypertension
Anticoagulant	Warfarin	Increased international normalized ratio (INR) and risk of bleeding
Anticonvulsant	Clobazam	Increased risk of benzodiazepine toxicity via cannabidol inhibition of CYP2C19
Antidepressant	Tricyclic: Desipramine	Case reports of tachycardia, lightheadedness, mood lability, and delirium with combination Cardiac complications reported in children and adolescents
	MAOI: Tranylcypromine	Caution: Cannabis increases serotonin levels and may result in a serotonin syndrome
Antifungal	Ketoconazole	Increased THC and cannabidol concentrations (by 2-fold) via CYP3A4 inhibition
Antipsychotic	Chlorpromazine, thioridazine	Drugs with anticholinergic and α_1-adrenergic properties can cause marked hypotension and increased disorientation
	Clozapine, olanzapine	Decreased efficacy via CYP1A2 induction
Antiretroviral Protease inhibitor	Indinavir, nelfinavir	Inhaled marijuana reported to reduce indinavir AUC by 17% and C_{max} of nelfinavir by 21%; no effect on viral load
Barbiturate		Additive effect causing anxiety and hallucinations
CNS depressant	Alcohol, benzodiazepines, hypnotics, opioids	Potentiation of CNS effects; increased impaired judgment
Disulfiram		Synergistic CNS stimulation reported, hypomania
Lithium		Clearance of lithium may be decreased
Methylxanthine	Theophylline	Increased clearance of theophylline by 40% via CYP1A2 induction
Opioid	Morphine	THC blocks excitation produced by morphine
Smoking (tobacco)		Additive effects on the induction of CYP1A2 isoenzyme; additive increase in heart rate and stimulant effects
Stimulant	Cocaine	Increased heart rate; blood pressure increased with high doses of both drugs; increased plasma level of cocaine and increased subjective reports of euphoria

KETAMINE

Class of Drug	Example	Interaction Effects
Antiretroviral Protease inhibitor	Nelfinavir, ritonavir	Elevated levels of ketamine possible due to inhibited metabolism
Benzodiazepine	Diazepam	Prolonged recovery with diazepam due to decreased metabolism Benzodiazepines may reduce the antidepressant effects of ketamine in the treatment of depression. Possible attenuation of ketamine response from concurrent use of benzodiazepines also suggested
NMDA receptor antagonist	Memantine	Do not combine, as adverse effects may be enhanced; additive effects of NMDA receptor blockade
Opioid	Morphine	Additive respiratory depression; ketamine is a respiratory depressant like morphine, though less potent
Stimulant	Amphetamine	Increased hallucinatory behavior

Hallucinogens and Cannabinoids (cont.)

LSD

Class of Drug	Example	Interaction Effects
Antidepressant	SSRI: fluoxetine	Grand mal seizures reported Recurrence or worsening of flashbacks reported with fluoxetine, sertraline, and paroxetine
Antiretroviral		
Protease inhibitor	Ritonavir	Elevated levels of LSD possible due to inhibited metabolism

MDA/MDMA

Class of Drug	Example	Interaction Effects
Alcohol		MDMA may reverse subjective feelings of alcohol sedation without reversing alcohol's effects on impulsivity or psychomotor skills
Antidepressant	SSRI: fluoxetine	Diminished pharmacological effects of MDA
Antiretroviral		
Protease inhibitor	Ritonavir	Case reports of increased plasma levels of MDMA due to inhibited metabolism via CYP2D6; death reported
Phosphodiesterase type 5 (PDE5) inhibitor	Sildenafil	Anecdotal reports of serious headaches and priapism requiring emergency treatment from the abuse of sildenafil and MDMA

Phencyclidine (PCP)

Class of Drug	Example	Interaction Effects
Acidifying agent	Cranberry juice, ammonium chloride	Increased excretion of PCP
Antiretroviral		
Protease inhibitor	Ritonavir	Elevated levels of PCP possible due to inhibited metabolism

Drug	Comments
CANNABIS Crushed leaves, stems, and flowers of female hemp plant (*Cannabis sativa*) Smoked (cigarettes or water pipe), swallowed Slang: Grass, pot, joint, hemp, weed, reefer, smoke, Mary Jane, Indian hay, ace, ganja, gold, J, locoweed, shit, herb, Mexican, ragweed, bhang, sticks, blunt, dope, sinsemilla, skunk, Hydro (hydroponic cannabis) **Hashish** – resin from flowers and leaves; more potent than cannabis plant Smoked, cooked, swallowed Slang: Hash, hash oil, weed oil, weed juice, honey oil, hash brownies, tea, black, solids, grease, smoke, boom, chronic, gangster, hemp	• Over 70 phytocannabinoids in cannabis; delta-9-tetrahydrocannabinol (THC) is the main psychoactive ingredient; high potency (> 20%) forms of cannabis (e.g., "skunk") increasingly common • Cannabidiol (CBD) is the second most common psychoactive cannabinoid ingredient in cannabis, typical range 0–13% • THC undergoes first-pass metabolism to form psychoactive metabolite 11-OH-THC. Half-life is 24–36 h for infrequent users and up to 10 days for frequent users. THC and CBD are metabolized primarily by CYP3A4; also by 2D6, 2C9, and 2C19. Weak inhibitor of 3A4, 2C9, and 2C19 • Induces CYP1A2 through activation of the aromatic hydrocarbon receptor • Effects occur rapidly and last up to several hours; accumulates in fat tissue for up to 4 weeks before being released back into bloodstream; effects may persist • Results of short-term controlled trials indicate that smoked cannabis reduces neuropathic pain, improves appetite and caloric intake, especially in patients with reduced muscle mass, and may relieve spasticity and pain in patients with multiple sclerosis[1] • THC may have beneficial effects in chemotherapy-induced nausea/vomiting (Cesamet) • Review of 2 trials suggests THC may have some benefit on the frequency and severity[2] of tics in Tourette's syndrome • Tolerance and psychological dependence may occur; reverse tolerance (supersensitivity) described • Combined with other drugs including PCP, opium, heroin, crack cocaine, or flunitrazepam to enhance effect • CNS effects: Most users experience euphoria with feelings of self-confidence and relaxation; some become dysphoric, anxious, agitated, and suspicious. Can cause psychotic symptoms with confusion, hallucinations, emotional lability (very prolonged or heavy use can cause serious and potentially irreversible psychosis) • Increased craving for sweets • Chronic use: Bronchitis, weight gain, bloodshot eyes, loss of energy, apathy, "fuzzy" thinking, slow reaction time, impaired judgment, decreased testosterone in males; increased risk of depression, anxiety, and schizophrenia • Link between cannabis use and early age at onset of psychosis suggested; results point to cannabis as a dangerous drug in young people at risk of developing psychosis[3] • Exogenous THC modulates release of neurotransmitters (including dopamine and glutamate) by interacting with specific cannabinoid receptors that are distributed in brain regions implicated in schizophrenia[4] • Cannabis cigarettes have a higher tar content than ordinary cigarettes and are potentially carcinogenic • Pregnancy: Can retard fetal growth and cause mild withdrawal reactions in the infant; developmental problems in children born to cannabis-dependent parents have been reported in some studies • Breastfeeding: Can reach high levels in breast milk
CANNABINOIDS, SYNTHETIC Psychoactive chemicals dissolved in solvent, applied or sprayed to plant material; usually smoked or prepared as a herbal infusion Slang: K2, Spice, Black Mamba (Turnera diffusa), Bombay Blue, Fake Weed, Genie, Zohai, Bliss, Blaze, JWH -018, -073, -250, Yucatan Fire, Skunk, Moon Rocks	• Synthetic designer drugs that mimic the effects of cannabis • Contain a mixture of herbs and synthetic cannabinoids, which may include: Cannabicyclohexanol, JWH-018, JWH-073, JWH-200, CP-47,497 or HU-210; chemicals are frequently changed and concentrations are unpredictable • Marketed as "synthetic marijuana," "herbal incense", "herbal smoking blends" or "potpourri" and sold online, in head shops, and some stores • Physical effects: 2–3 times more likely to be associated with sympathomimetic effects (i.e., tachycardia and hypertension) than THC; vomiting; high doses reported to cause convulsions, myocardial infarction[5] • Contaminant, (1-(5-fluoropentyl)-1H-indol-3-yl)(2,2,3,3-tetramethylcyclopropyl) methanone, has been associated with acute kidney injury • CNS effects: Elevated mood, relaxation, altered perception; anxiety, agitation, confusion, paranoia, and hallucinations reported; psychosis can be prolonged • Regular users may experience symptoms of addiction and withdrawal

Hallucinogens and Cannabinoids (cont.)

Drug	Comments
KETAMINE (Ketalar) General anesthetic in day surgery Taken orally as capsules, tablets, powder, crystals, and solution; injected, snorted, smoked Slang: K, special K, vitamin K, ket, green, jet, kit-kat, cat valiums, Ketalar SV	• NMDA receptor antagonist, prevents glutamate receptor activation, inhibits reuptake of monoamines (5-HT, NE, DA) • Used as a club drug at "raves" and involved in "date rapes"; most ketamine users are sporadic and polydrug users • Doses of 60–100 mg injected; consciousness maintained at this dose, but disorientation develops • Effects start within 60 sec (IV) and 10–20 min (PO); metabolized primarily by CYP2B6 and also by CYP3A4 and 2C9. Weak inhibitor of CYP3A4 • Physical effects: Increased heart rate and blood pressure, nausea, vomiting, increased muscle tone, nystagmus, stereotypic movements, impaired motor function, numbness; synthetic ketamine linked to serious urinary tract infections and bladder-control problems • CNS effects: Dream-like state, depersonalization, confusion, hostility, mild delirium, hallucinations, amnesia • Toxic effects: Severe delirium, respiratory depression, loss of consciousness, catatonia • IV infusions of ketamine have been found effective in patients with treatment-resistant depression (refer to Unapproved Treatments of Psychiatric Disorders chapter p. 445
LYSERGIC ACID DIETHYLAMIDE (LSD) Semi-synthetic drug derived from ergot (grain fungus) White powder used as tablet, capsule, liquid, liquid-impregnated paper, snorted, smoked, inhaled, injected Slang: Acid, cubes, purple haze, Raggedy Ann, sunshine, yellow sunshine, LBJ, peace pill, big D, blotters, domes, hits, tabs, doses, window-pane, microdot, boomers	• 5-HT$_{2A}$ receptor agonist • Effects occur in less than 1 h and last 2–18 h • Physical effects: Mydriasis, nausea, loss of appetite, muscle tension, hyperthermia, hypertension, weakness, numbness, tremors • CNS effects: Can cause agitation, visual hallucinations, suicidal, homicidal, and irrational behavior, and dysphoria; panic, psychotic reactions can last several days • Flashbacks occur without drug being taken • Tolerance develops rapidly; psychological dependence occurs • Combined with cocaine, mescaline, or amphetamine to prolong effects • Pregnancy: Increased risk of spontaneous abortions; congenital abnormalities have been reported
MESCALINE (3,4,5-trimethoxyphenethylamine) From cactus *Lophophora williamsii*, San Pedro cactus (*Echinopsis pachanoi*) and/or the Peruvian torch cactus (*Echinopsis peruviana*); pure product not readily available Cactus buttons are dried, then sliced, chopped, or ground; used as powder, capsule (masks bitter taste), tablet, solution, inhaled or injected Slang: Mesc, peyote, buttons, cactus	• Binds to 5-HT$_{2A}$ receptor as a partial agonist and acts on 5-HT$_{2C}$ receptor • Less potent than LSD, but cross-tolerance reported • Effects occur 1–2 h after ingestion and last 10–18 h • Physical effects: Euphoria, time distortion, brilliant colors, weightlessness, headache, dry skin, increased temperature and heart rate, hypotension or hypertension, numbness, tremors, dizziness, nausea, cardiac and respiratory depression • CNS effects: Anxiety, disorientation, impaired reality testing, and flashbacks • Dependence not reported but tolerance to effects occurs quickly
MORNING GLORY SEEDS Active ingredient is lysergic acid amide; 1/10th as potent as LSD Seeds eaten whole or ground, mushed, soaked, and solution injected Slang: Flying saucers, licorice drops, heavenly blue, pearly gates	• Effects occur after 30–90 min when seeds ingested and immediately when solution injected • Commercial seeds are treated with insecticides, fungicides, and other chemicals and can be poisonous

Drug	Comments
PHENCYCLIDINE General anesthetic used in veterinary medicine; often misrepresented as other drugs Powder, chunks, crystals used as tablets, capsules, liquid, inhaled, snorted, injected (IM or IV) Slang: PCP, angel dust, hog, horse tranquilizer, animal tranquilizer, peace pill, killer, weed, supergrass, crystal, "CJ", dust, rocket fuel, boat, love boat	• Antagonist at NMDA receptor • Effects occur in a few minutes and can last several days to weeks (half-life 18 h); metabolized primarily by CYP3A4 and also by CYP2C11. Weak inhibitor of CYP2B6 • Frequently sold on street as other drugs (easily synthesized); mis-synthesis yields a product that can cause abdominal cramps, vomiting, coma, and death • Physical effects: Intermittent vomiting, sialorrhea, loss of appetite, diaphoresis, miosis, nystagmus, hypertension, and ataxia can occur • CNS effects: Can cause apathy, estrangement, feelings of isolation, indifference to pain, delirium, disorientation with amnesia, schizophrenia-like psychosis, and violence (often self-directed); can feel intermittently anxious, fearful to euphoric • Toxic effects: Hypoglycemia, rhabdomyolysis, depression, delirium, CNS depression, coma; deaths have occurred secondary to uncontrollable seizures or to hypertension resulting in intracranial hemorrhage • Flashbacks occur • Psychological dependence occurs • Pregnancy: Signs of toxicity have been reported in newborns • Breastfeeding: Drug concentrates in milk and detectable for weeks after heavy use
PSILOCYBIN From *Psilocybe mexicana* mushroom Used as dried mushroom, white crystal, powder, capsule, injection; eaten raw, cooked or steeped as tea Slang: Magic mushrooms, sacred mushrooms, mushroom, shroom, purple passion	• Chemically related to LSD and DMT (see Tryptamines below); psilocybin is a prodrug for psilocin (4-HO-DMT, 4-hydroxy-dimethyltryptamine) which is rapidly produced in the body after ingestion • Effects occur within 30 min and last several hours • Partial agonist at 5-HT$_{1A}$ and 5-HT$_{2A}$ receptors • Effects: Nausea, vomiting, distorted time perceptions (users sometimes think they had a longer trip than the actual effect), nervousness, paranoia, and flashbacks • Tolerance develops rapidly; cross-tolerance occurs with LSD • Mistaken identity with "death-cap" (Amanita) mushroom can result in accidental poisoning
SALVIA DIVINORUM Member of the mint family Leaves chewed or crushed and the juice ingested as tea, smoked Slang: Diviner's sage, magic mint, Maria Pastora	• Main active ingredient is Salvinorin A; a potent kappa opioid receptor agonist • Effects, when taken orally, depend on the absorption of Salvinorin A through the oral mucosa as it is inactivated by the GI tract; when absorbed through oral mucosa, effects detected in 5–10 min, peak at 1 h and subside after 2 h. If inhaled, effects seen after 30 sec, peak in 5–10 min, and subside in 20–30 min; potency increased dramatically when smoked • Taken in combination with cannabis to prolong effect • Physical effects: Ataxia, incoherent speech, hysterical laughter, unconsciousness • CNS effects: Altered perception; can cause dramatic, and sometimes frightening, hallucinogenic experiences with doses higher than 1 mg
TRYPTAMINES **Dimethyltryptamine (DMT), alpha-methyltryptamine (AMT), 5-methyl-di-isopropyl-tryptamine (5-MeO-DIPT)** Oil or crystal smoked in a water pipe; oil soaked in parsley; dried and snorted or smoked, used as liquid (tea), injected Slang: Lunch-hour drug, businessman's trip, FOXY (= MeO-DIPT)	• Appear in nature in several plants in South America • Effects vary widely, depending on amount ingested; occur almost immediately with DMT and last 30–60 min (called "businessman's trip" due to its short duration of action) • Readily destroyed by stomach acids • Often mixed with cannabis • CNS effects: Anxiety and panic frequent due to quick onset of effects; produce intense visual hallucinations, loss of awareness of surroundings

DRUGS WITH HALLUCINOGENIC AND STIMULANT PROPERTIES

Drug	Comments
2,5-dimethoxy-4-methylamphetamine (STP/DOM) Chemically related to both mescaline and amphetamine Used orally Slang: Serenity, tranquility, peace	• Effects last 16–24 h • More potent than mescaline but less potent than LSD • "Bad trips" occur frequently; prolonged psychotic reactions reported in people with psychiatric history • Tolerance reported; no evidence of dependence • Anticholinergic effects, exhaustion, convulsions, excitement, and delirium reported

Hallucinogens and Cannabinoids (cont.)

Drug	Comments
3,4-methylene-dioxyamphetamine (MDA) Chemically related to both mescaline and amphetamine (synthetic drug) Used orally as liquid, powder, tablet; injection Slang: Love drug	• Also has stimulant-like properties • Typical doses: 60–120 mg • Effects occur after 30–60 min (orally), or sooner if injected, and last about 8 h • CNS effects: Hallucinations and perceptual distortions rare; feeling of peace and tranquility occurs • High doses: Hyperreactivity to stimuli, agitation, hallucinations, violent and irrational behavior, delirium, convulsions, and coma
3,4-methylene-dioxymethamphetamine (MDMA) Powder, usually in tablets or capsules; may also be snorted or smoked, "bumped" or cooked on lollypops or pacifiers Slang: Ecstasy, Molly, MDMA, "Adam", XTC, X, E, love drug, businessman's special, clarity, lover's speed, hugs, beans Herbal Ecstasy: MDMA mixed with ephedrine	• Also has stimulant-like properties • Increases levels of serotonin, norepinephrine and, to a lesser extent, dopamine • Many MDMA products are contaminated with other compounds including dextromethorphan, caffeine, phenylpropanolamine, ephedra, MDA, PMA, ketamine, methyl salicylate • Typical dose varies from 50–150 mg • Onset of effects 30–60 min; duration of action 3–6 h; half-life is about 8 h; metabolized primarily by CYP2D6 and also by CYP1A2, 2B6, and 3A4. May inhibit its own metabolism via CYP2D6; slow metabolizers of CYP2D6 may develop toxicity at moderate doses due to drug accumulation • Commonly used at "raves" • CNS effects: Wakefulness, increases energy and decreases fatigue and sleepiness; creates feelings of euphoria and well-being together with derealization, depersonalization, impaired memory and learning, and heightened tactile sensations (action believed to be mediated through release of serotonin) • Common physical effects include: Increased blood pressure and heart rate, increased endurance and sexual arousal, salivation, mydriasis, bruxism, trismus, increased tension, headache, restless legs, blurred vision, dry mouth, urinary retention, nausea, and suppressed appetite, thirst, and sleep • Severe physical reactions include: Hypertension, tachycardia, arrhythmia, hyperthermia, seizures; followed by hypotension, ischemic stroke, fatal brain hemorrhage, and coma; death can occur from excessive physical activity ("raves") that may result in disseminated intravascular coagulation, rhabdomyolysis, hyponatremia, acute renal and hepatic failure, and multiple organ failure • High doses can precipitate panic disorder, hallucinations, paranoid psychosis, aggression, and flashbacks • After-effects include: Anorexia, drowsiness, muscle aches, generalized fatigue, irritability, anxiety, and depression (last 1–2 days due to half-life of drug of about 8 h) • Tolerance to euphoric effects with chronic use • Chronic regular use may result in mood swings, depression, impulsivity, and lack of self-control, memory loss, and parkinsonism; can lead to psychological dependence • May also stress the immune system and increase susceptibility to infectious diseases
Benzylpiperazine (BZP) and 3-trifluoromethyphenylpiperazine (3-TFMPP) Slang: Peaq, Freq, PureRush, PureSpun	• Promoted as a special tonic and a "natural" alternative to more dangerous street drugs • Mechanism of action is believed to be similar to MDMA and the effects produced by BZP are comparable to those of amphetamine • Doses of 50–200 mg BZP ingested • Effects last 4–8 h • Metabolized via CYP2D6 and COMT • Physical effects: Nausea, hyperthermia, increased blood pressure, dilated pupils, tingling skin, and decreased appetite • CNS effects: Alertness, increased euphoria, and paranoia • With high doses: Hallucinations, respiratory depression, renal toxicity, and convulsions • Withdrawal effects include: Nausea, headache, fatigue, hangover, confusion, and insomnia
N-ethyl-3,4-methylene-dioxyamphetamine (MDE) Chemically related to MDMA (synthetic drug) Slang: Eve	• Effects as for MDMA (above) • Onset of effects within 30 min; duration of action 3–4 h

Drug	Comments
NBOMes (N-2-methoxy-benzyl substituted 2C class of hallucinogens) marketed online as "research chemicals" under various names: N-bumb, Smiles, Solaris, Cimbi-5, 25I,Bom-25, 2C-I-NBOMe, 25-I-NBOMe, 25I, Pandora, Diviniation, wizard, Smiley Paper Used sublingually, buccally, and snorted. 25I-NBOMe is often applied to sheets of blotter paper of which small portions (tabs) are held in the mouth to allow absorption through the oral mucosa. There are reports of intravenous injection of 25I-NBOMe solution and smoking the drug in powdered form	• 25I-NBOMe was originally synthesized as a radiotracer for positron emission tomography • Potent agonists of 5-HT$_{2A}$ receptor with stimulant and hallucinogenic properties – potency varies depending on product (easily synthesized) • 25I-NBOMe effects usually last 6–10 h if taken sublingually or buccally. When inhaled, effects usually last 4–6 h, but can be significantly longer depending on dosage; durations longer than 12 h reported • Effects similar to LSD, but more potent; tolerance reported • Physical effects: tachycardia, hyperpyrexia, mydriasis, increased sex drive • CNS effects: heightened senses, visual and auditory hallucinations, euphoria • Higher doses can cause: nausea, hypertension, confusion, paranoia, agitation, aggression, seizures, elevated white blood cell count, elevated creatine kinase, metabolic acidosis, acute kidney injury, death
NUTMEG Active ingredient related to trimethoxyamphetamine and to mescaline Seeds eaten whole, ground, powdered; sniffed	• Effects occur slowly and last several hours (duration of hallucinogenic effects is dose related) • Hallucinations are usually preceded by nausea, vomiting, diarrhea, and headache • Physical effects: Lightheadedness, drowsiness, thirst, and hangover can occur
Paramethoxyamphetamine (PMA) Synthetic drug Used as powder, capsules	• Often sold as MDMA but has more pronounced hallucinogenic and stimulant effects • Metabolized by CYP2D6 • Physical effects: Causes major increase in BP and pulse, hyperthermia, increased and labored breathing • Highly toxic; convulsions, coma, and death reported
Trimethoxyamphetamine (TMA) Synthetic drug related to mescaline Used orally, as powder, injection	• Effects occur after 2 h • Often misrepresented as MDA • More potent than mescaline • More toxic if injected or higher doses used • Can cause unprovoked anger and aggression

 Further Reading

References

1 American Medical Association. Use of cannabis for medicinal purposes. Report 3 of the Council on Science and Public Health (I-09). Retrieved from http://www.ama-assn.org/ama1/pub/upload/mm/443/csaph-report3-i09.pdf

2 Black N, Stockings E, Campbell G, et al. Cannabinoids for the treatment of mental disorders and symptoms of mental disorders: A systematic review and meta-analysis. Lancet Psychiatry. 2019;6(12):995–1010. doi:10.1016/S2215-0366(19)30401-8

3 Pardo M, Matalí JL, Sivoli J, et al. Early onset psychosis and cannabis use: Prevalence, clinical presentation and influence of daily use. Asian J Psychiatr. 2021;62:102714. doi:10.1016/j.ajp.2021.102714

4 Nielsen SM, Toftdahl NG, Nordentoft M, et al. Association between alcohol, cannabis, and other illicit substance abuse and risk of developing schizophrenia: A nationwide population based register study. Psychol Med. 2017;47(9):1668–1677. doi:10.1017/S0033291717000162

5 Forrester MB, Kleinschmidt K, Schwarz E, et al. Synthetic cannabinoids and marijuana exposures reported to poison centers. Hum Exp Toxicol. 2012;31:1006–1011. doi:10.1177/0960327111421945

Additional Suggested Reading

• Antoniou T, Bodkin J, Ho JM. Drug interactions with cannabinoids. CMAJ. 2020;192(9):E206. doi:10.1503/cmaj.191097

• Calvey T, Howells FM. An introduction to psychedelic neuroscience. Prog Brain Res. 2018;242:1–23. doi:10.1016/bs.pbr.2018.09.013

• Centre for Addiction and Mental Health (Toronto, Canada). Information about drugs and addiction: Hallucinogens. Retrieved from http://www.camh.net/About_Addiction_Mental_Health/Drug_and_Addiction_Information/hallucinogens_dyk.html

• Lindsey WT, Stewart D, Childress D. Drug interactions between common illicit drugs and prescription therapies. Am J Drug Alcohol Abuse. 2012;38(4):334–343. doi:10.3109/00952990.2011.643997

• Lopez-Gimenez JF, Gonzalez-Maeso J. Hallucinogens and Serotonin 5-HT2A receptor-mediated signalling pathways. Curr Top Behav Neurosci. 2018;36:45–73. doi:10.1007/7854_2017_478

Hallucinogens and Cannabinoids (cont.)

- Lucas CJ, Galettis P, Schneider J. The pharmacokinetics and the pharmacodynamics of cannabinoids. Br J Clin Pharmacol. 2018;84(11):2477–2482. doi:10.1111/bcp.13710
- Moulin V, Alameda L, Framorando D, et al. Early onset of cannabis use and violent behavior in psychosis. Eur Psychiatry. 2020;63(1):e78. doi:10.1192/j.eurpsy.2020.71
- National Institute on Drug Abuse. Drug Facts: MDMA (Ecstasy or Molly). Bethesda, MD: US Department of Health and Human Services/National Institutes of Health, 2018. Retrieved from http://www.drugabuse.gov/publications/drugfacts/mdma-ecstasy-or-molly
- Papaseit E, Pérez-Mañá C, Torrens M, et al. MDMA interactions with pharmaceuticals and drugs of abuse. Expert Opin Drug Metab Toxicol. 2020;16(5):357–369. doi:10.1080/17425255.2020.1749262

Opioids

 General Comments

- High rate of comorbidity, specifically depression, alcoholism, and antisocial personality disorder (often not clear if these are cause or effect)
- Prescription opioid abuse (e.g., codeine, oxycodone) in the general population is relatively high in North America
- Polydrug use and co-dependence on benzodiazepines appears particularly common among individuals injecting opioids
- High incidence of overdose and deaths reported through illicit use/abuse of prescription opioids (e.g., oxycodone, oxymorphone, fentanyl). Many "prescription" opioids (e.g., fentanyl) from illicit sources in Asia
- In many countries, naloxone kits (nasal spray or injectable) are available over the counter

 Pharmacological/ Psychiatric Effects

- Differ depending on type of drug taken, the dose, the route of administration, and whether combined with other drugs
- The elderly are more sensitive to effects and side effects of opioids

Physical
- Analgesia, "rush" sensation followed by relaxation, decreased tension, slow pulse and respiration, increased body temperature, dry mouth, constricted pupils, decreased GI motility

Mental
- Euphoria, state of gratification, sedation

High Doses
- Respiratory depression, cardiovascular complications, coma, and death
- Increased mortality associated with higher prescribed opioid doses in patients with chronic non-cancer pain[1]

Chronic Use
- General loss of energy, ambition, and drive, motor retardation, attention impairment, sedation, slurred speech
- Tolerance and physical dependence; withdrawal
- Cross-tolerance occurs with other opioids

D/C Discontinuation Syndrome

- Symptoms include: Yawning, runny nose, sneezing, lacrimation, dilated pupils, vasodilation, tachycardia, elevated BP, vomiting and diarrhea, restlessness, tremor, chills, piloerection, bone pain, abdominal pain and cramps, anorexia, anxiety, irritability, and insomnia
- Acute symptoms can last 10–14 days (longer with methadone)

 Treatment

- Opioid withdrawal states are generally not life-threatening; "cold turkey" is acceptable to some addicts
- Non-opioid alternatives (e.g., benzodiazepines, antipsychotics) usually do not work
- Drugs are prescribed for the following reasons:
  a) to reverse effects of toxicity by using opioid antagonists (e.g., naloxone – can precipitate withdrawal)
  b) to treat the immediate withdrawal reaction (e.g., clonidine, buprenorphine, methadone)
  c) to aid in detoxification, or for maintenance therapy in a supervised treatment program (e.g., methadone, buprenorphine)

 Drug Interactions

- Clinically significant interactions are listed below
- For more interaction information on any given combination, also see the corresponding chapter for the second agent

OPIOIDS (GENERAL)

Class of Drug	Example	Interaction Effects
Antibiotic	Clarithromycin, erythromycin	Increased plasma concentration of fentanyl, alfentanyl due to inhibited metabolism via CYP3A4, resulting in prolonged analgesia and adverse effects Increased level of oxycodone (AUC increased 2-fold in young patients and 2.3-fold in elderly patients) via CYP3A4 inhibition of clarithromycin
Anticonvulsant	Carbamazepine	Carbamazepine increases metabolism of codeine, fentanyl, oxycodone, and tramadol via CYP3A4 induction. May result in decreased analgesic effects of fentanyl, oxycodone, and tramadol, while potentially increasing analgesic effects of codeine via increased production of normorphine, a more potent metabolite of codeine
	Carbamazepine, phenobarbital, phenytoin	Opiate withdrawal symptoms may occur via CYP3A4 induction
	Phenytoin	Phenytoin is also a CYP3A4 inducer and may have similar interactions as carbamazepine. Phenytoin has been shown to increase production of norpethidine (AUC increased by 25%), a toxic metabolite of meperidine responsible for adverse effects (e.g., seizures, myoclonus, tremors) via CYP3A4 induction
Antidepressant	MAOI, RIMA	Increased excitation, sweating, and hypotension reported (especially with meperidine, pentazocine); may lead to development of encephalopathy, convulsions, coma, respiratory depression, and serotonin syndrome
	Doxepin, fluoxetine, imipramine, maprotiline, paroxetine, venlafaxine	Decreased efficacy of codeine due to inhibition of CYP2D6; must be metabolized to its active metabolite, morphine, (by CYP2D6) for its therapeutic effect
Antiemetic	Metoclopramide	Metoclopramide increases the rate of absorption of oral morphine, increasing its rate of onset and sedative effects. The gastric motility reduction of opioids may antagonize the gastric emptying effects of metoclopramide
	Ondansetron	Four of five controlled studies show ondansetron reduced the analgesic efficacy of tramadol. Tramadol may reduce pain via enhancing the effects of serotonin on presynaptic 5-HT$_3$ receptors in the spinal dorsal horn, while ondansetron reduces this effect via 5-HT$_3$ receptor antagonism
Antihistamine	Tripelennamine, cyclizine	"Opiate high" reported in combination with opium; euphoria
Antipsychotic	FGAs (haloperidol, perphenazine)	Decreased efficacy of codeine due to inhibition of CYP2D6; must be metabolized to its active metabolite, morphine, (by CYP2D6) for its therapeutic effect
	Quetiapine	Increased methadone concentrations via CYP2D6 and P-glycoprotein inhibition
Antiretroviral Protease inhibitor	Darunavir, nelfinavir, lopinavir/ritonavir	Opiate withdrawal symptoms may occur as a result of decreased methadone concentrations
	Ritonavir	Decreased clearance of opioid due to inhibited metabolism via CYP3A4, resulting in increased plasma level (caution with fentanyl, alfentanyl, meperidine, and propoxyphene)
Non-nucleoside reverse transcriptase inhibitor (NNRTI)	Efavirenz, nevirapine	Opiate withdrawal symptoms may occur as a result of decreased methadone concentrations
Antitubercular	Rifampin	Rifampin may increase the metabolism of codeine, fentanyl, morphine, oxycodone, and tramadol via CYP2D6 and/or CYP3A4 induction
CNS depressant	Alcohol, sedating antihistamines, benzodiazepines, muscle relaxants	Additive CNS effects; can lead to respiratory depression
Dextromethorphan		Decreased efficacy of codeine due to inhibition of CYP2D6; must be metabolized to its active metabolite, morphine, (by CYP2D6) for its therapeutic effect
H$_2$ antagonist	Cimetidine	Enhanced effect of opioid and increased adverse effects due to decreased metabolism; 22% decrease in clearance of meperidine
Opioid antagonist	Nalmefene, naloxone, naltrexone	Will precipitate withdrawal reaction
Stimulant	Cocaine	May potentiate cocaine euphoria

Opioids (cont.)

Opioids

Drug	Comments
HEROIN Diacetylmorphine – synthetic derivative of morphine Injected (IV – "mainlining", or SC – "skin popping"), smoked, inhaled on aluminum foil ("chasing the dragon"), taken orally Slang: "H", horse, junk, snow, stuff, lady, dope, shill, poppy, smack, scag, black tar, Lady Jane, white stuff, brown sugar, skunk, white horse	• Effects almost immediate following IV injection and last several hours; effects occur in 15–60 min after oral dosing • Risk of accidental overdose as street preparations contain various concentrations of heroin as well as other potent opioids like fentanyl • Physical dependence and tolerance occur within 2 weeks; withdrawal occurs within 8–12 h after last dose, peaks in 36–72 h, and can last up to 10 days • Physical effects: Pain relief, nausea, constipation, staggering gait, and respiratory depression • CNS effects: Euphoria, drowsiness, and confusion • Toxicity: Sinus bradycardia or tachycardia, hypertension or hypotension, palpitations, syncope, respiratory depression, coma, leukoencephalopathy, and death • Pregnancy: High rate of spontaneous abortions, premature labor and stillbirths – babies are often small and have an increased mortality risk; withdrawal symptoms in newborn reported • Breastfeeding: Tremors, restlessness, vomiting and poor feeding reported in infants
METHADONE (see p. 413) (Dolophine, Metadol, Methadose) Used as tablets, liquid, injected Slang: The kick pill, dolly, meth	• Drug used in withdrawal and detoxification from opioids, but subject to abuse • Effects occur 30–60 min after oral dosing and last 7–48 h • Chronic use causes constipation, blurred vision, sweating, decreased libido, menstrual irregularities, joint and bone pain, and sleep disturbances • Physical dependence and tolerance occur; withdrawal effects peak in 72–96 h, and can last up to 14 days • Pregnancy: Dosing needs should be reassessed (decreased between weeks 14 and 32 and increased prior to term); withdrawal effects reported in neonates • Breastfeeding: Small amounts of methadone enter milk; nurse prior to taking dose or 2–6 h after
MORPHINE Principal active component of opium poppy Taken as powder, capsule, tablet, liquid, injected Slang: "M", dreamer, sweet Jesus, junk, morph, Miss Emma, monkey, white stuff	• Effects as for heroin, but slower onset and longer-acting • Effects occur in 15–60 min after oral dosing and last 1–8 h for immediate-release products; metabolized primarily by UGT1A3 and 2B7; inhibits metabolism of UGT2B7 • Physical effects: Pain relief, nausea, constipation; with high doses, can get respiratory depression, unconsciousness, and coma • CNS effects: Drowsiness, confusion, and euphoria • High dependence liability (second to heroin) due to powerful euphoric and analgesic effects
OPIUM Resinous preparation from unripe seed pods of opium poppy; available as dark brown chunks or as powder Soaked, taken as solution, smoked Slang: Big O, black stuff, block, gum, hop	• Contains a number of alkaloids including morphine (6–12%) and codeine (0.5–1.5%) • Physical effects: Nausea common, constipation; with high doses, can get respiratory depression, unconsciousness, and coma • CNS effects: Drowsiness, confusion, and euphoria

OTHER FREQUENTLY ABUSED PRESCRIPTION OPIOIDS AND RELATED DRUGS

Drug	Comments
CODEINE Methylmorphine Used orally, liquid, injected Slang: Schoolboy, 3s, 4s, Captain Cody, Cody	• Naturally occurring alkaloid from opium poppy • Metabolized primarily by UGT2B7 and also by CYP2D6 and 3A4. Inhibits metabolism of UGT2B7 • Codeine must be metabolized to its active metabolite, morphine (by CYP2D6) for its therapeutic effect. A significant proportion of the population are poor or rapid metabolizers of CYP2D6, resulting in unpredictable opioid effects or adverse effects, including toxicity in ultra-rapid metabolizers

Drug	Comments
	• Common ingredient of both prescription and over-the-counter analgesics and antitussives (e.g., Fiorinal-C, Tylenol #1, etc.; not recommended for children) • Physical effects: Pain relief, constipation • CNS effects: Euphoria, drowsiness, and confusion • Toxic effects: Respiratory depression and arrest, decreased consciousness, coma, and death • Tolerance develops gradually; physical dependence is infrequent; withdrawal will occur with chronic high-dose use
DEXTROMETHORPHAN (Robitussin DM) Used orally Slang: Robo, robo-trip, poor man's PCP, candy, CCC, DM, DXM, skittles, triple C, velvet	• Higher doses can cause agitation, euphoria, altered perceptions, ataxia, nystagmus, hypertension, tachycardia, visual disturbances, and disorientation; may progress to panic attacks, delusions, psychotic/manic behavior, hallucinations, paranoia, and seizures • If combination product abused (e.g. cough/cold preparation) must consider toxic effects of other ingredients
FENTANYL (Duragesic, Sublimaze) Slang: Tango, cash, Apache, China girl, China white, dance fever, friend, goodfella, jackpot, murders, murder 8, TNT	• Effects almost immediate following IV injection and last 30–60 min; with IM use, onset slower and duration of action is up to 120 min; exposing application site of fentanyl patch to an external heat source (e.g., heating pad, hot tub) can increase drug absorption and result in increased drug effect • Metabolized primarily by CYP3A4; decreased metabolism with potent inhibitors of CYP3A4 • Physical effects: Dizziness, dry mouth, constipation, and GI distress • CNS effects: Primarily sedation, confusion, and euphoria occurs quickly • Overdoses have been reported in children who were accidentally exposed to patch due to improper storage or disposal. Toddlers may think the patch is a sticker, tattoo or bandage • High doses can produce muscle rigidity (including respiratory muscles) respiratory depression, unconsciousness, and coma • Risk of serotonin syndrome when used with various serotonergic agents (SSRIs, SNRIs, etc.) • Fentanyl analogues (e.g., carfentanyl) may be thousands of times more potent than morphine and hundreds of times more potent than fentanyl, producing significantly more respiratory depression • Fentanyl and its analogues often contaminate other illicit drugs (e.g., cocaine, heroin, methamphetamine) and are major contributors to overdose deaths
HYDROCODONE (e.g., Novahistex DH, Vicodin) Slang: vike, Watson-387	• Related to codeine but more potent • An ingredient in prescription antitussive preparations; sought by abusers due to easy availability and purity of product • Metabolized primarily by CYP2D6, 3A4, and by UGTs • Physical, CNS, and toxic effects as for codeine • Tolerance develops rapidly • Lethal dose: 0.5–1.0 g
HYDROMORPHONE (Dilaudid) Used orally Slang: Juice, dillies	• Semisynthetic opioid • Metabolized by UGT1A3 • At low doses, side effects less common than with other opioids; high doses more toxic due to strong respiratory depressant effect
LEVORPHANOL (Levo Dromoran)	• Synthetic opioid analgesic with effects similar to morphine • High doses can produce cardiac arrhythmias, hypotension, respiratory depression, and coma
MEPERIDINE/PETHIDINE (Demerol) Synthetic opioid derivative Used orally, injected Slang: Demmies, pain killer	• Metabolite (normeperidine) is highly toxic; may accumulate with chronic use and cause convulsions • High doses produce disorientation, hallucinations, respiratory depression, stupor, and coma • Risk of serotonin syndrome when used with various serotonergic agents (SSRIs, SNRIs, linezolid, etc.) and MAOIs

Opioids (cont.)

Drug	Comments
OXYCODONE (Percodan, Percocet, OxyNeo, OxyContin (US)) Semisynthetic derivative Used orally; tablets chewed, crushed and snorted, powder boiled for injection	• An ingredient in combination analgesic products and on its own • Metabolized by CYP2D6, 3A4, and UGTs • Very high abuse potential • Physical effects: Nausea, constipation; with high doses can get respiratory depression and coma • Mental effects: Drowsiness, disorientation, and euphoria
PENTAZOCINE (Talwin) Used orally, injected Slang: T's, big T, Tee, Tea	• Has both agonist and antagonist properties at opioid receptors • Repeated injections can result in tissue damage at injection site • Mixed with tripelennamine

Further Reading

References

[1] Dasgupta N, Funk MJ, Proescholdbell S, et al. Cohort study of the impact of high-dose opioid analgesics on overdose mortality. Pain Med. 2016;17(1):85–98. doi:10.1111/pme.12907. Erratum in: Pain Med. 2016;17(4):797–798. doi:10.1093/pm/pnw044

Additional Suggested Reading

• Beardsley PM, Zhang Y. Synthetic Opioids. Handb Exp Pharmacol. 2018;252:353–381. doi:10.1007/164_2018_149
• Busse JW, Craigie S, Juurlink DN, et al. Guideline for opioid therapy and chronic noncancer pain. CMAJ. 2017;189(18):E659–E666. doi:10.1503/cmaj.170363
• Dowell D, Haegerich T, Chou R. No shortcuts to safer opioid prescribing. N Engl J Med. 2019;380(24):2285–2287. doi:10.1056/NEJMp1904190
• McCance-Katz EF, Sullivan LE, Nallani S. Drug interactions of clinical importance among the opioids, methadone and buprenorphine, and other frequently prescribed medications: A review. Am J Addict. 2010;19(1):4–16. doi:10.1111/j.1521-0391.2009.00005.x
• Preda A. Opioid abuse. Medscape Reference [Article updated: December 1, 2014]. Retrieved from http://emedicine.medscape.com/article/287790-overview
• Volkow ND, Blanco C. The changing opioid crisis: Development, challenges and opportunities. Mol Psychiatry. 2021;26(1):218–233. doi:10.1038/s41380-020-0661-4
• Wang S. Historical Review: Opiate addiction and opioid receptors. Cell Transplant. 2019;28(3):233–238. doi:10.1177/0963689718811060

Inhalants/Aerosols

General Comments

• High rate of psychopathology, specifically alcoholism, depression, and antisocial personality disorder, has been demonstrated in individuals with a history of solvent use
• Considered "poor man's" drug of abuse, is inexpensive and readily available; primarily used by children and in third world countries to lessen hunger pain
• Use is often episodic, and "fads" determine current inhalant of choice; users often abuse/misuse other drugs
• Nitrite abuse often associated with "club" scene; amyl nitrite used to promote sexual excitement and orgasm; may cause a temporary loss of social inhibitions, thereby leading to higher-risk sexual practices

Slang

• Glue, gassing, sniffing, chemo, snappers
• Amyl and butyl nitrites: Pearls, poppers, rush, locker room, Bolt, Kix
• Nitrous oxides: Laughing gas, balloons, whippets

Substances Abused

• Volatile gases: Butane, propane, aerosol propellants
• Solvents: Airplane glue, gasoline, toluene, printing fluid, cleaning solvents, benzene, acetone, spray paint ("chroming"), amyl nitrite ("poppers"), etc.
• Aerosols: Deodorants, hair spray, freon
• Anesthetic gases: Nitrous oxide (laughing gas), chloroform, ether

Methods of Use	• "Bagging" – pouring liquid or discharging gas into plastic bag or balloon
	• "Sniffing" – holding mouth over container as gas is discharged
	• "Huffing" – holding a soaked rag over mouth or nose
	• "Torching" – inhaling fumes discharged from a cigarette lighter, then igniting the exhaled air

Pharmacological/ Psychiatric Effects
- Differ depending on type of drug taken
- Fumes sniffed, inhaled; use of plastic bag can lead to suffocation
- Inhaled product enters the bloodstream quickly via the lungs and CNS penetration is rapid – intoxication occurs within minutes and can last from a few minutes to an hour

Physical
- Drowsiness, dizziness, slurred speech, impaired motor function, muscle weakness, cramps, light sensitivity, headache, nausea or vomiting, salivation, sneezing, coughing, wheezing, decreased breathing and heart rate, hypotension, and cramps
- Fatalities can arise from cardiac arrest or inhalation of vomit while unconscious

Mental
- Changing levels of awareness, impaired judgment and memory, loss of inhibitions, hallucinations, euphoria, excitation, vivid fantasies, feeling of invincibility, and delirium

High Doses
- Loss of consciousness, convulsions, cardiac arrhythmia, seizures, and death

Chronic Use
- Fatigue, chronic headaches, encephalopathy, hearing loss, visual impairment, sinusitis, rhinitis, laryngitis, weight loss, kidney and liver damage, bone marrow damage, cardiac arrhythmias, and chronic lung disease
- Inability to think clearly, memory disturbances, depression, irritability, hostility, and paranoia
- Tolerance develops to desired effect; psychological dependence is frequent

Toxicity
- CNS: Acute and chronic effects reported (e.g., ataxia, peripheral neuropathy)
- Cardiac: An MI can occur, primarily with use of halogenated solvents
- Renal: Acidosis and hypokalemia
- Hepatic: Hepatitis and hepatic necrosis
- Hematological: Bone marrow suppression, primarily with benzene and nitrous oxide use
- Accidental suffocation from plastic bag used over the head

Use in Pregnancy◊
- Associated with increased risk of miscarriage, birth defects, low birth weight, and sudden infant death syndrome (SIDS); in a meta-analysis of 10 studies of maternal solvent exposure, 5 studies showed major malformations
- There is some evidence that prenatal exposure may cause long-term neurodevelopmental impairments, such as deficits in cognitive, speech, and motor skills
- Residual withdrawal symptoms reported in babies of mothers who used volatile substances during pregnancy. Symptoms in babies include excessive and high-pitched crying, sleeplessness, hyperreflexia, tremor, hypotonia, and poor feeding

Breast milk
- Risk of inhalants entering breast milk and exposing infant to adverse effects

Treatment
- Effects are usually short lasting; use calming techniques, reassurance

Drug Interactions
- Clinically significant interactions are listed below
- For more interaction information on any given combination, also see the corresponding chapter for the second agent

Class of Drug	Example	Interaction Effects
CNS depressant	Alcohol, benzodiazepines, hypnotics, opioids	Increased impairment of judgment, distortion of reality

◊ See p. 473 for further information on drug use in pregnancy and effects on breast milk

Inhalants/Aerosols (cont.)

Further Reading

Additional Suggested Reading
- Centre for Addiction and Mental Health (Toronto, Canada). Inhalants. Retrieved from https://www.camh.ca/en/health-info/mental-illness-and-addiction-index/inhalants
- Cruz SL, Bowen SE. The last two decades on preclinical and clinical research on inhalant effects. Neurotoxicol Teratol. 2021;87:106999. doi:10.1016/j.ntt.2021.106999

Gamma-hydroxybutyrate (GHB)/Sodium Oxybate

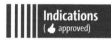

Indications (approved)

- 🔥 Narcolepsy: Oral treatment of cataplexy and excessive daytime sleepiness (Xyrem)

- Has been used in Europe to treat alcohol dependency at a dose of 50 mg/day
- Used for sedation and to treat opioid withdrawal

General Comments

- Prescribing and dispensing restrictions apply for use of Xyrem in patients with narcolepsy
- Xyrem is available as an oral solution containing 500 mg/mL
- Abused as a powder mixed in a liquid; usually sold in vials and taken orally; has a salty or soapy taste
- Used for its hallucinogenic and euphoric effects at raves
- Meta-analysis of GHB for alcohol dependence reported it was better than naltrexone and disulfiram in maintaining abstinence and had a better effect on alcohol cravings than disulfiram or placebo. Single studies suggest comparable efficacy to benzodiazepines in reducing alcohol withdrawal syndrome[1]
- Distributed as a "controlled drug" with generic name of sodium oxybate; improves nighttime sleep and reduces daytime sleep attacks and cataplexy at doses of 6–9 g/night; initial starting doses are recommended to be 4.5 g/night (divided into two doses of 2.25 g each). The second dose is taken 2.5–4 h after the first. Titrate to effect in increments of 1.5 g/night at weekly intervals (0.75 g at bedtime and 0.75 g taken 2.5–4 h later)
- Xyrem, being a CNS depressant, should not be used with alcohol or other CNS depressants. Patients should not drive or operate machinery for at least 6 h after taking Xyrem
- Originally researched as an anesthetic; shown to have limited analgesic effects and increased seizure risk
- Promoted illegally as a health food product, an aphrodisiac, and for muscle building
- Has been used in "date rapes" because it acts rapidly, produces disinhibition and relaxation of voluntary muscles, and causes anterograde amnesia for events that occur under the influence of the drug
- Products converted to GHB in the body include: Gammabutyrolactone (GBL – also called Blue Nitro Vitality, GH Revitalizer, GHR, Remforce, Renewtrient, and Gamma G – is sold in health food stores) and the industrial solvent butanediol (BD – also called tetramethylene glycol or Sucol B, and sold as Zen, NRG-3, Soma Solutions, Enliven, and Serenity)

Slang

- Liquid ecstasy, liquid X, liquid F, goop, GBH = Grievous Bodily Harm, Easy lay, Ghost Breath, G, Somatomax, Gamma-G, Growth Hormone Booster, Georgia home boy, nature's Quaalude, G-riffick, Soapy, Salty Water

Pharmacology

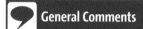

- Produced naturally in the body and is a metabolite of gamma aminobutyric acid (GABA); acts on $GABA_B$ receptor to potentiate GABAergic effects
- Reduces cataplexy
- Some effects of GHB are blocked by opioid receptor antagonists

Pharmacological/ Psychiatric Effects

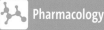

- Deep sleep reported with doses of 2.0 g
- At 10 mg/kg produces anxiolytic effect, muscle relaxation, and amnesia

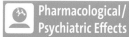

- At 20–30 mg/kg increases REM and slow-wave sleep
- Stimulates slow-wave sleep (stages 3 and 4) and decreases stage 1 sleep; with continued use, decreases REM sleep
- Caution: Doses above 60 mg/kg can result in anesthesia, respiratory depression, and coma
- Chronic use may result in tolerance and/or psychological dependence

 Pharmacokinetics

- Quickly absorbed orally; onset of action occurs within 30 min; peak plasma concentration reached in 20–60 min
- Food significantly decreases the bioavailability of Xyrem (sodium oxybate). Therefore, the first dose should be taken at least 2 h after eating. To minimize variability, the drug should be taken consistently in relation to meals
- Elimination half-life approximately 20–30 min; no longer detected in blood after 2–8 h and in urine after 8–12 h

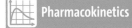 **Adverse Reactions**

Physical

- With high doses: High frequency of drop attacks – "victim" suddenly loses all muscular control and drops to the floor, unable to resist the "attacker"
- Drowsiness, dizziness, nausea, vomiting, headache, hypotension, bradycardia, hypothermia, ataxia, nystagmus, hypotonia, tremors, muscle spasms, seizures, decreased respiration; symptoms usually resolve within 7 h, but dizziness can persist up to 2 weeks
- Use of sodium oxybate in narcolepsy has been associated with headache, nausea, dizziness, sleepwalking, confusion and urinary incontinence; worsening of sleep apnea
- Use of high doses may lead to unconsciousness and coma (particularly dangerous in combination with alcohol)

Mental

- Feeling of well-being, lowered inhibitions, sedation, poor concentration, confusion, amnesia, euphoria, and hallucinations; can cause agitation and aggression

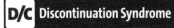 **Discontinuation Syndrome**

- Symptoms occur 1–6 h after abrupt cessation and can last for 5–15 days after chronic use
- Initial symptoms include nausea, vomiting, insomnia, anxiety, confusion, and/or tremor; after chronic use, symptoms can include mild tachycardia and hypertension, and can progress to delirium with auditory and visual hallucinations

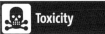 **Toxicity**

- Low therapeutic index; dangerous in combination with alcohol
- Overdoses can occur due to unknown purity and concentration of ingested product
- Symptoms: Bradycardia, seizures, apnea, sudden (reversible) coma with abrupt awakening and violence
- Coma reported in doses greater than 60 mg/kg (4 g)
- Several deaths reported secondary to respiratory failure

Management

- No known antidote

 Use in Pregnancy◊

- Schedule B drug

Breast milk

- Unknown

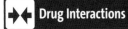 **Drug Interactions**

- Clinically significant interactions are listed below
- For more interaction information on any given combination, also see the corresponding chapter for the second agent

Class of Drug	Example	Interaction Effects
Antiretroviral		
Protease inhibitor	Ritonavir-saquinavir combination	GHB toxicity – may cause bradycardia, respiratory depression, and seizures
Benzodiazepine	Diazepam	Has been used to treat GHB withdrawal; theoretically may worsen respiratory depression
CNS depressant	Alcohol	Synergistic CNS depressant effects can occur, especially with high doses of GHB, leading to respiratory depression

◊ See p. 473 for further information on drug use in pregnancy and effects on breast milk

Gamma-hydroxybutyrate (GHB)/Sodium Oxybate (cont.)

Class of Drug	Example	Interaction Effects
Cannabis		Increased pharmacological effects
Stimulant	Amphetamines	Increased pharmacological effects

Further Reading

References

1 Leone MA, Vigna-Taglianti F, Avanzi G, et al. Gamma-hydroxybutyrate (GHB) for treatment of alcohol withdrawal and prevention of relapses. Cochrane Database Syst Rev. 2010;(2): CD006266. doi:10.1002/14651858.CD006266.pub2

Additional Suggested Reading

- Delic M. Inpatient management of GHB/GBL withdrawal. Psychiatr Danub. 2019;31(Suppl 3):354–356.
- Madah-Amiri D, Myrmel L, Brattebø G. Intoxication with GHB/GBL: Characteristics and trends from ambulance-attended overdoses. Scand J Trauma Resusc Emerg Med. 2017;25(1):98. doi:10.1186/s13049-017-0441-6
- National Institute on Drug Abuse. Drug facts: Club drugs (GHB, Rohypnol, ketamine, MDMA (Ecstasy), Methamphetamine, and LSD (Acid). Bethesda, MD: US Department of Health and Human Services/National Institutes of Health, 2020. Retrieved from https://nida.nih.gov/research-topics/commonly-used-drugs-charts

Flunitrazepam (Rohypnol)

General Comments

- Used as a sedative/tranquilizer in some European countries; not marketed in Canada or the USA
- Commonly used as a "date-rape" drug because it acts rapidly, produces disinhibition and relaxation of voluntary muscles, and causes anterograde amnesia for events that occur under the influence of the drug
- Alcohol potentiates the drug's effects

Slang

- Roofies, R-2s, Roches Dos, forget-me pill, Mexican Valium, roofinol, rope, rophies

Method of Use

- Purchased in doses of 1 and 2 mg (legal manufacturers have added blue or green dye to formulation to color beverages and make them murky); illegal manufacturing is common
- Ingested, snorted or injected
- Added to alcoholic beverages of unsuspecting victim

Pharmacology

- Fast-acting benzodiazepine, structurally related to clonazepam
- See p. 243

Pharmacokinetics

- Effects begin in 30 min, peak within 2 h, and last up to 8 h

Adverse Reactions

- These reactions are reported following restoration of consciousness

Physical

- Dizziness, impaired motor skills, "rubbery legs," weakness, unsteadiness, visual disturbances, blood-shot eyes, slurred speech, and urinary retention
- Decreased blood pressure and pulse, slowed breathing; may lead to respiratory depression and arrest

Mental

- Rapid loss of consciousness and amnesia; residual symptoms include drowsiness, fatigue, confusion, impaired memory and judgment, and reduced inhibition
- If some memory of the event remains, the "victim" may describe a disassociation of body and mind – a sensation of being paralyzed, powerless, and unable to resist

Toxicity	• See Benzodiazepines p. 245

Drug Interactions	• See Benzodiazepines pp. 246–248

Further Reading	**Additional Suggested Reading** • National Institute on Drug Abuse. Drug facts: Club drugs (GHB, Rohypnol, ketamine, MDMA (Ecstasy), Methamphetamine, and LSD (Acid). Bethesda, MD: US Department of Health and Human Services/National Institutes of Health, 2020. Retrieved from https://nida.nih.gov/research-topics/commonly-used-drugs-charts#rohypnol • Williams JF, Lundahl LH. Focus on adolescent use of club drugs and "other" substances. Pediatr Clin North Am. 2019;66(6):1121–1134. doi:10.1016/j.pcl.2019.08.013

Nicotine/Tobacco

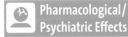 **General Comments**	• Slang: *E-cigarettes:* Vape pipes, hookah pens, e-hookahs *Waterpipe smoking:* Shisha, hookah, narghile, goza, hubble bubble *Chewing tobacco:* Snuff, spit tobacco, smokeless oral tobacco, chad, dip, snarl • Electronic cigarettes, also known as e-cigarettes or vapor cigarettes, are battery-operated devices that resemble traditional cigarettes. Instead of burning tobacco, they contain cartridges filled with nicotine and other chemicals. When the e-cigarette is used, the liquid chemicals in the cartridge are turned into a vapor or steam that is inhaled by the smoker. The liquid comes in a wide range of flavors, from tobacco and coffee to fruit flavors. Nicotine content varies widely among products and nicotine exposure depends on the user's inhalation and experience. There is limited research on their health risks • FDA has announced that e-cigarette use among youth has reach "epidemic proportions." Young people who use e-cigarettes are more likely to progress to smoking combustible cigarettes over time; those who use both e-cigarettes and combustible cigarettes may progress toward heavier use of both products, instead of substituting e-cigarettes from combustible ones • Increased rates and higher levels of smoking have been associated with a number of psychiatric disorders, including schizophrenia, depression, and anxiety disorders, resulting in high rates of morbidity and mortality[1] • Tobacco smoking is the leading cause of premature death in developed countries; tobacco smoke contains over 4,000 chemicals, approximately 50% are carcinogenic[2] • Smoking-related diseases include: Cancers (lung, cervix, pancreas, kidneys, bladder, stomach), cardiovascular disease, emphysema, pneumonia, COPD, aortic aneurysms, acute myeloid leukemia, cataracts, and gum disease
Pharmacological/ Psychiatric Effects	• Nicotine is an alkaloid found in the nightshade family of plants (Solanaceae), which constitutes approximately 0.6–3.0% of dry weight of tobacco. In low concentrations (an average cigarette yields about 1 mg of absorbed nicotine), the substance acts as a stimulant in mammals and is the main factor responsible for the dependence-forming properties of tobacco smoking • By binding to nicotinic acetylcholine receptors, nicotine stimulates the release of many chemical messengers including acetylcholine, norepinephrine, epinephrine, vasopressin, arginine, dopamine, autocrine agents, and β-endorphin. This release of neurotransmitters and hormones is responsible for most of nicotine's effects. Nicotine appears to enhance concentration and memory, due to the increase of acetylcholine. It also appears to enhance alertness, due to the increases of acetylcholine and norepinephrine. Arousal is increased by the increase of norepinephrine. Pain is reduced by the increases of acetylcholine and β-endorphin
Pharmacokinetics	• As nicotine enters the body, it is distributed quickly through the bloodstream and can cross the blood-brain barrier. On average, it takes about 7 sec for nicotine to reach the brain when inhaled • The amount of nicotine absorbed by the body from smoking depends on many factors, including the type of tobacco, whether the smoke is inhaled, and whether a filter is used. For chewing tobacco, dipping tobacco, snus (moist tobacco powder), and snuff (ground tobacco leaves used for

Nicotine/Tobacco (cont.)

inhalation), which are held in the mouth between the lip and gum, or taken in the nose, the amount released into the body tends to be much greater than from smoked tobacco
- Nicotine is metabolized in the liver by CYP450 enzymes (mostly CYP2A6 and also CYP2B6). A major metabolite is cotinine; other primary metabolites include nicotine *N'*-oxide, nornicotine, nicotine isomethonium ion, 2-hydroxynicotine, and nicotine glucuronide. Glucuronidation and oxidative metabolism of nicotine to cotinine are both inhibited by menthol, an additive to mentholated cigarettes, thus increasing the half-life of nicotine *in vivo*.
- Half-life of nicotine in the body is around 2 h

 Toxicity

- It is impossible to overdose on nicotine through smoking alone (though a person can overdose on nicotine through a combination of nicotine patches, nicotine gum, and/or tobacco smoking at the same time)
- Cases of poisoning have been reported in infants and young children with nicotine gum, nicotine patches, and E-cigarettes

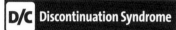 **Discontinuation Syndrome**

- Approximately 40% of smokers attempt to quit each year, but only 4–7% are likely to be successful on their first attempt; most relapse in the first week[3]. Motivational intervention techniques (practical counseling, support, encouragement) appear to be effective in increasing a patient's likelihood to try to quit and maintain abstinence
- Nicotine withdrawal symptoms peak within a few days and usually subside after a few weeks; however, some symptoms can last for months[4]:
  - Withdrawal symptoms, lasting a few days to a few weeks: Dizziness, restlessness, anxiety, insomnia, irritability, frustration, anger, difficulty concentrating, drowsiness, cough, dry throat or mouth, constipation, bloating, and bad breath
  - Withdrawal symptoms lasting weeks to months: Increased appetite, fatigue, "boredom," depressed mood, anhedonia, craving for tobacco, and exacerbation of an underlying psychiatric disorder
- Many behavioral factors can also affect the severity of withdrawal symptoms. For some people, the feel, smell, and sight of a cigarette and the ritual of obtaining, handling, lighting, and smoking the cigarette are all associated with the pleasurable effects of smoking and can make withdrawal or craving worse. Behavioral therapies can help smokers identify environmental triggers of craving so they can employ strategies to prevent or circumvent these symptoms and urges

 Use in Pregnancy◊

- Smoking (or exposure to second-hand smoke) during pregnancy results in babies with a lower-than-average birth weight and more health problems, as smoking exposes the baby to chemicals and carcinogens in tobacco and provides less oxygen and nutrients
- Smokers have a greater chance of having a miscarriage than nonsmokers. During birth, they are more likely to have complications
- Babies born to mothers who smoked may have more ear infections as well as more colds and respiratory problems; long-term effects on the offspring include impaired fertility, type 2 diabetes, obesity, hypertension, learning problems, sleep problems, and neurobehavioral defects[5]
- Children regularly exposed to second-hand smoke are at least 50% more likely to suffer damage to their lungs and to develop breathing problems such as asthma[6]

 Treatment

- Tobacco dependence is a chronic problem that often requires repeated interventions and multiple attempts to quit. Behavior therapies, counseling, and support have shown to improve outcomes
- Medications which have been found to be effective as first-line smoking cessation treatments include[3]:
  - Bupropion SR (see p. 19)
  - Nicotine replacement therapy (gum, lozenge, patch, inhaler; see p. 419)
  - Partial agonist/antagonist – varenicline (see p. 419)
  - Second-line treatments include: nortriptyline and clonidine

 Drug Interactions

- Polycyclic aromatic hydrocarbons are some of the major lung carcinogens found in tobacco smoke. They are potent inducers of CYP isoenzyme 1A2, and possibly 2E1
- NOTE: Both marijuana and tobacco smoking induce cytochrome CYP1A2 through activation of the aromatic hydrocarbon receptor, and the induction effect between the two products is additive[7]

◊ See p. 473 for further information on drug use in pregnancy and effects on breast milk

Class of Drug	Example	Interaction Effects
Alcohol		Positive correlation reported between cigarette smoking and alcohol use; alcohol potentiates rewarding effects of nicotine
Antidepressant	Fluvoxamine	Decreased plasma level of fluvoxamine by 25% due to increased metabolism via CYP1A2
	Tricyclic (amitriptyline, imipramine)	Increased clearance of antidepressant due to induction of CYP1A2
Antipsychotic	Clozapine, olanzapine	Decreased plasma level of antipsychotics due to increased metabolism via CYP1A2. Dosage modifications not routinely recommended but smokers may require higher doses for efficacy. Caution when patient stops smoking, as level of antipsychotic will increase (case report of serious clozapine toxicity following smoking cessation; serum increases of 72–261% reported); monitor clozapine levels and reduce antipsychotic dose as necessary
	Chlorpromazine, thioridazine	Decreased plasma level of chlorpromazine (by 24%) and thioridazine (by 46%) due to induction of metabolism via CYP1A2. Similar interaction with other phenothiazines possible. Caution when patient stops smoking as level of antipsychotic will increase; monitor antipsychotic levels and reduce dose as necessary
Benzodiazepine	Chlordiazepoxide, diazepam	Increased clearance of benzodiazepines due to enzyme induction
	Alprazolam	Alprazolam concentration reduced by 50%
Caffeine		Increased metabolism of caffeine
Cannabis		Additive CYP1A2 induction, additive increase in heart rate and stimulant effects
Corticosteroid	Inhaled puffers	Efficacy of corticosteroid for asthma reduced in smokers
Hormone	Oral contraceptives	Increased risk of serious cardiovascular effects in females over age 35 who smoke 15 or more cigarettes daily
Insulin		Faster onset of action and higher insulin levels in smokers
Theophylline		Decreased plasma level of theophylline due to increased metabolism via CYP1A2

 Further Reading

References

[1] Prochaska JJ, Das S, Young-Wolff KC. Smoking, mental illness, and public health. Annu Rev Public Health. 2017;38:165–185. doi:10.1146/annurev-publhealth-031816-044618

[2] Health Canada. Tobacco scientific facts. Retrieved from http://www.hc-sc.gc.ca/hc-ps/tobac-tabac/fact-fait/facts-faits-eng.php

[3] El Hajj MS, Jaam M, Sheikh Ali SAS, et al. Critical appraisal of tobacco dependence treatment guidelines. Int J Clin Pharm. 2021;43(1):85–100. doi:10.1007/s11096-020-01110-4

[4] US Preventive Services Task Force, Krist AH, Davidson KW, et al. Interventions for tobacco smoking cessation in adults, including pregnant persons: US Preventive Services Task Force recommendation statement. JAMA. 2021;325(3):265–279. doi:10.1001/jama.2020.25019

[5] Banderali G, Martelli A, Landi M, et al. Short and long term health effects of parental tobacco smoking during pregnancy and lactation: A descriptive review. J Transl Med. 2015;13:327. doi:10.1186/s12967-015-0690-y

[6] Public Health Agency of Canada. Smoking and Pregnancy. Retrieved from http://www.phac-aspc.gc.ca/hp-gs/know-savoir/smoke-fumer-eng.php

[7] Anderson GD, Chan LN. Pharmacokinetic drug interactions with tobacco, cannabinoids and smoking cessation products. Clin Pharmacokinet. 2016;55(11):1353–1368. doi:10.1007/s40262-016-0400-9

Additional Suggested Reading

- Hartmann-Boyce J, Livingstone-Banks J, Ordóñez-Mena JM, et al. Behavioural interventions for smoking cessation: An overview and network meta-analysis. Cochrane Database Syst Rev. 2021;1:CD013229. doi:10.1002/14651858.CD013229.pub2

- Jang S, Park S, Jang BH, et al. Study protocol of a pragmatic, randomised controlled pilot trial: clinical effectiveness on smoking cessation of traditional and complementary medicine interventions, including acupuncture and aromatherapy, in combination with nicotine replacement therapy. BMJ Open. 2017;7(5):e014574. doi:10.1136/bmjopen-2016-014574

- National Institute on Drug Abuse. Tobacco, nicotine, and e-cigarettes research report. Bethesda, MD: US Department of Health and Human Services/National Institutes of Health, 2022. Retrieved from https://nida.nih.gov/download/1344/tobacco-nicotine-e-cigarettes-research-report.pdf?v=4b566e8f4994f24caa650ee93b59ec41

- Patnode CD, Henderson JT, Coppola EL, et al. Interventions for tobacco cessation in adults, including pregnant persons: Updated evidence report and systematic review for the US Preventive Services Task Force. JAMA. 2021;325(3):280–298. doi:10.1001/jama.2020.23541

- Ren M, Lotfipour S. Nicotine gateway effects on adolescent substance use. West J Emerg Med. 2019;20(5):696–709. doi:10.5811/westjem.2019.7.41661

TREATMENT OF SUBSTANCE USE DISORDERS

≣ **Classification**	• Drugs available for treatment of substance use disorders may be classified as follows:

Substance Use Disorder	Approved Agent[A]	Page
Alcohol use disorder (AUD)	Acamprosate (Campral)	See p. 400
	Disulfiram[B], [D] (Antabuse)	See p. 402
	Naltrexone (Revia, Vivitrol[B])	See p. 405
Cannabis use disorder	No approved medication	
Cocaine use disorder	No approved medication	
Methamphetamine use disorder	No approved medication	
Opioid use disorder	Buprenorphine (Probuphine, Sublocade[B])	See p. 409
	Buprenorphine/Naloxone (Bunavail[B], Suboxone, Zubsolv[B])	See p. 409
	Methadone (Metadol-D[C], Methadose)	See p. 413
	Naltrexone (Revia, Vivitrol[B])	See p. 405
Tobacco use disorder	Bupropion (Zyban)	See p. 19
	Nicotine replacement therapies (nicotine patches, gum, lozenges, inhalers)	See p. 419
	Varenicline tartrate (Champix in Canada/Chantix in the USA)	See p. 419

[A] Generic preparations may be available, [B] Not marketed in Canada, [C] Not marketed in the USA, [D] Although no longer manufactured by a pharmaceutical company in Canada, it is available through specialty compounding pharmacies

Substance Use Disorder	Unapproved Agent Under Investigation	Comments
Alcohol use disorder	Baclofen	Controversial medication, recent studies and meta-analysis indicate some limited potential effect on increasing abstinence Uncertain whether baclofen improves withdrawal signs and symptoms and reduces side effects relative to placebo or other medications as studies do not show statistical significance
	Benzodiazepines	Considered standard in the treatment of alcohol withdrawal Benzodiazepines show a protective effect against alcohol withdrawal symptoms, in particular seizures, compared with placebo
	Gabapentin	Evidence suggests that gabapentin could be an effective treatment option for the management of alcohol use disorder, specifically in terms of management of alcohol withdrawal Gabapentin is safe and effective for mild alcohol withdrawal, but is not appropriate as monotherapy for severe withdrawal owing to risk of seizures
	Ondansetron	Some initial efficacy, specifically in a genetically defined subgroup. Appears to be selectively effective in two subsets of patients: Individuals who develop an AUD at ≤25 years of age (e.g., "early-onset" AUD) and those with a LL 5'-HTTLPR genotype in the SLC6A4 gene that codes for the serotonin transporter
	Pregabalin	A review of studies shows beneficial effects for alcohol relapse prevention; contradictory results seen for the treatment of withdrawal syndrome; greater benefits seen in patients with comorbid generalized anxiety disorder

Substance Use Disorder	Unapproved Agent Under Investigation	Comments
	Sodium oxybate	Sodium oxybate is the sodium salt of γ-hydroxybutyric acid (GHB). Used in Italy and Austria for withdrawal and abstinence support, with limited evidence, and an FDA black box warning for respiratory depression and dependence
	Topiramate	Evidence suggests that topiramate could be an effective treatment option for the management of alcohol use disorder, while there are limited results for its use to treat alcohol withdrawal syndrome
	Varenicline	Encouraging results for combined treatment of tobacco and alcohol dependence
Cannabis use disorder	Dronabinol	Agonist replacement, improved retention in treatment and reduction of withdrawal symptoms; however, no improvement over placebo regarding abstinence
	Gabapentin	Encouraging initial results for use in acute withdrawal, craving, relapse, and cognitive functioning
	N-acetylcysteine	Appears to have potential for cannabis craving and use, with some limited effect size
	Nabilone	Agonist replacement, no convincing studies as yet
	Nabiximols (Sativex)	Agonist replacement during cannabis withdrawal. Withdrawal symptoms decreased; however, no improvement over placebo regarding long-term reduction of cannabis use
Cocaine use disorder	Bupropion	Limited evidence in form of reports of increase in abstinence
	Mixed amphetamine salts	Mixed results, reduction in cocaine use, specifically in individuals with ADHD Recent positive study in combination with topiramate; higher doses appear to be associated with better outcomes
	N-acetylcysteine	May have potential to improve abstinence in individuals who have stopped using, with limited effect size
	Topiramate	Limited evidence in form of reports of increase in abstinence
Methamphetamine use disorder	Methylphenidate	Mixed results; most promising study with higher doses of methylphenidate
	Mirtazapine	Some RCT data suggesting efficacy specifically in cisgender men, transgender men, and transgender women who had sex with men
	N-acetylcysteine	A double-blind controlled, crossover study showed good efficacy in suppressing craving
	Naltrexone long-acting injection + bupropion	Some initial evidence that it may be effective
Opioid use disorder	Clonidine	May have a role as an adjunctive maintenance treatment with buprenorphine to increase abstinence duration Compared with placebo, clonidine was effective for reducing the severity of opioid withdrawal symptoms and increasing the probability of completing withdrawal management
	Injectable opioid agonist therapy (iOAT)	Specialist-led approach available in Canada for diacetylmorphine and hydromorphone through special access program. It is the highest intensity treatment option available for people with severe IV opioid use disorder who have been unsuccessful at reducing or ceasing illicit opioid use with the assistance of adequately dosed lower-intensity treatment options (i.e., oral opioid agonist therapy) For individuals who are treatment-refractory to methadone, prescription of diacetylmorphine or injectable hydromorphone administered in a highly-structured clinical setting may be beneficial in terms of reducing illicit substance use, criminal activity, incarceration, mortality, and treatment drop-out
	Lofexidine (Lucemyra)	Only approved for the mitigation of withdrawal symptoms to facilitate abrupt discontinuation of opioids in adults up to 14 days
	Slow-release oral morphine (SROM) (Kadian)	Potential option for individuals who respond poorly to buprenorphine/naloxone (Suboxone) and methadone and may require an alternative treatment approach. Health Canada's Non-Insured Health Benefits (NIHB) program includes SROM on its formulary as a treatment option for opioid dependence where methadone and buprenorphine are not appropriate or unavailable The highest dose described in the literature to date is 1,200 mg/day; however, clinical experience in fentanyl users suggests that some patients may require doses above 1,200 mg/day to manage cravings and withdrawals

Treatment of Substance Use Disorders (cont.)

Substance Use Disorder	Unapproved Agent Under Investigation	Comments
Tobacco use disorder	Clonidine	Well established for treatment of tobacco withdrawal
	Electronic cigarettes	The British National Institute for Health and Care Excellence supports electronic cigarettes for harm reduction; despite some safety concerns, electronic cigarettes may help with smoking cessation, though evidence is limited
	Nortriptyline	Equally effective and similar efficacy to bupropion and NRT

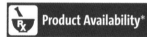 **General Comments**
- In patients with concurrent (also described as dual) disorders (a diagnosed psychiatric disorder and a substance use disorder) integrated treatment is suggested for both disorders, regardless of the status of the concurrent condition
- Given the lack of empirical evidence based on randomized clinical trials, treatment of concurrent conditions is often guided by clinical consensus and evidence established for individuals without concurrent disorders

Acamprosate

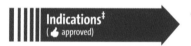 **Product Availability***

Generic Name	Chemical Class	Trade Name	Dosage Forms and Strengths
Acamprosate calcium	Calcium acetyl-homotaurine	Campral	Delayed-release enteric-coated tablets: 333 mg (equivalent to 300 mg acamprosate)

* Refer to Health Canada's Drug Product Database or the FDA's Drugs@FDA for the most current availability information.

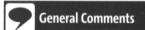 **Indications‡**
(👍 approved)

👍 Alcohol use disorder: Maintenance of abstinence; reduces alcohol cravings and prevents relapse

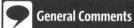 **General Comments**
- Individuals with moderate-to-severe AUD who do not benefit from, have contraindications to, or express a preference for an alternative to first-line medications may be offered topiramate or gabapentin
- Meta-analyses have shown that patients treated with acamprosate had significantly higher continuous abstinence rates than those on placebo
- Detoxification before an acamprosate trial and a goal of abstinence rather than controlled drinking improves outcome with acamprosate
- May not be effective in patients who are actively drinking at the start of treatment; it is not effective for acute withdrawal and does not treat delirium tremens. Initiate treatment as soon as possible after alcohol withdrawal; treatment should be continued during relapses
- Acamprosate treatment should be part of a comprehensive alcohol management program that includes psychosocial support
- Mixed results seen when combined with naltrexone as to increased efficacy and success of abstinence (see Drug Interactions p. 402); acamprosate appears more useful in maintaining abstinence as it reduces dysphoric effects that trigger some patients to resume drinking, while naltrexone controls alcohol consumption by reducing the pleasurable effects of alcohol
- Has been used in combination with disulfiram to increase abstinence
- Efficacy for promoting abstinence from alcohol has not been demonstrated in patients who abuse multiple substances[1]

‡ Indications listed here do not necessarily apply to all countries. Please refer to a country's regulatory database (e.g., US Food and Drug Administration, Health Canada Drug Product Database) for the most current availability information and indications

Pharmacology	• N-Methyl-D-aspartate (NMDA) receptor modulator, decreases activity at NMDA receptors • Decreases dopamine hyperexcitability • Restores glutamate tone and modulates neuronal hyperexcitability following withdrawal from alcohol, decreases activity of glutamate • Weak inhibitor of presynaptic GABA$_B$ receptors in the nucleus accumbens, increases GABA-ergic system
Dosing	• Adults over 60 kg: 666 mg tid; under 60 kg: 666 mg bid; to minimize GI effects, can initiate more gradually (i.e., 333 mg tid and increase dose by 1 tablet per week until target dose is reached) • Hepatic disorders: No dosage adjustment needed • Renal dysfunction: No dosage adjustment if CrCl between 50–80 mL/min; reduce dose to 333 mg tid if CrCl is 30–50 mL/min; avoid in patients with CrCl under 30 mL/min
Pharmacokinetics	• Bioavailability: 11%; food reduces bioavailability by 20%, not clinically significant • T_{max}: 3–9 h once steady state is reached • Steady state is reached in 5–7 days • Has low protein binding • Half-life is 20–33 h • Is not degraded by the liver and is primarily excreted as unchanged drug by the kidneys – not involved in CYP450 interactions
Adverse Effects	• Common: Nausea, flatulence, and diarrhea (dose related and decrease over time), headache, asthenia, and pruritus • Depression, anxiety, insomnia, and suicidal ideation reported • Less common: Vomiting, dizziness, fluctuations in libido, maculopapular rash, anorexia, xerostomia, hyperhidrosis, and metallic taste • Syncope, palpitations, peripheral edema • Weight gain, myalgia, diaphoresis • Acute renal failure reported
Precautions	• Use of acamprosate does not diminish withdrawal symptoms
Contraindications	• Avoid in severe renal insufficiency (CrCl less than 30 mL/min)
Toxicity	• Diarrhea reported after overdose of 56 g • Provide supportive treatment
Pediatric Considerations	• Not recommended
Geriatric Considerations	• Use caution and avoid in patients with renal impairment
Use in Pregnancy◊	• Safety in human pregnancy not established. May be used during pregnancy only after a careful benefit/risk assessment, when the patient cannot abstain from drinking alcohol without being treated with acamprosate and when there is consequently a risk of fetotoxicity or teratogenicity due to alcohol • Teratogenic effects ween in animal studies • Not recommended in humans during pregnancy
Breast Milk	• Not known if excreted in human milk

◊ See p. 473 for further information on drug use in pregnancy and effects on breast milk

Acamprosate (cont.)

 Nursing Implications
- Acamprosate treatment should be part of a comprehensive alcohol management program that includes psychosocial support
- Tablets are enteric-coated, they should not be broken or chewed but swallowed whole
- Monitor patients for symptoms of depression or suicidal thinking
- Diarrhea occurs commonly during therapy, is dose related and generally transient
- Compliance plays an important role in acamprosate efficacy

Patient Instructions
- For detailed patient instruction on acamprosate, see the Patient Information Sheet (details on p. 474)

Drug Interactions
- Clinically significant interactions are listed below
- For more interaction information on any given combination, also see the corresponding chapter for the second agent

Class of Drug	Example	Interaction Effects
Opioid antagonist	Naltrexone	Increased concentrations of acamprosate; C_{max} increased by 33% and AUC by 25%; no change in concentration of naltrexone or its metabolite, 6-β-naltrexone. No dosage adjustment needed

Disulfiram

 Product Availability*

Generic Name	Trade Name[A]	Dosage Forms and Strengths
Disulfiram[B], [D]	Antabuse	Tablets: 250 mg, 500 mg

* Refer to Health Canada's Drug Product Database or the FDA's Drugs@FDA for the most current availability information. [A] Generic preparations may be available, [B] Not marketed in Canada, [D] Although no longer manufactured by a pharmaceutical company in Canada, it is available through specialty compounding pharmacies

Indications‡
(👍 approved)
- 👍 Alcohol use disorder: Deterrent
- Comorbid alcohol use disorder and posttraumatic stress disorder: Has shown benefit in treatment

General Comments
- Does not target core of alcohol dependence
- Acts as an aversive agent or psychological deterrent; clinical efficacy is limited due to poor compliance
- Disulfiram does not directly influence the neural pathways linked to the rewarding effects of, cravings for, or motivation to drink alcohol
- Supervised disulfiram may have short-term efficacy; long-term effects on abstinence require evaluation
- Disulfiram is not recommended over other available pharmacotherapies for AUD that have been proven effective in preventing relapse and/or reducing alcohol consumption
- If disulfiram is used, it should be part of a comprehensive alcohol management program that includes psychosocial support[1]

‡ Indications listed here do not necessarily apply to all countries. Please refer to a country's regulatory database (e.g., US Food and Drug Administration, Health Canada Drug Product Database) for the most current availability information and indications

Pharmacology	• Inhibits alcohol metabolism by irreversibly inhibiting acetaldehyde dehydrogenase; the accumulating acetaldehyde as well as depletion of the potent vasoconstrictor norepinephrine caused by diethyldithiocarbamate, a metabolite of disulfiram, produces an unpleasant reaction consisting of headache, sweating, flushing, choking, nausea, vomiting, tachycardia, dizziness, and hypotension • Response is proportional to the dose and amount of alcohol ingested. Higher doses of disulfiram, if combined with alcohol, increase the risk of shock, circulatory failure, cerebral infarct, and death • Can occur 10–20 min after alcohol ingestion and may last for several hours; may last the entire time alcohol is in the blood • Increases brain dopamine concentrations by inhibiting dopamine catabolizing enzymes, dopamine-β-hydroxylase • Decreases norepinephrine, which may play a role in anti-craving
Dosing	• Initial dosage schedule: A maximum of 500 mg daily in a single dose for 1–2 weeks. However, doses above 300 mg/day increase the risk of adverse effects, even in the absence of alcohol • Maintenance regimen: Average maintenance dose is 250 mg daily (range: 125–500 mg daily), maintenance therapy may be required for months to years • No dosing adjustment provided for renal or hepatic impairment. Use with caution in acute or chronic nephritis or hepatic cirrhosis
Pharmacokinetics	• Highly lipid soluble; bioavailability 80% • Metabolized through multiple steps to active metabolites via CYP3A4/5, 1A2, 2B6, 2E1, and flavin monooxygenase • Selectively inhibits CYP2E1 with both acute and chronic administration; with chronic use, other enzymes (e.g., CYP1A2, 3A4, and P-gp) may also be inhibited
Onset & Duration of Action	• Onset of action: up to 12 h • Duration of action: Up to 14 days, due to slow restoration rate of acetaldehyde dehydrogenase
Adverse Effects	• Drowsiness and lethargy frequent, depression, disorientation, restlessness, excitation, psychosis • Physical effects: Neurological toxicity can occur proportional to dose and duration of therapy (e.g., central and peripheral neuropathy, movement disorders); optic neuritis, headaches, dizziness, skin eruptions, mild gastrointestinal disturbances, impotence, and garlic-like or metallic taste • Transient elevated liver function tests reported in up to 30% of individuals; hepatitis is rare. Baseline liver function test recommended and repeat periodically and at first symptoms or sign of liver dysfunction • Reversible encephalopathy and toxic encephalopathy with convulsions and coma may occur; is usually seen only in overdose
Precautions	• Do not give to intoxicated individuals or within 36 h of alcohol consumption • If alcohol reaction occurs, general supportive measures should be used; in severe hypotension, vasopressor agents may be required • Use cautiously in pulmonary disorders, liver disease, renal disorders, epilepsy, diabetes mellitus, and hypothyroidism • Patients with compromised liver function or unable to abstain from drinking are advised against taking disulfiram • Patients should not drink alcohol for two weeks after stopping disulfiram
Contraindications	• Coronary occlusion, myocardial disease, psychosis, hypersensitivity • Use of alcohol-containing products • Use of metronidazole
Toxicity	• Alcohol reaction is proportional to dose of drug and alcohol ingested; severe reactions may result in respiratory depression, cardiovascular collapse, arrhythmias, convulsions, and death
Lab Tests/Monitoring	• Liver function tests at baseline and after 10–14 days of commencing treatment • Monitor complete CBC and serum chemistries

Disulfiram (cont.)

 Pediatric Considerations
- For detailed information on the use of disulfiram in this population, please see the *Clinical Handbook of Psychotropic Drugs for Children and Adolescents*[2]

 Geriatric Considerations
- Cardiovascular tolerance decreases with age, thus increasing the severity of the alcohol reactions

 Use in Pregnancy◇
- Safety in pregnancy not established, limited data on maternal use during pregnancy

Breast Milk
- Unknown

 Nursing Implications
- The patient should be made aware of the purpose of this medication and educated about the consequences of drinking; informed consent to treatment is recommended
- The patient should avoid all products (food and drugs) containing alcohol, including tonics, cough syrups, mouth washes, and alcohol-based sauces; exposure to alcohol-containing rubs or organic solvents may also trigger a reaction
- Daily uninterrupted therapy must be continued until the patient has established a basis for self-control
- Medication should not be used alone, without proper motivation and supportive therapy; disulfiram will not cure alcohol use disorder but acts as a motivational aid
- Encourage patient to carry an identification card stating that they are taking disulfiram
- A disulfiram/alcohol reaction generally lasts 30–60 min but may be prolonged in severe reactions and may last the entire time alcohol is present in the blood

 Patient Instructions
- For detailed patient instructions on disulfiram, see the Patient Information Sheet (details on p. 474)

Drug Interactions
- Clinically significant interactions are listed below
- For more interaction information on any given combination, also see the corresponding chapter for the second agent

Class of Drug	Example	Interaction Effects
Alcohol		Dilsulfiram reaction (tachycardia, shortness of breath, hypotension, flushing); case reports of myocardial infarction
Antibiotic	Clarithromycin	Case of toxic epidermal necrolysis
	Metronidazole	Acute psychosis, ataxia, and confusional states reported
Anticoagulant	Warfarin	Increased INR response due to reduced metabolism
Anticonvulsant	Phenytoin	Increased phenytoin blood levels and toxicity due to reduced metabolism (carbamazepine and phenobarbital levels not significantly affected)
Antidepressant		
SSRI	Sertraline oral concentrate	Contains alcohol and may cause a disulfiram/alcohol reaction
Cyclic	Amitriptyline, desipramine	Increased plasma level of antidepressant due to reduced metabolism; neurotoxicity reported with combination
Irreversible MAOI	Tranylcypromine	Report of delirium, psychosis with combination
Antiparasitic	Tinidazole	May enhance adverse toxic effect of disulfiram

◇ See p. 473 for further information on drug use in pregnancy and effects on breast milk

Class of Drug	Example	Interaction Effects
Antiretroviral		
Protease inhibitor	Amprenavir solution	Toxicity reported – formulation contains propylene glycol; metabolism inhibited via aldehyde dehydrogenase
	Ritonavir solution	Alcohol-like reaction reported as formulation contains alcohol
	Tipranavir	Increased toxic effects of tipranavir
Antitubercular	Isoniazid	Unsteady gait, incoordination, behavioral changes reported due to reduced metabolism of isoniazid by CYP2E1
Benzodiazepine	Alprazolam, chlordiazepoxide, diazepam, triazolam	Increased activity of benzodiazepine due to decreased clearance (oxazepam, temazepam, and lorazepam not affected)
Caffeine		Reduced clearance of caffeine (by 24–30%) via weak CYP1A2 inhibition, which can cause irritability, insomnia, and anxiety; advise low caffeine intake
Cocaine		Increased plasma level (3–6-fold) and half-life (by 60%) of cocaine; increased risk of cardiovascular effects
Muscle relaxant	Tizanidine	Increased serum level of tizanidine which may cause hypotension, bradycardia, and excessive drowsiness
Stimulant	Dextroamphetamine	Disulfiram may inhibit the metabolism and excretion of dextroamphetamine; dextroamphetamine is contraindicated in patients with a history of alcohol abuse
	Methylphenidate	Case of psychotic-like episode with concurrent use, possibly via disulfiram's action in blocking dopamine-β-hydroxylase, whose low levels have been associated with ADHD and psychotic symptoms
Theophylline		Disulfiram (a weak CYP1A2 inhibitor) causes a dose-dependent negligible to slight decrease in clearance of theophylline, which may be clinically significant and require a dose reduction of theophylline due to its narrow therapeutic index

Naltrexone

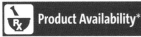

Product Availability*

Generic Name	Trade Name(A)	Dosage Forms and Strengths
Naltrexone	Revia	Tablets: 25 mg(B), 50 mg, 100 mg(B)
	Vivitrol(B)	Extended-release injection: 380 mg

* Refer to Health Canada's Drug Product Database or the FDA's Drugs@FDA for the most current availability information. (A) Generic preparations may be available, (B) Not marketed in Canada

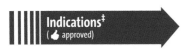

Indications‡
(👍 approved)

- 👍 Alcohol use disorder: As a component of a comprehensive psychotherapeutic or psychological alcoholism counselling program to support abstinence and reduce the risk of relapse
- 👍 Opioid dependence: Treatment adjunct following withdrawal
- Inconsistent results for naltrexone in treatment of bulimia nervosa
- Investigated in treatment of impulse-control disorders, e.g., trichotillomania, kleptomania, and compulsive sexual behaviors
- Adolescent sexual offenders – open trial suggests benefit in treatment with doses of 100–200 mg/day
- Used alone and combined with varenicline to decrease both alcohol use and smoking in heavy drinkers

‡ Indications listed here do not necessarily apply to all countries. Please refer to a country's regulatory database (e.g., US Food and Drug Administration, Health Canada Drug Product Database) for the most current availability information and indications

Naltrexone (cont.)

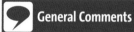

General Comments

- Naltrexone is an opioid antagonist and is contraindicated in patients prescribed opioid agonist therapy; thus, acamprosate should be considered as first-line for treating co-occurring AUD in this patient population
- Recommended to be used together with psychosocial interventions
- Meta-analyses have shown variable effects on abstinence: moderate decrease in the number of heavy drinking days has been shown; may be more effective in patients with high levels of alcohol craving[3] and in males with a family history of alcoholism; double-blind study suggests that it may not have long-term benefits in men with chronic severe alcohol dependence
- Safe to start while an individual is using alcohol; however, may be more effective with fewer side effects if started upon completion of withdrawal management (3–7 days of abstinence from alcohol use)
- Patient compliance plays a significant role in the efficacy of naltrexone
- Mixed results seen in combination with acamprosate regarding increased efficacy and success of abstinence (see Drug Interactions p. 408); naltrexone controls alcohol consumption while acamprosate is more useful in maintaining abstinence
- Does not attenuate craving for opioids or suppress withdrawal symptoms; patients must undergo detoxification before starting the drug
- Does not produce euphoria
- Pretreatment with oral naltrexone is not required prior to use of the extended-release injection[1]

Pharmacology

- Synthetic long-acting antagonist at various opioid receptor sites in the CNS; highest affinity for the μ-opioid receptor – inhibits the positive reinforcement of increased endorphins during alcohol use
- It is hypothesized to work by diminishing the rewarding effect of alcohol in the brain, as well as reducing cravings for alcohol in some individuals
- Blocks the "craving" mechanism in the brain, producing less of a high from alcohol; stops the reinforcing effect of alcohol by blocking the opioid system – promotes abstinence and reduces risk for relapse
- Blocks the effects of other opioid agonists

Dosing

Oral

- Alcohol dependence: 50 mg once daily
- Opioid dependence: Patient must undergo detoxification prior to starting naltrexone and be opioid-free for 7–10 days. Initiate dose at 12.5–25 mg/day and monitor for withdrawal signs; increase dose to 50 mg/day. For supervised administration, maintenance doses of 100 mg every other day or 150 mg every third day can be given

Injection

- The extended-release injection is formulated as microspheres and 380 mg is administered by IM injection into the gluteal muscle every 4 weeks
- Renal impairment: Mild – no dosing adjustments; moderate–severe – no dosing adjustments per manufacturer's labeling; however, has not been studied in moderate–severe renal failure
- Hepatic impairment: No dosing adjustments as per manufacturer's labeling; however, AUC increases 5–10-fold in patients with liver cirrhosis

Pharmacokinetics

Oral

- Rapidly and completely absorbed from the GI tract
- Undergoes extensive first-pass metabolism; only about 20% of drug reaches the systemic circulation
- Widely distributed; only 21–28% is protein bound
- Onset of effect occurs in 15–30 min in chronic morphine users
- Duration of effect is dose dependent; blockade of opioid receptors lasts 24–72 h
- Metabolized in liver (not via CYP450); major metabolite (6-β-naltrexone) is active as an opioid antagonist
- Elimination half-life is 96 h; excreted primarily by the kidneys

Injection	• Caution recommended in administering the drug to patients with renal impairment • Naltrexone AUC increased 5–10-fold in patients with liver cirrhosis • First peak occurs 2 h post injection; second peak occurs 2–3 days later; onset of effect seen within 48 h • Elimination half-life is 5–10 days and dependent on the erosion of the polymer; plasma concentrations are sustained for at least 30 days

 Adverse Effects

- Common with oral naltrexone: Nausea and vomiting (approximately 10% – more common in females; may be reduced with slower dose titration), dysphoria
- Common with extended-release injection: Nausea, headache, fatigue, pain; and tenderness at injection site, swelling, bruising, pruritus or indurations; cellulitis, hematoma, abscess, and necrosis have been reported
- GI effects: Abdominal pain, cramps, dyspepsia, anorexia, and weight loss; women are more sensitive to GI side effects
- CNS effects: Insomnia, anxiety, depression, confusion, nervousness, fatigue; case reports of naltrexone-induced panic attacks, suicidal thoughts, and attempted suicide
- Physical effects: Headache (6.6%), joint and muscle pain or stiffness
- Dose-related elevated enzymes and hepatocellular injury reported
- Eosinophilia, cases of eosinophilic pneumonia
- Cases of allergic pneumonia reported with injection

 D/C Discontinuation Syndrome

- No data available

 Precautions

- Since naltrexone is an opioid antagonist, do not give to patients who have used opioids (including tramadol) in the previous 10 days – may result in symptoms of opioid withdrawal
- Do not use in patients with liver disorders
- Attempts to overcome blockade of naltrexone with high doses of opioid agonists (e.g., morphine) may lead to respiratory depression and death
- Patients need to monitor injection site for swelling, tenderness, induration, bruising, pruritus, or redness that worsens or does not improve over 2 weeks
- FDA has received many reports of injection site reactions such as cellulitis, induration, hematoma, abscess, and necrosis
- Patients who have been treated with naltrexone may respond to lower opioid doses (than previously used) when naltrexone is discontinued. This could potentially lead to accidental overdose

 (STOP) Contraindications

- Patients receiving opioids or those in acute opioid withdrawal
- Acute hepatitis or liver failure
- History of sensitivity to naltrexone

 Toxicity

- No experience in humans; 800 mg dose for 1 week showed no evidence of toxicity
- Risk for serious injection site reaction increased if injected subcutaneously or into fatty tissue rather than muscle

 Lab Tests/Monitoring

- Baseline liver function tests recommended
- Repeat liver function tests monthly for 6 months
- May cause false positives with opioid immunoassays

Pediatric Considerations

- Has been studied in children for aggression, self-injurious behavior, autism, and mental retardation (dose: 0.5–2 mg/kg/day)
- Effects noted within first hour of administration
- For detailed information on the use of naltrexone in this population, please see the *Clinical Handbook of Psychotropic Drugs for Children and Adolescents*[2]

Naltrexone (cont.)

Geriatric Considerations	• No data

Use in Pregnancy◊	• No adequate and well-controlled studies in pregnant women • Should be used in pregnancy only when the potential benefits justify the potential risk to the fetus • Shown to have embryocidal and fetotoxic effects in animal studies when given 30 and 60 times the human dose
Breast Milk	• Naltrexone and its primary metabolite 6-β-naltrexone are excreted into breast milk in very low concentrations • Effects on the nursing infant unknown. Due to the potential for tumorigenicity shown for naltrexone in animal studies, and for the potential of serious adverse reactions in nursing infants, a decision should be made to discontinue nursing or discontinue the drug, taking into account the importance of the drug to the mother

Nursing Implications	• Naltrexone should be used in conjunction with established psychotherapy or self-help programs • As naltrexone does not attenuate craving for opioids or suppress withdrawal symptoms, compliance problems may occur; individuals must undergo opioid detoxification prior to starting drug • Patients should be advised to carry documentation stating that they are taking naltrexone • Advise patients receiving extended-release injections of naltrexone that administration of large doses of opioids may lead to serious adverse effects, coma or death • Advise patients to report shortness of breath, coughing, wheezing or significant redness and discomfort at the injection site to their physician • Vivitrol injection must be diluted only with the supplied diluent and administered with needle provided in kit. Store kit in the refrigerator; can be kept at room temperature for no more than 7 days. Once diluted, the injection should be administered IM right away (alternating buttocks); pain on injection possible; monitor patients for rash or indurations at injection site • Should a patient miss a scheduled appointment for receiving injectable naltrexone, the next dose of injection can be given as soon as possible • Monitor for signs of depression or suicidal ideation • Naltrexone may cause false positives with opioid immunoassays

Patient Instructions	• For detailed patient instructions on naltrexone, see the Patient Information Sheet (details on p. 474)

Drug Interactions	• Clinically significant interactions are listed below • For more interaction information on any given combination, also see the corresponding chapter for the second agent

Class of Drug	Example	Interaction Effects
Acamprosate		Increased concentrations of acamprosate; C_{max} increased by 33% and AUC by 25%; no clinically significant adverse events reported with this combination
Insulin		Case report of increased insulin requirements when given naltrexone (unknown mechanism or clinical significance)
Opioid	Codeine, methadone, morphine, etc.	Decreased efficacy of opioid, may result in opioid withdrawal

◊ See p. 473 for further information on drug use in pregnancy and effects on breast milk

Buprenorphine

 Product Availability*

Generic Name	Trade Name[(A)]	Dosage Forms and Strengths
Buprenorphine	Buprenex[(B), (D)]	Injection: 0.3 mg/mL
	Butrans[(D)]	Transdermal patch: 5, 10, 15, 20 micrograms/h
	Sublocade	Long-acting injection (pre-filled syringe): 100 mg/0.5 mL, 300 mg/1.5 mL
	Subutex[(B)]	Sublingual tablets: 2 mg, 8 mg
	Probuphine	Subdermal implant: 80 mg
Buprenorphine HCl/Naloxone HCl	Bunavail[(B)]	Buccal film: 2.1 mg/0.3 mg, 4.2 mg/0.7 mg, 6.3 mg/1 mg
	Suboxone	Sublingual tablets: 2 mg/0.5 mg, 8 mg/2 mg, 12 mg/3 mg[(C)], 16 mg/4 mg[(C)]
	Suboxone SL Film	Sublingual film: 2 mg/0.5 mg, 4 mg/1 mg, 8 mg/2 mg, 12 mg/3 mg
	Zubsolv[(B)]	Sublingual tablets: 0.7 mg/0.18 mg, 1.4 mg/0.36 mg, 2.9 mg/0.71 mg, 5.7 mg/1.4 mg, 8.6 mg/2.1 mg, 11.4 mg/2.9 mg

* Refer to Health Canada's Drug Product Database or the FDA's Drugs@FDA for the most current availability information. [(A)] Generic preparations may be available, [(B)] Not marketed in Canada, [(C)] Not marketed in the USA, [(D)] Indicated for pain only

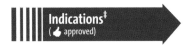 **Indications‡**
(👍 approved)

- 👍 Opioid use disorder; used alone or together with naloxone – sublingual tablets, extended-release once-monthly injection, and buprenorphine hydrochloride subdermal implant in patients clinically stabilized on no more than 8 mg of sublingual buprenorphine in combination with counseling and psychosocial support
- Analgesic for moderate to severe pain – transdermal patch or injection

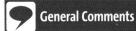 **General Comments**

- Suboxone contains buprenorphine and naloxone in a 4:1 ratio – intended to deter intravenous abuse by attenuating the effect of buprenorphine and producing withdrawal symptoms if taken IV by those physically dependent on opioids
- Sublocade is indicated for treatment of moderate–severe opioid use disorder in patients who have initiated treatment with a transmucosal buprenorphine-containing product, followed by dose adjustment for a minimum of 7 days
- Probuphine is indicated in the management of opioid dependence in patients clinically stabilized on no more than 8 mg of sublingual buprenorphine in combination with counseling and psychosocial support. Must be inserted and removed only by healthcare professionals who have successfully completed a live training program, the PROBUPHINE Education Program
- Reduces use and craving for opioids; should be combined with concurrent behavior therapies and psychosocial programs
- Considered as effective as moderate doses of methadone; methadone is considered the treatment of choice in patients with higher levels of physical dependence
- May be preferred for less dependent users, less chaotic lifestyles or codeine dependency
- Improvement noted in psychosocial adjustment and social functioning
- Causes minimal withdrawal symptoms due to partial agonist activity
- Other formulations of buprenorphine (i.e., injection, patch) are not approved for the treatment of opioid addiction
- Transdermal patch and buccal film have a warning regarding QTc prolongation in higher doses which is not reported with sublingual tablets[4]

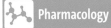 **Pharmacology**

- Buprenorphine is a partial μ-opioid receptor agonist and κ-opioid receptor antagonist (naloxone is an opioid antagonist)
- Opioid agonist effects increase linearly with increasing doses of buprenorphine, to a plateau or "ceiling effect"; less risk of respiratory depression and fatal overdose

‡ Indications listed here do not necessarily apply to all countries. Please refer to a country's regulatory database (e.g., US Food and Drug Administration, Health Canada Drug Product Database) for the most current availability information and indications

Buprenorphine (cont.)

- When buprenorphine is taken by those physically dependent on opioids, its partial opioid activity will precipitate opioid withdrawal symptoms. However, if taken while in opioid withdrawal, buprenorphine's partial agonist effects will be experienced as relief from withdrawal symptoms
- If switching to buprenorphine from methadone maintenance, it is recommended that the methadone dose be tapered down to 30 mg or less prior to starting buprenorphine, to minimize precipitated withdrawal symptoms[3] Alternatively, more novel approaches such as the Bernese model can be utilized. Small, repetitive doses of buprenorphine with sufficient dosing intervals (i.e., 12–24 h) would be administered while patient is maintained on methadone or other μ-opioid receptor agonists. Buprenorphine will begin to accumulate at the receptor due to its high receptor affinity and long binding time and, as a result, an increasing amount of μ-opioid receptor agonist will be gradually replaced by buprenorphine at which time μ-opioid receptor agonist can be discontinued

 Dosing

- 4–24 mg (buprenorphine) sublingually given once daily; due to long half-life, some patients can be dosed every 2 days or 3 times per week
- Phases of treatment:
  - Induction Phase: Individual needs to abstain from opioids for 12–24 h, depending on the duration of action of the opioid used, to be exhibiting at least mild to moderate withdrawal symptoms prior to first dose to prevent precipitated withdrawal: 2–4 mg buprenorphine administered sublingually initially, with another dose later in the day if needed on day 1, and then dose titrated from there based on effect
  - Stabilization Phase: Buprenorphine dose adjusted in increments/decrements of 2–4 mg to a level that suppresses both cravings and withdrawal effects (4–24 mg/day)
  - Maintenance Phase: Patient is on a stable dose of buprenorphine; the patient may require indefinite maintenance therapy
  - Renal impairment: No dosing adjustments required
  - Hepatic impairment: No dosing adjustments required for mild–moderate impairment. For severe impairment, use with caution – reduce initial dose and titration increments. Watch for adverse effects and toxicity
- Buprenorphine extended-release subcutaneous injection (Sublocade): Recommended dosing is 2 monthly initial doses of 300 mg followed by 100 mg monthly maintenance doses. Increasing the maintenance dose to 300 mg may be considered for patients in which the benefits outweigh the risk
- Buprenorphine subdermal implants (Probuphine): Each dose consists of 4 Probuphine implants inserted subdermally in the inner side of the upper arm. Probuphine subdermal implants are intended to be in place for 6 months of treatment. Remove Probuphine implants at the end of the 6-month period. Each Probuphine is a sterile, single, off-white, soft, flexible, rod-shaped ethylene vinyl acetate (EVA) implant, 26 mm in length and 2.5 mm in diameter, containing 74.2 mg of buprenorphine (equivalent to 80 mg of buprenorphine hydrochloride)
- Buprenorphine-naloxone micro-induction (commonly referred to as the "Bernese method"):
  - Rapid micro-induction (micro-dosing) that involves the administration of small, frequent doses of buprenorphine/naloxone; removes the need for a period of withdrawal prior to the start of treatment[5]
    - Prescribers may find the Bernese method more convenient than the classic induction method, since treatment can be initiated immediately without waiting for the patient to be in withdrawal first. There may be a role for micro-dosing in the treatment of opioid use disorder, especially in individuals who previously had difficulty starting or continuing buprenorphine. Further randomized, systematic studies are required to determine whether the Bernese method is associated with better tolerability and treatment outcomes compared with conventional induction methods, as well as to establish an optimal dose titration schedule
    - Micro-dosing buprenorphine/naloxone is one way to start opioid agonist treatment when an individual cannot stop their opioid use
    - An example of an outpatient micro-dosing induction schedule for buprenorphine-naloxone[6]:
      · Day 1: 0.5 mg loading dose
      · Day 2: 0.5 mg bid
      · Day 3: 1 mg bid
      · Day 4: 2 mg bid
      · Day 5: 3 mg bid
      · Day 6: 4 mg bid
      · Day 7: 12 mg (discontinue other opioids)

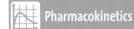

Pharmacokinetics	• Sublingual buprenorphine provides moderate bioavailability while sublingual naloxone bioavailability is poor; therefore, buprenorphine's opioid agonist effects predominate
	• Peak effects seen in 3–4 h after dosing; C_{max} and AUC increase in a linear fashion with dose increases
	• Buprenorphine is highly bound to plasma proteins (96%) – primarily to α and β globulin
	• Buprenorphine half-life is 24–60 h (37 h mean); naloxone half-life is 1–2 h (mean)
	• Metabolized by CYP3A4 to active metabolite, norbuprenorphine, and other inactive glucuronidated metabolites
	• Buprenorphine is essentially eliminated in feces by biliary excretion of the glucuroconjugated metabolites (approximately 70%), the rest being eliminated in urine
	• Buprenorphine extended-release subcutaneous injection (Sublocade):
	  – After injection, an initial buprenorphine peak was observed and median T_{max} occurred 24 h after injection. After the initial buprenorphine peak, plasma buprenorphine concentrations decreased slowly to a plateau. Steady-state was achieved at 4–6 months
	  – Apparent terminal plasma half-life of buprenorphine extended-release subcutaneous injection ranged between 43 and 60 days as a result of the slow release of buprenorphine from the subcutaneous depot
	• Buprenorphine subdermal implants (Probuphine): After insertion, an initial buprenorphine peak was observed and median T_{max} occurred at 12 h after insertion. After the initial buprenorphine peak, the plasma buprenorphine concentrations decreased slowly and steady-state plasma buprenorphine concentrations were reached by approximately week 4

Adverse Effects	• Most common in first 2–3 days of therapy and are dose related • After the first dose, patient may experience some withdrawal symptoms, see pharmacology section p. 410 • Common: Headache, dizziness, insomnia, somnolence, nausea, vomiting, constipation, sweating, CNS depression, orthostatic hypotension, and various pains • Increase in liver enzymes; cases of hepatitis, acute hepatic injury reported in the context of misuse, particularly IV use; monitor liver function tests periodically • Lower risk of respiratory depression and overdose than methadone due to the ceiling effect • Injection and implant site pain are the two most common adverse effects reported in clinical trials of Sublocade and Probuphine
D/C Discontinuation Syndrome	• Withdrawal syndrome reported in patients on chronic therapy and with naloxone combination • Causes milder withdrawal than full opioid antagonists (e.g., methadone), onset may be delayed • Symptoms include: Nausea/vomiting, diarrhea, muscle aches/cramps, sweating, lacrimation, rhinorrhea, dilated pupils, yawning, craving, mild fever, dysphoric mood, insomnia, and irritability
Precautions	• Buprenorphine can precipitate withdrawal in opioid-dependent individuals (see pharmacology section p. 410) • Chronic administration produces opioid-type dependence, characterized by withdrawal upon abrupt discontinuation or rapid taper • Buprenorphine can be abused; if sublingual combination tablets are crushed and injected by opioid-dependent individual, naloxone may exert effects and precipitate a withdrawal syndrome • Use with caution in patients with compromised respiratory function or liver disorder, opioid naïve, severe hepatic impairment, or acute alcoholism and delirium tremens • Buprenorphine detoxification can occur faster than methadone detoxification; decrease dose by 2–4 mg every 2 weeks

Toxicity	• Very high doses can cause respiratory depression, which may be delayed in onset and more prolonged than with other opioids; reversal with naloxone is more difficult due to buprenorphine's very tight binding to opioid receptors[3]
	• Safer in overdose than pure agonists due to poor bioavailability and ceiling effect of agonist action
	• Symptoms include: Pinpoint pupils, sedation, and hypotension; respiratory depression and deaths have been reported, particularly when buprenorphine was misused intravenously or in combination with alcohol or other opioids
	• Treatment: Symptomatic
	  – Monitor for respiratory depression
	  – Naloxone may not be effective in reversing respiratory depression

Buprenorphine (cont.)

 Pediatric Considerations
- Not recommended in children under age 16
- Canadian labeling does not approve use in patients under age 18

 Geriatric Considerations
- Elderly patients are more likely to experience confusion and drowsiness
- Respiratory depression occurs more frequently
- Long-term use not recommended

 Use in Pregnancy◇
- Expression of CYP3A4 and CYP2D6 increases in the liver, intestine, and central nervous system in pregnant women. Buprenorphine is metabolized by CYP3A4, therefore increased expression of CYP3A4 will result in lower plasma concentrations. Thus, multiple-day dosing may be needed in pregnant women even if buprenorphine is prescribed at a low dose. As pregnancy progresses, a higher dose of buprenorphine may also be required
- Teratogenic effects reported in animal studies; effects in humans unknown
- Evidence comparing buprenorphine with methadone indicates that buprenorphine is an acceptable treatment for opioid use disorder in pregnant women
- Neonatal abstinence syndrome may occur with onset generally within a day or two after birth and lasting a mean of 4 days
- Buprenorphine/naloxone combination not recommended during pregnancy

Breast Milk
- Buprenorphine passes into mother's milk; breastfeeding is not recommended

 Nursing Implications
- Buprenorphine is an opioid and considered to be a controlled substance
- Buprenorphine should be used in conjunction with behavior/psychosocial therapies
- The tablets should not be handled, but tipped directly into the mouth from a medicine cup; they should be placed (all together) under the tongue until dissolved (takes 2–10 min); drinking fluids prior to taking the tablets may speed up the dissolution process[3]; chewing or swallowing them reduces the bioavailability of the drug; the patient should not drink for at least 5 min so as to allow the drug to be absorbed
- Buprenorphine subdermal implants (Probuphine) are inserted subdermally in the inner side of the upper arm. The implants are intended to be in place for 6 months of treatment, then removed
- Educate patient about not increasing his/her dose without physician approval; misuse/abuse may result in toxicity
- Serious CNS consequences may occur if buprenorphine is combined with benzodiazepines, hypnotics or alcohol

 Patient Instructions
- For detailed patient instructions on buprenorphine, see the Patient Information Sheet (details p. 474)

 Drug Interactions
- Potentially clinically significant interactions are listed below

Class of Drug	Example	Interaction Effects
Antibiotic	Clarithromycin, erythromycin	Increased levels of buprenorphine possible due to inhibited metabolism via CYP3A4
Antidepressant		
SSRI	Citalopram	May enhance QTc prolongation
Tricyclic	Amitriptyline	May cause additive psychomotor performance impairment and enhanced respiratory depressant effects
Reversible MAOI	Moclobemide	May enhance adverse or toxic effects of MAOIs

◇ See p. 473 for further information on drug use in pregnancy and effects on breast milk

Class of Drug	Example	Interaction Effects
Anticonvulsant	Carbamazepine, phenytoin, phenobarbital	Decreased levels of buprenorphine possible due to increased metabolism via CYP3A4
Antifungal	Ketoconazole	Increased C_{max} and AUC of buprenorphine reported due to inhibited metabolism via CYP3A4
Antiretroviral Non-nucleoside reverse transcriptase inhibitor (NNRTI)	Efavirenz	Decreased level of buprenorphine (50% AUC) via CYP3A4 induction, possible clinical significance
Protease inhibitor	Atazanavir	Increased level of buprenorphine and decreased level of atazanavir
	Indinavir, ritonavir, saquinavir	Increased level of buprenorphine possible due to inhibited metabolism via CYP3A4
Antipsychotic	Quetiapine	May enhance QTc prolongation
Antitubercular	Rifampin	Decreased level of buprenorphine (70% AUC, 38% C_{max}) via CYP3A4 induction, monitor for opiate withdrawal
Anxiolytic	Benzodiazepine	Respiratory depression, coma, and death reported when intravenous or high doses of buprenorphine used in combination
CNS depressant	Alcohol, antipsychotics, gabapentinoids	CNS depression; deaths have been reported in combination
Opioid	Morphine, meperidine, fentanyl	Low doses of buprenorphine antagonize analgesic effects High doses are synergistic; increase risk of CNS and respiratory depression
	Methadone	Can precipitate withdrawal

Methadone

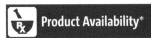 **Product Availability***

Generic Name	Trade Name(A)	Dosage Forms and Strengths
Methadone		Bulk powder Oral solution: 5 mg/5 mL, 10 mg/5 mL Injection(B): 10 mg/mL
	Dolophine(B),(D)	Tablets: 5 mg, 10 mg
	Metadol-D(C),(D)	Oral solution: 1 mg/mL, 10 mg/mL Tablets: 1 mg, 5 mg, 10 mg, 25 mg
	Methadose	Oral solution: 10 mg/mL Tablets(B): 5 mg, 10 mg, 40 mg (dispersible)

* Refer to Health Canada's Drug Product Database or the FDA's Drugs@FDA for the most current availability information. (A) Generic preparations may be available, (B) Not marketed in Canada, (C) Not marketed in the USA, (D) Indicated for pain only

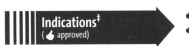 **Indications‡**
(👍 approved)

- 💧 Detoxification and maintenance treatment in opioid use disorder
- 💧 Treatment of severe pain

‡ Indications listed here do not necessarily apply to all countries. Please refer to a country's regulatory database (e.g., US Food and Drug Administration, Health Canada Drug Product Database) for the most current availability information and indications

Methadone (cont.)

 General Comments

- Methadone is recommended for opioid agonist treatment if induction with buprenorphine/naloxone is challenging or not preferred
- Useful drug in opioid-dependent patients who desire maintenance opioid therapy:
  - Effective orally and can be administered once daily, due to its long half-life
  - Suppresses withdrawal symptoms of other opioids
  - Suppresses chronic craving for opioids without developing tolerance
  - When taken orally at appropriate doses, reduced euphoria due to slow onset
- Patients receiving methadone remain in treatment longer, demonstrate a decreased use of illicit opioids, and maintain social stability
- Methadone is an opioid and its prescribing, dispensing, and usage is governed by Federal regulations (regulations vary in different countries). When used for opioid dependence, most patients receive their methadone from the pharmacy on a daily basis and are required to drink the contents of the bottle in the presence of the pharmacist. Stable patients may be permitted to carry premeasured individual doses of methadone once the first dose of each new prescription has been witnessed

 Pharmacology

- A synthetic opioid acting on the μ-opioid receptor
- Analgesic and sedative properties – similar to other opioids, but with a longer duration of action
- Relieves opioid withdrawal symptoms while blocking euphoric effects including those of other administered opioids

 Dosing

- Initial dose: 20–30 mg (lower if risk factors for toxicity), given once daily; may give additional 5–10 mg if withdrawal symptoms are not suppressed or reappear. Do not exceed a total of 40 mg on the first day
- During initiation, individuals should be seen at least weekly to carefully monitor treatment response
- Levels accumulate over the first few days, therefore do not increase doses too quickly. Increase by 5–10 mg every 3–5 days to a stable maintenance dose
- Slower dose escalation is recommended for individuals who may be at higher risk of opioid toxicity, including individuals with recent loss of tolerance
- Doses between 60 mg and 100 mg are often more effective than lower doses
- When doses are greater than 80 mg, increase by 5–10 mg every 5–7 days
- Dosing adjustments are made based on cravings and withdrawal symptoms. Titrate to a dose where opiate withdrawal symptoms do not occur for 24 h
- Usual maintenance range: 60–120 mg daily
- Oral methadone doses are approximately twice the intravenous dose (due to decreased bioavailability)
- Patients vary in dosage requirements; dosage is adjusted to control abstinence symptoms without causing marked sedation or respiratory depression
- In rare cases, patients who are rapid metabolizers of methadone may require a divided (split) dose rather than one single daily dose; this situation should be carefully evaluated and monitored for toxicity and respiratory depression
- When tapering off methadone, decrease the dose by less than 10% every 10–14 days

 Pharmacokinetics

- Bioavailability: 36–100%
- Peak plasma level: 2–3 h
- 85–90% protein bound
- Half-life: 8–59 h (average: 25 h); half-life increases with repeated dosing. Note: $T_{1/2}$ is longer than methadone's duration of action (4–8 h)
- Half-life of analgesic effect is 4–8 h with a single dose but may be prolonged with repeated doses
- Metabolized by the liver, primarily via CYP3A4 and 2B6, with minor elimination via CYP2C19, CYP2D6, other enzymes may contribute to methadone metabolism – see Drug Interactions pp. 416–418
- Inhibits P-gp
- Urine testing must be done to detect illicit drug use and/or compliance with methadone

Onset & Duration of Action

- Onset of effect: 30–60 minutes
- Duration of action increases with chronic use

Adverse Effects

CNS Effects

- Drowsiness, insomnia, euphoria, dysphoria, confusion, cognitive impairment, depression, seizures, and weakness; tolerance develops to sedating and analgesic effects
- With chronic use: Sleep disturbances, impairment in psychomotor and cognitive performance tests
- Headache

Anticholinergic Effects

- Sweating, flushing
- Chronic constipation

Cardiovascular Effects

- Dizziness, lightheadedness, hypotension
- Cases of QT prolongation and torsades de pointes – increased risk with higher doses (more than 150 mg/day), drug accumulation, in patients with pre-existing heart disease, in combination with drugs that increase the QT interval or with drugs that decrease the metabolism of methadone via CYP3A4 (see Drug Interactions pp. 416–418) [baseline ECG recommended; repeat periodically and if dose increased above 150 mg/day]

Endocrine & Metabolic Effects

- Amenorrhea, decreased libido
- Hypokalemia, hypomagnesemia, and weight gain

GI Effects

- Nausea, vomiting, and decreased appetite
- Constipation

Urogenital & Sexual Effects

- Impotence, ejaculatory problems

Musculoskeletal Effects

- Pain in joints and bones

Other Adverse Effects

- Rarely, pulmonary edema and respiratory depression

Discontinuation Syndrome

- Rapid withdrawal can result in opioid withdrawal syndrome, which includes CNS effects: Restlessness, agitation, insomnia, headache; autonomic effects: Increased blood pressure, heart rate, body temperature and respiration, lacrimation, perspiration, congestion, itching, "gooseflesh"; neurological effects: Muscle twitching, cramps, tremors; GI effects: Nausea, vomiting, diarrhea, anorexia
- Symptoms may begin 24–48 h after the last dose, peak in 72 h, and may last for 6–7 weeks
- If no dosing changes occurred, consider drug interaction as a potential cause of withdrawal symptoms

Management

- Reinstitute dose to previous level (if stopped for more than 3 days, titrate back up slowly); restabilize patient and monitor while tapering dose at a slower rate
- Clonidine may ameliorate withdrawal symptoms

Precautions

- Methadone has a high physical and psychological dependence liability, therefore withdrawal symptoms will occur on abrupt discontinuation – decrease the dose slowly
- Prior to prescribing methadone, a baseline ECG should be done; repeat within 30 days of treatment and annually, or if patient has unexplained syncope or seizures. Consider discontinuing or reducing the dose if QTc interval is greater than 500 ms. Avoid methadone in patients with a history of structural heart disease, arrhythmia or syncope
- Due to its long half-life, methadone can accumulate to dangerous levels if dose is increased too quickly, without allowing maximal effects to be assessed at steady state. Peak respiratory depressant effects occur later and persist longer than peak analgesic effects
- Methadone detoxification may be a lengthy process of approximately 12 weeks; decrease dose by less than 10% every 10–14 days depending on patient response; can use clonidine to decrease withdrawal symptoms

Methadone (cont.)

Toxicity	• With excessive doses, can develop shallow breathing, pinpoint pupils, flaccidity of skeletal muscles, low blood pressure, slowed heart rate, cold and clammy skin; can progress to cyanosis, coma, severe respiratory depression, circulatory collapse, and cardiac arrest
Pediatric Considerations	• For detailed information on the use of methadone in this population, please see the *Clinical Handbook of Psychotropic Drugs for Children and Adolescents*[2] • Has been used for postoperative pain in children at doses of 0.2 mg/kg; longer duration of action than with morphine. Drug must be tapered (by 5–10% every 1–2 days) if used for longer than 5–7 days; the patient must be continually assessed for withdrawal symptoms
Geriatric Considerations	• Methadone has a high potential for drug interactions and is associated with QT interval prolongation. In addition, methadone is difficult to titrate because of its large inter-individual variability in pharmacokinetics, particularly in the frail elderly, with a risk for accumulation due to a long elimination half-life
Use in Pregnancy◊	• Methadone treatment throughout pregnancy reduces risk of perinatal and infant mortality in heroin-dependent women and is not associated with adverse postnatal development • Dosing needs should be assessed during pregnancy: Decreased between weeks 14 and 32, increased prior to term, reduced following birth, and reassessed regularly • Short-term withdrawal effects reported in approximately 60% of infants (not dose related); no long-term effects demonstrated
Breast Milk	• A small amount of methadone enters breast milk; nurse prior to a dose of methadone or 2–6 h after dose
Nursing Implications	• Methadone must be prescribed in sufficient doses, on a maintenance basis, to prevent relapse; long-term treatment may be required. Premature withdrawal may lead to relapse • Methadone is an opioid and must be prescribed according to Federal regulations. Many patients pick up their methadone from the pharmacy on a daily basis and drink the medication in the presence of the pharmacist. Stable patients may be permitted to carry premeasured individual doses of methadone once the first dose of each new prescription has been witnessed • Each time the patient is to be medicated, he/she should be assessed for impairment (i.e., drowsiness, slurred speech, forgetfulness, lack of concentration, disorientation, and ataxia); patients should not be medicated if they appear impaired or smell of alcohol – the physician should be contacted as to management of the patient • Encourage patients to carry a card in their wallet stating that they are taking methadone • If a patient misses one or more appointments to receive his/her dose of methadone, this may indicate clinical instability and possible relapse; use caution due to possible loss of tolerance to drug • Contact the prescriber if more than 2 methadone doses have been missed or the patient has ingested other substances
Patient Instructions	• For detailed patient instructions on methadone, see the Patient Information Sheet (details on p. 474)
Drug Interactions	• Clinically significant interactions are listed below • For more interaction information on any given combination, also see the corresponding chapter for the second agent

◊ See p. 473 for further information on drug use in pregnancy and effects on breast milk

Class of Drug	Example	Interaction Effects
Alcohol		Acute alcohol use can decrease methadone metabolism and increase the plasma level – may result in intoxication and respiratory depression Chronic alcohol use can induce methadone metabolism and decrease the plasma level May enhance CNS depressant effect
Antacid	Al/Mg antacids	Decreased absorption of methadone
Antiarrhythmic	Quinidine	Possible risk of QT prolongation
Antibiotic	Ciprofloxacin	Case report of increased methadone adverse reactions (sedation, confusion, and respiratory depression) due to inhibition of CYP1A2 and CYP3A4
Anticonvulsant	Barbiturates, carbamazepine, phenytoin	Decreased plasma level of methadone due to enhanced metabolism via CYP3A4 and CYP2B6 (phenytoin and barbiturates), via CYP3A4 (carbamazepine). Phenytoin levels may increase by 50%
Antidepressant		
Cyclic	Amitriptyline, desipramine	Increased plasma level of desipramine (by about 108%) due to decreased metabolism via CYP2D6 inhibition Increased giddiness, euphoria; suspected potentiation of methadone's "euphoric" effects – abuse with amitriptyline reported
SSRI	Fluvoxamine	Increased plasma level of methadone by (10–100%) with fluvoxamine, due to (1) increased clearance, (2) reduced metabolism via CYP3A4 inhibition, and (3) competitive inhibition via CYP2D6
Antifungal	Fluconazole	Increase in methadone peak and trough plasma levels by 27% and 48%, respectively; clearance decreased by 24% via inhibition of CYP3A4, may enhance QTc prolongation
	Itraconazole	Case report of prolonged rate-corrected QT interval leading to torsades de pointes following two doses of itraconazole (200 mg). May increase serum concentration of methadone
	Ketoconazole	May increase serum concentration of methadone
	Voriconazole	Increase in methadone plasma levels (47% increased AUC); case reports of torsades de pointes
Antipsychotic	Risperidone	Case reports of precipitation of opioid withdrawal symptoms (mechanism unclear)
Antiretroviral		
Non-nucleoside reverse transcriptase inhibitor (NNRTI)	Delavirdine	Likely to increase methadone levels via inhibition by CYP3A4
	Efavirenz, nevirapine	Increased clearance of methadone and decreased total concentration (AUC) (by up to 60% with efavirenz and nevirapine) via enzyme induction – withdrawal symptoms reported within 7–10 days
Nucleoside reverse transcriptase inhibitor (NRTI)	Abacavir	Abacavir levels decreased by 34%, however, clearance remained the same Methadone plasma level decreased by 23% – may result in withdrawal
	Didanosine, stavudine	Decreased bioavailability of antiretrovirals due to increased degradation in GI tract by methadone (C_{max} and AUC decreased by 66% and 63%, respectively, for didanosine, and by 44% and 25% for stavudine)
	Zidovudine	Inhibited metabolism of AZT by methadone (AUC increased by 43%)
Protease inhibitor	Amprenavir	AUC, C_{max}, and C_{min} of amprenavir decreased by 30%, 27%, and 25%, respectively Methadone levels decreased an average of 35% with amprenavir/abacavir combination
	Indinavir	Variable effects reported on C_{max} of indinavir Reduced AUC of methadone (by 40%)
	Lopinavir/ritonavir	Methadone AUC decreased by 36% due to increased clearance (attributed to lopinavir) – may result in withdrawal
	Nelfinavir	AUC of nelfanavir metabolite decreased by 53% – significance unknown
	Ritonavir	Variable effects on clearance of methadone reported
	Ritonavir/saquinavir	Displacement from protein binding of methadone and decrease in AUC of both R-methadone and S-methadone

Methadone (cont.)

Class of Drug	Example	Interaction Effects
Antitubercular	Isoniazid	Increased plasma level of methadone due to decreased metabolism via CYP3A4
	Rifampin	Decreased plasma level of methadone (by up to 50%) due to enhanced metabolism via CYP2D6 and CYP3A4 – may cause withdrawal symptoms
Benzodiazepine	Clonazepam, diazepam	Enhanced risk of respiratory depression Combined use suggested to negatively influence treatment outcomes but by lowering anxiety there may be opportunity to lower methadone dose
	Diazepam	"Opiate high" reported with combined use
Buprenorphine		Decreased metabolism of methadone through inhibition of CYP3A4
Disulfiram		Decreased clearance of methadone
Grapefruit juice		Decreased metabolism of methadone through inhibition of CYP3A4 and P-gp
H₂ antagonist	Cimetidine	Decreased clearance of methadone; case reports of apnea with the combination
Hypnotic	Zolpidem	Decreased metabolism of methadone through inhibition of CYP3A4
Opioid	Butorphanol, nalbuphine, pentazocine	Occurrence of withdrawal symptoms due to partial antagonist effects of these opioids
	Morphine	Efficacy of opioid analgesic reduced; dosage may need to be increased
Opioid antagonist	Naltrexone	Diminished analgesic effect and may precipitate withdrawal
QTc prolonging agents		For high-risk combinations, may need to discontinue methadone and initiate buprenorphine treatment
St. John's wort		Decreased plasma level of methadone; symptoms of withdrawal reported buprenorphine treatment
Stimulant	MDMA	Decreased metabolism of methadone through inhibition of CYP2D6
Urine acidifier	Ascorbic acid	Increased elimination of methadone
Urine alkalizer	Sodium bicarbonate	Decreased elimination of methadone

Pharmacotherapy for Nicotine/Tobacco Use Disorder

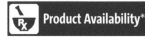 **Product Availability***

Generic Name	Pharmacological Class	Trade Name(A)	Dosage Forms and Strengths
Bupropion	Antidepressant	Zyban	Tablets: 150 mg
Nicotine	Nicotine replacement	Commit, Thrive	Lozenges: 2 mg, 4 mg
		Nicoderm, Habitrol(B)	Transdermal patch: 7 mg/24 h, 14 mg/24 h, 21 mg/24 h
		Nicorette, Nicorette DS(B), Thrive gum	Gum: 2 mg, 4 mg
		Nicorette QuickMist	Sublingual spray: 1 mg/spray
		Nicorette, Nicotrol(B)	Cartridges: 10 mg (delivers 4 mg nicotine)
		Nicotrol NS	Inhalation system: 0.5 mg/spray
		Electronic cigarettes	
Varenicline	Nicotinic receptor partial agonist	Champix(C), Chantix(B)	Tablets: 0.5 mg, 1 mg

* Refer to Health Canada's Drug Product Database or the FDA's Drugs@FDA for the most current availability information.   (A) Generic preparations may be available,   (B) Not marketed in Canada,   (C) Not marketed in the USA

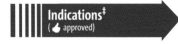 **Indications‡**
(👍 approved)

🚬 Aid in smoking cessation

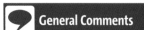 **General Comments**

- Choice of treatment should be guided by the individual's preference, contraindications and precautions for use, potential adverse drug reactions, drug interactions, convenience, individual's previous experience, availability, and cost
- Regardless of smoking cessation option selected, 12-month abstinence rates are usually 25% or less
- Improved outcomes are seen with combining behavioral counseling and pharmacotherapy
- Several combinations of first-line drugs have been shown to be effective in maintaining abstinence (see Precautions p. 422), including[7, 8]:
  - Long-term (more than 14 weeks) nicotine patch + nicotine gum, lozenge or spray
  - Nicotine patch (6–14 weeks) + nicotine inhaler (up to 6 months)
  - Nicotine patch (6–14 weeks) + bupropion SR (up to 14 weeks)
- Combining nicotine patch with acute dosing forms shown to be more beneficial when compared to the use of a single form of nicotine product
- Long-term use (up to 6 months) of medications may be helpful for smokers who experience persistent withdrawal symptoms or who have relapsed in the past after stopping treatment
- There is evidence that electronic cigarettes help smokers to stop smoking long-term compared with placebo electronic cigarettes

‡ Indications listed here do not necessarily apply to all countries. Please refer to a country's regulatory database (e.g., US Food and Drug Administration, Health Canada Drug Product Database) for the most current availability information and indications

Pharmacotherapy for Nicotine/Tobacco Use Disorder (cont.)

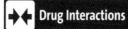 **Drug Interactions**

DRUG INTERACTIONS WITH NRT

Class of Drug	Example	Interaction Effects
Analgesic	Acetaminophen, pentazocine	Increased levels of analgesic due to inhibition of metabolism, on smoking cessation
	Propoxyphene	First-pass metabolism decreased; may require a lower dose
Adrenergic agonist	Isoproterenol, phenylephrine	May require an increase in dose due to a decrease in circulating catecholamine, on smoking cessation
Adrenergic blocker	Labetalol, prazosin	May require a decrease in dose due to a decrease in circulating catecholamines, on smoking cessation
Antidepressant	Imipramine	Increased level of antidepressant due to inhibition of metabolism, on smoking cessation
Antipsychotic	Clozapine, olanzapine	Smoking induces the CYP1A2 enzyme, resulting in lower clozapine and olanzapine levels. Smoking cessation or reduction may therefore result in higher levels of these drugs. Monitor for side effects related to higher levels of clozapine and olanzapine
β-blocker	Propranolol	Increased level of β-blocker due to inhibition of metabolism, on smoking cessation
Caffeine		Increased caffeine levels due to inhibition of metabolism, on smoking cessation
Insulin		May require a decrease in insulin dosage on smoking cessation
Nicotinic receptor partial agonist	Varenicline	Combination can increase adverse effects including nausea, headache, vomiting, dizziness, dyspepsia, and fatigue
Theophylline		Increased level of theophylline due to inhibition of metabolism, on smoking cessation

For DRUG INTERACTIONS WITH BUPROPION, see pp. 19–25

DRUG INTERACTIONS WITH VARENICLINE

Class of Drug	Example	Interaction Effects
Alcohol		Alcohol intake may increase the risk of patients experiencing psychiatric adverse effects
H₂ antagonist	Cimetidine, ranitidine	Increased serum concentration of varenicline by 29% due to decreased renal clearance
NRT	Transdermal nicotine	Combination can increase adverse effects including nausea, headache, vomiting, dizziness, dyspepsia, and fatigue

Comparison of Treatments for Nicotine/Tobacco Use Disorder

	Bupropion SR	Nicotine Replacement Therapy (NRT)	Varenicline
General Comments	Relieves craving and withdrawal symptoms Effective in patients with a history of depression May be used in combination with NRT May minimize weight gain following smoking cessation Can be used in patients with cardiovascular disease	Does not deliver nicotine to the circulation as fast as smoking Variable plasma levels occur if gum or lozenge chewed/sucked too quickly or too slowly *Nicotine inhaler:* mimics hand-to-mouth smoking action (coping mechanism) *Nasal spray:* Fastest nicotine delivery system Does not counter the habit/satisfaction of smoking Adherence rate highest with nicotine patch, moderate with nicotine gum, lozenge and inhaler, and low with nicotine nasal spray	Relieves craving and withdrawal symptoms Significant decrease in smoking satisfaction and psychological reward from smoking reported Meta-analysis suggests varenicline may increase the odds of quitting over NRT and bupropion
Pharmacology	Blocks reuptake of dopamine and noradrenaline Noncompetitive inhibitor of brain nicotine receptors	Replaces nicotine through various delivery systems Delivers nicotine that binds to the nicotinic acetylcholine receptor	Partial agonist activity at the $\alpha_4\beta_2$ nicotinic acetylcholine receptor (i.e., agonist activity to a lesser degree than nicotine), while simultaneously preventing nicotine binding (i.e., antagonist activity)
Pharmacokinetics	See p. 20	*Gum and lozenge:* Rate of absorption depends on rate of chewing the gum or sucking the lozenge; time to peak plasma level = 25 min; blood nicotine levels stabilize with repeated use every 30 min Metabolized by liver, and partly by kidney and lung; plasma half-life = 120 min. Higher levels reported in renal insufficiency *Inhaler:* Peak plasma levels = after continuous inhalation for over 20 min; half-life of primary metabolite, cotinine: 15–20 h *Patch:* Eliminates variability of GI absorption; reduces nicotine first-pass metabolism; effects wear off in 20–24 h. Delivers nicotine slowly and passively over time *Spray:* Absorbed very quickly *E-cigarettes:* Can deliver levels of nicotine that are comparable to or higher than cigarettes; the average peak plasma level with E-cigarettes appears to be lower than that reported from tobacco cigarette use	Peak plasma levels occur in 3–4 h; bioavailability not affected by food Steady state reached after 4 days Protein binding = 20% Elimination half-life = 17–24 h 92% excreted unchanged in urine
Dosing	150 mg q a.m. x 3 days, then 150 mg bid (given at least 8 h apart) for 7–12 weeks; consider for long-term therapy (up to 6 months after quitting)	*Gum:* 2–4 mg q 1–2 h for 6 weeks (max. 30 pieces/day of the 2 mg gum (60 mg) or 20 pieces/day of the 4 mg gum (80 mg)); 2 mg if smoking < 25 cigarettes/day *Lozenge:* At least 9 lozenges/day for 6 weeks (max. 20/day); 2 mg if smoking first cigarette more than 30 min after waking *Inhaler:* 6–16 cartridges/day up to 6 months; each cartridge delivers 4 mg nicotine over 80 inhalations *Patch:* 28 mg/24 h for heavy smokers or 14 mg/24 h for light smokers for 6–8 weeks; step-down dosage: 21 mg/24 h x 4 weeks, then 14 mg/24 h x 2 weeks, then 7 mg/24 h x 2 weeks. Studies have been done using up to 42 mg nicotine patch *Spray:* 1 spray in each nostril 1–2 times/h. Max.: 5 times/h or 40 times/day (total of 80 sprays/day), each spray delivers 1 mg of nicotine; use initial dose for 8 weeks, then taper over 4–6 weeks *QuickMist:* 1–2 sprays/h	0.5 mg daily x 3 days, then 0.5 mg bid x 4 days, then 1 mg bid (morning and supper) for 3 months Some studies have found 0.5 mg bid as effective as 1 mg bid If CrCl < 30 mL/min: 0.5 mg/day, max. dose 0.5 mg bid

Comparison of Treatments for Nicotine/Tobacco Use Disorder (cont.)

	Bupropion SR	Nicotine Replacement Therapy (NRT)	Varenicline
Dosing comments	Start 1–2 weeks prior to quit date. Target quit date should be after at least 1 week of treatment	With nicotine gum, lozenge or inhaler, do not eat or drink anything but water for 15 min before or after use; acidic beverages decrease absorption *Gum:* Bite gum, then chew until "tingle," then park in cheek for 30–60 sec; repeat for 30 min *Lozenge:* Suck lozenge and allow to dissolve slowly; do not chew or swallow lozenge; use tongue to move lozenge from one side of mouth to the other; it should take 20–30 min to dissolve *Spray:* Spray into nostrils. The nicotine is quickly absorbed into the nasal membranes	Start 1 week prior to quit date Take with food to reduce nausea Take second dose at supper to minimize insomnia Total course may be 3–6 months
Abstinence Rate After 6 Months	16.5%	13–17%	26%
Adverse Effects	See p. 20 Insomnia, agitation, headache, dry mouth (10%), disturbed concentration, dizziness, and nausea Changes in behavior, hostility, agitation, depressed mood and suicidal ideation and acts reported	*Gum or lozenge:* Jaw pain, throat irritation, taste perversion, stomatitis, gingivitis, hiccups (10%), dyspepsia, nausea, headache (11%), dizziness, and insomnia *Inhaler:* Mouth and throat irritation (small puffs less irritating than long puffs), sneezing, rhinitis, and pharyngitis *Patch:* Local skin irritation, insomnia, vivid dreams, and headache *Spray:* Nose and throat irritation, cough, sneezing, and watery eyes Over 100 trials confirm NRT is not associated with increased cancer risk	Nausea (30%), vomiting, headaches (15%), insomnia (18%), abnormal dreams (13%), somnolence, loss of consciousness, flatulence, constipation, dry mouth, dizziness, falls, abnormal spasms and movement; rare hypersensitivity reactions including angioedema, Stevens-Johnson syndrome, and erythema multiforme Changes in behavior, confusion, anxiety, hostility, agitation, restlessness, psychosis, depressed mood and suicidal ideation and acts reported Possible link to heart attacks, seizures, and diabetes
Discontinuation	Commonly discontinued after 7–12 weeks. Some patients require up to 12 months of treatment	Taper use of NRT gradually to minimize withdrawal symptoms Taper dose of nicotine inhaler during final 3 months of use	Commonly discontinued after 12 weeks
Precautions		Caution in patients with recent MI, serious arrhythmias, and unstable angina Caution in endocrine disorders (e.g., diabetes, hyperthyroidism) due to release of catecholamines Avoid nicotine spray in patients with severe reactive airway disease; potential for dependence Smoking whilst using NRT can lead to nicotine toxicity with: Headache, nausea, vomiting, abdominal pain, diarrhea, salivation, sweating, flushing, and palpitations Nicotine addiction may be transferred from cigarettes to gum	Caution in patients with underlying psychiatric disorder or those operating machinery Reduce dosage in patients with kidney impairment Black Box Warning: Serious neuropsychiatric events (including depression, suicidal thoughts, and suicide) have been reported

	Bupropion SR	Nicotine Replacement Therapy (NRT)	Varenicline
Contraindications	Anorexia, bulimia, seizures, heavy alcohol use, and use of MAOIs	Unstable cardiac conditions Skin diseases that may complicate patch application	Unstable cardiac conditions Should not be used by pilots, air traffic controllers, truckers, and bus drivers due to risk of impairment
Use in Adolescents	Reports of efficacy in adolescents	Little evidence that nicotine replacement is effective in adolescents	Sparse data
Use in Pregnancy◇	Not recommended	Guidelines suggest that nicotine replacement may be used during pregnancy and breastfeeding[9]. These agents are considered much safer than smoking in pregnancy (use suggested even over oral medications for smoking cessation) Nicotine patch should be removed overnight	Not recommended

◇ See p. 473 for further information on drug use in pregnancy and effects on breast milk

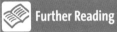 **Further Reading**

References

1 Kranzler HR, Soyka M. Diagnosis and pharmacotherapy of alcohol use disorder: A review. JAMA. 2018;320(8):815–824. doi:10.1001/jama.2018.11406

2 Elbe D, Black TR, McGrane IR, et al. Clinical handbook of psychotropic drugs for children and adolescents. (4th ed.). Boston, MA: Hogrefe Publishing, 2019.

3 Work Group on Substance Use Disorders, Kleber HD, Weiss RD, et al. Treatment of patients with substance use disorders, second edition. American Psychiatic Association. Am J Psychiatry. 2006;163(8 Suppl):5–82.

4 Coe MA, Lofwall MR, Walsh SL. Buprenorphine pharmacology review: Update on transmucosal and long-acting formulations. J Addict Med. 2019;13(2):93–103. doi:10.1097/ADM. 0000000000000457

5 Wong JSH, Nikoo M, Westenberg JN, et al. Comparing rapid micro-induction and standard induction of buprenorphine/naloxone for treatment of opioid use disorder: Protocol for an open-label, parallel-group, superiority, randomized controlled trial. Addict Sci Clin Pract. 2021;16(1):11. doi:10.1186/s13722-021-00220-2

6 Randhawa PA, Brar R, Nolan S. Buprenorphine-naloxone "microdosing": An alternative induction approach for the treatment of opioid use disorder in the wake of North America's increasingly potent illicit drug market. CMAJ. 2020;192(3):E73. doi:10.1503/cmaj.74018

7 Caldwell BO, Crane J. Combination nicotine metered dose inhaler and nicotine patch for smoking cessation: A randomized controlled trial. Nicotine Tob Res. 2016;18(10):1944–1951. doi:10.1093/ntr/ntw093

8 Hollands GJ, McDermott MS, Lindson-Hawley N, et al. Interventions to increase adherence to medications for tobacco dependence. Cochrane Database Syst Rev. 2015;2:CD009164. doi:10.1002/14651858.CD009164.pub2

9 National Institute for Health and Clinical Excellence (NICE). Tobacco: Preventing uptake, promoting quitting and treating dependence. London, UK: NICE, 2021. Retrieved from https://www.nice.org.uk/guidance/ng209

Additional Suggested Reading

• Bogen DL, Perel JM, Helsel JC, et al. Pharmacologic evidence to support clinical decision making for peripartum methadone treatment. Psychopharmacology (Berl). 2013;225(2):441–451. doi:10.1007/s00213-012-2833-7

• Brezing CA, Levin FR. The current state of pharmacological treatments for cannabis use disorder and withdrawal. Neuropsychopharmacology. 2018;43(1):173–194. doi:10.1038/npp.2017. 212

• Canadian Action Network for the Advancement, Dissemination and Adoption of Practice-informed Tobacco Treatment (CAN-ADAPTT), Centre for Addiction and Mental Health. Canadian smoking cessation clinical practice guideline. Toronto, ON: Author, 2011. Retrieved from https://www.nicotinedependenceclinic.com/English/CANADAPTT/Guideline/Introduction.aspx

• Chan B, Freeman M, Kondo K, et al. Pharmacotherapy for methamphetamine/amphetamine use disorder: A systematic review and meta-analysis. Addiction 2019;114(12):2122–2136. doi:10.1111/add.14755

• Chan B, Kondo K, Freeman M, et al. Pharmacotherapy for cocaine use disorder: A systematic review and meta-analysis. J Gen Intern Med. 2019;34(12):2858–2873. doi:10.1007/s11606-019-05074-8

• Cleary BJ, Reynolds K, Eogan M, et al. Methadone dosing and prescribed medication use in a prospective cohort of opioid-dependent pregnant women. Addiction. 2013;108(4):762–770. doi:10.1111/add.12078

• Crockford D, Addington D. Canadian schizophrenia guidelines: Schizophrenia and other psychotic disorders with coexisting substance use disorders. Can J Psychiatry. 2017;62(9):624–634. doi:10.1177/0706743717720196

424

Treatment of Substance Use Disorders (cont.)

- Dematteis M, Acuriacombe M, D'Agnone O, et al. Recommendations for buprenorphine and methadone therapy in opioid use disorder: A European consensus. Expert Opin Pharmacother. 2017;18(18):1987–1999. doi:10.1080/14656566.2017.1409722
- Ebbert JO, Hatsukami DK, Croghan IT, et al. Combination varenicline and bupropion SR for tobacco-dependence treatment in cigarette smokers: A randomized trial. JAMA. 2014;311(2):155-163. doi:10.1001/jama.2013.283185
- Farhoudian A, Baldacchino A, Clark N, et al. COVID-19 and Substance Use Disorders: Recommendations to a comprehensive healthcare response. An International Society of Addiction Medicine (ISAM) practice and policy interest group position paper. BCN. 2020;11(2):129–146. doi:10.32598/bcn.11.covid19.1
- Hollands GJ, Naughton F, Farley A, et al. Interventions to increase adherence to medications for tobacco dependence. Cochrane Database Syst Rev. 2019;8(8):CD009164. doi:10.1002/14651858.CD009164.pub3
- Iacobucci G. Doctors should advise smokers on using e-cigarettes, says NICE. BMJ. 2018;360:k1449. doi:10.1136/bmj.k1449
- Kalra G, De Sousa A, Shrivastava A. Disulfiram in the management of alcohol dependence: A comprehensive clinical review. Open J Psychiatr. 2014;4(1):43–52. doi:10.4236/ojpsych.2014.41007
- Leggio L, Falk DE, Ryan ML, et al. Medication development for alcohol use disorder: A focus on clinical studies. Hadb Exp Pharmacol. 2020;258:443–462. doi:10.1007/164_2019_295
- Lingford-Hughes AR, Welch S, Peters L, et al. BAP updated guidelines: Evidence-based guidelines for the pharmacological management of substance abuse, harmful use, addiction and comorbidity: Recommendations from BAP. J Psychopharmacol. 2012;26(7):899–952. doi:10.1177/0269881112444324
- Mattick RP, Breen C, Kimber J, et al. Buprenorphine maintenance versus placebo or methadone maintenance for opioid dependence. Cochrane Database Syst Rev. 2014;(2):CD002207. doi:10.1002/14651858.CD002207.pub4
- Murphy L, Isaac P, Janecek E, et al. Buprenorphine for the treatment of opioid dependence. Pharmacy Connection. 2012;Winter:21–29. Retrieved from http://www.ocpinfo.com/client/ocp/OCPHome.nsf/web/Buprenorphine
- O'Malley SS, Zweben A, Fucito LM, et al. Effect of varenicline combined with medical management on alcohol use disorder with comorbid cigarette smoking: A randomized clinical trial. JAMA Psychiatry. 2018;75(2):129–138. doi:10.1001/jamapsychiatry.2017.3544
- Paulus MP, Stewart JL. Neurobiology, clinical presentation, and treatment of methamphetamine use disorder: A Review. JAMA Psychiatry. 2020;77(9):959–966. doi:10.1001/jamapsychiatry.2020.0246
- Reus VI, Fochtmann LJ, Bukstein O, et al. The American Psychiatric Association practice guideline for the pharmacological treatment of patients with alcohol use disorder. Am J Psychiatry. 2018;175(1):86–90. doi:10.1176/appi.ajp.2017.1750101
- Rose AK, Jones A. Baclofen: Its effectiveness in reducing harmful drinking, craving, and negative mood. A meta-analysis. Addiction. 2018;113(8):1396–1406. doi:10.1111/add.14191
- Soghoian S, Wiener SW, Diaz-Alcala JE. Disulfiram toxicity. eMedicine; 2016. Retrieved from http://emedicine.medscape.com/article/814525-overview
- Vaz LR, Leonardi-Bee J, Aveyard P, et al. Factors associated with smoking cessation in early and late pregnancy in the Smoking, Nicotine, and Pregnancy Trial: A trial of nicotine replacement therapy. Nicotine Tob Res. 2014;16(4):381–389. doi:10.1093/ntr/ntt156

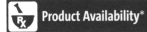

Product Availability* Several drugs traditionally used to treat medical conditions have been helpful in ameliorating or preventing symptoms of certain psychiatric disorders. This section presents a summary of some of these drugs and their uses. **As a general rule, unapproved treatments should be reserved for patients highly resistant to conventional therapies. Clinicians should be cognizant of medicolegal issues when prescribing drugs for non-approved indications.**

	Anxiety Disorders	Bipolar Disorder	Dementia	Depression	Psychosis	Substance Use Disorders
Adrenergic agents						
β-blockers (atenolol, propranolol) (p. 426)	+/C					
Doxazosin (p. 427)	PR (PTSD)					PR (alcohol)
Prazosin (p. 427)	C (PTSD)					PR/S/C (alcohol)
Thyroid hormones (p. 428)		C/S		+/S		
Anti-inflammatory agents						
Celecoxib (p. 430)	PR/S	S/C		+/S	S/C (SCZ)	
Cytokine inhibitors (e.g., adalimumab, etanercept, infliximab, tocilizumab) (p. 431)				PR		
Glucocorticoid (p. 431)	C (PTSD)					
Minocycline (p. 432)				S/C	+/S/C (SCZ)	
Pioglitazone, rosiglitazone (p. 433)				S/C	PR	
Statins (p. 434)				PR/S/C		
Cannabinoids (e.g., nabilone, dronabinol, nabiximols) (p. 434)	+ (PTSD)					+/S (cannabis withdrawal)
Dopaminergic agents						
Armodafinil (p. 435)		+/S				
Modafinil (p. 436)		PR/S		+/S		
Pramipexole (p. 436)		+/S		+/S		
GABA agents/anticonvulsants						
Baclofen (p. 437)						C (alcohol)
Pregabalin (p. 438)	+/S					+/C (alcohol)
Sodium oxybate (p. 439)						+/S (alcohol)
Hormones						
Estrogen/progesterone (p. 440)			C	+/S/C	+/S (females) (SCZ)	
Raloxifene (p. 442)					+/S/C (SCZ)	
Tamoxifen (p. 442)		PR/S (mania)				
Testosterone (p. 443)			C	S/C		

Unapproved Treatments of Psychiatric Disorders (cont.)

	Anxiety Disorders	Bipolar Disorder	Dementia	Depression	Psychosis	Substance Use Disorders
NMDA agents						
D-cycloserine (p. 444)	S/C					
Dextromethorphan-quinidine (p. 445)			+PR			
Ketamine (p. 445)	+			+/S		
Pregnenolone (p. 446)					S/C (SCZ, SCZ-affective)	
Riluzole (p. 447)	S/C (OCD, GAD)			S/C		
5-HT₃ antagonists (granisetron, ondansetron, tropisetron) (p. 448)	+/S (OCD)				+/S (SCZ)	
Miscellaneous						
ACE inhibitors/ARBs (p. 449)	C (PTSD)			PR/C		
Allopurinol (p. 449)		S/C (mania)				
Nalmefene (p. 450)						+/S/C (alcohol)
Pimavanserin (p. 450)			PR (psychosis)	PR/S	+ (PD) PR (SCZ, DLB)	

* Refer to Health Canada's Drug Product Database or the FDA's Drugs@FDA for the most current availability information
C = contradictory results, P = partial improvement, + = positive, PR = preliminary data, S = synergistic effect; DLB = dementia with Lewy bodies, PD = Parkinson's disease, SCZ = schizophrenia, SCZ-affective = schizoaffective disorder

Adrenergic Agents

β-blockers	β-blockers (e.g., propranolol) have membrane-stabilizing effect and GABA-mimetic activity; presynaptic 5-HT₁ₐ antagonists
Anxiety Disorders	• Suggested to inhibit memory consolidation by interfering with protein synthesis; anxiolytic properties may result from its peripheral (autonomic) rather than its central activity – propranolol aids in breaking a vicious cycle of anxiety in which catastrophic misappraisal of bodily sensations of orthosympathetic origin, such as palpitations or increased ventilation, fuel the occurrence of panic attacks • Propranolol dose: Up to 320 mg/day; atenolol 50 mg/day • Propranolol and atenolol beneficial for somatic or autonomically mediated symptoms of anxiety (e.g., tremor, palpitations) as seen in performance anxiety and acute panic • Efficacy reported in adults and children with PTSD – propranolol treatment after the traumatic event reported not to alter PTSD incidence, although physiological responses are generally attenuated; early administration reported to treat intrusive memories and reduce severity of later symptoms; recent double-blind, placebo-controlled, randomized clinical trial in 60 adults diagnosed with long-standing PTSD reported positive results with propranolol administered 90 min before a brief memory reactivation session, once a week for 6 consecutive weeks. Inconclusive whether propranolol was more effective than placebo in reducing probability of experiencing PTSD at 3 months after the traumatic event • Meta-analysis suggests limited data on the benefit of propranolol in long-term treatment of anxiety disorders; no advantage over benzodiazepines reported in the treatment of panic disorders with or without agoraphobia • Retrospective data on 92 military patients prescribed atenolol for mental health-related issues showed 86% of patients reported a positive effect and continued to take atenolol, including 87% of those diagnosed with PTSD, 100% of those with other specified trauma- and stressor-related disorders, and 81% of those with anxiety disorders. Data also suggest that atenolol may be more effective and better tolerated than propranolol

- Caution in patients with a history (or family history) of cardiovascular problems, alcohol use, and asthma (propranolol)

Argolo FC, Cavalcanti-Ribeiro P, Netto LR, et al. Prevention of posttraumatic stress disorder with propranolol: A meta-analytic review. J Psychosom Res. 2015;79(2):89–93. doi:10.1016/j.jpsychores.2015.04.006

Armstrong C, Kapolowicz MR. A preliminary investigation on the effects of atenolol for treating symptoms of anxiety. Mil Med. 2020;185(11–12):e1954–e1960. doi:10.1093/milmed/usaa170

Bertolini F, Robertson L, Bisson JI, et al. Early pharmacological interventions for universal prevention of post-traumatic stress disorder (PTSD). Cochrane Database Syst Rev. 2022;2(2): CD013443. doi:10.1002/14651858.CD013443.pub2

Brunet A, Saumier D, Liu A, et al. Reduction of PTSD symptoms with pre-reactivation propranolol therapy: A randomized controlled trial. Am J Psychiatry. 2018;175(5):427–433. doi:10.1176/appi.ajp.2017.17050481

Steenen SA, van Wijk AJ, van der Heijden GJMG, et al. Propranolol for the treatment of anxiety disorders: Systematic review and meta-analysis. J Psychopharmacol. 2016; 30(2):128–139. doi:10.1177/0269881115612236

Doxazosin

α_1-adrenergic antagonist

Posttraumatic Stress Disorder

- Dose: 4–16 mg/day (has longer half-life than prazosin, 16–30 h, and can be used once daily)
- A retrospective chart review of patients with PTSD and/or borderline personality disorder showed a significant reduction in trauma-associated nightmares when treated with doxazosin; 25% of patients treated for 12 weeks had full remission of nightmares
- A pilot study in VA veterans suggested benefit with doxazosin XL

Calegaro VC, Mosele PHC, Duarte e Souza I, et al. Treating nightmares in PTSD with doxazosin: A report of three cases. Braz J Psychiatry. 2019; 41(2): 189–190. doi:10.1590/1516-4446-2018-0292

Roepke S, Danker-Hopfe H, Repantis D, et al. Doxazosin, an α-1-adrenergic-receptor antagonist, for nightmares in patients with posttraumatic stress disorder and/or borderline personality disorder: A chart review. Pharmacopsychiatry. 2017;50(1):26–31. doi:10.1055/s-0042-107794

Rodgman C, Verrico CD, Holst M, et al. Doxazosin XL reduces symptoms of posttraumatic stress disorder in veterans with PTSD: A pilot clinical trial. J Clin Psychiatry. 2016;77(5):e561–e565. doi:10.4088/JCP.14m09681

Smith C, Koola MM. Evidence for using doxazosin in the treatment of posttraumatic stress disorder, Psychiatr Ann. 2016;46(9):553–555. doi:10.3928/00485713-20160728-01

Alcohol Use Disorder

- Dose: Titrate up to 16 mg/day
- Stress physiology is disrupted with chronic alcohol use, particularly during early alcohol abstinence; α_1 antagonists may help to normalize these stress system changes seen in AUD
- A small meta-analysis of 6 studies with a total of 319 participants tested the effectiveness of drugs acting on adrenergic receptors for AUD and found a significant treatment effect of prazosin and doxazosin on alcohol consumption but not abstinence
- Doxazosin appears to have a better response in patients with a family history of AUD and higher pretreatment standing blood pressure, and this may represent a biomarker of doxazosin's response)

Burnette EM, Nieto SJ, Grodin EN, et al. Novel agents for the pharmacological treatment of alcohol use disorder. Drugs. 2022;82(3):251–274. doi:10.1007/s40265-021-01670-3

Vanderkam P, Solinas M, Ingrand I, et al. Effectiveness of drugs acting on adrenergic receptors in the treatment for tobacco or alcohol use disorders: Systematic review and meta-analysis. Addiction. 2021;116(5):1011–1020. doi:10.1111/add.15265

Prazosin

α_1-adrenergic antagonist

Posttraumatic Stress Disorder

- Dose: Titrate gradually up to 20 mg/day; doses up to 48 mg/day have been used (requires dosing 2–4 times/day due to short half-life)
- High noradrenergic activity may be associated with hyperarousal, trauma nightmares, and sleep disturbances in individuals with PTSD, probably through the stimulation of α_1 adrenergic receptors in the brain prefrontal cortex
- Data contradictory, though in a recent meta-analysis, pooled effect estimates show that prazosin has a statistically significant benefit on PTSD symptoms and sleep disturbances; in another meta-analysis, statistically significant improvement in nightmares was demonstrated
- Daytime prazosin reported to decrease distress related to trauma cues
- Case series reports successful outcome using high-dose (up to 30 and 45 mg) prazosin for PTSD with comorbid treatment-resistant mood disorders

Unapproved Treatments

Adrenergic Agents (cont.)

- A retrospective chart review reported that prazosin was well tolerated and associated with improvements in nightmares and sleep in youth (mean age 13.4 ± 2.9 years; 82% female) with PTSD of whom 76% had a history of sexual abuse and 65% had at least one comorbid psychiatric disorder; dose ranges of 1–4 mg daily used in children
- In a randomized placebo-controlled trial of 304 military veterans with chronic PTSD, prazosin (up to 20 mg/day in males and 12 mg/day in females) did not alleviate distressing dreams or improve sleep quality
- Pretreatment blood pressure (BP) predicts therapeutic response of prazosin in PTSD patients
- Main side effects reported include hypotension, headache, drowsiness, and nausea
- The US Department of Veterans Affairs and the Department of Defense guidelines for PTSD suggest against prazosin as monotherapy or augmentation therapy for global symptoms of PTSD based on lack of demonstrated efficacy. The guidelines also found insufficient evidence to recommend for or against the use of prazosin as mono- or augmentation therapy for nightmares or sleep disturbance associated with PTDS

Akinsanya A, Marwaha R, Tampi RR. Prazosin in children and adolescents with posttraumatic stress disorder who have nightmares: A systematic review. J Clin Psychopharmacol. 2017;37(1):84–88. doi:10.1097/JCP.0000000000000638

George KC, Kebejian L, Ruth LJ, et al. Meta-analysis of the efficacy and safety of prazosin versus placebo for the treatment of nightmares and sleep disturbances in adults with posttraumatic stress disorder. J Trauma Dissociation. 2016;17(4):494–510. doi:10.1080/15299732.2016.1141150

Keeshin BR, Ding Q, Presson AP, et al. Use of prazosin for pediatric PTSD-associated nightmares and sleep disturbances: A retrospective chart review. Neurol Ther. 2017;6(2):247–257. doi:10.1007/s40120-017-0078-4

Raskind MA, Peskind ER, Chow B, et al. Trial of prazosin for post-traumatic stress disorder in military veterans. N Engl J Med. 2018;378(6):507–517. doi:10.1056/NEJMoa1507598

Reist C, Streja E, Tang CC, et al. Prazosin for treatment of post-traumatic stress disorder: A systematic review and meta-analysis. CNS Spectr. 2021;26(4):338–344. doi:10.1017/S1092852920001121

VA/DOD clinical practice guideline for the management of posttraumatic stress disorder and acute stress disorder. 2017;Version 3.0. Retrieved from https://www.healthquality.va.gov/guidelines/MH/ptsd/VADoDPTSDCPGFinal012418.pdf

Zhang Y, Ren R, Sanford LD, et al. The effects of prazosin on sleep disturbances in post-traumatic stress disorder: A systematic review and meta-analysis. Sleep Med. 2020;67:225–231. doi:10.1016/j.sleep.2019.06.010

Alcohol Use Disorder

- Dose: Titrate up to 16 mg/day
- Stress physiology is disrupted with chronic alcohol use, particularly during early alcohol abstinence; α_1 antagonists may help normalize these stress system changes seen in AUD
- Postulated that alcohol withdrawal is a significant predictor of alcohol-related prefrontal-striatal dysfunction, and prazosin treatment reversed these effects, which in turn contributed to improved alcohol treatment outcomes
- A 12-week RCT of prazosin with 100 patients found that an individual's degree of alcohol withdrawal symptoms predicted clinical response, such that participants with high levels of withdrawal symptoms benefited most from treatment (e.g., reduced craving and heavy-drinking days; improved anxiety and mood symptoms)
- Two placebo-controlled studies evaluated prazosin for co-occurring alcohol use disorder and PTSD, with mixed results. Combination therapy with naltrexone and propranolol have also been proposed

Burnette EM, Nieto SJ, Grodin EN, et al. Novel agents for the pharmacological treatment of alcohol use disorder. Drugs. 2022;82(3):251–274. doi:10.1007/s40265-021-01670-3

Verplaetse TL, McKee SA, Petrakis IL. Pharmacotherapy for co-occurring alcohol use disorder and post-traumatic stress disorder; targeting the opioidergic, noradrenergic, serotonergic, and GABAergic/glutamatergic systems. Alcohol Res. 2018;39(2):193–205.

Thyroid Hormones

Modulate adrenergic receptor function and permit a given concentration of catecholamines to be more effective; metabolic enhancers

Depression

- Levothyroxine (T_4) therapy leads to a significant decline in the level of inflammatory cytokines which may play a role in the pathogenesis of depression
- Dose: liothyronine (T_3): 5–50 micrograms/day, levothyroxine (T_4) 5–500 micrograms/day
- Augmentation with T_3 suggested to be more efficient than with T_4 because of individual differences in thyroid hormone metabolism

- In refractory depression, may potentiate effects of antidepressants; positive effects seen in up to 60% of refractory patients within 2 weeks – may be more beneficial in women than in men; suggested that treatment be discontinued if no response seen after 3 weeks
- Meta-analysis of 8 studies (4 double-blind) of T_3 augmentation showed an absolute response rate of 23% in patients refractory to tricyclics; evidence suggests limited benefit for augmentation of SSRIs
- Case series using higher T_3 dose (100 micrograms/day) long term, improved symptoms in 14 of 17 treatment-refractory patients
- Suggested T_3 may actually be treating subclinical hypothyroidism; free thyroid hormone concentrations are associated with depression severity and have an impact on treatment outcome
- Double-blind study suggests that liothyronine may prevent ECT-induced memory impairment in patients with MDD
- Negative results reported when T_3 added to T_4 therapy in hypothyroid patients with depressive symptoms
- Transitory side effects can include: Sweating, shaking, anxiety, and tachycardia
- May exacerbate mania

Dwyer JB, Aftab A, Radhakrishnan R, et al. Hormonal treatments for major depressive disorder: State of the art. Am J Psychiatry. 2020;177(8):686–705. doi:10.1176/appi.ajp.2020.19080848

Mohagheghi A, Arfaie A, Amiri S, et al. Preventive effect of liothyronine on electroconvulsive therapy-induced memory deficit in patients with major depressive disorder: A double-blind controlled clinical trial. Biomed Res Int. 2015;2015:503918. doi:10.1155/2015/503918

Nuñez NA, Joseph B, Pahwa M, et al. Augmentation strategies for treatment resistant major depression: A systematic review and network meta-analysis. J Affect Disord. 2022;302:385–400. doi:10.1016/j.jad.2021.12.134

Tang R, Wang J, Yang L, et al. Subclinical hypothyroidism and depression: A systematic review and meta-analysis. Front Endocrinol (Lausanne). 2019;10:340. doi:10.3389/fendo.2019.00340

Tayde PS, Bhagwat NM, Sharma P, et al. Hypothyroidism and depression: Are cytokines the link? Indian J Endocrinol Metab. 2017; 21(6):886–892. doi:10.4103/ijem.IJEM_265_17

Bipolar Disorder	

- Administration of supraphysiologic thyroid hormone has been suggested to improve depressive symptoms by modulating function in components of the anterior limbic network
- Dose: liothyronine (T_3): average dose: 90.4 micrograms/day, range: 13–188 micrograms/day; levothyroxine (T_4): 300–500 micrograms/day
- Controversial results seen; response to treatment is usually evident within the first 2 weeks
- Studies of specific subgroups of bipolar disorder (rapid cycling, mixed, or depressive bipolar) have reported associations with thyroid antibodies; conflicting results seen. May be treating unidentified hypothyroidism; association reported between elevated T_3 hormone and bipolar affective disorder and that patients with bipolar affective disorder are 2.55 times more commonly associated with thyroid dysfunction
- High dose of T_4 reported to be an effective adjunctive maintenance treatment of prophylaxis-resistant mood disorder
- Double-blind study of 32 treatment-resistant rapid-cycling patients on lithium, comparing the effects of T_3 and T_4 therapy against placebo, demonstrated a benefit of adjunctive T_4 in alleviating resistant depression, reducing time in mixed states, and increasing time in euthymic state. Adjunctive T_3 did not show statistically significant benefit over placebo in reducing time spent in the disturbed mood states
- Reported to alleviate symptoms and increase cycle length primarily in rapid-cycling female patients; controversial results reported in males; adjunctive to other therapies of bipolar disorder
- Review of T_3 in bipolar depression reported: 1) improvement in 56%, 75%, and 79% of patients in three open studies, respectively, 2) improvement in 89% of cases in a retrospective chart review, and 3) improvement in 66% of patients in a mirror-image design study. In the comparative study, T_3 performed significantly better than placebo. The only randomized double-blind study did not show any substantial difference between T_3 and placebo
- Recommended to regularly assess bone mineral density in postmenopausal women on chronic T_4 therapy

Bauer M, Whybrow PC. Role of thyroid hormone therapy in depressive disorders. J Endocrinol Invest. 2021;44(11):2341–2347. doi:10.1007/s40618-021-01600-w

Parmentier T, Sienaert P. The use of triiodothyronine (T3) in the treatment of bipolar depression: A review of the literature. J Affect Disord. 2018;229:410–414. doi:10.1016/j.jad.2017.12.071

Pilhatsch M, Stamm TJ, Stahl P, et al. Treatment of bipolar depression with supraphysiologic doses of levothyroxine: A randomized, placebo-controlled study of comorbid anxiety symptoms. Int J Bipolar Disord. 2019;7(1):21. doi:10.1186/s40345-019-0155-y

Walshaw PD, Gyulai L, Bauer M, et al. Adjunctive thyroid hormone treatment in rapid cycling bipolar disorder: A double-blind placebo-controlled trial of levothyroxine (L-T4) and triiodothyronine (T3). Bipolar Disord. 2018;20(7):594—603. doi:10.1111/bdi.12657

Anti-inflammatory Agents

Celecoxib	Evidence suggests that inflammatory processes and immune responses are involved in the pathophysiology of depression as well as schizophrenia. Several studies have reported high levels of peripheral pro-inflammatory markers, notably C-reactive protein (CRP), interleukin-6 (IL-6), tumor necrosis factor (TNF-α), and interleukin-1 receptor antagonist (IL-1ra) in patients with MDD. COX-2 inhibitors influence the serotonergic system in the CNS, both directly and through immune mechanisms in the CNS

Anxiety

- A pilot study was conducted in patients with a primary diagnosis of an anxiety disorder, with stabilised symptoms, who underwent either 6 weeks of celecoxib augmentation of continued treatment (18 patients) or "treatment as usual" (9 patients). As compared to controls, celecoxib augmentation was associated with beneficial effects on anxiety and depressive symptoms as well as mental well-being and overall illness severity. There were no significant changes in blood levels of inflammatory cytokines in either group

Depression

- Dose: 200–400 mg daily
- Open and double-blind studies show benefit of adjunctive celecoxib in treating mild–moderate depression in patients with concurrent medical illness; NSAIDs have poor clinical benefit as antidepressant monotherapy
- Four studies demonstrated improved antidepressant treatment effects for celecoxib add-on treatment compared to antidepressants + placebo; one study found that higher levels of the pro-inflammatory marker IL-6 predicted better antidepressant response to adjunctive celecoxib; negative results reported in combination with vortioxetine in a 6-week double-blind, placebo-controlled randomized trial

Baune BT, Sampson E, Louise J, et al. No evidence for clinical efficacy of adjunctive celecoxib with vortioxetine in the treatment of depression: A 6-week double-blind placebo controlled randomized trial. Eur Neuropsychopharmacol. 2021;53:34–46. doi:10.1016/j.euroneuro.2021.07.092

Colpo GD, Leboyer M, Dantzer R, et al. Immune-based strategies for mood disorders: Facts and challenges. Expert Rev Neurother. 2018;18(2):139–152. doi:10.1080/14737175.2018.1407242

Faridhosseini F, Sadeghi R, Farid L, et al. Celecoxib: A new augmentation strategy for depressive mood episodes. A systematic review and meta-analysis of randomized placebo-controlled trials. Hum Psychopharmacol. 2014;29(3):216–223. doi:10.1002/hup.2401

Köhler O, Krogh J, Mors O, et al. Inflammation in depression and the potential for anti-inflammatory treatment. Curr Neuropharmacol. 2016;14(7):732–742. doi:10.2174/1570159X14666151208113700

Majd M, Hashemian F, Hosseini SM, et al. A randomized, double-blind, placebo-controlled trial of celecoxib augmentation of sertraline in treatment of drug-naive depressed women: A pilot study. Iran J Pharm Res. 2015;14(3):891–899. Retrieved from https://www.ncbi.nlm.nih.gov/pmc/articles/PMC4518118/s

Bipolar disorder

- The effect of NSAIDs in bipolar depression remains unclear as clinical studies have yielded mixed results. Several small studies suggest that adjunctive use of anti-inflammatory agents, including celecoxib, might improve depressive symptoms in bipolar disorder. A large multi-centre double-blind, 12-week, randomized, placebo-controlled trial found no evidence that adjunctive celecoxib was superior to placebo for the treatment of bipolar depression
- Adjunctive NSAIDs in the treatment of mania have yielded mixed results with anti-manic effects yet to be consistently demonstrated. Regardless of illness phase, early results suggest that anti-inflammatory agents are likely most beneficial in the subgroup of BD with immune dysregulation

Husain MI, Chaudhry IB, Khoso AB, et al. Minocycline and celecoxib as adjunctive treatments for bipolar depression: A multicentre, factorial design randomised controlled trial. Lancet Psychiatry. 2020;7(6):515–527. doi:10.1016/S2215-0366(20)30138-3

Rosenblat JD, McIntyre RS. Bipolar disorder and immune dysfunction: Epidemiological findings, proposed pathophysiology and clinical implications. Brain Sci. 2017;7(11):pii:E144. doi:10.3390/brainsci7110144

Schizophrenia

- Neuroinflammation has been implicated in the neurobiological pathways of schizophrenia. Systematic quantitative reviews and meta-analysis suggest cytokine imbalances in people with schizophrenia relative to controls; IL-6 is one of the most consistently disturbed cytokines in schizophrenia; other cytokines include IL-1, TNF, and IFN
- Meta-analysis of 5 randomized DBPC studies of NSAID augmentation (4 used celecoxib, 1 used ASA) of antipsychotic drugs showed NSAIDs can potentially decrease symptom severity in schizophrenia; recent reviews do not encourage the use of aspirin (1000 mg/day)
- Two meta-analyses (2016 and 2017) of 8 and 6 RCTs, respectively, report that adjunctive celecoxib appears to be an efficacious and safe treatment in improving psychotic symptoms, particularly in first-episode schizophrenia
- A 2019 meta-analysis found heterogeneous results, ranging from strong positive to strong negative effects of celecoxib as augmentation therapy. The effects of celecoxib on symptom severity was not significant and heterogeneity was high

Çakici N, van Beveren NJM, Judge-Hundal G, et al. An update on the efficacy of anti-inflammatory agents for patients with schizophrenia: A meta-analysis. Psychol Med. 2019;49(14):2307–2319. doi:10.1017/S0033291719001995

Marini S, De Berardis D, Vellante F, et al. Celecoxib adjunctive treatment to antipsychotics in schizophrenia: A review of randomized clinical add-on trials. Mediators Inflamm. 2016;2016:3476240. doi:10.1155/2016/3476240

Zheng W, Cai DB, Yang XH, et al. Adjunctive celecoxib for schizophrenia: A meta-analysis of randomized, double-blind, placebo-controlled trials. J Psychiatr Res. 2017;92:139–146. doi:10.1016/j.jpsychires.2017.04.004

Cytokine Inhibitors	Tumor necrosis factor-α (TNF-α) is a key cytokine that induces mood symptoms in the context of sickness behavior; molecules with anti-TNF-α activity may have antidepressant action. Interleukin-17 (IL-17) is a pro-inflammatory cytokine that has been implicated in the pathophysiology of depression and antidepressant response

Depression

- A systematic review and meta-analysis of antidepressant activity of anti-cytokine treatment using clinical trials of chronic inflammatory conditions where depressive symptoms were measured as a secondary outcome, demonstrated that adalimumab, etanercept, infliximab, and tocilizumab all showed statistically significant improvements in depressive symptoms
- In a 12-week study in 60 patients moderately resistant to previous antidepressant therapy, infliximab (5 mg/kg at week 0, 2 weeks, and 6 weeks) had an antidepressant effect only in individuals who had elevated levels of inflammatory markers. Studies have suggested that alterations in proinflammatory cytokines play an important role in the pathophysiology of treatment-resistant depression, as well as a significant relationship between the number of failed treatments and the levels of TNF-α and C-reactive protein
- Brodalumab, an anti-IL-17 receptor antibody and ixekizumab, an anti-IL-17-A monoclonal antibody have both shown efficacy in depression in patients with psoriasis. Similarly, sirukumab and siltuximab, two anti-IL-6 antibodies, have been shown to be effective in reducing depressive symptom severity among patients with rheumatoid arthritis and multicentric Castleman disease even after controlling for symptom severity of primary illnesses
- A potential limiting factor of anti-TNF-α strategies is the significant risk of opportunistic infections associated with them; medications targeting the TNF-α pathway may trigger psychiatric effects, including anxiety, depression, suicidal ideation, and manic episode, in patients with or without affective disorders

Bavaresco DV, Rodrigues Uggioni ML, Dagostin Ferraz S, et al. Efficacy of infliximab in treatment-resistant depression: A systematic review and meta-analysis. Pharmacol Biochem Behav. 2020;188:172838. doi:10.1016/j.pbb.2019.172838

Colpo GD, Leboyer M, Dantzer R, et al. Immune-based strategies for mood disorders: Facts and challenges. Expert Rev Neurother. 2018;18(2):139–152. doi:10.1080/14737175.2018.1407242

Jha MK. Anti-inflammatory treatments for major depressive disorder: What's on the horizon? J Clin Psychiatry. 2019;80(6):18ac12630. doi:10.4088/JCP.18ac12630

Kappelmann N, Lewis G, Dantzer R, et al. Antidepressant activity of anti-cytokine treatment: A systematic review and meta-analysis of clinical trials of chronic inflammatory conditions. Mol Psychiatry. 2018;23(2):335–343. doi:10.1038/mp.2016.167

Miola A, Dal Porto V, Meda N, et al. Secondary mania induced by TNF-α inhibitors: A systematic review. Psychiatry Clin Neurosci. 2022;76(1):15–21. doi:10.1111/pcn.13302

Roman M, Irwin MR. Novel neuroimmunologic therapeutics in depression: A clinical perspective on what we know so far. Brain Behav Immun. 2020;83:7–21. doi:10.1016/j.bbi.2019.09.016

Glucocorticoid	Suggested to restrict retrieval of previous aversive learning episodes. Decreased levels of 24-h urinary cortisol have been linked with the pathophysiology of PTSD. Initiating therapy within the first 6 h of a trauma is thought to be crucial to impeding the disruption to memory consolidation that occurs within this period

Posttraumatic Stress Disorder

- Hydrocortisone: Dose: 30–40 mg ½ to 1 h before exposure-based treatment
- Hydrocortisone given in supplementary fashion before exposure-based treatment in PTSD patients had varied outcomes. A randomized, double-blind, placebo-controlled trial in 60 veterans showed that patients with higher baseline glucocorticoid sensitivity showed a greater reduction in avoidance symptoms with hydrocortisone augmentation of prolonged exposure therapy
- A systematic review identified 19 RCTs, with 16 included in the meta-analysis, and found some evidence for the potential efficacy of hydrocortisone in the prevention of PTSD in adults
- Double-blind study suggests that low-dose hydrocortisone (20 mg bid), administered within 24 h of a trauma, may be a promising approach to the prevention of PTSD in acutely injured trauma patients
- Hydrocortisone augmentation of prolonged exposure therapy showed greater reduction in PTSD symptoms. Subgroup analyses of 8 studies revealed a significant effect of hydrocortisone when it was administered in a preventative context, but not when it was administered in a curative context

Anti-inflammatory Agents (cont.)

- Perioperative administration of IV dexamethasone, compared with placebo, during cardiac surgery did not positively or negatively affect the prevalence of PTSD and depression
- 54 male veterans with combat-related PTSD received either 4-weekly dexamethasone or placebo administrations, paired with a 45-second trauma memory reactivation task; significantly more veterans in the dexamethasone group lost their diagnosis of PTSD at one month posttreatment compared to the placebo group, but the difference was not maintained at three or six months. There was no effect on depressive symptoms

Astill Wright L, Sijbrandij M, Sinnerton R, et al. Pharmacological prevention and early treatment of post-traumatic stress disorder and acute stress disorder: A systematic review and meta-analysis. Transl Psychiatry. 2019;9(1):334. doi:10.1038/s41398-019-0673-5

Bertolini F, Robertson L, Bisson JI, et al. Early pharmacological interventions for universal prevention of post-traumatic stress disorder (PTSD). Cochrane Database Syst Rev. 2022;2(2): CD013443. doi:10.1002/14651858.CD013443.pub2

Medici CR, Gradus JL, Pedersen L, et al. No impact of preadmission anti-inflammatory drug use on Risk of depression and anxiety after critical illness. Crit Care Med. 2017;45(10):1635–1641. doi:10.1097/CCM.0000000000002571

Surís A, Holliday R, Adinoff B, et al. Facilitating fear-based memory extinction with dexamethasone: A randomized controlled trial in male veterans with combat-related PTSD. Psychiatry. 2017;80(4):399–410. doi:10.1080/00332747.2017.1286892

Minocycline	Anti-infective drug with anti-inflammatory and neuroprotective properties (including increased neurogenesis and antioxidation, anti-glutamate excitotoxicity, and down-regulation of pro-inflammatory agents); blocks the neurotoxicity of N-methyl-D-aspartate (NMDA) antagonists and may exert a differential effect on NMDA signaling pathways; modulates kynurenine pathways; may protect against gray matter loss and modulate fronto-temporal areas involved in the pathophysiology of schizophrenia. Minocycline has the advantage of good penetration into the central nervous system (CNS) through the blood-brain barrier, which accounts for its important neuroprotective ability

Depression	• Dose: 200 mg/day

- Minocycline has broad anti-inflammatory properties due to its inhibitory actions on the mechanisms relevant to inflammation-induced depression, like the kynurenine (KYN) and the p38 pathways
- Double-blind study reported that 100 mg minocycline bid was safe and effective in improving mild–moderate depressive symptoms in HIV/AIDS patients with mild–moderate depression
- A multi-site, 12-week, double-blind, placebo-controlled, pilot trial of adjunctive minocycline in treatment-resistant patients showed positive improvements in HAMD and CGI scores
- Data contradictory as to efficacy, as a recent meta-analysis of RCTs showed no significant effect on depressive and manic symptoms in either bipolar depression or MDD. Eighteen clinical studies (including published and unpublished RCTs, open label studies, ongoing clinical trials and a case report) were reviewed; 3 RCTs were analyzed and demonstrated a large antidepressant effect for minocycline compared to placebo, with good tolerability
- In a study comparing the effects of minocycline and ASA on bipolar depression, participants with higher baseline levels of IL-6 responded better to minocycline administration than patients with lower levels of inflammation; the minocycline-treated participants who showed a greater decrease in IL-6 levels between baseline and visit 7 also showed a larger reduction in depressive symptoms over the trial
- A 4-week, placebo-controlled, randomized clinical trial of minocycline (200 mg/day) added to antidepressants in 39 treatment-resistant patients confirmed efficacy only in patients with low-grade inflammation defined as CRP ≥ 3 mg/L

Bai S, Guo W, Feng Y, et al. Efficacy and safety of anti-inflammatory agents for the treatment of major depressive disorder: A systematic review and meta-analysis of randomised controlled trials. J Neurol Neurosurg Psychiatry. 2020;91(1):21–32. doi:10.1136/jnnp-2019-320912

Emadi-Kouchak H, Mohammadinejad P, Asadollahi-Amin A, et al. Therapeutic effects of minocycline on mild-to-moderate depression in HIV patients: A double-blind, placebo-controlled, randomized trial. Int Clin Psychopharmacol. 2016;31(1):20–26. doi:10.1097/YIC.0000000000000098

Husain MI, Chaudhry IB, Husain N, et al. Minocycline as an adjunct for treatment-resistant depressive symptoms: A pilot randomised placebo-controlled trial. J Psychopharmacol. 2017;31(9):1166–1175. doi:10.1177/0269881117724352

Rosenblat JD, McIntyre RS. Efficacy and tolerability of minocycline for depression: A systematic review and meta-analysis of clinical trials. J Affect Disord. 2018;227:219–225. doi:10.1016/j.jad.2017.10.042

Savitz JB, Teague TK, Misaki M, et al. Treatment of bipolar depression with minocycline and/or aspirin: An adaptive, 2×2 double-blind, randomized, placebo-controlled, phase IIA clinical trial. Transl Psychiatry. 2018;8(1):27. doi:10.1038/s41398-017-0073-7

Soczynska JK, Kennedy SH, Alsuwaidan M, et al. A pilot, open-label, 8-week study evaluating the efficacy, safety and tolerability of adjunctive minocycline for the treatment of bipolar I/II depression. Bipolar Disord. 2017;19(3):198–213. doi:10.1111/bdi.12496

Zheng W, Zhu XM, Zhang QE, et al. Adjunctive minocycline for major mental disorders: A systematic review. J Psychopharmacol. 2019;33(10):1215–1226. doi:10.1177/0269881119858286

Schizophrenia/Psychosis	

- Dose: 200 mg/day
- Data contradictory as to benefit of adjunctive minocycline for positive or negative symptoms in recent-onset schizophrenia; suggested that the mechanisms underlying negative symptoms and comorbid depression in psychosis might be very different from those present in MDD and targeted by minocycline
- Improvement in negative symptoms with addition of 200 mg minocycline to risperidone therapy was significantly correlated with the reduction of serum levels of pro-inflammatory cytokines IL-1β and IL-6; visual learning/memory and executive function were the cognitive domains that significantly improved with adjunctive minocycline according to a meta-analysis
- An open-label study of 5 patients showed that adjunctive minocycline (200 mg/day for 8 weeks) attenuated both methamphetamine-induced positive and negative symptoms and also improved neuropsychological functions, particularly auditory working memory
- Two meta-analyses of 8 and 6 RCTs, respectively, revealed a significant superiority of adjunctive minocycline treatment over placebo for both positive and negative symptoms
- Improvement in attention and memory reported in one study, as well as a decrease in extrapyramidal side effects
- Well tolerated with few side effects

Çakici N, van Beveren NJM, Judge-Hundal G, et al. An update on the efficacy of anti-inflammatory agents for patients with schizophrenia: A meta-analysis. Psychol Med. 2019;49(14):2307–2319. doi:10.1017/S0033291719001995

Chaves C, Marque CR, Maia-de-Oliveira JP, et al. Effects of minocycline add-on treatment on brain morphometry and cerebral perfusion in recent-onset schizophrenia. Schizophr Res. 2015;161(2–3):439–445. doi:10.1016/j.schres.2014.11.031

Ľupták M, Michaličková D, Fišar Z, et al. Novel approaches in schizophrenia – From risk factors and hypotheses to novel drug targets. World J Psychiatry. 2021;11(7):277–296. doi:10.5498/wjp.v11.i7.277

Solmi M, Veronese N, Thapa N, et al. Systematic review and meta-analysis of the efficacy and safety of minocycline in schizophrenia. CNS Spectr. 2017;22(5):415–426. doi:10.1017/S1092852916000638

Xiang YQ, Zheng W, Wang SB, et al. Adjunctive minocycline for schizophrenia: A meta-analysis of randomized controlled trials. Eur Neuropsychopharmacol. 2017;27(1):8–18. doi:10.1016/j.euroneuro.2016.11.012

Zhang L, Zheng H, Wu R, et al. Minocycline adjunctive treatment to risperidone for negative symptoms in schizophrenia: Association with pro-inflammatory cytokine levels. Prog Neuropsychopharmacol Biol Psychiatry. 2018;85:69–76. doi:10.1016/j.pnpbp.2018.04.004

Pioglitazone/Rosiglitazone	**Selective agonists of the nuclear transcription factor peroxisome proliferator-activated receptor-gamma (PPAR-γ) – have anti-inflammatory properties**

Depression	

- Dose: Pioglitazone 30 mg/day; rosiglitazone 8 mg/day
- Four double-blind randomized controlled trials suggest that pioglitazone, either alone or as add-on therapy to conventional treatments, was found to be more effective than placebo and could induce remission of MDD. Improvement in depression scores was associated with improvement in 3 biomarkers of insulin resistance (homeostatic model assessment [HOMA-IR], oral glucose tolerance test, and fasting plasma glucose) and 1 biomarker of inflammation (interleukin-6) among 21 biomarkers studied
- Younger patients may have better response
- Negative results reported in a double-blind placebo-controlled study of pioglitazone 15–45 mg/day for treatment of bipolar depression
- Pioglitazone has been associated with several side effects, including an increased risk for fractures, weight increase, and cardiovascular events

Colle R, de Larminat D, Rotenberg S, et al. Pioglitazone could induce remission in major depression: A meta-analysis. Neuropsychiatr Dis Treat. 2016;13:9–16. doi:10.2147/NDT.S121149

Colle R, de Larminat D, Rotenberg S, et al. PPAR-γ agonists for the treatment of major depression: A review. Pharmacopsychiatry. 2017;50(2):49–55. doi:10.1055/s-0042-120120

Lin KW, Wroolie TE, Robakis T, et al. Adjuvant pioglitazone for unremitted depression: Clinical correlates of treatment response. Psychiatry Res. 2015;230(3):846–852. doi:10.1016/j.psychres.2015.10.013

Köhler O, Krogh J, Mors O, et al. Inflammation in depression and the potential for anti-inflammatory treatment. Curr Neuropharmacol. 2016;14(7):732–742. doi:10.2174/1570159X14666151208113700

Anti-inflammatory Agents (cont.)

Schizophrenia	
	• In a randomized, double-blind, placebo-controlled trial of 40 patients with chronic schizophrenia on risperidone and a minimum score of 20 on the negative subscale of the Positive and Negative Syndrome Scale (PANSS), patients in the pioglitazone (30 mg/day) group showed significantly more improvement in PANSS negative subscale scores as well as PANSS total scores compared with the placebo group

Çakici N, van Beveren NJM, Judge-Hundal G, et al. An update on the efficacy of anti-inflammatory agents for patients with schizophrenia: A meta-analysis. Psychol Med. 2019;49(14):2307–2319. doi:10.1017/S0033291719001995

Iranpour N, Zandifar A, Farokhnia M, et al. The effects of pioglitazone adjuvant therapy on negative symptoms of patients with chronic schizophrenia: A double-blind and placebo-controlled trial. Hum Psychopharmacol. 2016;31(2):103–112. doi:10.1002/hup.2517

Statins

Statins are also known as HMG-CoA reductase inhibitors and modulate the inflammatory response by various mechanisms, including decreasing cholesterol synthesis in the liver

Depression	
	• Dose: Lovastatin 30 mg/day; simvastatin 20 mg/day, atorvastatin 20 mg/day
	• Statin use is associated with either antidepressant or depressogenic effects; use of higher doses of statins related to an overrepresentation of MDD and antidepressant prescription
	• Early data contradictory as to benefit of statin add-on therapy for treating depression; a meta-analysis suggests lipophilic statins are more effective than hydrophilic statins; positive effects seen after 2 weeks and response seen after 8–12 weeks of therapy
	• A meta-analysis of 13 studies comparing atorvastatin with placebo reported that it significantly reduced the severity of depressive symptoms

Bai S, Guo W, Feng Y, et al. Efficacy and safety of anti-inflammatory agents for the treatment of major depressive disorder: A systematic review and meta-analysis of randomised controlled trials. J Neurol Neurosurg Psychiatry. 2020;91(1):21–32. doi:10.1136/jnnp-2019-320912

De Giorgi R, De Crescenzo F, Rizzo Pesci N, et al. Statins for major depressive disorder: A systematic review and meta-analysis of randomized controlled trials: PLoS One. 2021;16(3): e0249409. doi:10.1371/journal.pone.0249409

Kim SW, Kang HJ, Jhon M , et al. Statins and inflammation: New therapeutic opportunities in psychiatry. Front Psychiatry. 2019;10:103. doi:10.3389/fpsyt.2019.00103

Lee MC, Peng TR, Chen BL, et al. Effects of various statins on depressive symptoms: A network meta-analysis: J Affect Disord. 2021;293:205–213. doi:10.1016/j.jad.2021.06.034

Yatham MS, Yatham KS, Ravindran AV, et al. Do statins have an effect on depressive symptoms? A systematic review and meta-analysis. J Affect Disord. 2019;257:55–63. doi:10.1016/j.jad.2019.07.002

Cannabinoids

Nabilone

Nabilone and dronabinol are synthetic cannabinoids that activate cannabinoid receptor type 1 (CB1) cell receptors (abundantly expressed in the CNS). Nabiximols is partially purified medicinal cannabis extract containing $\triangle^9$-THC and CBD at a 1:1 ratio (see information on hallucinogens and cannabinoids in Drugs of Abuse chapter p. 377)

Cannabis Withdrawal	
	• Approximately 30% of regular cannabis users report withdrawal symptoms on cessation of prolonged use, such as irritability, insomnia, decreased appetite, depressed mood, anxiety, and restlessness. Among highly dependent and/or in-treatment users, the withdrawal incidence can be up to 50–95%
	• Dose: Nabilone 0.5 mg/day for 7 days, then 1 mg/day for 7 days, then 1.5 mg/day for 7 days, then 2 mg/day for 4 weeks before tapering the medication over the final 3 weeks by reversing the titration schedule
	• A review of 10 trials demonstrated that the use of dronabinol, nabilone, or nabiximols, either alone or in combination with other drugs, shows promise in reducing cannabis withdrawal symptoms, probably with a dose-dependent effect; nabiximols was used in spray form in 4 studies with an average dose of 28.9 sprays/day (equivalent to 77.5 mg THC or 71.7 mg CBD) to 40 sprays/day (equivalent to 108 mg THC or 100 mg CBD), and all trials reported lower withdrawal rates, better tolerance, and higher retention rates in the experimental group
	• Side effects reported include nausea, vomiting, and sedation

Hill KP, Palastro MD, Gruber SA, et al. Nabilone pharmacotherapy for cannabis dependence: A randomized, controlled pilot study. Am J Addict. 2017;26(8):795–801. doi:10.1111/ajad.12622

Khan R, Naveed S, Mian N, e al. The therapeutic role of cannabidiol in mental health: A systematic review. J Cannabis Res. 2020;2(1):2. doi:10.1186/s42238-019-0012-y

Werneck MA, Kortas GT, de Andrade AG, et al. A systematic review of the efficacy of cannabinoid agonist replacement therapy for cannabis withdrawal symptoms. CNS Drugs. 2018;32(12):1113–1129. doi:10.1007/s40263-018-0577-6

Posttraumatic Stress Disorder	

- Cohort studies and reviews suggest that different medicinal cannabinoids (cannabidiol (CBD), Δ^9-tetrahydrocannabinol (Δ^9-THC), and nabilone) at distinct doses and formulations could represent promising treatment strategies for the improvement of overall PTSD symptomatology as well as specific symptom domains (e.g., sleep disorders, arousal disturbances, suicidal thoughts), also influencing quality of life, pain, and social impact
- Dose: Nabilone 0.5–6 mg/day; dronabinol 7.5–10 mg; nabiximols spray
- An RCT and an open label study of nabilone demonstrated positive outcomes in the treatment of PTSD-related symptoms. In the open trial, 72% of study participants reported total cessation or lessening of severity of recurrent nightmares and some noted reduction in PTSD-related flashbacks and improved sleep time
- In 4 of 5 studies, dronabinol induced significant changes in extinction-related autonomic or behavioral responses, with medium to large effect sizes (i.e., from 0.55–0.81)
- Most commonly reported adverse effects were sedation, dry mouth, and feeling "stoned." Psychosis was reported in two individuals with a previous medical history of psychosis

Cowling T, MacDougall D. Nabilone for the treatment of post-traumatic stress disorder: A review of clinical effectiveness and guidelines [internet]. Ottawa (ON): Canadian Agency for Drugs and Technologies in Health; 2019. CADTH Rapid Response Reports. Retrieved from https://www.ncbi.nlm.nih.gov/books/NBK546995/

Rehman Y, Saini A, Huang S, et al. Cannabis in the management of PTSD: A systematic review. AIMS Neurosci. 2021;8(3):414–434. doi:10.3934/Neuroscience.2021022

Steardo L Jr, Carbone EA, Menculini G, et al. Endocannabinoid system as therapeutic target of PTSD: A systematic review. Life (Basel). 2021;11(3):214. doi:10.3390/life11030214

Dopaminergic Agents

Armodafinil

R-enantiomer of modafinil. See modafinil section for mechanism of action

Bipolar Disorder	

- Dose: 150–200 mg/day
- Double-blind placebo-controlled studies in patients with bipolar I depression found that adjunctive armodafinil improved symptoms and outcome measures of depression; a review of the literature shows odds ratio of 1.47 for armodafinil/modafinil
- A meta-analysis of RCTs of bipolar disorder I patients showed that augmentation with armodafinil was associated with significantly greater rates of treatment response
- A meta-analysis of 6 studies provides some evidence in support of modafinil and armodafinil (as well as lisdexamfetamine) as adjunctive agents in bipolar depression. They were more likely to induce remission from an episode of resistant bipolar depression than placebo, but did not differ statistically from placebo in terms of response (response rate ranged from 16% to 38% in the placebo arm and from 30% to 55% in the active treatment arm)
- Side effects included headache, nausea, diarrhea, anxiety, and insomnia
- Weak inducer of CYP1A2 and CYP3A4; weak inhibitor of CYP2C19. Drug interaction reported with carbamazepine via mutual induction of CYP3A4

Bartoli F, Cavaleri D, Bachi B, et al. Repurposed drugs as adjunctive treatments for mania and bipolar depression: A meta-review and critical appraisal of meta-analyses of randomized placebo-controlled trials. J Psychiatr Res. 2021;143:230–238. doi:10.1016/j.jpsychires.2021.09.018

Darwish M, Bond M, Yang R, et al. Evaluation of the potential for pharmacokinetic drug-drug interaction between armodafinil and carbamazepine in healthy adults. Clin Ther. 2015;37(2):325–337. doi:10.1016/j.clinthera.2014.09.014

McIntyre RS, Lee Y, Zhou AJ, et al. The efficacy of psychostimulants in major depressive episodes: A systematic review and meta-analysis. J Clin Psychopharmacol. 2017;37(4):412–418. doi:10.1097/JCP.0000000000000723

Nunez NA, Singh B, Romo-Nava F, et al. Efficacy and tolerability of adjunctive modafinil/armodafinil in bipolar depression: A meta-analysis of randomized controlled trials. Bipolar Disord. 2020;22(2):109–120. doi:10.1111/bdi.12859

Dopaminergic Agents (cont.)

Szmulewicz AG, Angriman F, Samamé C, et al. Dopaminergic agents in the treatment of bipolar depression: A systematic review and meta-analysis. Acta Psychiatr Scand. 2017;135(6):527–538. doi:10.1111/acps.12712

Tsapakis EM, Preti A, Mintzas MD, et al. Adjunctive treatment with psychostimulants and stimulant-like drugs for resistant bipolar depression: A systematic review and meta-analysis. CNS Spectr. 2020:1–12. doi:10.1017/S109285292000156X

Modafinil

The exact mechanism of action is unclear. Studies have shown it to increase the levels of dopamine in the striatum and nucleus accumbens, norepinephrine in the hypothalamus and ventrolateral preoptic nucleus, and serotonin in the amygdala and frontal cortex. Modafinil and armodafinil both activate glutamatergic, GABAergic, histaminergic, and orexin/hypocretin pathways, and mechanistically function, in part, as dopamine reuptake inhibitors

Depression

- Dose: 100–400 mg/day
- Review of double-blind, open label, and retrospective studies suggests modafinil may improve residual fatigue and sedation in patients receiving antidepressants; may enhance executive function, decrease sleepiness, and improve concentration, mood, and motivation
- Double-blind and open-label studies showed benefit in patients with atypical depression
- A meta-analysis concluded significant benefits of modafinil augmentation on improvements in overall depression scores and remission rates in patients with unipolar major depressive disorder and bipolar depression; a significant positive effect was seen on fatigue symptoms
- Main side effects include headache and nausea; weight loss reported
- Has a low abuse potential
- Weak inducer of CYP1A2, 2B6, and 3A4; may decrease levels of drugs metabolized by these enzymes

Kleeblatt J, Betzler F, Kilarski LL, et al. Efficacy of off-label augmentation in unipolar depression: A systematic review of the evidence. Eur Neuropsychopharmacol. 2017;27(5):423–441. doi:10.1016/j.euroneuro.2017.03.003

Nuñez NA, Joseph B, Pahwa M, et al. Augmentation strategies for treatment resistant major depression: A systematic review and network meta-analysis. J Affect Disord. 2022;302:385–400. doi:10.1016/j.jad.2021.12.134

Vaccarino SR, McInerney SJ, Kennedy SH, et al. The potential procognitive effects of modafinil in major depressive disorder: A systematic review. J Clin Psychiatry. 2019;80(6):19r12767. doi:10.4088/JCP.19r12767

Bipolar Disorder

- A meta-analysis of 6 studies provides some evidence in support of modafinil and armodafinil (as well as lisdexamfetamine) as adjunctive agents in bipolar depression. They were more likely to induce remission from an episode of resistant bipolar depression than placebo, but did not differ statistically from placebo in terms of response (response rate ranged from 16%–38% in the placebo arm and from 30%–55% in the active treatment arm)
- Placebo-controlled trials suggest modafinil plus a mood stabilizer may be more effective for treating bipolar depression without increasing the risk of mania
- Case report of modafinil-induced psychosis in a patient with bipolar I depression, after 2 days on 100 mg dose

Bartoli F, Cavaleri D, Bachi B, et al. Repurposed drugs as adjunctive treatments for mania and bipolar depression: A meta-review and critical appraisal of meta-analyses of randomized placebo-controlled trials. J Psychiatr Res. 2021;143:230–238. doi:10.1016/j.jpsychires.2021.09.018

Tsapakis EM, Preti A, Mintzas MD, et al. Adjunctive treatment with psychostimulants and stimulant-like drugs for resistant bipolar depression: A systematic review and meta-analysis. CNS Spectr. 2020:1–12. doi:10.1017/S109285292000156X

Pramipexole

D_2/D_3 dopamine receptor agonist; neuroprotective and exerts beneficial effects on sleep architecture

Depression

- Dose: 0.375–3 mg/day
- A systematic review of 5 RCTs, 3 open-label trials, and 5 observational studies of pramipexole, with 504 participants with unipolar or bipolar depression, found an overall short-term response rate of 52.2% and remission rate of 36.1%, and an overall long-term response rate of 62.1% and remission rate of 39.6%. In the RCTs, patients treated with pramipexole had a superior response rate compared with placebo and similar to SSRIs

- A review of open and one double-blind studies suggests efficacy in bipolar and unipolar depression, used alone or in combination with TCAs or SSRIs; has a large effect size (0.6–1.1) with a low short-term rate of manic switching in bipolar patients (1% mania and 5% hypomania)
- Pramipexole reported to augment antidepressants in 116 treatment-refractory patients; 37 (32%) with bipolar disorder and 79 (68%) with major depressive disorder (MDD), who failed to respond to at least 2 antidepressant trials of different classes. 74.1% of patients responded ($\geq 50\%$ reduction of baseline Hamilton Depression Rating Scale total score) and 66.4% remitted (Hamilton Depression Rating Scale total score < 7). Global Assessment of Functioning score significantly increased from 53 (50–60) at baseline to 80 (71–81) at 24 weeks. Ten patients (8.6%) dropped out (8 due to side effects and 2 for lack of efficacy) and one experienced an induced hypomanic switch
- Positive response reported in a comparative retrospective study assessing the efficacy and safety of pramipexole in the treatment of 14 patients with resistant depression, in combination with ECT or after a partial response to ECT; one patient became hypomanic
- Several controlled studies and meta-analyses have shown pramipexole to be effective for depression in patients with Parkinson's disease; however, caution should be taken when prescribing dopamine agonists as they can predispose to impulse control problems
- High incidence of nausea; sedation and dizziness reported; reports of compulsive behaviors and psychosis

Escalona R, Fawcett J. Pramipexole in treatment-resistant depression, possible role of inflammatory cytokines. Neuropsychopharmacology. 2017;42(1):363. doi:10.1038/npp.2016.217

Fawcett J, Rush AJ, Vukelich J, et al. Clinical experience with high-dosage pramipexole in patients with treatment-resistant depressive episodes in unipolar and bipolar depression. Am J Psychiatry. 2016;173(2):107–111. doi:10.1176/appi.ajp.2015.15060788

Gauthier C, Souaiby L, Advenier-Iakovlev E, et al. Pramipexole and electroconvulsive therapy in treatment-resistant depression. Clin Neuropharmacol. 2017;40(6):264–267. doi:10.1097/WNF.0000000000000253

Tundo A, de Filippis R, De Crescenzo F. Pramipexole in the treatment of unipolar and bipolar depression. A systematic review and meta-analysis. Acta Psychiatr Scand. 2019;140(2):116–125. doi:10.1111/acps.13055

Bipolar Disorder

- A comprehensive appraisal of the comparative efficacy of adjunctive pharmacotherapies for acute bipolar depression reported that adjunctive pramipexole outperformed placebo; pramipexole was more effective in reducing depression severity in BD-II
- Case report of benefit in the treatment of refractory depression, in combination with mood stabilizers, in a patient with rapid cycling bipolar disorder
- Double-blind study showed improvement in 60% of bipolar II depressed patients when pramipexole added to lithium therapy

Bahji A, Ermacora D, Stephenson C, et al. Comparative efficacy and tolerability of adjunctive pharmacotherapies for acute bipolar depression: A systematic review and network meta-analysis. Can J Psychiatry. 2021;66(3):274–288. doi:10.1177/0706743720970857

Bartoli F, Cavaleri D, Bachi B, et al. Repurposed drugs as adjunctive treatments for mania and bipolar depression: A meta-review and critical appraisal of meta-analyses of randomized placebo-controlled trials. J Psychiatr Res. 2021;143:230–238. doi:10.1016/j.jpsychires.2021.09.018

Hegde A, Singh A, Ravi M, et al. Pramipexole in the treatment of refractory depression in a patient with rapid cycling bipolar disorder. Indian J Psychol Med. 2015; 37(4):473–474. doi:10.4103/0253-7176.168614

GABA Agents/Anticonvulsants

Baclofen

GABA$_B$ receptor agonist

Alcohol Use Disorder

- Usual dose: 30 mg; up to 400 mg/day used in refractory patients (Caution: A daily dose higher than 180 mg is proposed as a limit beyond which additional precautions should be taken, such as close monitoring; CNS and respiratory depression are the main symptoms following acute baclofen overdose with prolonged coma and seizures, with some deaths reported)
- Contradictory results reported in the treatment of alcohol dependence; superiority over placebo not demonstrated in some studies nor in a recent meta-analysis. Out of 16 RCTs in which the effect of baclofen was studied, 7 showed a significant positive effect of baclofen on (one or more of the) primary outcome measures; more effective in promoting abstinence than reducing heavy drinking
- Recommended as second-line therapy, at a dose of 300 mg to prevent relapse and reduce drinking, in the 2015 Recommendations of the French Alcohol Society, issued in partnership with the European Federation of Addiction Societies; approved for treatment of AUD in France

GABA Agents/Anticonvulsants (cont.)

- The marked heterogeneity in response to baclofen in the treatment of alcohol dependence is suggested to be due to high pharmacokinetic variability (GABBR1 rs29220 polymorphism which may also predict adverse effects to baclofen)
- May be particularly useful in patients with liver disease, for whom certain other pharmacologic interventions are relatively contraindicated
- Caution due to possible mood elevating properties and abuse potential
- Main adverse effects include drowsiness, dizziness, euphoria, depression, headache, paraesthesias, speech disorders, ataxia, and insomnia – increased with higher doses

Burnette EM, Nieto SJ, Grodin EN, et al. Novel agents for the pharmacological treatment of alcohol use disorder. Drugs. 2022;82(3):251–274. doi:10.1007/s40265-021-01670-3

Ghosh S, Bhuyan D. Baclofen abuse due to its hypomanic effect in patients with alcohol dependence and comorbid major depressive disorder. Clin Psychopharmacol Neurosci. 2017;15(2):187–189. doi:10.9758/cpn.2017.15.2.187

Liu J, Wang LN. Baclofen for alcohol withdrawal. Cochrane Database Syst Rev. 2017;(8):CD008502. doi:10.1002/14651858.CD008502.pub5

Minozzi S, Saulle R, Rösner S. Baclofen for alcohol use disorder. Cochrane Database Syst Rev. 2018;26(11):CD012557. doi:10.1002/14651858.CD012557.pub2

Neven A, Dumont GJH. [The efficacy of baclofen in alcohol dependence] (Article in Dutch). Tijdschr Psychiatr. 2019;61(8):544–553.

Palpacuer C, Duprez R, Huneau A, et al. Pharmacologically controlled drinking in the treatment of alcohol dependence or alcohol use disorders: A systematic review with direct and network meta-analyses on nalmefene, naltrexone, acamprosate, baclofen and topiramate. Addiction. 2018;113(2):220–237. doi:10.1111/add.13974

Reynaud M, Aubin HJ, Trinquet F, et al. A randomized, placebo-controlled study of high-dose baclofen in alcohol-dependent patients – the ALPADIR study. Alcohol Alcohol. 2017;52(4):439–446. doi:10.1093/alcalc/agx030

Rolland B, Paille F, Gillet C, et al. Pharmacotherapy for alcohol dependence: The 2015 recommendations of the French Alcohol Society, issued in partnership with the European Federation of Addiction Societies. See comment in PubMed Commons below CNS Neurosci Ther. 2016;22(1):25–37. doi:10.1111/cns.12489

Pregabalin

Pregabalin binds to the $\alpha_2\delta$ subunit of the voltage-dependent calcium channel and thus reduces calcium influx into the nerve terminals; also decreases the release of glutamate, noradrenaline, and substance P; it increases neuronal GABA levels by producing a dose-dependent increase in glutamic acid decarboxylase activity (the enzyme that converts glutamic acid to GABA)

Anxiety Disorders

- Dose: 150–700 mg/day; suggested that plateau reached at 300 mg
- Meta-analysis suggests benefit in generalized anxiety disorder; considered effective against psychological and somatic anxiety symptoms and improves sleep maintenance; considered a first-line agent for the long-term treatment of GAD by the World Federation of Societies of Biological Psychiatry. Patients with early response to pregabalin are more likely to respond significantly at endpoint
- Meta-analysis suggests that pregabalin is significantly more effective than placebo across a range of disorders within the anxiety spectrum, including generalized anxiety disorder, social anxiety disorder, and pre-operative anxiety; benefit seen as augmentation drug for OCD and PTSD
- Double-blind studies suggest that perioperative pregabalin (1 or 2 doses of 150 mg) can decrease preoperative anxiety, improve sleep quality, and reduce postoperative pain scores and analgesic usage
- A retrospective study of 33 patients with anxiety secondary to major neurocognitive disorders showed that pregabalin doses of 50–700 mg/day decreased concomitant benzodiazepine use from 78.8% to 33.3%. No pregabalin treatment was discontinued for lack of efficacy or for tolerance
- Onset of action occurs in about 1 week and is maintained long term
- Efficacy comparable to benzodiazepines and venlafaxine, with less cognitive and psychomotor impairment than benzodiazepines
- Transient sedation and dizziness reported; weight gain
- Mild withdrawal symptoms observed – withdraw gradually, over at least a week
- **Caution: Can produce euphoria; reports of misuse, abuse or dependence in substance-seeking individuals**

Hong JSW, Atkinson LZ, Al-Juffali N, et al. Gabapentin and pregabalin in bipolar disorder, anxiety states, and insomnia: Systematic review, meta-analysis, and rationale. Mol Psychiatry. 2022;27(3):1339–1349. doi:10.1038/s41380-021-01386-6

Montgomery SA, Lyndon G, Almas M, et al. Early improvement with pregabalin predicts endpoint response in patients with generalized anxiety disorder: An integrated and predictive data analysis. Int Clin Psychopharmacol. 2017;32(1):41–48. doi:10.1097/YIC.0000000000000144

Novais T, Doutone A, Gombault C, et al. Description of the treatment course by pregabalin for anxiety in patients with a major neurocognitive disorder. J Clin Psychopharmacol. 2019;39(3):261–263. doi:10.1097/JCP.0000000000001029

Schjerning O, Rosenzweig M, Pottegård A, et al. Abuse potential of pregabalin: A systematic review. CNS Drugs. 2016;30(1):9–25. doi:10.1007/s40263-015-0303-6

Alcohol Use Disorder	

- Dose: 150–600 mg/day; higher doses used in withdrawal treatment studies
- A review of studies shows beneficial effects for alcohol relapse prevention; contradictory results seen for the treatment of withdrawal syndrome; greater benefits seen in patients with comorbid generalized anxiety disorder
- A double-blind, placebo-controlled trial reported decreased heavy drinking days, decreased total alcohol consumption, and increased sober days in the pregabalin group (dose 150 mg/day); no significant differences seen between the two groups in the scores on alcohol craving, depression, and anxiety scales
- A double-blind comparison study with naltrexone demonstrated that pregabalin showed greater benefit on symptoms of anxiety, hostility, psychosis, and abstinence; better outcomes were seen in patients with comorbid psychiatric disorders
- Limited evidence supports a role of pregabalin in the treatment of physical dependence and accompanying withdrawal symptoms associated with opioids, benzodiazepines, nicotine, cannabinoids, and alcohol
- Trial of pregabalin in detoxification from alcohol showed reduced symptoms of withdrawal and of craving; improvement in psychiatric symptoms reported
- Common adverse effects include drowsiness, fogginess, dizziness, and insomnia
- **Caution: Potential for misuse, abuse, dependence, and withdrawal in predisposed individuals**

Evoy KE, Morrison MD, Saklad SR. Abuse and misuse of pregabalin and gabapentin. Drugs. 2017;77(4):403–426. doi:10.1007/s40265-017-0700-x

Freynhagen R, Backonja M, Schug S, et al. Pregabalin for the treatment of drug and alcohol withdrawal symptoms: A comprehensive review. CNS Drugs. 2016;30(12):1191–1200. doi:10.1007/s40263-016-0390-z

Gimeno C, Dorado ML, Roncero C, et al. Treatment of comorbid alcohol dependence and anxiety disorder: Review of the scientific evidence and recommendations for treatment. Front Psychiatry. 2017;8:173. doi:10.3389/fpsyt.2017.00173

Schjerning O, Rosenzweig M, Pottegård A, et al. Abuse potential of pregabalin: A systematic review. CNS Drugs. 2016;30(1):9–25. doi:10.1007/s40263-015-0303-6

Sodium Oxybate

The active metabolite of sodium oxybate is gamma-hydroxybutyric acid (GHB) and acts as an agonist at the $GABA_B$ receptor complex and the GHB receptor

Alcohol Use Disorder	

- Dose: 50 mg/kg tid
- Approved for treatment of AUD in Austria and Italy
- Results of randomized controlled trials indicate that sodium oxybate is at least as effective as diazepam and clomethiazole in patients with alcohol withdrawal syndrome, rapidly alleviating symptoms, and at least as effective as naltrexone or disulfiram in the maintenance of abstinence in alcohol-dependent patients
- Report on 7 patients treated with sodium oxybate, in combination with nalmefene 18 mg/day, described that during the first month of combined treatment, two patients were able to achieve alcohol abstinence, 5 were able to suppress and 2 to reduce episodes of heavy drinking days, while one patient had decreased cravings
- Data from published studies suggest sodium oxybate may be more effective for patients with very high drinking rate level; abstinence rates improved as compared to placebo
- May be more effective when used in combination with other pharmacotherapies, including disulfiram, nalmefene, or naltrexone/escitalopram
- Not effective against hallucinations in alcohol withdrawal
- Caution: Craving and dependence may limit use. Patients with alcohol dependence and borderline personality disorder or who are in remission from heroin or cocaine addiction, may not be suitable candidates for sodium oxybate therapy because of an increased risk of abuse

Caputo F, Maremmani AG, Addolorato G, et al. Sodium oxybate plus nalmefene for the treatment of alcohol use disorder: A case series. J Psychopharmacol. 2016;30(4):402–409. doi:10.1177/0269881116629126

Mannucci C, Pichini S, Spagnolo EV, et al. Sodium oxybate therapy for alcohol withdrawal syndrome and keeping of alcohol abstinence. Curr Drug Metab. 2018;19(13):1056–1064. doi:10.2174/1389200219666171207122227

Skala K, Caputo F, Mirijello A, et al. Sodium oxybate in the treatment of alcohol dependence: From the alcohol withdrawal syndrome to the alcohol relapse prevention. Expert Opin Pharmacother. 2014;15(2):245–257. doi:10.1517/14656566.2014.863278

van den Brink W, Addolorato G, Aubin HJ, et al. Efficacy and safety of sodium oxybate in alcohol-dependent patients with a very high drinking risk level. Addict Biol. 2018;23(4):969–986. doi:10.1111/adb.12645

Hormones

Estrogens & Progesterone	*Estrogens* increase central bioavailability of norepinephrine, serotonin, and acetylcholine; may increase binding sites on platelets for antidepressants; estrogens also alter dopamine synthesis, increase its turnover, and modulate dopamine receptor sensitivity. Estrogens, especially 17β-estradiol, have immunomodulatory effects by regulating innate immune signaling pathways and modulating inflammatory elements such as cytokines. *Phytoestrogens* (naturally occurring, polyphenolic, non-steroidal plant compounds that are structurally similar to 17β-estradiol and have estrogenic and/or antiestrogenic effects) act as estrogen agonists without any currently known detrimental effects. *Progesterone* enhances serotonergic activity (chronic estrogen use augments activity of progesterone in CNS)

Depression	• Dose: Transdermal estrogen 100 micrograms/day; conjugated estrogens 0.625 mg/day for 21 days followed by progesterone 5 mg/day; phytoestrogens 25–100 mg/day

- A number of studies report estrogen therapy to be effective in improving mood in perimenopausal women; negative results seen in a randomized, double-blind, parallel study. Efficacy for overt depression or during postmenopause is questionable
- A double-blind study showed that for recently postmenopausal women, hormone replacement therapy did not alter cognition as hypothesized; however, beneficial mood effects with small–medium effect size were noted after 4 years of use of conjugated equine estrogens, but not after 4 years of transdermal estradiol
- A double-blind study demonstrated that 12 months of transdermal estradiol (0.1 mg/day) plus oral micronized progesterone (200 mg/day for 12 days given every 3 months) were more effective than placebo in preventing the development of clinically significant depressive symptoms among initially euthymic perimenopausal and early postmenopausal women
- A systematic review and meta-analysis reports that phytoestrogens can relieve depressive symptoms among postmenopausal women who take low doses (25 mg/day ≤ dose ≤ 100 mg/day) for a long-term duration
- A review and meta-analysis reports that longer exposure to endogenous estrogens (i.e., later menopause and a longer reproductive period) is associated with a lower risk of depression in later life; growing evidence from basic and clinical research suggests that fluctuations in ovarian hormones and derived neurosteroids result in alterations in regulation of the HPA axis by GABA, generating greater vulnerability to depression
- Maximum clinical effect may take up to 4 weeks

Dwyer JB, Aftab A, Radhakrishnan R, et al. Hormonal treatments for major depressive disorder: State of the art. Am J Psychiatry. 2020;177(8):686–705. doi:10.1176/appi.ajp.2020.19080848

Georgakis MK, Thomopoulos TP, Diamantaras AA, et al. Association of age at menopause and duration of reproductive period with depression after menopause: A systematic review and meta-analysis. JAMA Psychiatry. 2016;73(2):139–149. doi:10.1001/jamapsychiatry.2015.2653

Gleason CE, Dowling NM, Wharton W, et al. Effects of hormone therapy on cognition and mood in recently postmenopausal women: Findings from the randomized, controlled KEEPS-cognitive and affective study. PLoS Med. 2015;12(6):e1001833. doi:10.1371/journal.pmed.1001833

Gordon JL, Rubinow DR, Eisenlohr-Moul TA, et al. Efficacy of transdermal estradiol and micronized progesterone in the prevention of depressive symptoms in the menopause transition: A randomized clinical trial. JAMA Psychiatry. 2018;75(2):149–157. doi:10.1001/jamapsychiatry.2017.3998

Kleeblatt J, Betzler F, Kilarski LL, et al. Efficacy of off-label augmentation in unipolar depression: A systematic review of the evidence. Eur Neuropsychopharmacol. 2017;27(5):423–441. doi:10.1016/j.euroneuro.2017.03.003

Li J, Li H, Yan P, et al. Efficacy and safety of phytoestrogens in the treatment of perimenopausal and postmenopausal depressive disorders: A systematic review and meta-analysis. Int J Clin Pract. 2021;75(10):e14360. doi:10.1111/ijcp.14360

Slopien R, Slopien A, Warenik-Szymankiewicz A. Serum prolactin concentration and severity of depression symptoms in climacteric women. Clin Exp Obstet Gynecol. 2015;42(6):749–751.

Dementia	• Estrogen promotes cholinergic activity, reduces neuronal loss, improves blood flow, has anti-inflammatory properties, and reduces cholesterol. Estradiol serves as a neurotrophomodulatory substance for basal forebrain cholinergic neurons thought to be involved in learning and memory

- Postmenopausal women treated with estrogens alone, or in combination with progestin, were found to have higher resting cortisol concentrations than controls matched for time of day. Basal cortisol was a modest predictor of learning and memory; higher cortisol was associated with better recall and fewer memory errors
- A meta-analysis confirmed that estrogen replacement therapy decreases the risk of onset and/or development of not only AD but also PD. Some findings, however, put in doubt the use of estrogens not only in the prevention of AD but also in hormone replacement therapy; an increased risk of AD and PD was observed in elderly women treated with estrogens and increased mortality was also indicated

- Recent reviews indicate that the positive outcome of HRT in AD may depend on such factors as age of starting hormone treatment, the duration of hormone administration, and an individual's risk of developing cancer and/or stroke
- Emerging results seem to suggest that timing of estrogen use may be important; short-term hormone replacement near menopause onset may offer a reasonable strategy to impede development of dementia. Timing of hormone treatment initiation was significantly associated with mini mental status, with higher scores for women who initiated hormone therapy within 5 years of menopause compared with those initiating hormone treatment 6-or-more years later. Longer endogenous estrogen exposure was also associated with higher cognitive status in late life
- The association between endogenous sex hormones and both objective and subjective measures of cognitive function was studied in 3,044 women who were followed up to 23 years in a prospective cohort study. Plasma levels of estrone, estrone sulfate, estradiol, androstenedione, testosterone, dehydroepiandrosterone (DHEA), and dehydroepiandrosterone sulfate (DHEA-S) were measured between 1989 and 1990, neuropsychologic testing was done between 1999 and 2008, and patients were asked about subjective cognition in 2012; there were no clear associations of endogenous hormone levels at midlife and cognition in later life, although a suggested finding of higher levels of plasma estrone was associated with better cognitive function
- A retrospective analysis of 489,105 Finnish women on postmenopausal hormone therapy (HT) showed that risk of death from vascular dementia was reduced by 37–39% (less than 5 or $\geq$ 5 years of exposure) with the use of any systemic HT (estradiol only or estradiol-progestin combination), as compared to non-users. Risk of death from Alzheimer's disease was not reduced with systemic HT use less than 5 years, but was slightly reduced (15%) if HT exposure exceeded 5 years. Age at systemic HT initiation (under 60 vs. $\geq$ 60 years) did not affect the death risk reductions

Engler-Chiurazzi EB, Singh M, Simpkins JW. From the 90's to now: A brief historical perspective on more than two decades of estrogen neuroprotection. Brain Res. 2016;1633:96–100. doi:10.1016/j.brainres.2015.12.044

Hampson E, Duff-Canning SJ. Salivary cortisol and explicit memory in postmenopausal women using hormone replacement therapy. Psychoneuroendocrinology. 2016;64:99–107. doi: 10.1016/j.psyneuen.2015.11.009

Li J, Li H, Yan P, et al. Efficacy and safety of phytoestrogens in the treatment of perimenopausal and postmenopausal depressive disorders: A systematic review and meta-analysis. Int J Clin Pract. 2021;75(10):e14360. doi:10.1111/ijcp.14360

Matyi JM, Rattinger GB, Schwartz S, et al. Lifetime estrogen exposure and cognition in late life: The Cache County Study. Menopause. 2019;26(12):1366–1374. doi:10.1097/GME. 0000000000001405

Mikkola TS, Savolainen-Peltonen H, Tuomikoski P, et al. Lower death risk for vascular dementia than for Alzheimer's disease with postmenopausal hormone therapy users. J Clin Endocrinol Metab. 2017;102(3):870–877. doi:10.1210/jc.2016-3590

Pike CJ. Sex and the development of Alzheimer's disease. J Neurosci Res. 2017; 95(1–2):671–680. doi:10.1002/jnr.23827

Uchoa MF, Moser VA, Pike CJ. Interactions between inflammation, sex steroids, and Alzheimer's disease risk factors. Front Neuroendocrinol. 2016;43:60–82. doi:10.1016/j.yfrne.2016.09. 001

Wu M, Li M, Yuan J, et al. Postmenopausal hormone therapy and Alzheimer's disease, dementia, and Parkinson's disease: A systematic review and time-response meta-analysis. Pharmacol Res. 2020;11:104693. doi:10.1016/j.phrs.2020.104693

Schizophrenia

- Dose: Conjugated estrogens 0.625 mg/day; estradiol oral 50–200 micrograms/day; 17β-estradiol transdermal 100–200 micrograms/day
- Estrogens regulate important pathophysiological pathways and have neuroprotective effects in schizophrenia, including dopamine activity, COMT, mitochondrial function, and the stress response system
- The observation that women have a later onset and lesser symptoms of schizophrenia, and that there is a spike in diagnosis after menopause, has led to the hypothesis that estrogens may have a protective role; premenopausal women generally require lower doses of an antipsychotic during high estrogenic phases of the menstrual cycle as estrogens increase the availability and efficacy of antipsychotics; a decline in antipsychotic efficacy has been noted after menopause
- A literature review showed that estrogen augmentation demonstrated significant benefits in patients with schizophrenia for overall, positive, and negative symptoms. Subgroup analyses yielded significant results for estrogens in premenopausal women for overall, positive, and negative symptoms
- A review of the literature suggests that add-on hormone therapy during the perimenopause in women with schizophrenia ameliorates psychotic and cognitive symptoms, and may also help affective symptoms. Vasomotor, genitourinary, and sleep symptoms are also reduced
- A randomized study of 180 female participants (aged 18–45 years) with schizophrenia and ongoing symptoms of psychosis (PANSS score higher than 60) despite a stable dose of antipsychotic medication, found a fluctuating but overall trend towards improvement of comorbid depressive symptoms in women taking transdermal estrogen 200 micrograms compared with estrogen 100 micrograms or placebo

Hormones (cont.)

- Transdermal estradiol (200 micrograms) was reported to be an effective add-on treatment for women of childbearing age with schizophrenia; significant improvements in the primary outcome measure, PANSS positive subscale, occurred almost entirely in 100 participants older than 38 years; adjunctive transdermal estradiol showed promise as a treatment for women with comorbid depression and schizophrenia
- Side effects included breast tenderness. Consider the risk of breast cancer, thromboembolic events, and cardiovascular disease

Çakici N, van Beveren NJM, Judge-Hundal G, et al. An update on the efficacy of anti-inflammatory agents for patients with schizophrenia: A meta-analysis. Psychol Med. 2019;49(14):2307–2319. doi:10.1017/S0033291719001995

Lascurain MB, Camuñas-Palacín A, Thomas N, et al. Improvement in depression with oestrogen treatment in women with schizophrenia. Arch Womens Ment Health. 2020;23(2):149–154. doi:10.1007/s00737-019-00959-3

McGregor C, Riordan A, Thornton J. Estrogens and the cognitive symptoms of schizophrenia: Possible neuroprotective mechanisms. Front Neuroendocrinol. 2017;47:19–33. doi:10.1016/j.yfrne.2017.06.003

Searles S, Makarewicz JA, Dumas JA. The role of estradiol in schizophrenia diagnosis and symptoms in postmenopausal women. Schizophr Res. 2018;196:35–38. doi:10.1016/j.schres.2017.05.024

Trifu SC, Istrate D, Miruna DA. Gaps or links between hormonal therapy and schizophrenia? (Review). Exp Ther Med. 2020;20(4):3508–3512. doi:10.3892/etm.2020.9017

Weiser M, Levi L, Zamora D, et al. Effect of adjunctive estradiol on schizophrenia among women of childbearing age: A randomized clinical trial. JAMA Psychiatry. 2019;76(10):1009–1017. doi:10.1001/jamapsychiatry.2019.1842

Raloxifene

Selective estrogen receptor modulator. Binds estrogen receptor alpha (ESR-α), improves memory and attention, and normalizes cortical and hippocampal activity

Schizophrenia

- Dose: 60–120 mg/day
- Review of published studies of adjunctive raloxifene in males and females with schizophrenia shows mixed results in restoring cognition or reducing symptom severity; benefits may be related to patient's age, dosage, and duration of treatment. Menopause status (pre-menopausal, peri-menopausal or post-menopausal) as well as menstrual cycle irregularities may influence results on cognition
- Adjunctive raloxifene treatment shown to have beneficial effects on attention/processing speed and memory for both men and women with schizophrenia; negative results reported in a 24-week, double-blind, randomized, placebo-controlled study of raloxifene (60 mg/day) as an adjuvant treatment for cognitive symptoms in postmenopausal women with schizophrenia
- Double-blind placebo-controlled studies report contradictory results with raloxifene (120 mg/day) augmentation of antipsychotics in postmenopausal women: Negative results seen in severely decompensated patients with schizophrenia, while positive results reported in refractory schizophrenia
- Consideration: Small increase in the risk of venous thromboembolism and endometrial cancer

Gurvich C, Hudaib A, Gavrilidis E, et al. Raloxifene as a treatment for cognition in women with schizophrenia: The influence of menopause status. Psychoneuroendocrinology. 2019;100:113–119. doi:10.1016/j.psyneuen.2018.10.001

Kulkarni J, Gavrilidis E, Gwini SM, et al. Effect of adjunctive raloxifene therapy on severity of refractory schizophrenia in women: A randomized clinical trial. JAMA Psychiatry. 2016;73(9):947–954. doi:10.1001/jamapsychiatry.2016.1383

Weiser M, Levi L, Burshtein S, et al. Raloxifene plus antipsychotics versus placebo plus antipsychotics in severely ill decompensated postmenopausal women with schizophrenia or schizoaffective disorder: A randomized controlled trial. J Clin Psychiatry. 2017 Jul;78(7):e758–e765. doi:10.4088/JCP.15m10498

Zhu XM, Zheng W, Li XH, et al. Adjunctive raloxifene for postmenopausal women with schizophrenia: A meta-analysis of randomized, double-blind, placebo-controlled trials. Schizophr Res. 2018;197:288–293. doi:10.1016/j.schres.2018.01.017

Tamoxifen

Selective estrogen receptor modulator. Competitively binds to estrogen receptors and inhibits the intracellular action of protein kinase C

Bipolar Disorder

- A review of 5 placebo-controlled RCTs of tamoxifen used alone or in combination with lithium or valproate for the treatment of mania reported benefit over placebo in symptom reduction at 4–6 weeks

Bartoli F, Cavaleri D, Bachi B, et al. Repurposed drugs as adjunctive treatments for mania and bipolar depression: A meta-review and critical appraisal of meta-analyses of randomized placebo-controlled trials. J Psychiatr Res. 2021;143:230–238. doi:10.1016/j.jpsychires.2021.09.018

Palacios J, Yildiz A, Young AH, et al. Tamoxifen for bipolar disorder: Systematic review and meta-analysis. J Psychopharmacol. 2019;33(2):177–184. doi:10.1177/0269881118822167

Testosterone	**Testosterone is a modulator of GABA$_A$ receptors and inhibits 5-HT$_3$ receptors centrally**

Depression

- Testosterone concentrations (total, free, and bioavailable) reported to be lower in males over the age of 45 with MDD; no association found in elderly females
- Dose: 400 mg IM every 2 weeks; testosterone transdermal gel 1% (10 mg/day), dehydroepiandrosterone (DHEA) 30–50 mg/day; route of administration may play a role in treatment response
- High rate (i.e., 56%) of depression and depressive symptoms diagnosed in men referred for borderline testosterone levels
- A systematic review investigated the effect of testosterone replacement therapy (TRT) on depressive symptoms in patients with late-onset testosterone deficiency. TRT improved depressive symptoms in most trials, except in patients with MDD
- A prospective longitudinal study of 3,179 older men, free of clinically significant depressive symptoms at baseline, showed that low serum total testosterone, but not calculated free testosterone, was associated with incident depression over 8.4–10.9 years
- Meta-analysis of data showed a significant positive impact of testosterone on mood; effect more significant in men under age 60, and the effect size was larger in subthreshold depression compared with major depression
- Data suggests benefit as augmentation strategy in men with low-normal serum testosterone refractory to SSRIs
- A study of 103 women showed an association between postpartum depression and persistently high serum testosterone levels 24–28 h following childbirth (as compared to controls); estradiol and progesterone levels did not show significant differences; in the context of menopause, a high testosterone-to-estradiol ratio is associated with higher frequency of depressive symptoms
- An 8-week randomized, double-blind, placebo-controlled trial of adjunctive testosterone cream in 101 women, aged 21–70 years with antidepressant-resistant major depression, reported that testosterone, although well tolerated, was not more effective than placebo in improving symptoms of depression, fatigue, or sexual dysfunction

Aswathi A, Rajendiren S, Nimesh A, et al. High serum testosterone levels during postpartum period are associated with postpartum depression. Asian J Psychiatr. 2015;17:85–88. doi: 10.1016/j.ajp.2015.08.008

Caldiroli A, Capuzzi E, Tagliabue I, et al. Augmentative pharmacological strategies in treatment-resistant major depression: A comprehensive review. Int J Mol Sci. 2021;22(23):13070. doi:10.3390/ijms222313070

Dwyer JB, Aftab A, Radhakrishnan R, et al. Hormonal treatments for major depressive disorder: State of the art. Am J Psychiatry. 2020;177(8):686–705. doi:10.1176/appi.ajp.2020.19080848

Giltay EJ, van der Mast RC, Lauwen E, et al. Plasma testosterone and the course of major depressive disorder in older men and women. Am J Geriatr Psychiatry. 2017;25(4):425–437. doi:10.1016/j.jagp.2016.12.014

Kleeblatt J, Betzler F, Kilarski LL, et al. Efficacy of off-label augmentation in unipolar depression: A systematic review of the evidence. Eur Neuropsychopharmacol. 2017;27(5):423–441. doi:10.1016/j.euroneuro.2017.03.003

Vartolomei MD, Kimura S, Vartolomei L, et al. Systematic review of the impact of testosterone replacement therapy on depression in patients with late-onset testosterone deficiency. Eur Urol Focus. 2020;6(1):170–177. doi:10.1016/j.euf.2018.07.006

Dementia

- Normal age-related testosterone loss in men is associated with increased risk for several diseases; limited preclinical and clinical evidence suggests that testosterone can be involved in the pathogenesis of age-dependent cognitive impairment
- A meta-analysis of 27 studies with 18,599 participants revealed inconsistent findings on the association between testosterone levels and the risk of all-cause dementia or AD; overall, an increased risk of all-cause dementia with decreasing total testosterone (total-T; 4,572 participants). Some studies also found an increased risk of AD with lower levels of total-T, free testosterone, and bioavailable testosterone
- Testosterone administration in hypogonadal men with AD and cognitive impairment has shown variable results. Several studies showed that testosterone administration improved memory and cognition in AD while others did not find any benefit
- Levels of testosterone, dihydrotestosterone, estradiol, estrone, SHBG, LH, and FSH were measured in men aged 70 years and older at baseline (2005–2007; 1,705 participants), 2-year follow-up (2007–2009; 1,367 participants), and 5-year follow-up (2010–2013; 958 participants); a change in all the studied hormones, except for estradiol was significantly associated with cognitive decline. Men who had dementia at baseline had significantly greater decline in serum testosterone levels

Hormones (cont.)

Ford AH, Yeap BB, Flicker L, et al. Sex hormones and incident dementia in older men: The health in men study. Psychoneuroendocrinology. 2018;98:139–147. doi:10.1016/j.psyneuen.2018.08.013

Pike CJ. Sex and the development of Alzheimer's disease. J Neurosci Res. 2017; 95(1–2): 671–680. doi:10.1002/jnr.23827

Uchoa MF, Moser VA, Pike CJ. Interactions between inflammation, sex steroids, and Alzheimer's disease risk factors. Front Neuroendocrinol. 2016;43:60–82. doi:10.1016/j.yfrne.2016.09.001

Zhang Z, Kang D, Li H. Testosterone and cognitive impairment or dementia in middle-aged or aging males: Causation and intervention, a systematic review and meta-analysis. J Geriatr Psychiatry Neurol. 2021;34(5):405–417. doi:10.1177/0891988720933351

NMDA Agents (Glutamatergic Modulators)

D-Cycloserine	Acts as a "super agonist" at NMDA receptors containing GluN2C subunits and, under certain conditions, may act as an antagonist at NMDA receptors containing GluN2B subunits
Anxiety Disorders	• Studies in animals and clinical trials in patients with anxiety disorders have demonstrated that single or intermittent dosing with D-cycloserine enhances memory consolidation • Dose: 50–500 mg/day • Mixed results seen. Individual studies have reported promising results but meta-analyses question the benefit of D-cycloserine in augmenting the effects of cognitive and behavioral therapies in the treatment of anxiety disorders in adults, children, and adolescents, including PTSD, panic disorder, social anxiety disorder, specific phobia, and OCD; efficacy is not moderated by the concurrent use of antidepressants • A meta-analysis of studies suggests that D-cycloserine may increase the speed or efficiency of exposure treatment; administering D-cycloserine more than 60 min before exposures, and giving more doses (this advantage leveled off at 9 doses) appear to be related to better outcomes • Early data suggests intermittent therapy may decrease anxiety, improve negative symptoms of schizophrenia, and enhance learning when combined with cognitive behavioral therapy for delusions or with cognitive remediation • May help maintain social skills training in autism spectrum disorder • Adverse effects include sedation, headache, increased anxiety, and restlessness

Bürkner PC, Bittner N, Holling H, et al. D-cycloserine augmentation of behavior therapy for anxiety and obsessive-compulsive disorders: A meta-analysis. PLoS One. 2017;12(3):e0173660. doi:10.1371/journal.pone.0173660

Garakani A, Murrough JW, Freire RC, et al. Pharmacotherapy of anxiety disorders: Current and emerging treatment options. Front Psychiatry. 2020;11:595584. doi:10.3389/fpsyt.2020.595584

Goff DC. D-cycloserine in schizophrenia: New strategies for improving clinical outcomes by enhancing plasticity. Curr Neuropharmacol. 2017;15(1):21–34. doi:10.2174/1570159X14666160225154812

Hofmeijer-Sevink MK, Duits P, Rijkeboer MM, et al. No effects of D-cycloserine enhancement in exposure with response prevention therapy in panic disorder with agoraphobia: A double-blind, randomized controlled Trial. J Clin Psychopharmacol. 2017;37(5):531–539. doi:10.1097/JCP.0000000000000757

Mataix-Cols D, Fernández de la Cruz L, Monzani B, et al. D-cycloserine augmentation of exposure-based cognitive behavior therapy for anxiety, obsessive-compulsive, and posttraumatic stress disorders: A systematic review and meta-analysis of individual participant data. JAMA Psychiatry. 2017;74(5):501–510. doi:10.1001/jamapsychiatry.2016.3955

McGuire JF, Wu MS, Piacentini J, et al. A meta-analysis of D-cycloserine in exposure-based treatment: Moderators of treatment efficacy, response, and diagnostic remission. J Clin Psychiatry. 2017;78(2):196–206. doi:10.4088/JCP.15r10334

Wink LK, Minshawi NF, Shaffer RC, et al. D-cycloserine enhances durability of social skills training in autism spectrum disorder. Mol Autism. 2017;8:2. doi:10.1186/s13229-017-0116-1

Dextromethorphan-Quinidine (DM-Q)	Dextromethorphan is an NMDA receptor antagonist. Quinidine inhibits the rapid first-pass metabolism of DM, thus increasing its plasma level and CNS bioavailability; approved in the USA (Nuedexta) for treatment for pseudobulbar affect (PBA: uncontrollable episodes of crying and/or laughing)
Dementia	• Agitation and aggression scores were significantly reduced in a double-blind placebo-controlled study of patients with probable Alzheimer's disease; scores also reduced when patients on placebo were provided active drug • Open-label study showed DM-Q significantly reduced pseudobulbar affect symptoms in patients with dementia • Adverse events included falls, headache, urinary tract infection, and diarrhea; the medication was not associated with cognitive impairment, sedation, or clinically significant QTc prolongation Aftab A, Lam JA, Liu F, et al. Recent developments in geriatric psychopharmacology. Expert Rev Clin Pharmacol. 2021;14(3):341–355. doi:10.1080/17512433.2021.1882848 Doody RS, D'Amico S, Cutler AJ, et al. An open-label study to assess safety, tolerability, and effectiveness of dextromethorphan/quinidine for pseudobulbar affect in dementia: PRISM II results. CNS Spectr. 2016;21(6):450–459. doi:10.1017/S1092852915000620 Tampi RR, Joshi P, Marpuri P, et al. Evidence for using dextromethorphan-quinidine for the treatment of agitation in dementia. World J Psychiatry. 2020;10(4):29–33. doi:10.5498/wjp.v10.i4.29

Ketamine	NMDA receptor non-competitive antagonist; has a complex pharmacological profile, including anti-inflammatory action, and affects numerous receptors; antidepressant effects appear to involve the facilitation of glutamatergic neurotransmission in the prefrontal cortex; elevated baseline levels of cytokine IL-6 predicts better treatment response to ketamine Ketamine is controlled under Schedule I of the Controlled Drugs and Substances Act in Canada; spray must be compounded intranasal esketamine (Spravato – the S(+) enantiomer of ketamine) is approved for adults with treatment-resistant depression or major depression with acute suicidal ideation or behaviour (see p. 80)
Anxiety Disorders	• A double-blind, psychoactive-controlled ascending dose study (12 participants) was conducted in patients with treatment-resistant generalized anxiety and social anxiety disorder who were not currently depressed. Ascending doses of ketamine (0.25, 0.5, and 1 mg/kg) were administered at weekly intervals, and midazolam 0.01 mg/kg (the control) was randomly inserted into the ketamine dose sequence. Dose-response improvements in anxiety ratings occurred within an hour of ketamine dosing and persisted for up to 1 week. A dose-response effect was also noted for dissociative side effects as well as changes in blood pressure and heart rate • In a maintenance treatment study of 20 patients with treatment-refractory generalized anxiety disorder and/or social anxiety disorder who received 3 months of weekly ketamine (1 mg/kg injected subcutaneously 2 times/week). Fear Questionnaire ratings decreased by approximately 50%, as did Hamilton Anxiety ratings. 18 patients reported improved social functioning and/or work functioning during maintenance treatment. The most common adverse events were nausea, dizziness, and blurred vision; post-dose dissociative symptoms tended to reduce after repeated dosing • A double-blind RCT of intravenously administered ketamine at 0.5 mg/kg, compared with saline placebo, showed benefit in patients with social anxiety disorder measured using the Liebowitz Social Anxiety Scale • Ketamine via IV infusion reported to significantly improve obsessive-compulsive symptomatology, with effects that are rapid (occurring in hours to minutes) but short-lasting (days to weeks); concurrent cognitive behavior therapy or deep brain stimulation may prolong the effects of ketamine Glue P, Neehoff S, Sabadel A, et al. Effects of ketamine in patients with treatment-refractory generalized anxiety and social anxiety disorders: Exploratory double-blind psychoactive-controlled replication study. J Psychopharmacol. 2020;34(3):267–272. doi:10.1177/0269881119874457 Glue P, Neehoff SM, Medlicott NJ, et al. Safety and efficacy of maintenance ketamine treatment in patients with treatment-refractory generalised anxiety and social anxiety disorders. J Psychopharmacol. 2018;32(6):663–667. doi:10.1177/0269881118762073
Depression	• Dose: Ketamine 0.1–0.75 mg/kg administered over 2–100 min (use as a single sub-anesthetic intravenous infusion); intranasal dose: 50–80 mg q 2–3 days; sublingual syrup 8–16 mg/day; other routes include: oral, transmucosal, intramuscular, and subcutaneous • One study that compared esketamine (0.25 mg/kg) and RS-ketamine (0.5 mg/kg) found no differences in efficacy, tolerability, or psychotomimetic profile between the two agents • Evidence supports rapid antidepressant effects of ketamine as a single or augmentation treatment in major depressive disorder; in bipolar depression and in depression with suicidal ideation; ketamine has demonstrated efficacy in the rapid reduction of suicidal symptoms • Appears to directly target core depressive symptoms such as sad mood, suicidality, helplessness, and worthlessness rather than inducing a nonspecific mood-elevating effect; when compared to ECT, ketamine reported to improve neurocognitive functioning, especially attention and executive functions, whereas ECT was related to a small overall decrease in cognitive performance • Has been used, in combination with propofol, during ECT treatment with variable response

NMDA Agents (Glutamatergic Modulators) (cont.)

- Antidepressant effects are transient (observed within hours of administration, peak after about a day, and relapse reported within 3–21 days after single or multiple use); benefits can be maintained for weeks to months by continuation of ketamine sessions at 2- to 4-day intervals; case series suggests that D-cycloserine may prolong the initial clinical response after ketamine
- Repeated infusions of IV ketamine (up to 0.75 mg/kg) have been used to augment current therapy for treatment-resistant depression with some short-lived response reported; time to relapse after varying doses (0.1, 0.5, or 1.0 mg/kg) of a single administration of IV ketamine was dose related; suggested that repeated infusions may offer better response than single infusion
- Data from a trial of ketamine, given as 4 infusions over 1–2 weeks to 105 treatment-resistant women, reported rapid antidepressant response in 26% of postmenopausal women and 30% of premenopausal women, and an overall remission rate of 13%; postmenopausal women experienced anti-suicidal effects more rapidly than premenopausal women, while premenopausal women experienced improvement in social function more rapidly
- Side effects include transient increase in blood pressure and heart rate, light-headedness, sedation, confusion, emotional blunting, and dissociative symptoms; acute impairments of working, episodic, and semantic memory have been reported in recreational users as well as healthy volunteers and may persist with chronic use. Case report of mania in patient with unipolar major depression. Anxiety-related experiences induced by ketamine reported to be significantly higher in nonresponders
- Drugs that induce CYP2B6 and CYP3A4 may reduce exposure to ketamine whilst drugs that inhibit these enzymes may increase exposure to ketamine; concurrent benzodiazepines may diminish the antidepressant benefits of ketamine, drugs that inhibit glutamatergic signaling (such as lamotrigine) may reduce the adverse effects of ketamine
- Concerns exist regarding the potential for abuse of ketamine; case report of MDD following chronic abuse of ketamine

Andrade C. Ketamine for depression, 5: Potential pharmacokinetic and pharmacodynamic drug interactions. J Clin Psychiatry. 2017;78(7):e858–e861. doi:10.4088/JCP.17f11802

Basso L, Bönke L, Aust S, et al. Antidepressant and neurocognitive effects of serial ketamine administration versus ECT in depressed patients. J Psychiatr Res. 2020;123:1–8. doi:10.1016/j.jpsychires.2020.01.002

Caldiroli A, Capuzzi E, Tagliabue I, et al. Augmentative pharmacological strategies in treatment-resistant major depression: A comprehensive review. Int J Mol Sci. 2021;22(23):13070. doi:10.3390/ijms222313070

Cusin C, Ionescu DF, Pavone KJ, et al. Ketamine augmentation for outpatients with treatment-resistant depression: Preliminary evidence for two-step intravenous dose escalation. See comment in PubMed Commons below Aust N Z J Psychiatry. 2017;51(1):55–64. doi:10.1177/0004867416631828

Dean RL, Hurducas C, Hawton K, et al. Ketamine and other glutamate receptor modulators for depression in adults with unipolar major depressive disorder. Cochrane Database Syst Rev. 2021;9(9):CD011612. doi:10.1002/14651858.CD011612.pub3

Henter ID, Park LT, Zarate CA Jr. Novel glutamatergic modulators for the treatment of mood disorders: Current status. CNS Drugs. 2021;35(5):527–543. doi:10.1007/s40263-021-00816-x

McIntyre RS, Rosenblat JD, Nemeroff CB, et al. Synthesizing the evidence for ketamine and esketamine in treatment-resistant depression: An international expert opinion on the available evidence and implementation. Am J Psychiatry. 2021;178(5):383–399. doi:10.1176/appi.ajp.2020.20081251

Swainson J, McGirr A, Blier P, et al. The Canadian Network for Mood and Anxiety Treatments (CANMAT) Task Force Recommendations for the use of racemic ketamine in adults with major depressive disorder: Recommandations Du Groupe De Travail Du Réseau Canadien Pour Les Traitements De L'humeur Et De L'anxiété (Canmat) concernant l'utilisation de la kétamine racémique chez les adultes souffrant de trouble dépressif majeur. Can J Psychiatry. 2021;66(2):113–125. doi:10.1177/0706743720970860

Pharmacy Connection. Intranasal ketamine and esketamine for treatment resistant depression [internet]. Toronto (ON): The Ontario College of Pharmacists; 2021. The Official Digital Publication of the Ontario College of Pharmacists. Retrieved from https://pharmacyconnection.ca/intranasal-ketamine-and-esketamine-for-treatment-resistant-depression-winter-2021/

Pregnenolone	Neurosteroid; modulates excitatory glutaminergic NMDA receptors (reduces the response of the GABA$_A$ receptor). It is precursor for other steroid hormones and exerts its own effect as an anti-inflammatory molecule to maintain immune homeostasis in various inflammatory conditions
Schizophrenia	• Dose: 30–50 mg/day • Data contradictory; early studies suggested promise as an adjunctive treatment in schizophrenia and schizoaffective disorder; improvement noted in both positive and negative symptoms • Low-dose (30 mg/day) augmentation also demonstrated significant amelioration of EPS and improvement in attention and working memory performance; visual learning/memory and attention were the cognitive domains that significantly improved in a meta-analysis

- A double-blind study using pregnenolone 50 mg with L-theanine 400 mg (vs. placebo) to augment current antipsychotics in patients with chronic schizophrenia or schizoaffective disorder demonstrated significant improvement in negative symptoms such as blunted affect, alogia, and anhedonia. Add-on pregnenolone/L-theanine also was significantly associated with a reduction of anxiety scores related to such as anxious mood, tension, and cardiovascular symptoms as well as an increase in general functioning
- Four trials assessed the effect of add-on pregnenolone therapy in 101 patients with schizophrenia. Add-on pregnenolone therapy was more effective than antipsychotic monotherapy in reducing PANSS total scores, while its effect on positive and negative symptom scores was not statistically significant
- Negative results reported in a randomized double-blind clinical trial of 82 female inpatients with chronic schizophrenia

Cai H, Cao T, Zhou X, et al. Neurosteroids in schizophrenia: Pathogenic and therapeutic implications. Front Psychiatry. 2018;9:73. doi:10.3389/fpsyt.2018.00073

Kardashev A, Ratner Y, Ritsner MS. Add-on pregnenolone with L-theanine to antipsychotic therapy relieves negative and anxiety symptoms of schizophrenia: An 8-week, randomized, double-blind, placebo-controlled trial. Clin Schizophr Relat Psychoses. 2015 Jul 28. [Epub ahead of print]. doi:10.3371/CSRP.KARA.070415

Kashani L, Shams N, Moazen-Zadeh E, et al. Pregnenolone as an adjunct to risperidone for treatment of women with schizophrenia: A randomized double-blind placebo-controlled clinical trial. J Psychiatr Res. 2017;94:70–77. doi:10.1016/j.jpsychires.2017.06.011

Ľupták M, Michaličková D, Fišar Z, et al. Novel approaches in schizophrenia – From risk factors and hypotheses to novel drug targets. World J Psychiatry. 2021;11(7):277–296. doi:10.5498/wjp.v11.i7.277

Riluzole

Riluzole (1) inactivates voltage-dependent sodium channels on glutamatergic nerve terminals, thereby blocking glutamatergic neurotransmission, (2) blocks some of the postsynaptic effects of glutamic acid by noncompetitive blockade of the NMDA receptors, and (3) blocks GABA reuptake

Anxiety Disorders

- Dose: 50–100 mg bid
- Quantitative analysis of 7 RCTs revealed positive but nonsignificant effects of riluzole (as compared to placebo) on OCD and depression. Open-label study, case series, and double-blind study suggest benefit of riluzole augmentation in adults with treatment-refractory OCD; data contradictory as in another double-blind study, clinical improvement was not found to be statistically significant though a trend towards benefit was seen in secondary analysis. No benefit reported when used, at a maximum dose of 100 mg/day, to augment therapy in children with OCD
- Augmentation of an SSRI or SNRI may selectively improve hyperarousal symptoms in patients with PTSD without changes in overall PTSD symptoms, depression, anxiety, or disability
- Open-label studies have shown efficacy as sole treatment or augmenting agent in GAD
- Riluzole is well tolerated by adults and children; common side effects include headache, nausea, fatigue, and sedation. Elevations in transaminase levels reported but none resulted in drug discontinuation; pancreatitis reported in children
- Increased riluzole serum levels reported in co-therapy with CYP1A2 inhibitors (e.g., fluvoxamine)

de Boer JN, Vingerhoets C, Hirdes M, et al. Efficacy and tolerability of riluzole in psychiatric disorders: A systematic review and preliminary meta-analysis. Psychiatry Res. 2019;278:294–302. doi:10.1016/j.psychres.2019.06.020

Emamzadehfard S, Kamaloo A, Paydary K, et al. Riluzole in augmentation of fluvoxamine for moderate to severe obsessive-compulsive disorder: Randomized, double-blind, placebo-controlled study. Psychiatry Clin Neurosci. 2016;70(8):332–341. doi:10.1111/pcn.12394

Grant P, Farmer C, Song J, et al. Riluzole serum concentration in pediatric patients treated for obsessive-compulsive disorder. J Clin Psychopharmacol. 2017;37(6):713–716. doi:10.1097/JCP.0000000000000797

Mechler K, Häge A, Schweinfurth N, et al. Glutamatergic agents in the treatment of compulsivity and impulsivity in child and adolescent psychiatry: A systematic review of the literature. Z Kinder Jugendpsychiatr Psychother. 2018;46(3):246–263. doi:10.1024/1422-4917/a000546

Pittenger C, Bloch MH, Wasylink S, et al. Riluzole augmentation in treatment-refractory obsessive-compulsive disorder: A pilot randomized placebo-controlled trial. J Clin Psychiatry. 2015;76(8):1075–1084. doi:10.4088/JCP.14m09123

Depression

- Dose: 50–200 mg/day
- Quantitative analysis of 7 RCTs revealed positive but nonsignificant effects of riluzole (as compared to placebo) on OCD and depression
- No change in severity of depressive symptoms reported in a double-blind placebo-controlled study of patients with bipolar depression receiving riluzole compared with placebo. In a recent meta-analysis of 7 RCTs, riluzole showed no antidepressant efficacy compared to placebo in monotherapy or riluzole–ketamine combined therapy; there was some difference in depression severity change in riluzole–citalopram therapy
- Increased riluzole serum levels reported with co-therapy with CYP1A2 inhibitors (e.g., fluvoxamine)

NMDA Agents (Glutamatergic Modulators) (cont.)

de Boer JN, Vingerhoets C, Hirdes M, et al. Efficacy and tolerability of riluzole in psychiatric disorders: A systematic review and preliminary meta-analysis. Psychiatry Res. 2019;278:294–302. doi:10.1016/j.psychres.2019.06.020

Park LT, Lener MS, Hopkins M, et al. A double-blind, placebo-controlled, pilot study of riluzole monotherapy for acute bipolar depression. J Clin Psychopharmacol. 2017;37(3):355–358. doi:10.1097/JCP.0000000000000693

Yao R, Wang H, Yuan M, et al. Efficacy and safety of riluzole for depressive disorder: A systematic review and meta-analysis of randomized placebo-controlled trials. Psychiatry Res. 2020;284:112750. doi:10.1016/j.psychres.2020.112750

5-HT$_3$ Antagonists

Granisetron, Ondansetron, Tropisetron	**5-HT$_3$ receptor antagonists cause increased release of norepinephrine (NE), acetylcholine (ACh), and serotonin (5-HT) within various brain circuits**

Anxiety Disorders

- Dose: Ondansetron 1–8 mg/day; granisetron 1 mg bid
- Ondansetron has been used to augment SSRIs for OCD in several therapeutic studies, and granisetron in one trial. Both drugs showed some efficacy in open studies and superiority to placebo in double-blind studies. Superiority of ondansetron over granisetron was seen in a randomized, placebo-controlled, double-blind study

Andrade C. Ondansetron augmentation of serotonin reuptake inhibitors as a treatment strategy in obsessive-compulsive disorder. J Clin Psychiatry. 2015;76(1):e72–e75. doi:10.4088/JCP.14f09704

Serata D, Kotzalidis GD, Rapinesi C, et al. Are 5-HT3 antagonists effective in obsessive-compulsive disorder? A systematic review of literature. Hum Psychopharmacol. 2015;30(2):70–84. doi:10.1002/hup.2461

Schizophrenia

- Granisetron 1 mg bid, ondansetron 4–16 mg, or tropisetron 5–20 mg used in combination with antipsychotic
- Meta-analysis of 5-HT$_3$ antagonist studies in stable schizophrenia patients shows that augmentation is associated with significant reduction in negative symptoms, general psychopathology, and total symptom ratings without reduction in positive symptom ratings
- 5 RCTs that included 149 patients on ondansetron (4–8 mg/day) and 155 patients on placebo were analyzed. Adjunctive ondansetron outperformed placebo in the reduction of Positive and Negative Syndrome Scale total score as well as negative and general psychopathology symptom scores, but not in positive and depressive symptom scores. Ondansetron was also superior over placebo in improving extrapyramidal symptoms
- A systematic review reported that ondansetron and tropisetron (a 5-HT$_3$ antagonist and α_7 nicotinic receptor partial agonist) improved sensory gating in patients with schizophrenia. Tropisetron also improved sustained visual attention in nonsmoking patients
- Primary side effect was constipation with combination therapy

Andrade C. Nonsteroidal anti-inflammatory drugs and 5-HT3 serotonin receptor antagonists as innovative antipsychotic augmentation treatments for schizophrenia. J Clin Psychiatry. 2014;75(7):e707–e709. doi:10.4088/JCP.14f09292

Garay RP, Bourin M, de Paillette E, et al. Potential serotonergic agents for the treatment of schizophrenia. See comment in PubMed Commons below Expert Opin Investig Drugs. 2016;25(2):159–170. doi:10.1517/13543784.2016.1121995

Zheng W, Cai DB, Zhang QE et al. Adjunctive ondansetron for schizophrenia: A systematic review and meta-analysis of randomized controlled trials. J Psychiatr Res. 2019;113:27–33. doi:10.1016/j.jpsychires.2019.02.024

| **ACE inhibitors/ARBs** | **The renin-angiotensin pathway is suggested to be involved in mediating stress and anxiety, and possibly depression (in addition to its effect on cardiovascular regulation)** |

Anxiety Disorders

- The renin-angiotensin system has been directly implicated in the PTSD-CVD link due to its involvement in sympathetic arousal; may be important in PTSD, as ACE-inhibitor/ARB usage has been associated with lower symptoms. Individuals with the CC rs4311 genotype appear to benefit more with ACE-Inhibitors/ARBs
- Meta-analysis of 11 studies reported that when compared with placebo or other antihypertensive medications, ARBs and ACE inhibitors were associated with improved overall quality of life, positive wellbeing, and decreased anxiety
- Negative results reported in a placebo-controlled trial of losartan (flexibly titrated from 25 to 100 mg/day) for 10 weeks in 149 men and women meeting DSM-5 PTSD criteria

Brownstein DJ, Salagre E, Köhler C, et al. Blockade of the angiotensin system improves mental health domain of quality of life: A meta-analysis of randomized clinical trials. Aust N Z J Psychiatry. 2018;52(1):24–38. doi:10.1177/0004867417721654

Nylocks KM, Michopoulos V, Rothbaum AO, et al. An angiotensin-converting enzyme (ACE) polymorphism may mitigate the effects of angiotensin-pathway medications on posttraumatic stress symptoms. Am J Med Genet B Neuropsychiatr Genet. 2015;168B(4):307–315. doi:10.1002/ajmg.b.32313

Depression

- Preliminary evidence suggests a role for the renin-angiotensin system (RAS) in the pathophysiology of MDD; ACE inhibitors and ARBs suggested to reduce oxidative and inflammatory stress and enhance neurogenesis; findings strongly suggest that a hyperactive RAS seems to play a role in the pathophysiology of mood disorders; its relationship with the risk of suicide is unclear
- Case reports and observational studies show that ACE inhibitors and ARBs may have positive effects on depression, whereas other antihypertensive agents do not; no placebo-controlled double-blind studies to date
- Data contradictory; in a randomised placebo-controlled trial of citalopram in 284 coronary heart disease patients with MDD, the use of ACE inhibitors predicted a worse response to citalopram
- Patients with the ACE2 genetic variant (G8790A) showed a significantly better response to sertraline in a randomized controlled trial

Mohite S, Sanches M, Teixeira AL. Exploring the evidence implicating the renin-angiotensin system (RAS) in the physiopathology of mood disorders. Protein Pept Lett. 2020;27(6):449–455. doi:10.2174/0929866527666191223144000

| **Allopurinol** | **Xanthine oxidase inhibitor – suggested to increase adenosine, a neuromodulator of dopaminergic and glutamatergic systems. May have neuroprotective effect due to antioxidant properties** |

Bipolar Disorder

- Dose: 300 mg once daily or bid
- There is evidence of increased uric acid levels in drug-naïve subjects with bipolar disorder during their first manic episode; association between manic symptoms, uric acid excretion, hyperuricemia, and gout has been described
- A review of meta-analyses of randomized placebo-controlled trials reported that allopurinol demonstrates higher efficacy than placebo for symptom reduction and remission of mania, at 4–8 weeks, with low quality of evidence
- In patients with acute mania, the probability of remission after 4 weeks was 23 times higher in the treatment group (i.e., sodium valproate 15–20 mg/kg + 300 mg allopurinol twice a day) compared to the control group (i.e., sodium valproate 15–20 mg/kg + placebo)
- Two meta-analyses were done of 5 studies; suggest that allopurinol may have some efficacy as an adjunct in reducing mania symptoms during acute manic episodes, particularly in patients with a more severe form of mania
- A meta-analysis of 4 RCTs of allopurinol plus lithium vs. placebo plus lithium demonstrated no benefit in adults with bipolar disorder
- Negative results reported in double-blind study. In some studies, subjects with restricted caffeine use showed a greater effect size compared to caffeine users

Bartoli F, Cavaleri D, Bachi B, et al. Repurposed drugs as adjunctive treatments for mania and bipolar depression: A meta-review and critical appraisal of meta-analyses of randomized placebo-controlled trials. J Psychiatr Res. 2021;143:230–238. doi:10.1016/j.jpsychires.2021.09.018

Bartoli F, Crocamo C, Clerici M, et al. Allopurinol as add-on treatment for mania symptoms in bipolar disorder: Systematic review and meta-analysis of randomised controlled trials. Br J Psychiatry. 2017;210(1):10–15. doi:10.1192/bjp.bp.115.180281

Miscellaneous (cont.)

Butler M, Urosevic S, Desai P et al. Treatment for bipolar disorder in adults: A systematic review. Rockville (MD): Agency for Healthcare Research and Quality (US);2018;Report No.:18-EHC012-EF. AHRQ Comparative Effectiveness Reviews. Retrieved from https://www.ncbi.nlm.nih.gov/pubmed/30329241

Chen AT, Malmstrom T, Nasrallah HA. Allopurinol augmentation in acute mania: A meta-analysis of placebo-controlled trials. J Affect Disord. 2018;226:245–250. doi:10.1016/j.jad.2017.09.034

Nalmefene	**Opioid antagonist (a mu and delta receptor antagonist and partial agonist and a kappa-opioid receptor agonist/antagonist)**

Alcohol Use Disorder

- Dose: 18–20 mg/day prn
- Treatment is based on as-needed concept: Patients take one tablet (18 mg) each day they perceive a risk of drinking alcohol, preferably 1–2 h prior to anticipated time of drinking, but otherwise as soon as drinking has started. Maximum of 1 tablet per day
- Approved in the European Union to reduce alcohol consumption in alcohol-dependent adults with a high drinking risk level; currently approved for use as an injectable opioid antagonist in the USA
- As-needed use significantly reduced both the number of heavy drinking days and total alcohol consumption in alcohol-dependent patients with at least a high drinking risk level at screening and randomization; a single dose of nalmefene reduces the neuronal response to alcohol-associated stimuli in the ventral striatum and seems to influence neuronal brain responses responsible for reward-associated behavior
- An indirect meta-analysis indicates an advantage of nalmefene over naltrexone; another meta-analysis suggests limited efficacy of nalmefene; an RCT reported that alcohol-dependent patients who selectively benefit from nalmefene have prognostic factors, such as non-smoking status, no family history of problem drinking, and a late onset of problem drinking
- A case series suggests that the combination of nalmefene plus sodium oxybate may improve response
- Nalmefene must not be used in patients taking opioid medicines, in patients who have a current or recent addiction to opioids, patients with acute opioid withdrawal symptoms, or in patients suspected to have used opioids recently. It must also not be used in patients with severe liver or kidney impairment or a recent history of acute alcohol withdrawal syndrome (including hallucinations, seizures (fits), and tremors)
- Side effects include nausea, fatigue, and drowsiness/sleepiness. A patient with schizoaffective disorder showed decompensation of psychotic symptoms (consisting of auditory hallucinations, delusions, and ideas of persecution) after two doses of medication; the symptoms improved two days after treatment discontinuation

Brodtkorb TH, Bell M, Irving AH, et al. The cost effectiveness of nalmefene for reduction of alcohol consumption in alcohol-dependent patients with high or very high drinking-risk levels from a UK societal perspective. CNS Drugs. 2016;30(2):163–177. doi:10.1007/s40263-016-0310-2

Burnette EM, Nieto SJ, Grodin EN, et al. Novel agents for the pharmacological treatment of alcohol use disorder. Drugs. 2022;82(3):251–274. doi:10.1007/s40265-021-01670-3

Caputo F, Maremmani AG, Addolorato G, et al. Sodium oxybate plus nalmefene for the treatment of alcohol use disorder: A case series. J Psychopharmacol. 2016;30(4):402–409. doi:10.1177/0269881116629126

Castera P, Stewart E, Großkopf J, et al. Nalmefene, given as needed, in the routine treatment of patients with alcohol dependence: An interventional, open-label study in primary care. Eur Addict Res. 2018;24(6):293–303. doi:10.1159/000494692

Mann K, Torup L, Sørensen P, et al. Nalmefene for the management of alcohol dependence: Review on its pharmacology, mechanism of action and meta-analysis on its clinical efficacy. Eur Neuropsychopharmacol. 2016;26(12):1941–1949. doi:10.1016/j.euroneuro.2016.10.008

Palpacuer C, Laviolle B, Boussageon R, et al. Risks and benefits of nalmefene in the treatment of adult alcohol dependence: A systematic literature review and meta-analysis of published and unpublished double-blind randomized controlled trials. PLoS Med. 2015;12(12):e1001924. doi:10.1371/journal.pmed.1001924

Pimavanserin	**A 5-HT$_{2A}$ antagonist and inverse receptor agonist in the mesolimbic system; has minimal affinity for dopaminergic, muscarinic, histaminergic, and adrenergic receptors**

Depression

- 207 patients with MDD and an inadequate response to an SSRI or SNRI were randomized to receive augmentation with placebo or pimavanserin for 5 weeks; nonresponders to the placebo were re-randomized to receive placebo or pimavanserin for a further 5 weeks. At week 5 of Stage 1, LS mean (SE) difference for pimavanserin vs. placebo was significant for changes on the HDRS-17 and SDS with effect sizes of 0.626 and 0.498, respectively; adjunctive pimavanserin was associated with a significant improvement in anxious depression in patients with MDD. Pimavanserin augmentation also significantly improved sleep/wakefulness disturbance of MDD and alleviated sexual side effects of SSRIs and SNRIs

- In an 8-week, single-arm, open-label study, pimavanserin as monotherapy or adjunctive therapy was well tolerated and associated with early and sustained improvement of depressive symptoms in patients with PD
- Most common adverse events with pimavanserin were dry mouth, nausea, and headache
- Caution in renal impairment, pre-existing QT-interval prolongation or history of cardiac arrhythmia, and in combination with CYP3A4 inhibitors

Fava M, Dirks B, Freeman MP, et al. A phase 2, randomized, double-blind, placebo-controlled study of adjunctive pimavanserin in patients with major depressive disorder and an inadequate response to therapy (CLARITY). J Clin Psychiatry. 2019;80(6):19m12928. doi:10.4088/JCP.19m12928

| Dementia |

- In a phase 3, double-blind, randomized, placebo-controlled discontinuation trial involving patients with psychosis related to Alzheimer's disease, Parkinson's disease dementia, dementia with Lewy bodies, frontotemporal dementia, or vascular dementia, patients received open-label pimavanserin for 12 weeks. Those who had a reduction from baseline of at least 30% in the score on the Scale for the Assessment of Positive Symptoms–Hallucinations and Delusions were assigned to either continued pimavanserin or placebo for up to 26 weeks. A relapse occurred in 12 of 95 patients (13%) in the pimavanserin group and in 28 of 99 (28%) in the placebo group
- Efficacy reported in reducing delusions and hallucinations in Alzheimer's disease

Aftab A, Lam JA, Liu F, et al. Recent developments in geriatric psychopharmacology. Expert Rev Clin Pharmacol. 2021;14(3):341–355. doi:10.1080/17512433.2021.1882848

| Schizophrenia |

- Dose: 34 mg/day
- Approved in the USA for treatment of hallucinations and delusions associated with Parkinson's disease psychosis
- Unclear results reported in a retrospective cohort study comparing patients with PD or dementia with Lewy bodies initiated on quetiapine including 45 patients or pimavanserin with 47 patients for psychosis. Time-to-treatment discontinuation analysis, which accounted for efficacy, safety, and tolerability, revealed a lower early pimavanserin discontinuation rate and a higher late pimavanserin discontinuation rate
- A phase 2, 26-week, randomized, double-blind, placebo-controlled study of pimavanserin in stable outpatients with schizophrenia aged 18–55 years with predominant negative symptoms showed a significant reduction in negative symptoms

Bugarski-Kirola D, Arango C, Fava M, et al. Pimavanserin for negative symptoms of schizophrenia: Results from the ADVANCE phase 2 randomised, placebo-controlled trial in North America and Europe. Lancet Psychiatry. 2022;9(1):46–58. doi:10.1016/S2215-0366(21)00386-2

NATURAL HEALTH PRODUCTS

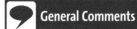

General Comments

Although pharmacotherapy is generally the first line of treatment for psychiatric disorders, an increasing number of patients are turning to natural health products (NHPs). Most NHP use is self-prescribed (60%) and undisclosed to health care providers (20–90%). In one study, 34% of users took NHPs to treat a mood disorder, while almost half of the users also took concurrent prescription medication. Another study found that 63% of patients hospitalized for psychiatric indications had used complementary alternative medicine (CAM) within the past year, with 79% of patients not disclosing their use to their psychiatrist. The widespread use of NHPs for mental illnesses makes it necessary for health care providers to understand their benefits and risks and look for relevant drug–NHP interactions.

In addition, clinical research has found that many mental health disorders are associated with an increase in central and peripheral markers of oxidative stress and inflammation. This makes it plausible that NHPs with antioxidant and anti-inflammatory properties may be of benefit in managing these conditions.

This chapter looks at the evidence and safety of some commonly used NHPs that are used for a variety of conditions. Although, in most cases, the optimum dose of the natural health product (herb or supplement) is not known, the most frequently studied dose is provided, along with the proposed mechanism of action.

Drug	ADHD	Alzheimer's Disease	Anxiety	Bipolar Disorder	Depression	Schizophrenia	Sleep Disorders
Ginkgo Biloba (p. 452)		C/+	PR/+			PR/S/+	
Kava Kava (p. 454)			C/+				
Melatonin (p. 455)							C/+
Omega-3 Fatty Acids (p. 457)	C/+	PR/+		C/S/+	C/S/+	C	
S-Adenosyl-L-Methionine (p. 459)					C/S/+		
St. John's wort (p. 460)			PR/C		+†		
Valerian (p. 462)			C/+				C/+
Vitamins (p. 463)							
Vitamin B		PR			PR/S	PR/+	
Vitamin B₉		PR			PR/S		
Vitamin C		PR/+				PR	
Vitamin D		PR			PR/C		
Vitamin E		C				PR/S	

† Mild to moderate depression only;
C = contradictory results, + = positive findings, PR = preliminary data, S = synergistic/adjunctive effect, SC = significant safety concerns

Ginkgo Biloba

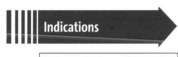

Indications

Alzheimer's Disease/Dementia

- Ginkgo has not been shown to prevent or slow down the progression of dementia or the risk of developing Alzheimer's disease (AD), but it may help to improve symptoms

- A 2022 meta-analysis concluded that 14 of the 20 (70%) clinical studies evaluated showed that ginkgo biloba extract (GBE) was able to improve cognitive ability of AD patients. Highlights:
  - GBE may be more effective in 'younger' populations (60–70 years), where AD-related damage is relatively mild
  - Using a higher dose (240 mg/day) for at least 24 weeks was shown to be more effective than using lower doses for a shorter period of time
  - Methodological quality of trials ranged from 3–7 (out of 9, using the CAMARADES list)
  - This meta-analysis supports a review done in 2020 which concluded that the optimal therapeutic effect of GBE was in patients taking ginkgo for at least 24 weeks at a minimum dose of 240 mg/day. It also concluded that EGb may be able to improve cognitive function in patients suffering from mild dementia
- Dementia prevention:
  - Ginkgo evaluation of memory study followed 3,069 participants above age 72 for over 6 years, who received EGb 761 (120 mg bid) or placebo; assessed cognitive decline, functional disability, incidence of CVD and stroke, and total mortality, and showed that ginkgo did not result in less cognitive decline and was ineffective in reducing the development of dementia and Alzheimer's disease
  - Patients complaining of cognitive decline were given EGb 761 (120 mg bid) or matched placebo and followed for 5 years. The risk of progression to Alzheimer's disease was comparable in both groups
- Compared to conventional therapy:
  - Although ginkgo has been shown to be as efficacious and tolerable as donepezil in the treatment of mild to moderate Alzheimer's disease, (160 mg EGb 761 extract; 20 participants) after 6 months, larger patient samples are required to confirm these findings
  - Patients suffering from Alzheimer's dementia were given ginkgo (120 mg/day) or rivastigmine (4.5 mg/day) for six months. Only patients taking the cholinesterase inhibitor reported significant improvements in Mini-Mental State Examination (MMSE) and Short Mental Test (SMT) scores

Anxiety Disorders	• A double-blind RCT (107 participants) using ginkgo extract EGb 761 for 4 weeks showed that participants' HAM-A total scores decreased significantly compared to placebo
Schizophrenia	• A review and meta-analysis suggested that the addition of ginkgo to antipsychotic therapy (haloperidol, chlorpromazine, clozapine) produces significant moderate improvement in total and negative symptoms of chronic schizophrenia (average length of study = 8 weeks) • Reported to be effective in reducing symptoms of tardive dyskinesia in patients with schizophrenia (AIMS total score reduced in 51.3% of patients)

General Comments

- Earliest use of ginkgo dates back to China 5,000 years ago
- Available by prescription in many parts of Europe
- Has been safely used for up to 6 years
- One of the most popular natural products used by the geriatric population

Pharmacology

- The constituents flavonoids and terpenoids are believed to be responsible for ginkgo's neuroprotective effects in AD, which include: antioxidation, anti-inflammation, protection against mitochondrial dysfunction and β-amyloid aggregation, and phosphorylation of the tau protein
- Also appears to increase vascular circulation and inhibit binding of platelet activating factor, decreasing blood coagulation
- Popular extract from ginkgo leaves (EGb 371) has exhibited neuroprotective effects, including protecting hippocampal neurons against cell death induced by β-amyloid

Dosing

- Alzheimer's disease:
  - Doses studied: 120–240 mg/day divided in 2–3 doses; best results seen at the higher doses
  - May take 6–8 weeks to see a clinical effect
- Anxiety: 240–480 mg/day used
- Schizophrenia:
  - Doses studied: 120–360 mg/day (given tid)
  - Most studies use ginkgo extracts EGb 761 or LI 1370. Both are similar and contain approximately 24–25% flavone glycosides and 6% terpene lactones

Ginkgo Biloba (cont.)

Adverse Effects

- Adverse effects are rare and may include: mild GI upset, headache, dizziness, palpitations, constipation, and allergic skin reactions
- Serious cases of bleeding reported; hence CAUTION with patients on anticoagulant/anti-platelet drugs; may increase bleeding times; clinical significance is controversial
- To avoid GI side effects, start at 120 mg

Drug Interactions

- Interactions: Inhibitor of CYP2C9 and inducer of CYP2C19 and CYP1A2; may interact with drugs metabolized by these isoenzymes: Decreases levels of omeprazole, ritonavir, and tolbutamide; may inhibit metabolism of warfarin; may potentiate drugs that lower the seizure threshold. Avoid with talinolol – shown to increase levels by 36% in one study

Further Reading

References
- Liu H, Ye M, Guo H. An updated review of randomized clinical trials testing the improvement of cognitive function of ginkgo biloba extract in healthy people and Alzheimer's patients. Front Pharmacol. 2020;10:1688. doi:10.3389/fphar.2019.01688
- Yuan Q, Wang C, Shi J, et al. Effects of Ginkgo biloba on dementia: An overview of systematic reviews. J Ethnopharmacol. 2017;195:1–9. doi:10.1016/j.jep.2016.12.005
- Xie L, Zhu Q, Lu J. Can we use ginkgo biloba extract to treat Alzheimer's disease? Lessons from preclinical and clinical studies. Cells. 2022;11(3):479. doi:10.3390/cells11030479

Kava Kava

Indications

Anxiety Disorders

- A number of meta-analyses over the years conclude that kava extract is an effective symptomatic treatment for anxiety when compared to placebo as shown by decreased HAM-A scores. A number of studies also suggest that kava extract must be taken for more than 5 weeks in order to see a benefit
- In a 2018 meta-analysis of 5 trials kava was reported to have been shown to be an effective treatment for short-term anxiety relief and that this may be more pronounced in patients who are younger (early–mid 40s) and female
- Kava was shown to be an effective treatment for short-term anxiety relief and that this may be more pronounced in patients who are younger (early–mid 40s) and female
- In 2020, a 16-week double-blind, randomized, placebo-controlled trial found that kava was no more effective than placebo in treating generalized anxiety disorder (GAD). The authors concluded that kava's therapeutic application as an anxiolytic may be more effective prior to a potential situational anxiogenic event, rather than as a clinical treatment option
- Compared to placebo, kava extract WS 1490 (200 mg daily) significantly improved sleep disturbances associated with anxiety in a 4-week randomized, placebo-controlled, double-blind study

General Comments

- Made from the rhizome, roots, and stem of *Piper methysticum*; active constituent kavalactones
- Used throughout the Pacific Islands as a ceremonial drink to induce relaxation and sleep and to decrease anxiety; may have anticonvulsant and muscle-relaxant activity
- Has been used safely in trials up to 24 weeks; however, more recent evidence suggests that use be limited to a maximum of 8 weeks

Pharmacology

- CNS effects appear to be mediated by the blockage of voltage-gated sodium and calcium channels, ultimately suppressing glutamate release
- The kavalactones desmethoxyyangonin and methysticin are believed to block MAO-B metabolism, producing psychotropic effects
- Sedative and antianxiety properties may result from kava's effects on facilitating GABA transmission by increasing the number of GABA sites

Dosing	• Most clinical trials have used kava extract standardized to 70% kavalactones; 300 mg divided in three doses (delivering 210 mg kavalactones/day)

Adverse Effects	• Adverse effects at lower doses are rare and transient. They include gastric discomfort, dizziness, and, with chronic use, yellow skin discoloration • Doses above 400 mg/day: Dry flaking skin, red eyes, facial puffiness, muscle weakness, dystonic reactions, dyskinesias, and choreoathetosis • Does not adversely affect cognition, mental acuity or coordination • **Caution:** There is some concern of hepatotoxicity with long-term use; it appears to be safe to use for short periods (under 8 weeks)

Drug Interactions	• Avoid concurrent use with CNS depressants (including alcohol and benzodiazepines), shown to increase side effects and toxicity • Preliminary evidence reports that Kava kava can inhibit CYP1A2, 2C9, 2C19, 2D6, 2E1, and 3A4, and may interact with levodopa, alprazolam, and paroxetine

Further Reading	**References** • Natural Medicines Database: Kava monograph. Retrieved from http://www.naturaldatabase.com • Sarris J, Byrne GJ, Bousman CA, et al. Kava for generalised anxiety disorder: A 16-week double-blind, randomised, placebo-controlled study. Aust N Z J Psychiatry. 2020;54(3):288–297. doi:10.1177/0004867419891246 • Smith K, Leiras C. The effectiveness and safety of Kava Kava for treating anxiety symptoms: A systematic review and analysis of randomized clinical trials. Complement Ther Clin Practice. 2018;33:107–117. doi:10.1016/j.ctcp.2018.09.003

Melatonin

 Indications

Sleep Disorders

- The circadian resetting effects of melatonin are well documented; however, exogenous melatonin on its own is not able to reset a patient's self-selected light/dark schedule. Rather, the timing of melatonin and light act in combination to achieve the desired resetting effect
- Effective for treating delayed sleep phase syndrome (DSPS) and improving non-24-hr sleep-wake disorder
- A 2022 meta-analysis (23 studies) reported on the use of melatonin for improving sleep quality (as assessed by the Pittsburgh Sleep Quality Index) in different disease states. Highlights:
  - Melatonin intervention significantly improved sleep quality in patients with primary sleep disorders, respiratory diseases, and metabolic disorders, but failed to find significance in patients with psychiatric disorders, neurodegenerative diseases, and other diseases
  - A high degree of heterogeneity was seen between studies, but was expected due to different health conditions, doses, and duration
- A 2019 meta-analysis demonstrated that melatonin significantly improved sleep in patients with primary sleep disorders compared to placebo:
  - Reduced sleep-onset latency by ~ 7–9 min
  - Increased total sleep time: 8.25 min
  - Improved sleep quality
  - Trials with longer duration and higher doses reported greater effects
- In primary insomnia, melatonin has been shown to decrease sleep latency over the short term (4 weeks or less) by approximately 15 min. Clinical significance is questionable
- An observational cohort study of 100 inpatients found that melatonin was as effective as zolpidem when rating sleep effectiveness and disturbance
- Fast-release melatonin (0.5 mg) given 1 h before bedtime, combined with behavioral sleep–wake scheduling, was more effective than placebo in helping people with DSPS. In a study with 104 participants, the melatonin group fell asleep on average 34 min earlier and had significant decreases in self-reported sleep disturbance, severity of insomnia, and interference with daily life compared to placebo
- May be more useful in the elderly (who sometimes have decreased nocturnal secretion of melatonin); found not to be effective in patients with sleep disturbances and dementia

Melatonin (cont.)

- May be helpful for medically ill patients with insomnia for whom conventional hypnotics may be problematic
- Case reports suggest melatonin may facilitate withdrawal from benzodiazepines (which can decrease nocturnal melatonin production)
- Early data suggest it may be beneficial in children with ADHD and in multi-disabled children (with neurological or behavioral disorders) with severe insomnia in doses of 2–10 mg, and in autism spectrum disorder

 General Comments

- Hormone produced by the pineal gland involved in regulation of circadian rhythms
- Circulating melatonin levels are consistently reduced in the metabolic syndrome, ischemic and non-ischemic cardiovascular diseases, and neurodegenerative disorders like Alzheimer's and Parkinson's disease[2]
- Effects may be larger when endogenous melatonin levels are low
- Also used for jet lag
- There is no well-known standardization for melatonin and many brands have been found to contain impurities as well as dissimilar amounts of actual hormone (http://www.consumerlab.com/ is a useful reference to look for brand quality)

 Pharmacology

- Synthesis and release of melatonin is stimulated by darkness and inhibited by light
- Acts on MT_1 and MT_2 receptors in the hypothalamic suprachiasmatic nuclei (master circadian clock site)
- Acts to reset the circadian clock and "trigger" the onset of sleep
- Melatonin levels typically peak between 2 and 4 a.m.; physiologically, levels are highest between 1 and 3 years of age

 Dosing

- Insomnia: 0.3–10 mg/day (0.3 mg = physiological dose) taken 30–120 min before bedtime; exogenous melatonin does not appear to affect endogenous production or secretion of melatonin. Lowest possible dose recommended
- Peak plasma concentrations achieved within 60 min; metabolized by the liver; elimination half-life = 20–50 min
- Immediate-release products may help individuals having difficulty falling asleep, while sustained-release or long-acting formulation is better for people having trouble staying asleep

 Adverse Effects

- Adverse effects are rare (likely safe when used for short duration at doses of 5 mg/day or less)
- Drowsiness is one of the most common side effects; patients should not drive or operate machinery after taking melatonin
- At higher doses: Abdominal cramps, headache, dizziness, daytime fatigue, and increased irritability
- At very high doses (more than 75 mg) can exacerbate depression, cause coagulation abnormalities, and inhibit ovulation

 Drug Interactions

- Caution in patients taking warfarin or other agents that affect coagulation; may increase sedative effects of CNS depressants (including benzodiazepines and alcohol)
- Drugs that inhibit CYP1A2 can increase plasma levels of melatonin; also, drugs that are metabolized by CYP1A2 can increase plasma levels of melatonin via competitive metabolism

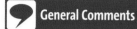 **Further Reading**

References
- Burgess HJ, Emens JS. Drugs used in circadian sleep-wake rhythm disturbances. Sleep Med Clin. 2020:15(2):301–310. doi:10.1016/j.jsmc.2020.02.015
- Cardinali DP. Melatonin and healthy aging. Vitam Horm. 2021;115:67–88. doi:10.1016/bs.vh.2020.12.004
- Fatemeh G, Sajjad M, Niloufar R, et al. Effect of melatonin supplementation on sleep quality: A systematic review and meta-analysis of randomized controlled trials. J Neurol. 2022;269(1):205–216. doi:10.1007/s00415-020-10381-w
- Sletten TL, Magee M, Murray JM, et al. Efficacy of melatonin with behavioural sleep-wake scheduling for delayed sleep-wake phase disorder: A double-blind randomized clinical trial. PLOS Medicine. 2018;15(6):e1002587. doi:10.1371/journal.pmed.1002587
- Stoianovici R, Brunetti L, Adams CD. Comparison of melatonin and zolpidem for sleep in an academic community hospital: An analysis of patient perception and inpatient outcomes. J Pharm Pract. 2019;897190019851888. doi:10.1177/0897190019851888

Omega-3 Polyunsaturated Fatty Acids

Indications

ADHD

- Suggested that relative deficiencies in PUFA (mainly EPA) may be implicated in some of the behavioral and learning problems associated with ADHD
- A meta-analysis of 5 studies that examined omega-6 to omega-3 ratio (n6/n3) and arachidonic acid to eicosapentaenoic acid ratio (AA/EPA) found that an elevated n6/n3 and, more specifically, AA/EPA ratio may represent the underlying disturbance in essential fatty acid levels in patients with ADHD
- Review of 13 trials (n = 1011) concluded that there is very little evidence that fish oils alone provide benefit for children/adolescents with ADHD
- A randomized study (90 participants) that compared omega-3/6, long-acting methylphenidate or the combination for 12 months found that ADHD symptoms decreased in all treatment arms; significant differences favoring omega-3/6 + methylphenidate over omega-3/6 alone were found for ADHD total and hyperactivity–impulsivity subscales; adverse events were numerically less frequent with omega-3/6 or methylphenidate + omega-3/6 than with methylphenidate alone

Alzheimer's Disease

- Evidence from observational studies shows that regular consumption of omega-3 PUFA-rich foods in healthy populations (without pre-existing AD or dementia) offers a protective effect against future AD
- Epidemiological evidence supports the idea that omega-3 polyunsaturated fatty acids may play a role in maintaining adequate cognitive functioning in predementia syndromes, but not when the AD process has already taken over
- A systematic review of 7 articles concluded that omega-3 fatty acid supplementation may be beneficial at disease onset, when there is slight impairment of brain function; however, there is not enough evidence to support omega-3 fatty acid supplementation in the treatment of Alzheimer's disease

Bipolar Disorder

- Preliminary double-blind study suggests that patients with BD who took supplements of fish oil, in addition to their usual medication, had a significantly longer period of remission than those on placebo
- However, a 2021 RCT found no difference in the number of mood episode relapses, the number of hospital admissions, or time to relapse. Authors concluded that there is little evidence that supplementing with omega-3 PUFAs is of prophylactic benefit in BD
- Epidemiological data suggest a relationship between consumption of seafood and decreased lifetime prevalence of depression, bipolar I and II disorder, and bipolar spectrum disorder; contradictory data reported as to efficacy and dosage in depressed and rapid-cycling BD
- Systematic review identified 5 studies of highly variable methodological quality. Only one 12-week study was of sufficient quality and showed positive effects for treating depression (not mania) when omega-3 PUFAs (1 g ethyl-EPA/day) were used as an adjunct to conventional mood stabilizers
- In another RCT, patients with bipolar disorder and rapid cycling took EPA 6 mg/day in addition to their conventional treatment (for 4 months), there were no significant differences in depression or manic symptoms compared to treatment plus placebo

Depression

- Epidemiological studies suggest that high fish consumption is correlated with decreased depression
- A 2021 meta-analysis of 36 studies found that omega-3 PUFAs had a small/modest positive effect in MDD compared with placebo. The authors conclude that this effect is unlikely to be meaningful to people who have MDD. The same analysis reported that omega-3 PUFAs appeared to be as effective as fluoxetine in one study
- A meta-analysis of 26 studies involving 2160 patients reported that omega-3 PUFAs with EPA $\geq 60\%$ at a dosage of ≤ 1 g/day had beneficial effects on depression. EPA is the component that appears to reduce symptoms of depression
- The clinical guidelines (2019) issued by the International Society for Nutritional Psychiatry Research indicate that omega-3 fatty acids, when given in 1-2 g per day (as pure EPA or a 2:1 ratio of EPA:DHA) for at least 8 weeks, can increase the effects of an antidepressant when both are started at the same time; furthermore, omega-3 therapy may improve the effects of an antidepressant when results have been inadequate
- Evidence suggests that low levels of omega-3 fatty acids are correlated with depressive symptoms during pregnancy and after delivery; however, one study showed it was ineffective for the treatment of MDD in pregnant women
- CANMAT 2016 guidelines state that omega-3 fatty acids have level 1 evidence of efficacy but, because of the inconsistency in the evidence, are recommended as second-line monotherapy for mild to moderate MDD and adjunctive to antidepressants for moderate to severe MDD

Omega-3 Polyunsaturated Fatty Acids (cont.)

Schizophrenia	• In a 2022 meta-analysis of 6 studies, use of omega-3 PUFAs was associated with reduced PANSS scores in schizophrenia, but the results were not significant

- In a 2022 meta-analysis of 6 studies, use of omega-3 PUFAs was associated with reduced PANSS scores in schizophrenia, but the results were not significant
- A 2021 systematic review reported that the effectiveness of omega-3 supplementation on symptoms of schizophrenia varies among the different phases of illness. Specifically, it appeared to significantly improve positive and negative symptoms during the prodromal phase, improve mainly the negative symptoms in patients in their first episode, and only partly improve symptoms in patients with chronic schizophrenia
- Preliminary data suggest a relationship between high consumption of omega-3 fatty acids and less severe symptoms of schizophrenia; ethyl-EPA suggested to inhibit phospholipase A_2, an enzyme found to be overactive in patients with schizophrenia and may be responsible for depletion of arachidonic acid from brain and red cell phospholipids in these patients
- In a small double-blind placebo-controlled randomized 6-month study, an intervention with omega-3 fatty acids (using 2.2 g EPA + DHA per day) significantly improved the level of functioning (measured by PANSS) in first-episode schizophrenia patients compared to placebo
- A meta-analysis of 6 studies concluded that EPA did not improve the symptoms of schizophrenia
- Supplementation of a mixture of EPA/DHA (180:120 mg) in combination with vitamins E and C (400 units:500 mg) bid for 4 months reported to significantly reduce psychopathology in patients with schizophrenia
- Review of double-blind studies suggests ethyl-EPA (at a dose of 2 g/day) can augment effects of clozapine in treatment-refractory patients

 General Comments

- N-3 fatty acid deficiencies have been reported in people with a wide range of mental disorders by several studies
- The human body is not able to synthesize omega-3 polyunsaturated fatty acids (PUFAs)
- N-3 PUFAs are responsible for approximately 20% of the brain's dry weight and 33% of all fats in the CNS
- Best source for PUFAs is fatty fish (e.g., mackerel, halibut, salmon), as this contains eicosapentaenoic acid (EPA) and docosahexaenoic acids (DHA)
- Other sources are green leafy vegetables, nuts, flaxseed oil, and canola oil; all contain alpha-linolenic acid (ALA), which can be converted (only 5–10%) to EPA and DHA

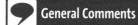 **Pharmacology**

- Positive effects on depressive illnesses are believed to be a result of changes to cell membrane structure and function, impacting particularly cellular communication, inflammatory processes, and neurotransmitter activities

 Dosing

- Bipolar disorder: 1–2 g/day (EPA)
- Depression: 1–4 g/day (EPA + DHA)
- Schizophrenia: 1–4 g/day (EPA + DHA)
- Alzheimer's disease: 1–4 g/day (EPA + DHA)
- The ratio of EPA:DHA is important; over 60% (EPA) has been shown to be better in clinical trials
- One serving of fish (100 g or 3.5 oz) contains approximately 1 g EPA/DHA. Fresh fish is always best but patients may need to supplement in order to get higher doses

 Adverse Effects

- Well tolerated in adults and children at doses of 3–4 g/day; mild gastrointestinal effects
- Fishy aftertaste, belching (take with meals or freeze to help with this)
- May increase bleeding risk at higher doses (more than 3 g/day)
- Risk of hypomania noted in a few cases, but no such instances reported in systematic reviews or meta-analyses in bipolar depression

 Drug Interactions

- Hypotensive agents: can lower blood pressure, resulting in additive effects
- High doses (more than 3 g/day) may increase LDL cholesterol levels by 5–10%

 Further Reading

References
- Appleton KM, Voyias PD, Sallis HM, et al. Omega-3 fatty acids for depression in adults. Cochrane Database Syst Rev. 2021;11(11):CD004692. doi:10.1002/14651858.CD004692.pub5
- Barragan E, Breuer D, Dopfner M. Efficacy and safety of Omega-3/6 fatty acids, methylphenidate, and a combined treatment in children with ADHD. J Atten Disord. 2017;21(5):433–441. doi:10.1177/1087054713518239

- Canhada S, Castro K, Schweigert Perry I, et al. Omega-3 fatty acids' supplementation in Alzheimer's disease: A systematic review. Nutr Neurosci. 2018;21(8):529–538. doi:10.1080/1028415X.2017.1321813
- Ciappolino V, Delvecchio G, Agostoni C, et al. The role of n-3 polyunsaturated fatty acids (n-3PUFAs) in affective disorders. J Affect Disord. 2017;224:32–47. doi:10.1016/j.jad.2016.12.034
- Guu TW, Mischoulon D, Sarris J, et al. International society for nutritional psychiatry research practice guidelines for omega-3 fatty acids in the treatment of major depressive disorder. Psychother Psychosom. 2019;88(5):263–273. doi:10.1159/000502652
- Hallahan B, Ryan T, Hibbeln JR, et al. Efficacy of omega-3 highly unsaturated fatty acids in the treatment of depression. Br J Psychiatry. 2016;209(3):192–201. doi:10.1192/bjp.bp.114.160242
- Hsu MC, Ouyang WC. A systematic review of effectiveness of omega-3 fatty acid supplementation on symptoms, social functions, and neurobiological variables in schizophrenia. Biol Res Nurs. 2021;23(4):723–737. doi:10.1177/10998004211020121
- LaChance L, McKenzie K, Taylor VH, et al. Omega-6 to Omega-3 fatty acid ratio in patients with ADHD: A meta-analysis. J Can Acad Child Adolesc Psychiatry. 2016;25(2):87-96. PMCID:27274774
- Liao Y, Xie B, Zhang H, et al. Efficacy of omega-3 PUFAs in depression: A meta-analysis. Transl Psychiatry. 2019;9(1):190. doi:10.1038/s41398-019-0515-5
- McPhilemy G, Byrne F, Waldron M, et al. A 52-week prophylactic randomised control trial of omega-3 polyunsaturated fatty acids in bipolar disorder. Bipolar Disord. 2021;23(7):697–706. doi:10.1111/bdi.13037
- Ravindran AV, Balneaves LG, Faulkner G, et al. Canadian Network for Mood and Anxiety Treatments (CANMAT) 2016 clinical guidelines for the management of adults with major depressive disorder: Section 5. Complementary and alternative medicine treatments. Can J Psychiatry. 2016;61(9):576–587. doi:10.1177/0706743716660290
- Xu X, Shao G, Zhang X, et al. The efficacy of nutritional supplements for the adjunctive treatment of schizophrenia in adults: A systematic review and network meta-analysis. Psychiatry Res. 2022;311:114500. doi:10.1016/j.psychres.2022.114500

S-Adenosyl-L-Methionine (SAMe)

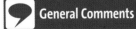

Indications

Depression

- Systematic review of 6 studies suggests comparable efficacy to tricyclic antidepressants and more effective than placebo for mild to moderate depression (trials lasted up to 8 weeks)
- A 12-week, 3-armed trial of SAMe (1600–3200 mg), escitalopram (10–20 mg) or placebo showed no significant differences in response rates
- In a 2016 Cochrane review of 8 RCTs, SAMe was compared to placebo, desipramine, escitalopram, and imipramine:
  – There were no changes in symptoms from baseline to end of treatment with SAMe or placebo
  – No difference in effectiveness between SAMe and imipramine or escitalopram
  – SAMe was more effective than placebo when used as an add-on to SSRIs
- In another review (2017), 12 of 19 placebo-controlled trials showed SAMe was significantly more effective than placebo and comparable to TCAs
- CANMAT 2016 guidelines state that SAM-e is recommended as second-line adjunctive treatment for use in mild to moderate MDD
- More high-quality studies are needed to demonstrate the efficacy of SAMe in more severe depression or as monotherapy

General Comments

- Low serum and CSF levels of SAMe reported in patients with MDD
- Can be found in protein food sources (e.g., beef)
- Widely prescribed as an antidepressant in Europe but sold over the counter in North America
- Used most commonly for treatment of depression and osteoarthritis

Pharmacology

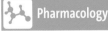

- SAMe is an amino acid that acts as a methyl donor needed in the synthesis of monoamine transmitters (dopamine, norepinephrine, and serotonin) and membrane phospholipids
- Several anti-inflammatory effects have been identified
- Abnormal methylation has been implicated as a potential pathogenic mechanism in depression and dementia
- May increase membrane fluidity and influence monoamine and phospholipid metabolism; may increase the turnover of serotonin, norepinephrine, and dopamine

S-Adenosyl-L-Methionine (SAMe) (cont.)

 Dosing

- For mild to moderate MDD, the lowest dose shown to be effective is 800 mg/day, and for severe MDD 1600 mg/day (in 2–3 divided doses)
- Usual starting dose is 400 mg/day for the first 1–2 weeks, then increased by 200–400 mg/day every 5–7 days to a maximum dose of 800 mg bid
- Best absorbed when taken at least 20 min before breakfast or lunch
- Rapid onset reported (~ 10 days); response may depend on folate and vitamin B_{12} levels
- Although tosylate salt is the most commercially available, the butanedisulfonate salt has been shown to be the most stable and to have superior bioavailability

 Adverse Effects

- Generally well tolerated
- May lead to insomnia if taken in the afternoon
- Higher doses can cause GI effects, headache, tachycardia, anxiety, restlessness, insomnia, and fatigue
- No weight gain reported
- **Contraindication:** Bipolar disorder, due to case reports of the induction of mania through SAMe treatment

 Drug Interactions

- Antidepressant drugs (avoid due to possible serotonin syndrome)
- SAMe may methylate levodopa, leading to a decreased response

 Further Reading

References

- Galizia I, Oldani L, Macritchie K, et al. S-adenosyl methionine (SAMe) for depression in adults. Cochrane Database Syst Rev. 2016;(10):CD011286. Retrieved from doi:10.1002/14651858.CD011286.pub2
- Mischoulon D, Price LH, Carpenter LL, et al. A double-blind, randomized, placebo-controlled clinical trial of S-adenosyl-L-methionine (SAMe) versus escitalopram in major depressive disorder. J Clin Psychiatry. 2014;75(4):370–376. doi:10.4088/JCP.13m08591
- Ravindran AV, Balneaves LG, Faulkner G, et al. Canadian Network for Mood and Anxiety Treatments (CANMAT) 2016 clinical guidelines for the management of adults with major depressive disorder: Section 5. Complementary and alternative medicine treatments. Can J Psychiatry. 2016;61(9):576–587. doi:10.1177/0706743716660290
- Sharma A, Gerbarg P, Bottiglieri T, et al. S-adenosylmethionine for neuropsychiatric disorders: A clinician-oriented review of research. J Clin Psychiatry. 2017;78(6):e656–e667. doi:10.4088/JCP.16r11113

St. John's Wort

 Indications

Depression

- Overall, this well-researched herb has been shown to have the most robust evidence in the treatment of depression, proving to be superior to placebo and as effective as SSRIs for major depression (mild to moderate)
- A meta-analysis of 27 trials that ranged from 4 to 12 weeks (3,088 participants) in patients with mild to moderate depression, St. John's wort (SJW) demonstrated comparable response and remission rates to SSRIs. In addition, patients treated with SJW had a significantly lower discontinuation/dropout rate compared to SSRIs
- CANMAT 2016 guidelines recommend St. John's wort as first-line monotherapy in mild to moderate MDD and as second-line adjunctive treatment for moderate to severe MDD
- St. John's wort does not seem to be effective in severe depression
- No studies to date on use as adjuvant therapy with conventional therapies

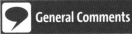

General Comments	• Despite high-quality evidence of efficacy, there is a general lack of knowledge about the practicality of using SJW for depression among physicians • Extracts of Hypericum perforatum L. (St. John's wort) have been used historically to treat depressive disorders; some formulations are only available by prescription in Europe • This extract is the best-known "natural" antidepressant and is now used to treat depression, anxiety, and sleep disorders
Pharmacology	• Both hypericum and hyperforin have been shown to be active in several animal studies; however, it is believed that at least 7 constituents contribute to its overall effect • Inhibits reuptake of serotonin, norepinephrine, dopamine, GABA, and L-glutamate • Downregulates monoamine receptors (weaker effect)
Dosing	• Most clinical trials have used 300 mg of standardized 0.3% hypericin or 2–5% hyperforin taken 3 times per day; dose has been increased to 1200–1800 mg after 2 weeks if no response • Effect is usually seen after 10–14 days (with significant clinical response seen at 4–6 weeks)

Adverse Effects	• In general, better tolerability and fewer adverse effects than with conventional antidepressants:
	  – Gastrointestinal discomfort, confusion, fatigue
	  – Photosensitivity (in large doses: 2–4 g/day); fair-skinned individuals should use protective measures against sunlight
	  – May cause insomnia (decrease dose or take in the morning)
	  – May induce hypomania (in depression) and mania (in occult bipolar disorder)
	• **Contraindications:** Pregnancy, lactation, Alzheimer's disease, schizophrenia (case reports of inducing psychosis), and bipolar disorder (case reports of hypomania or mania)

Drug Interactions	• Hypericum has many possible major drug interactions – best to avoid using this natural product if taking other medications • Potent inducer of CYP3A4 (and, to a lesser extent, CYP2C9 and CYP1A2), and the P-glycoprotein transporter; reported to decrease plasma level of drugs metabolized by these systems, including cyclosporine (30–70% decrease has resulted in rejection of transplanted organ); also reported to decrease plasma level of indinavir (57% decrease in AUC), digoxin (up to 25% decrease in AUC), theophylline, imatinib, irinotecan, amitriptyline, barbiturates, alprazolam, methadone, opioids, phenytoin, and warfarin; breakthrough bleeding and cases of pregnancy reported in patients on oral contraceptives; may interact with other drugs metabolized by these enzymes • Several cases of serotonin syndrome reported in combination with serotonergic drugs
Further Reading	**References** • Chrubasik-Hausmann S, Vlachojannis J, McLachlan AJ. Understanding drug interactions with St John's wort (Hypericum Perforatum L.): Impact of hyperforin content. J Pharm Pharmcol. 2019;71(1):129–138. doi:10.1111/jphp.12858 • Natural Medicines Database: St. John's wort monograph. Retrieved from http://www.naturaldatabase.com • Ng QX, Venkatanarayanan N, Ho CY. Clinical use of Hypericum perforatum (St. John's wort) in depression: A meta-analysis. J Affect Disord. 2017;210:211–221. doi:10.1016/j.jad.2016.12.048 • Ravindran AV, Balneaves LG, Faulkner G, et al. Canadian Network for Mood and Anxiety Treatments (CANMAT) 2016 clinical guidelines for the management of adults with major depressive disorder: Section 5. Complementary and alternative medicine treatments. Can J Psychiatry. 2016;61(9):576–587. doi:10.1177/0706743716660290 • Warnick SJ, Mehdi L, Kowalkowski J. Wait – there's evidence for that? Integrative medicine treatments for major depressive disorder. Int J Psychiatry Med. 2021;56(5):334–343. doi:10.1177/00912174211046353

Valerian

Indications

Anxiety Disorders

- A 2020 systematic review and meta-analysis of valerian in the treatment of anxiety (8 studies) found an overall effect size of 0.71 (–1.66, 3.07) when analyzing the studies using either the whole root or extract
- Placebo-controlled RCT compared valerian (mean dose 81.3 mg/day), diazepam (6.5 mg/day) and placebo for 4 weeks. Patients receiving valerian and diazepam had significant improvement in HAM-A scores (but not total anxiety scores)
- Use in benzodiazepine withdrawal questionable:
  - 19 patients with chronic insomnia were tapered off benzodiazepines over a 2-week period
  - 2 weeks after initiating placebo or 300 mg/day valerian, sleep latency was superior in the placebo group

Sleep Disorders

- A 2020 systematic review and meta-analysis of valerian sought to understand the reasons behind the inconsistent outcomes in its effectiveness to improve subjective sleep quality (10 studies). Major findings include:
  - Of the different dosage forms, studies using the whole root/rhizome had superior results compared with other dosage forms (e.g., extracts)
  - Repeated administration of valerian (whole root/rhizome) was more effective in alleviating sleep problems compared with single use of the herb
  - Authors speculate that the limited shelf life of one of the constituents, valepotriates, may be one reason for negative outcomes observed in trials (this supports the idea of using the raw herb)
- 18 RCTs (1,093 participants) found that most studies had significant methodological problems. In 6 studies, subjective improvement in sleep quality when outcome was measured as a dichotomous variable (yes or no), but there was evidence of publication bias in this summary
- A meta-analysis of 14 RCTs found no improvement in sleep onset latency, duration, efficiency or quality compared to placebo
- Several placebo-controlled crossover studies show improvement in sleep quality, decrease in sleep latency, and a decrease in the number of awakenings; response better in females and individuals less than 40 years of age; some studies did not show benefit

General Comments

- Valerian consists of the roots, rhizomes (underground stems), and stolons from the plant Valeriana officinalis
- Therapeutic uses for insomnia described by Hippocrates and Galen (2nd century)
- Traditionally used for insomnia, anxiety, seizures, and migraine
- Well studied but majority of studies are of poor quality; often combined with other herbal combinations such as hops and St. John's wort

Pharmacology

- Active ingredients associated with sedative properties thought to be valepotriates, mono- and sesquiterpenes (e.g., valerenic acid), and pyridine alkaloids
- Has benzodiazepine-like effects
- May enhance GABA release and decrease uptake
- Able to alter binding at benzodiazepine receptor and cause CNS depression (mechanism of action unclear)

Dosing

- Dose: 200–1200 mg/day
- Usual dose 400–900 mg taken 2 h before bedtime

Adverse Effects

- Well tolerated for up to 6 weeks
- Adverse effects include nausea, excitability, blurred vision, headache
- Advise against stopping suddenly: withdrawal symptoms including delirium, visual hallucinations, and cardiac complications reported after abrupt discontinuation of chronic use
- No detrimental effects on driving performance were seen after taking valerian (compared to placebo)
- Contraindications:
  - Liver dysfunction reported; use with caution in patients with a history of liver disease – periodic liver function tests recommended

- Surgery: discontinue 2 weeks prior to surgery (due to CNS depressant effects)
- Pregnancy and breastfeeding

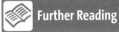

Drug Interactions
- Avoid using in combination with benzodiazepines or other CNS depressants
- Will potentiate the effects of other CNS drugs

Further Reading

References
- Leach MJ, Page AT. Herbal medicine for insomnia: A systematic review and meta-analysis. Sleep Med Rev. 2015;24:1–12. doi:10.1016/j.smrv.2014.12.003
- Natural Medicines Comprehensive Database: Valerian monograph. Retrieved from http://www.naturaldatabase.com
- Shinjyo N, Waddell G, Green J. Valerian root in treating sleep problems and associated disorders – A systematic review and meta-analysis. J Evid Based Integr Med. 2020;25:1–31. doi: 10.1177/2515690X20967323
- Thomas K, Canedo J, Perry P, et al. Effects of valerian on subjective sedation, field sobriety testing and driving simulator performance. Accid Anal Prev. 2016;92:240–244. doi:10.1016/j.aap.2016.01.019

Vitamins

Indications

Alzheimer's Disease (AD)
- Vitamin B_9 (folate):
  - In an RCT (121 participants), folic acid (1.25 mg/day) augmentation of donepezil resulted in a slight increase in Mini-Mental State Examination (MMSE) scores compared to the control group. The investigators concluded that folic acid is beneficial in patients with AD
  - Vitamin B supplementation was successful at lowering serum homocysteine (a potential risk factor for cognitive impairment) in 4 RCTs, but no significant changes in MMSE scores were found
  - A longitudinal study in elderly people found that taking high doses of folic acid (more than the recommended daily amount) significantly reduced the risk of developing AD
  - Further investigations are necessary in order to ascertain whether folate is associated with the onset or progression of AD
- Vitamin C:
  - Many population studies have shown an association between higher ascorbic acid (AA) intake and reduced relative risk for AD. It is also known that AA levels in plasma are decreased in patients with AD
  - However, there have also been several studies reporting that AA supplementation did not appear to have any neuroprotective effects against developing AD
  - Vitamin C in the diet or taken as supplements may help prevent AD due to its antioxidant properties
- Vitamin D:
  - Several systematic reviews and meta-analyses have suggested that there is a relationship between vitamin D and neuropsychological functioning: higher levels of serum 25 (OH) have been associated with a lower risk of dementia and AD. Similarly, a link between low serum concentrations of vitamin D and the emergence of cognitive disorders has been reported
- Vitamin E:
  - Shown to reduce cell death associated with β-amyloid protein
  - Meta-analysis suggests there is no evidence of efficacy of vitamin E in the prevention or treatment of people with AD or mild cognitive impairment; however, there is some evidence that it may slow the progression of AD by 6 months when used in high doses (2000 IU/day)
  - The evidence remains inconclusive and the clinical safety of vitamin E remains controversial. More research in this area is needed

Depression
- Vitamin B_9 (folate) and L-methylfolate:
  - Small overall benefits for unipolar depression; however, large doses (15 mg/day) of L-methylfolate (the active form of folate) as adjunctive therapy in MDD was found to have moderate-to-large benefits for depressive symptoms vs. placebo in a few small RCTs

Vitamins (cont.)

- Despite a known link between folate deficiency and depression, it has been poorly studied (most studies look at multivitamin complexes)
- Small systematic review: RCTs suggest that folic acid, in combination with antidepressants, may reduce residual symptoms of depression, especially in individuals with low folate levels; greater response rate reported in women
- A meta-analysis of 11 RCTs suggests that treatment with folate and vitamin B_{12} does not decrease severity of depressive symptoms over a short period of time but may be helpful in long-term management of special populations; there was high heterogeneity between studies
- Vitamin D:
  - Vitamin D was found to significantly reduce depressive symptoms in patients with clinical depression in 3 double-blind RCTs
  - A meta-analysis or 9 RCTs with 4,923 participants did not find a significant reduction in depression after vitamin D supplementation; however, most of the studies focused on individuals with low levels of depression and sufficient serum vitamin D at baseline
  - A 2020 RCT involving 18,353 patients showed that in adults over 50 years of age, vitamin D supplementation did not significantly reduce depressive symptoms or reduce depression

Schizophrenia	- Vitamin B:
	  - Low levels of vitamin B have been reported in patients with schizophrenia
	  - Vitamin B_6 may act as an antioxidant and free radical scavenger and reactive carbonyl compounds are believed to contribute to the pathogenesis of schizophrenia
	  - A systematic review and meta-analysis of 18 RCTs showed that vitamin B supplementation (B_6, B_8, and B_{12}) reduced symptoms significantly more than control conditions. However, no effects of B vitamins were observed in individual domains of positive and negative symptoms. Meta-regression analyses indicated that shorter illness duration was associated with greater vitamin B effectiveness
	- Vitamin C:
	  - Reports that ascorbic acid in doses up to 8 g/day may antagonize dopamine neurotransmission and potentiate the activity of the antipsychotic (may antagonize the metabolism of the antipsychotic). Supplementation of vitamin C with atypical antipsychotics reported to increase ascorbic acid levels, reduce oxidative stress, and improve BPRS scores
	- Vitamin D deficiencies have been reported in patients with schizophrenia. At this point there is only suggestive evidence that vitamin D may play a role in improving psychotic symptoms
	- Vitamin E:
	  - Most studied antioxidant for improving tardive dyskinesia (TD); 40 trials conducted over the past 30 years – evidence is limited and contradictory. May protect against further deterioration or reduce the risk of development. Patients with TD for less than 5 years might respond better

General Comments	- Vitamin B_9 (folate):
	  - A naturally occurring water-soluble B vitamin found in leafy vegetables, fruits, and legumes
	  - Available as folic acid (synthetic form), 5-MTHF (5-methyltetrahydrofolate), and folinic acid
	  - Folate deficiency has been associated with depression, poor cognitive function, and schizophrenia
	  - Low folate levels have been linked to atrophy of the cerebral cortex, more notably in people with neocortical lesions related to Alzheimer's disease

Pharmacology	- Vitamin B_9 (folate):
	  - Reduces the level of homocysteine, an amino acid believed to exacerbate some psychiatric symptoms
	  - Folic and folinic acid are converted to L-methylfolate, which crosses the blood/brain barrier and activates enzymes needed to synthesize dopamine, norepinephrine, and serotonin
	  - Participates in methylation of homocysteine and synthesis of methionine and SAMe
	- Vitamin B_{12}:
	  - Acts as a cofactor in the synthesis of serotonin
	- Vitamin C:
	  - Required for the biosynthesis of collagen, L-carnitine, and certain neurotransmitters
	  - Important antioxidant that has been shown to regenerate other antioxidants including alpha-tocopherol (vitamin E)
	  - Limits the damaging effects of free radicals, hence, considered to be helpful in mitigating oxidative stress associated with age-related diseases

- Vitamin D:
  - Fat-soluble vitamin involved in the modulation of cell growth, neuromuscular and immune function, and reduction of inflammation
  - Many genes encoding proteins that regulate cell proliferation, differentiation, and apoptosis are modulated in part by vitamin D
- Vitamin E:
  - Fat-soluble antioxidant that stops the production of reactive oxygen species formed when fat undergoes oxidation
  - May help prevent or delay the chronic diseases associated with free radicals
  - Lower α-tocopherol levels have been shown to have a strong association with AD

 Dosing

- Alzheimer's disease: unclear at this time
  - Folic acid 1.25 mg/day based on one RCT where it was used to augment donepezil
- Depression:
  - Folic acid 200–500 micrograms/day has been used to enhance response to antidepressants
  - Vitamin D 1,500–7,143 units/day have been studied
- Schizophrenia:
  - Vitamin E was used in doses of 1200–1600 units/day for treatment of tardive dyskinesia

 Further Reading

References

- Almeida OP, Ford AH, Flicker L. Systematic review and meta-analysis of randomized placebo-controlled trials of folate and vitamin B12 for depression. Int Psychogeriatr. 2015;27(5):727–737. doi:10.1017/S1041610215000046
- Brown HE, Roffman JL. Emerging treatments in schizophrenia: Highlights from recent supplementation and prevention trials. Harv Rev Psychiatry. 2016;24(2):e1–e7. doi:10.1097/HRP.0000000000000101
- Fenech M. Vitamins associated with brain aging, mild cognitive impairment, and Alzheimer disease: Biomarkers, epidemiological and experimental evidence, plausible mechanisms, and knowledge gaps. Adv Nutr. 2017;8(6):958–970. doi:10.3945/an.117.015610
- Firth J, Stubbs B, Sarris J, et al. The effects of vitamin and mineral supplementation on symptoms of schizophrenia: A systematic review and meta-analysis. Psychol Med. 2017;47(9):1515–1527. doi:10.1017/S0033291717000022
- Gowda U, Mutowo MP, Smith BJ, et al. Vitamin D supplementation to reduce depression in adults: Meta-analysis of randomized controlled trials. Nutrition. 2015;31(3):421–429. doi:10.1016/j.nut.2014.06.017
- Okereke OI, Reynolds CF, Mischoulon D, et al. Effect of long-term vitamin D3 supplementation vs placebo on risk of depression or clinically relevant depressive symptoms and on change in mood scores: A randomized clinical trial. JAMA. 2020;324(5):471–480. doi:10.1001/jama.2020.10224
- Roberts E, Carter B, Young AH. Caveat emptor: Folate in unipolar depressive illness, a systematic review and meta-analysis. J Psychopharmacol. 2018;32(4):377–384. doi:10.1177/0269881118756060
- Roy NM, Al-Harthi L, Sampat N, et al. Impact of vitamin D on neurocognitive function in dementia, depression, schizophrenia and ADHD. Front Biosci (Landmark Ed). 2021;26(3):566–611. doi:10.2741/4908
- Soares-Weiser K, Maayan N, Bergman H. Vitamin E for antipsychotic-induced tardive dyskinesia. Cochrane Database Syst Rev. 2018;1:CD000209. doi:10.1002/14651858.CD000209.pub3
- Stubbs JF, Sarris J, Rosenbaum S, et al. The effects of vitamin and mineral supplementation on symptoms of schizophrenia: A systematic review and meta-analysis. Psychol Med. 2017;47(9):1515–1527. doi:10.1017/S0033291717000022
- Yu JT, Xu W, Tan CC, et al. Evidence-based prevention of Alzheimer's disease: Systematic review and meta-analysis of 243 observational prospective studies and 153 randomised controlled trials. J Neurol Neurosurg Psychiatry. 2020;91(11):1201–1209. doi:10.1136/jnnp-2019-321913
- Zhang DM, Ye JX, Mu JS, et al. Efficacy of vitamin B supplementation on cognition in elderly patients with cognitive-related diseases. J Geriatr Psychiatry Neurol. 2017;30(1):50–59. doi:10.1177/0891988716673466

PHARMACOGENETIC INFORMATION FOR COMMON PSYCHOTROPIC DRUGS

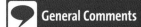 **General Comments**

- Responses to psychotropic drugs are influenced by an array of factors including age, sex, ethnicity, nutritional status, smoking and alcohol or other drug use. In addition, there is now strong evidence for the role of genetic variability in individual responses to psychotropic drugs.[1] With genetic testing becoming more widely available in the clinical setting (e.g., see [2]), it is important that prescribers have access to pharmacogenetic information. A brief summary of common genetic variations associated with the metabolism of commonly prescribed psychotropic drugs is provided below. A number of sources are available for further information, e.g., the US Food and Drug Administration (FDA)[3], the Clinical Pharmacogenetics Implementation Consortium (CPIC)[4, 5], the Dutch Pharmacogenetics Working Group (DPWG)[6], and the PharmGKB database[7]
- Information on pharmacokinetic effects of CYP2C19 and CYP2D6 enzymes responsible for the metabolism of a substantial majority of psychotropic drugs that is provided here pertains to highly polymorphic genes encoding these enzymes. For more details on CYP polymorphisms, refer to the Pharmacogene Variation (PharmVar) Consortium (https://www.pharmvar.org/) and PharmGKB (https://www.pharmgkb.org/) databases
- The information below is derived from the FDA biomarker table(https://www.fda.gov/media/124784/download), consult this for further details

Pharmacogenetic Effects

CYP2C19 poor metabolizer OR taking CYP2C19 inhibitors (e.g., benzodiazepines, cimetidine, modafinil)

Drug Class	Generic Name	Effects/Recommendations
Antidepressant SSRI	Citalopram	In CYP2C19 poor metabolizers, citalopram steady-state C_{max} and AUC was increased by 68% and 107%, respectively. Citalopram 20 mg/day is the maximum recommended dose in CYP2C19 poor metabolizers or patients taking another CYP2C19 inhibitor due to risk of QT prolongation
	Escitalopram	Escitalopram 30 mg given once daily resulted in mean C_{max} 1.7-fold higher than the mean C_{max} for the maximum recommended therapeutic dose of escitalopram monotherapy at steady state (20 mg). Exposure under supratherapeutic 30 mg dose is similar to the steady-state concentrations expected in CYP2C19 poor metabolizers following a therapeutic dose of 20 mg

CYP2D6 poor metabolizer OR taking CYP2D6 inhibitors (e.g., bupropion, fluoxetine, fluvoxamine, mirabegron, paroxetine, quinidine, viloxazine)

Drug Class	Generic Name	Effects/Recommendations
ADHD drug Selective norepinephrine reuptake inhibitor	Atomoxetine	CYP2D6 poor metabolizers have a 10-fold higher AUC and a 5-fold higher peak concentration to a given dose of atomoxetine compared with extensive metabolizers. Higher blood levels in poor metabolizers lead to a higher rate of some adverse effects of atomoxetine Initiate at 0.5 mg/kg/day and only increase to usual target dose of 1.2 mg/kg/day if symptoms fail to improve after 4 weeks and the initial dose is well tolerated
	Viloxazine	In a multiple-dose study with viloxazine 900 mg once daily in healthy volunteers, steady-state C_{max} and AUC(0–24h) were 21% and 26% higher, respectively, in CYP2D6 poor metabolizers compared to extensive metabolizers

Drug Class	Generic Name	Effects/Recommendations
Antidepressant		
SNRI	Duloxetine	Concomitant administration of duloxetine 40 mg twice daily with fluvoxamine 100 mg, a potent CYP1A2 inhibitor, to 14 CYP2D6 poor metabolizer subjects resulted in a 6-fold increase in duloxetine AUC and C_{max}
SNRI	Venlafaxine	CYP2D6 poor metabolizers have increased levels of venlafaxine and reduced levels of the active metabolite O-desmethylvenlafaxine compared to CYP2D6 extensive metabolizers
SMS	Vortioxetine	Maximum recommended dose is 10 mg/day in known CYP2D6 poor metabolizers. Reduce dose by one half if patient is taking a strong CYP2D6 inhibitor concomitantly. Increased dose to original level when CYP2D6 inhibitor is discontinued
Nonselective cyclic	Amitriptyline, clomipramine, desipramine, imipramine, nortriptyline, protriptyline, trimipramine	CYP2D6 poor metabolizers have higher than expected plasma concentrations of tricyclic antidepressants when given usual doses. The increase in plasma concentration may be small, or quite large (8-fold increase in plasma AUC of tricyclic antidepressant)
	Doxepin	CYP2C19 and CYP2D6 poor metabolizers may have higher doxepin plasma levels than more extensive metabolizers
Antipsychotic		
FGA	Perphenazine	CYP2D6 poor metabolizers demonstrate higher plasma concentrations of perphenazine at usual doses, which may correlate with emergence of side effects
	Pimozide	Children: At doses above 0.05 mg/kg/day, CYP2D6 genotyping should be performed. Pimozide dose in CYP2D6 poor metabolizers should not exceed 0.05 mg/kg/day, and doses should not be increased earlier than 14 days Adults: At doses above 4 mg/day, CYP2D6 genotyping should be performed. Pimozide dose in CYP2D6 poor metabolizers should not exceed 4 mg/day, and doses should not be increased earlier than 14 days
SGA	Clozapine	Dose reduction may be necessary in patients who are CYP2D6 poor metabolizers. Clozapine plasma concentrations may be increased in these patients
TGA	Aripiprazole	Based on simulation, a 4.5-fold increase in mean C_{max} and AUC values at steady state is expected when CYP2D6 extensive metabolizers are administered with both strong CYP2D6 and CYP3A4 inhibitors. A 3-fold increase in mean C_{max} and AUC values at steady state is expected in CYP2D6 poor metabolizers administered with strong CYP3A4 inhibitors Dosage reduction recommended in patients who are known CYP2D6 poor metabolizers and in patients taking concomitant CYP3A4 or CYP2D6 inhibitors. When the coadministered drug is withdrawn from the combination therapy, adjust aripiprazole dosage to its original level Dosage adjustment may be necessary in patients who are taking concomitant CYP3A4 inducers. When the coadministered CYP3A4 inducer is withdrawn, reduce aripiprazole dosage to original level over 1–2 weeks In patients who may be receiving a combination of strong, moderate, and weak inhibitors of CYP3A4 and CYP2D6, the dosing may be reduced to one quarter (25%) of the usual dose initially and then adjusted to achieve a favorable clinical response
	Brexpiprazole	Based on simulation, a 5.1-fold increase in AUC values at steady state is expected when CYP2D6 extensive metabolizers are administered with both strong CYP2D6 and CYP3A4 inhibitors. A 4.8-fold increase in mean AUC values at steady state is expected in CYP2D6 poor metabolizers administered with strong CYP3A4 inhibitors Dosage reduction recommended in patients who are known CYP2D6 poor metabolizers and in patients taking concomitant CYP3A4 or CYP2D6 inhibitors. When the coadministered drug is withdrawn from the combination therapy, adjust brexpiprazole dosage to its original level Dosage adjustment may be necessary in patients who are taking concomitant CYP3A4 inducers. When the coadministered CYP3A4 inducer is withdrawn, reduce brexpiprazole dosage to the original level over 1–2 weeks
H₃ receptor inverse agonist	Pitolisant	In patients known to be CYP2D6 poor metabolizers, initiate at 8.9 mg once daily and titrate to a maximum dose of 17.8 mg once daily after 7 days

Pharmacogenetic Effects (cont.)

Drug Class	Generic Name	Effects/Recommendations
VMAT2 inhibitor	Deutetrabenazine	Clinically relevant QT prolongation may occur in some patients treated with deutetrabenazine who are CYP2D6 poor metabolizers or who are co-administered a strong CYP2D6 inhibitor. In patients who are CYP2D6 poor metabolizers, total daily dosage should not exceed 36 mg (maximum single dose of 18 mg)
	Valbenazine	Increased exposure (C_{max} and AUC) to valbenazine's active metabolite is anticipated in CYP2D6 poor metabolizers and may increase the risk of adverse reactions. Valbenazine may cause an increase in the corrected QT interval in patients who are CYP2D6 poor metabolizers or who are taking a strong CYP2D6 or CYP3A4 inhibitors Consider dose reduction

References

[1] Ravyn D, Ravyn V, Lowney R, et al. CYP450 pharmacogenetic treatment strategies for antipsychotics: A review of the evidence. Schizophrenia Res. 2013.149(1–3):1–14. doi:10.1016/j.schres.2013.06.0351

[2] Shuldiner AR, Palmer K, Pakyz RE, et al. Implementation of pharmacogenetics: The University of Maryland personalized anti-platelet pharmacogenetics program. Am J Med Genet C Semin Med Genet. 2014;166(1):76–84. doi:10.1002/ajmg.c.31396

[3] FDA. Table of pharmacogenomic associations. Retrieved from: https://www.fda.gov/medical-devices/precision-medicine/table-pharmacogenetic-associations

[4] Relling MV, Klein TE. CPIC: Clinical Pharmacogenetics Implementation Consortium of the Pharmacogenomics Research Network. Clin Pharmacol Ther. 2011;89(3):464–467. doi:10.1038/clpt.2010.279

[5] Hicks JK, Bishop JR, Sangkuhl K, et al. Clinical Pharmacogenetics Implementation Consortium (CPIC) guideline for CYP2D6 and CYP2C19 genotypes and dosing of selective serotonin reuptake inhibitors. Clin Pharmacol Ther. 2015;98(2):127–134. doi:10.1002/cpt.147

[6] Swen JJ, Nijenhuis M, de Boer A, et al. Pharmacogenetics: From bench to byte – an update of guidelines. Clin Pharmacol Ther. 2011;89(5):662–673. doi:10.1038/clpt.2011.34

[7] Whirl-Carrillo M, McDonagh EM, Hebert JM, et al. Pharmacogenomics knowledge for personalized medicine. Clin Pharmacol Ther. 2012;92(4):414–417. doi:10.1038/clpt.2012.96

Additional Suggested Reading

- Baskys A. Application of pharmacogenetics in clinical practice: Problems and solutions. J Neural Transm (Vienna). 2019;126(1):109–113. doi:10.1007/s00702-018-1894-0

GLOSSARY

ACE	Angiotensin-converting enzyme
ACE inhibitors	Angiotensin-converting enzyme inhibitors. Vein-relaxing medications that help lower blood pressure
ADHD	Attention deficit hyperactivity disorder
ADL	Activities of daily living
Agranulocytosis	Reduction of neutrophil white blood cells to very low levels
Akathisia	Inability to relax, compulsion to change position, motor restlessness
Akinesia	Absence of voluntary muscle movement
AKRs	Aldo-keto reductases, enzymes involved in phase II drug metabolism
Alopecia	Hair loss
ALT/SGPT	Alanine aminotransferase/serum glutamic pyruvic transaminase
Amenorrhea	Absence of menstruation
ANC	Absolute neutrophil count
Anorexia	Lack of appetite for food
Anterocollis	Forward spasm of the neck
Anticholinergic	Block effects of acetylcholine
Antiemetic	Helps prevent nausea and vomiting
ARB	Angiotensin receptor blocker
Arrhythmia	Any variation of the normal rhythm (usually of the heart beat)
Arteriosclerosis	Hardening and degeneration of the arteries due to fibrous tissue formation
Arthralgia	Pain in the joints
ASA	Acetylsalicylic acid
AST/SGOT	Aspartate aminotransferase/serum glutamic oxaloacetic transaminase
Asterixis	Abnormal tremor consisting of involuntary jerking movements, especially in the hands, frequently occurring with impending hepatic coma and other forms of metabolic encephalopathy; also called flapping tremor
Asthenia	Weakness, fatigue
Ataxia	Incoordination, especially the inability to coordinate voluntary muscular action
Atherosclerosis	Degeneration of the walls of the arteries due to fatty deposits
Atypical depression	As per DSM-5, patient has mood reactivity and at least 2 of the following symptoms: increased appetite or weight, hypersomnia, leaden paralysis and a long-standing pattern of extreme sensitivity to perceived interpersonal rejection
AUC	Area under the concentration vs. time curve (on graph depicting drug in the plasma after a single dose) – represents the extent of systemic exposure of the body to the drug
Autonomic	The part of the nervous system that is functionally independent of thought control (involuntary)
BAD	Bipolar affective disorder
BD	Bipolar disorder
Ballismus	Jerking, twisting
Bioavailability	The fraction of an administered dose of unchanged drug that reaches the systemic circulation
Bipolar I disorder	Cyclical mood disorder with depression alternating with mania or mixed mania
Bipolar II disorder	Cyclical mood disorder with depression alternating with hypomania
Blepharospasm	Forceful sustained eye closure
BMI (body mass index)	Weight (in kg) divided by height (in m^2)
BPH	Benign prostatic hyperplasia
BPRS	Brief Psychiatric Rating Scale
Bradycardia	Abnormally slow heart beat
Brugada syndrome	Cardiac conduction disorder that can lead to sudden cardiac death
Bruxism	Teeth clenching, grinding
BUN	Blood urea nitrogen
Cataplexy	Loss of muscle tone and collapse
CBC	Complete blood count
CBT	Cognitive-behavioral therapy
Centiloid	Unit of a 0–100 scale developed to standardize analysis methods of PET scans for amyloids in Alzheimer's disease patients
CHD	Coronary heart disease
CHF	Congenital heart failure
Choreiform	Purposeless, uncontrolled sinuous movements,
Choreoathetosis	Slow, repeated, involuntary sinuous movements or twitching of muscles
Chronic brain syndrome	Irreversible damage to brain cells = dementia
CI	Confidence interval
Clearance	Rate at which drug is removed from the body (depends on rate of metabolism by liver and elimination from body)
CNS	Central nervous system
CNS depression	Drowsiness, ataxia, incoordination, slowing of respiration which in severe cases may lead to coma and death
COPD	Chronic obstructive pulmonary disorder

Glossary (cont.)

Cortex	The external layer (superficial gray matter) of the brain
Coryza	"Head cold," acute catarrhal inflammation of nasal mucosa
CrCl	Creatinine clearance
CRP	C-reactive protein
CSF	Cerebrospinal fluid
CVD	Cardiovascular disease
Cycloplegia	Paralysis of accommodation of the eye
CYP	Cytochrome P450 enzymes, involved in drug metabolism
DA	Dopamine
DBPC	Double-blind placebo-controlled
DDAVP	Desmopressin acetate
Dermatitis	Inflammation of the skin
Diaphoresis	Perspiration
Diplopia	Double vision
DLPFC	Dorsolateral prefrontal cortex
DRESS	Drug reaction with eosinophilia and systemic symptoms
Dysarthria	Impaired, difficult speech
Dysgeusia	Unpleasant taste
Dyspepsia	Pain or discomfort in upper abdomen or chest (gas, feeling of fullness, or burning pain)
Dysphagia	Difficulty in swallowing
Dyskinesia	Abnormal movements, i.e., twitching, grimacing, spasm
Dystonia	Disordered muscle tone leading to spasms or postural change
ECG	Electrocardiogram (tracing of electrical activity of the heart muscle)
ECT	Electroconvulsive therapy, "shock therapy"
EEG	Electroencephalogram (tracing of electrical activity of the brain)
Edema	Swelling of body tissues due to accumulation of fluid
eGFR	Estimated glomerular filtration rate, a measure for the kidneys' elimination function
Elimination	Excretion or removal of drug (and/or metabolites) from the body, usually by the kidneys
Emesis	Vomiting
Endocrine	A gland that secretes internally, a ductless gland
Enzyme	Organic compound that acts upon specific fluids, tissues, or chemicals in the body to facilitate chemical action
Enuresis	Involuntary discharge of urine
Eosinophilia myalgia syndrome (EMS)	Connective tissue disease with eosinophilia and myalgia (Eosinophils are blood cells that are usually in low quantities)
Epigastric	Referring to the upper middle region of the abdomen
Epistaxis	Nose bleed

EPS	Extrapyramidal side effects
ER	Extended release
Exacerbation	Increase in severity of symptoms or disease
Extrapyramidal	Refers to certain nuclei of the brain close to the pyramidal tract
Extrapyramidal syndrome	Parkinsonian-like effects of drugs
FAS	Fetal alcohol syndrome
Fasciculation	Twitching of muscles
FASD	Fetal alcohol spectrum disorder
Fibrosis	Formation of fibrous or scar tissue
First-pass effect	Drugs absorbed from the intestine first pass through the liver; a portion of the drug is metabolized before it can act on receptors
FSH	Follicle-stimulating hormone
GABA	Gamma-amino butyric acid; an inhibitory neuro-transmitter
GAD	Generalized anxiety disorder
Galactorrhea	Excretion of milk from breasts
GERD	Gastroesophageal reflux disease
GFR	Glomerular filtration rate
GI	Gastrointestinal
Glaucoma	Increased pressure within the eye
Glomerular	Pertaining to small blood vessels of the kidney that serve as filtering structures in the excretion of urine
Glossodynia	Burning mouth syndrome – a persistent tingling or burning sensation in the lips, tongue or entire mouth
GnRH	Gonadotropin-releasing hormone
Gynecomastia	Increase in breast size in males
Half-life	Time required to decrease the plasma concentration of a drug by 50% (depends on drug clearance and volume of distribution)
HAM-A	Hamilton Anxiety Rating Scale
HAM-D	Hamilton Depression Rating Scale
HDL	High-density lipoprotein
Histological	Pertaining to microscopic tissue anatomy
Hypercalcemia	An excessive amount of calcium in the blood
Hyperkinetic	Abnormal increase in activity
Hyperparathyroidism	Increased secretion of the parathyroid
Hyperreflexia	Increased action of the reflexes
Hypertension	High blood pressure
Hyperthyroid	Excessive activity of the thyroid gland
Hypertrophy	Enlargement
Hypesthesia	Diminished sensitivity to tactile stimuli
Hypnotic	Inducing sleep

Hypospadias	Developmental abnormality in males in which the urethra opens on the under surface of the penis or in the perineum
Hypotension	Low blood pressure
Hypothyroid	Insufficiency of thyroid secretion
Induration	Area of hardened tissue
INR	International normalized ratio; measures coagulation of blood
IR	Immediate release
Jaundice	Yellow skin caused by excess of bile pigment
Kindling	Epileptogenesis caused by adaptive changes in neurons producing repeated electrical discharges
LDH	Lactate dehydrogenase (an enzyme)
LDL	Low-density lipoprotein
LFTs	Liver function tests
LH	Luteinizing hormone
LHRH	Luteinizing hormone-releasing hormone
Libido	Drive or energy usually associated with sexual interest
Limbic system	A system of brain structures common to the brains of all mammals (deals with emotions)
Leukocytosis	Increase in the white blood cells in the blood
Leukopenia	Decrease in the white blood cells in the blood
Macrosomia	Birth weight of infant more than 4 kg
MADRS	Montgomery Åsberg Depression Rating Scale
Manic depressive psychosis	Conspicuous mood swings ranging from normal to elation or depression, or alternating of the two; in DSM-IV, called bipolar affective disorder
MAOI	Monoamine oxidase (an enzyme) inhibitor
MDD	Major depressive disorder
Metabolic syndrome	An interrelated cluster of CVD risk factors that include abdominal obesity, dyslipidemia, hypertension, and impaired glucose tolerance (also called insulin resistance syndrome, syndrome X, or dysmetabolic syndrome); see p. 157 for diagnostic criteria
Metabolism	Chemical processes living organisms utilize to maintain life. Drug metabolism is the biochemical process by which living organisms modify pharmaceutical substances. For example, drug metabolism often converts fat-soluble drugs into more water-soluble drugs, which can more readily be excreted by the kidneys. Most psychotropic drugs are metabolized by cytochrome P450 enzymes
Metabolites	Resultant by-products of metabolism; metabolites can be either active substances or nonactive agents
MI	Myocardial infarction
Micrographia	Decrease in size of hand writing; may be a form of akinesia
Miosis	Constricted pupils
MMSE	Mini-Mental State Examination
MRI	Magnetic resonance imaging

MTHFR	Methylenetetrahydrofolatereductase, metabolic enzyme with polymorphism that may be a factor in various conditions
Myalgia	Tenderness or pain in muscles
Mydriasis	Dilated pupils
Narcolepsy	Condition marked by an uncontrollable desire to sleep
Nephritis	Inflammation of the kidneys
NMDA	N-methyl-D-aspartate
NMS	Neuroleptic malignant syndrome – rare disorder characterized by autonomic dysfunction (e.g., tachycardia and hypertension), hyperthermia, altered consciousness, and muscle rigidity with an increase in creatine kinase (CK) and myoglobinuria
NRT	Nicotine replacement therapy
Nystagmus	Involuntary movement of the eyeball or abnormal movement on testing
OCD	Obsessive-compulsive disorder
OC	Oral contraceptive
Oculogyric crisis	Rolling up of the eyes and the inability to focus
Occipital	In the back part of the head
ODT	Oral disintegrating tablets
Ophthalmoplegia	Paralysis of the extraocular eye muscles
Opisthotonus	Arching (spasm) of the body due to contraction of back muscles
Oral hypoesthesia	Diminished oral sensitivity
OROS	Osmotic-controlled release oral delivery system
Orthostatic hypotension	Faintness caused by suddenly standing erect (leading to a drop in blood pressure)
Osteomalacia	Rickets
PANSS	Positive and negative syndrome scale used in the diagnosis and monitoring of symptoms of schizophrenia
Palinopsia	Visual perseveration, "tracking" or shimmering
Papilledema	Edema of the optic disc
Paresthesia	Feeling of "pins and needles," tingling or stiffness in distal extremities
Parkinsonism	A condition marked by mask-like facial appearance, tremor, change in gait and posture (resembles Parkinson's disease)
PD	Panic disorder (with/without agoraphobia)
Perioral	Around the mouth
Peripheral neuropathy	Pathological changes in the peripheral nervous system
PET	Positron emission tomography; a functional imaging technique that uses a radioactive tracer drug to show metabolic and other physiological activities in the body
Petechiae	Small purplish hemorrhagic spots on skin
P-gp	P-glycoprotein; a protein that transports molecules through cell membranes (e.g., in and out of specific body organs)
Photophobia	Sensitivity of the eyes to light
Photosensitivity	Light sensitive

Clinical Handbook of Psychotropic Drugs, 25th edition, © 2023 Hogrefe Publishing

Glossary (cont.)

PI	Protease inhibitor
Piloerection	"Goose-bumps" or hair standing up
Pisa syndrome	A condition where an individual leans to one side
PMS	Premenstrual syndrome
Polydipsia	Excessive drinking
Polyuria	Excessive urination
"Poop-out" syndrome	Tolerance to effects (tachyphylaxis)
Postural hypotension	Lowered blood pressure caused by a change in position
Priapism	Abnormal, continued erection of the penis
Prostatic hypertrophy	Enlargement of the prostate gland
Pruritus	Itching
PSA	Prostate-specific antigen
Psychosis	A major mental disorder of organic or emotional origin in which there is a departure from normal patterns of thinking, feeling and acting; commonly characterized by loss of contact with reality
Psychomotor excitement	Physical and emotional overactivity
Psychomotor retardation	Slowing of physical and psychological reactions
PT	Prothrombin time; used to determine the blood's coagulation tendency (extrinsic pathway)
PTSD	Posttraumatic stress disorder
Pyloric	Referring to the lower opening of the stomach
Rabbit syndrome	Tremor of the lower lip
RCT	Randomized controlled trial
RDBCT	Randomized double-blind controlled trial
Retardation	Slowing
Retrocollis	Spasm of neck muscles causing the head to twist up and back
Schizophrenia	A severe disorder of psychotic depth characterized by a retreat from reality with delusions and hallucinations
Sedative	Producing calming of activity or excitement
Serotonin syndrome	Hypermetabolic syndrome resulting from serotonergic excess; symptoms include: Disorientation, confusion, agitation, tremor, myoclonus, hyperreflexia, twitching, shivering, ataxia, hyperactivity
SIADH	Syndrome of inappropriate secretion of antidiuretic hormone
Sialorrhea	Excessive flow of saliva
SIDS	Sudden infant death syndrome
SL	Sublingual
Social AD	Social anxiety disorder
Somnambulism	Sleepwalking
SR	Sustained release
Stereotypic	Rhythmic and repetitive

SULTs	Sulfotransferases, enzymes involved in phase II drug metabolism
SUVr	Standard uptake value ratio – compares data from two different areas of the same PET image
Syncope	A sudden loss of strength or fainting
T2DM	Type 2 diabetes mellitus
Tachycardia	Abnormally rapid heart rate
Tachyphylaxis	Tolerance to effects
Tardive dyskinesia	Persistent dyskinetic movements that appear late in neuroleptic therapy
Tardive dystonia	Persistent abnormal muscle tone that appears late in neuroleptic therapy
TCA	Tricyclic antidepressant
TD	Tardive dyskinesia
Therapeutic index	Ratio of median lethal dose of a drug to its median effective dose: i.e., $$\text{therapeutic index} = \frac{\text{median lethal dose}}{\text{median effective dose}}$$
TIA	Transient ischemic attack
Tinnitus	A noise in the ears (ringing, buzzing, or roaring)
Torticollis	Spasm on one side of the neck causing the head to twist
Tortipelvis	Twisting of pelvis due to muscle spasm
Tracking	A reaction in which the medication leaves the original injection site and moves to another
TRH	Thyrotropin-releasing hormone, releases TSH and prolactin
Trismus	Severe spasm of the muscles of the jaw resembling tetanus (lock jaw); jaw clenching
TSH	Thyroid-stimulating hormone
UGT	Uridine diphosphate glucuronosyltransferase, enzyme involved in drug metabolism
Ulceration	An open lesion on the skin or mucous membrane
Vasoconstrictor	Causes narrowing of the blood vessels
VMAT2 inhibitors	Agents that inhibit the vesicular monoamine transporter 2, a cell membrane protein, thus decreaasing dopamine release
Volume of distribution (Vd)	The theoretical volume that a drug would have to occupy to provide the same concentration as it currently is in blood plasma
WBC	White blood cell count
Wernicke-Korsakoff syndrome	Syndrome characterized by confusion, ataxia, ophthalmoplegia, recent memory impairment, and confabulation
XR	Extended release
Z-drugs	Nonbenzodiazepine hypnotics whose names largely begin with z

DRUG USE IN PREGNANCY AND EFFECTS ON BREAST MILK

Drug labeling

- The FDA requires prescription drug labeling to include the following three detailed subsections, as outlined in the Pregnancy and Lactation Labeling Rule (2014):
  - **Pregnancy:** This subsection provides information relevant to the use of the drug in pregnant women, such as dosing and potential risks to the developing fetus, as well as information about whether there is a registry that collects and maintains data on how pregnant women are affected when they use the drug or biological product. Information in drug labeling about the existence of any pregnancy registries was previously recommended but not required
  - **Lactation:** This subsection provides information about using the drug while breastfeeding, such as the amount of drug in breast milk and potential effects on the breastfed child
  - **Females and Males of Reproductive Potential:** This subsection includes information about pregnancy testing, contraception, and infertility as it relates to the drug. This information was previously included in labeling, but there was no consistent placement for it
- The "Pregnancy" and "Lactation" subsections include three subheadings: "risk summary," "clinical considerations," and "data." These subheadings provide more detailed information regarding, for example, human and animal data on the use of the drug, and specific adverse reactions of concern for pregnant or breastfeeding women

Pregnancy exposure registries and studies

- If any psychotropic medication is used during pregnancy, consider patient enrollment or registration in any relevant studies or pregnancy exposure registries (e.g., in the US: FDA list of pregnancy registries at https://www.fda.gov/ScienceResearch/SpecialTopics/WomensHealthResearch/ucm134848.htm)
- In the US, the National Pregnancy Registry for Psychiatric Medications is dedicated to gathering information on psychotropic medications to improve the evidence base. It maintains registries for antidepressants, atypical antipsychotics, and ADHD medications at https://womensmentalhealth.org/research/pregnancyregistry

---

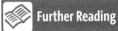 **Further Reading**

Additional Suggested Resources

Print resources

- Betcher HK, Wisner KL. Psychotropic treatment during pregnancy: Research synthesis and clinical care principles. J Womens Health (Larchmt). 2020;29(3):310–318. doi:10.1089/jwh.2019.7781
- Briggs GG, Freeman RK, Towers CV, et al. Briggs drugs in pregnancy and lactation: A reference guide to fetal and neonatal risk. (12th ed.) New York, NY: Wolters Kluwer, 2021.
- Creeley CE, Denton LK. Use of prescribed psychotropics during pregnancy: A systematic review of pregnancy, neonatal, and childhood outcomes. Brain Sci. 2019;(9):235. doi:10.3390/brainsci9090235
- Hale TW, Krutsch K. Hale's medications and mothers' milk 2023. (20th ed.) New York, NY: Springer, 2022.
- Larsen ER, Damkier P, Pedersen LH, et al. Use of psychotropic drugs during pregnancy and breast-feeding. Acta Psychiatr Scand Suppl. 2015;445(1):1–28. doi:10.1111/acps.12479
- McAllister-Williams RH, Baldwin DS, Cantwell R, et al. British Association for Psychopharmacology consensus guidance on the use of psychotropic medication preconception, in pregnancy and postpartum 2017. J Psychopharmacol. 2017;31(5):519–552. doi:10.1177/0269881117699361
- Raffi ER, Nonacs R, Cohen LS. Safety of psychotropic medications during pregnancy. Clin Perinatol. 2019;46(2):215–234. doi:10.1016/j.clp.2019.02.004

Online resources (freely accessible)

- Exposure to psychotropic medications and other substances during pregnancy and lactation: A handbook for health care providers [A Canadian resource developed by the Centre for Addiction and Mental Health in Toronto and the Motherisk Program]. http://www.camhx.ca/Publications/Resources_for_Professionals/Pregnancy_Lactation/index.html
- LactMed [A US National Library of Medicine database of drugs and other chemicals to which breastfeeding mothers may be exposed. Includes information on the levels of such substances in breast milk and infant blood, and the possible adverse effects in the nursing infant]. https://www.ncbi.nlm.nih.gov/books/NBK501922/
- MotherToBaby [A US and Canadian nonprofit service that provides evidence-based information about medications and other exposures during pregnancy and while breastfeeding]. https://mothertobaby.org

Online resources (subscription required)

- HalesMeds.com [electronic version (online/app) of Hale's medications and mothers' milk]. https://www.halesmeds.com/
- REPROTOX [A database developed by the Reproductive Toxicology Center in Washington, DC, USA for its members, which contains summaries on the effects of medications, chemicals, infections, and physical agents on pregnancy, reproduction, and development]. http://www.reprotox.org
- TERIS - Teratogen Information System [Developed by the University of Washington, Seattle, WA, USA; provides current information on the teratogenic effects of drugs and environmental agents]. http://depts.washington.edu/terisweb/teris/index.html

PATIENT INFORMATION SHEETS

The Patient Information Sheets contain information that may be passed on to patients about some of the most frequently used psychotropic medications as well as three nonpharmacological interventions. The sheets are designed to be easily understood by patients, give details on such matters as the uses of the drug, how quickly it starts working, how long it should be taken, side effects and what to do if they occur, what to do if a dose is forgotten, drug interactions, and precautions. Information sheets such as these, of course, cannot replace a proper consultation with and advice from the physician or other medical professional, but can serve as a useful tool to increase compliance, improve efficacy, and enhance safety.

The authors and the publisher welcome feedback and suggestions from readers (for contact addresses, see the front of the book).

Printable pdf files of Patient Information Sheets on the drugs and classes of drugs listed on the right can be downloaded free of charge once you have registered on the Hogrefe website.

How to proceed:

1. Go to **www.hgf.io/media** and create a user account. If you already have one, please log in).

2. Go to **My supplementary materials** in your account dashboard and enter the code below. You will automatically be redirected to the download area, where you can access and download the Patient Information Sheets.

Code: B-2YRI3G

To ensure that you have permanent direct access to the Patient Information Sheets, we recommend that you download them and save them on your device.

The Patient Information Sheets may be reproduced by users of the *Clinical Handbook of Psychotropic Drugs* for their own clinical practice but not for any commercial use.

The following Patient Information Sheets are available:

1. Acamprosate
2. Anticonvulsant Mood Stabilizers
3. Antiparkinsonian Agents for Treating Extrapyramidal Side Effects
4. Antipsychotics
5. Anxiolytics and Benzodiazepines
6. Atomoxetine
7. Bright Light Therapy
8. Buprenorphine
9. Bupropion
10. Buspirone
11. Clonidine and Guanfacine
12. Clozapine
13. Cyclic Antidepressants
14. Dextromethorphan/Bupropion Combination
15. Deutetrabenazine
16. Disulfiram
17. Drugs for Treatment of Dementia
18. Electroconvulsive Therapy
19. Esketamine
20. Hypnotics/Sedatives
21. Lithium
22. MAOI Antidepressants
23. Methadone
24. Mirtazapine
25. Moclobemide
26. Naltrexone
27. Pimavanserin
28. Psychostimulants
29. Repetitive Transcranial Magnetic Stimulation
30. SARI Antidepressants
31. Selegiline Transdermal
32. Sex-Drive Depressants
33. SNRI Antidepressants
34. SSRI Antidepressants
35. Valbenazine
36. Vilazodone
37. Viloxazine
38. Vortioxetine

INDEX OF DRUGS*

* Page numbers in **bold type** indicate main entries.

Do you want print <u>and</u> online?
Deal with adults <u>and</u> children?

Then combine CHPD publications and save

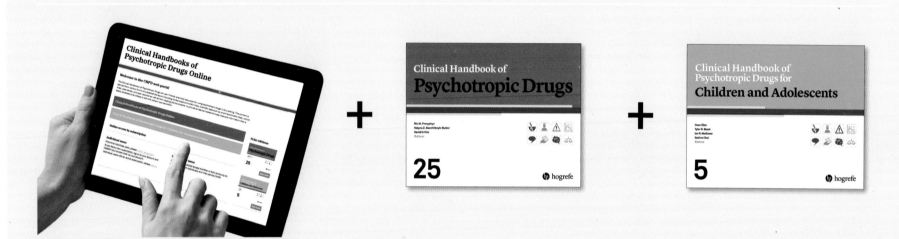

The *Clinical Handbook of Psychotropic Drugs* is available as a print edition and as an online version, for adults and for children and adolescents. Save money with product combinations. Each print edition and each online subscription (2 years) costs US $99.80.

Buy any two CHPD products and save nearly US $50.
Buy all four CHPD products and get 33% discount off the combined list prices!

More information at **https://hogrefe.com/us/chpd**

 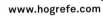
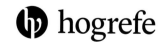

Clinical Handbook of Psychotropic Drugs
25th edition

The *Clinical Handbook of Psychotropic Drugs* has become a standard reference and working tool for psychiatrists, psychologists, physicians, pharmacists, nurses, and other mental health professionals.

· Independent, unbiased, up to date

· Packed with unique, easy-to-read comparison charts and tables (dosages, side effects, pharmacokinetics, interactions...) for a quick overview of treatment options

· Succinct, bulleted information on all classes of medication: on- and off-label indications, side effects, interactions, pharmacodynamics, precautions in the young, the elderly, and pregnancy, nursing implications, and much more – all you need to know for each class of drug

· Potential interactions and side effects summarized in comparison charts

· With instantly recognizable icons and in full color throughout, allowing you to find at a glance all the information you seek

This book is a must for everyone who needs an up-to-date, easy-to-use, comprehensive summary of all the most relevant information about psychotropic drugs.

DOWNLOAD
Clearly written patient information sheets can be downloaded as printable PDF files from the Hogrefe website after registration

Hogrefe Publishing Group

Göttingen · Berne · Vienna · Oxford · Paris
Boston · Amsterdam · Prague · Florence
Copenhagen · Stockholm · Helsinki · Oslo
Madrid · Barcelona · Seville · Bilbao
Zaragoza · São Paulo · Lisbon

www.hogrefe.com

New in this edition:

· Antidepressants chapter includes a new section on the NMDA receptor antagonist/CYP2D6 inhibitor combination product (dextromethorphan/bupropion)

· Antipsychotics updates include revised clozapine monitoring tables which now also contain monitoring requirements for patients with or without non-benign ethnic neutropenia

· Mood Stabilisers sections on Lithium and Anticonvulsants extensively revised

· Dementia chapter includes a new section on lecanemab, a new fast-track FDA-approved treatment for Alzheimer's disease

· Treatment of Substance Use Disorders chapter includes revisions to buprenorphine dosing section that include a rapid micro-induction method (Bernese method) that allows treatment to start without waiting for patient to be in withdrawal

· Unapproved Treatments of Psychiatric Disorders, Natural Health Products, and Pharmacogenetics chapters all substantially revised

· New formulations and trade names include:
  – Auvelity (dextromethorphan/bupropion extended-release tablets)
  – Invega Hafyera (paliperidone 6-monthly IM injection)
  – Leqembi (lecanemab infusion)
  – Subutex (buprenorphine sublingual tablets)
  – Quviviq (daridorexant tablets)

Also available: CHPD Online

Recent praise for the *Clinical Handbook*:

"A powerhouse of practical information ... Unrivalled in scope ... This outstanding and unique handbook is as rich in useful content as many full textbooks."
Barbara Jovaisas, PharmD, in *Canadian Pharmacists Journal*

"This is a very important book that provides valuable information which otherwise would be scattered among different publications. With the increasing rate of prescription of psychotropic drugs, this volume should be on the desk of every physician. The information is crucial for understanding side effects, vulnerabilities, and interactions of psychotropic drug treatment."
Giovanni A. Fava, MD, in *Psychotherapy and Psychosomatics*

"The handbook is easy to use, comprehensive in scope, and up to date – a winner!"
Catherine Chiles, MD, in *Journal of Clinical Psychiatry*

"Comprehensive ... clearly organized ... an ideal resource for rapid and straightforward retrieval of essential clinical information ... a 'must have' for those who work in mental health care."
Marshall Cates, PharmD, in *Annals of Pharmacotherapy*

"Should be available at all nursing stations."
C. Lindsay DeVane, PharmD, in *American Journal of Health Systems Pharmacy*

ISBN 978-0-88937-632-8